Oral Microb
and
Infectious Disease

SECOND STUDENT EDITION

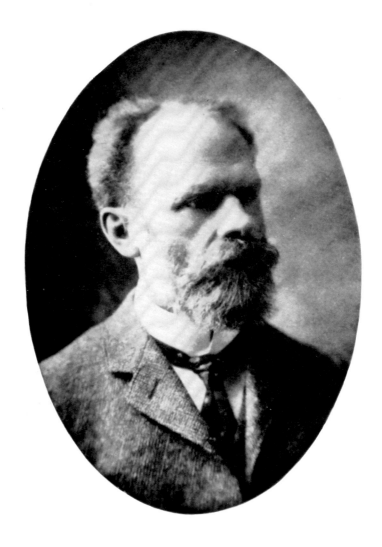

WILLOUGHBY D. MILLER, A.B., D.D.S., M.D., Ph.D., Sc.D.,
(1853–1907)

The father of oral microbiology. As the formulator of the chemico-parasitic theory of dental caries he was the first to apply a basic science to the solution of dental disease. Dr. Miller was a great leader as an investigator, practicing dentist, teacher, and prolific author in all phases of dentistry. He wrote the first comprehensive textbook of oral microbiology. *Die Mikroorganismen der Mundhöhle*, published in Germany in 1889 and in the United States in 1890 as *The Micro-Organisms of the Human Mouth*. (From School of Dentistry, University of Michigan.)

Oral Microbiology and Infectious Disease

SECOND STUDENT EDITION

edited by
GEORGE S. SCHUSTER,
D.D.S., Ph.D.

Professor of Oral Biology, School of Dentistry;
Associate Professor of Cell and Molecular Biology,
School of Medicine; Coordinator of Microbiology
for Dentistry, Medical College of Georgia,
Augusta, Georgia

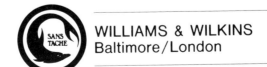

WILLIAMS & WILKINS
Baltimore/London

Made in the United States of America

First Edition, 1957
    Reprinted, 1958
    Reprinted, 1959
    Reprinted, 1961
Second Edition, 1962
    Reprinted, 1963
    Reprinted, 1965
    Reprinted, 1966
Third Edition, 1968
    Reprinted, 1972
Fourth Edition, 1976
Student Edition, 1978
    Reprinted, 1980

Library of Congress Cataloging in Publication Data

Main entry under title:

Oral microbiology and infectious disease.

    Rev. ed. of: Oral microbiology and infectious disease / George W. Burnett. George S. Schuster. Student ed. 1978.
    Includes index.
    1. Mouth—Microbiology. 2. Medical microbiology. I. Schuster, George S., 1940–. II. Burnett, George Wesley, 1914–   . Oral microbiology and infectious disease. [DNLM: 1. Communicable diseases. 2. Mouth—Microbiology. 3 Mouth diseases. QW 65062]
QR47.069 1983   617'.522   82-2026
ISBN 0-683-07611-6   AACR2

Composed and printed at the
Waverly Press, Inc.
Mt. Royal and Guilford Aves.
Baltimore, Md. 21202, U.S.A.

To the Memory of
WILLOUGHBY DAYTON MILLER
Founder of Oral Microbiology
His Concepts Have Never Been Superseded,
Only Amplified

Preface to the Second Student Edition

Oh that one would hear me!
behold, my desire is,
that the Almighty would
answer me,
and that mine adversary
had written a book.
　　　　　Job XXXI:35

Previous editions of *Oral Microbiology and Infectious Disease* were prepared as reference-texts, to serve as a textbook for the dental student and as a reference book to the field of oral microbiology. Subsequently, such editions became too large and too costly for typical student use, and as a result the student edition evolved. In that form the book was reduced in size and content. This was accomplished by reductions in text and illustrations and elimination of certain topics. At the same time the essential character of previous editions was preserved, i.e. a book not limited to oral diseases but also providing the student with a sound background in the principles of microbiology and systemic infectious disease. A similar philosophy is being followed in preparing the second student edition.

Students enter dentistry with considerable variation in science background, and as a result dentistry, as other educational areas, has developed a basic core of material to be mastered. Unfortunately, in many areas the minimum standards become the norm, a practice that should be unacceptable in a health science profession. While the basic information should be available to the students who enter with minimal predental science requirements, those with more background or a desire to go deeper into a subject should be able to derive enough information that they can intelligently review and evaluate the literature. To meet this need, a book should maintain a balance between providing the essential information in a form useful to the neophyte and providing an adequate level for the better prepared or motivated student. Following the precedent set by previous editions,

we have attempted to achieve such a balance.

While maintaining the character of previous editions of *Oral Microbiology and Infectious Disease*, there is a significant departure in this second edition from previous versions: That is the use of multiple authors. All are individuals who are active in the field of oral microbiology and are involved in dentally oriented research and teaching. This adds depth and strength to the coverage of a field that is obviously more complex than previously imagined. Thus, the strengths of the previous editions have been added to and reinforced in the new.

While a broad knowledge of microbiology and infectious disease is important to the dentist, he must be particularly knowledgeable in the specific relationships of these to the oral cavity. Therefore, as before, examples involving the oral microbiota are used whenever possible, and special attention has been given to oral infectious diseases, diseases with oral manifestations and those general infections with particular implications to dental personnel.

All chapters have been completely rewritten or revised and new literature references have been added. By these changes we hope to provide the dentist with a sound background in microbiology and infectious disease and a foundation on which to add more in-depth knowledge. It is only when the practitioner has such a foundation and the ability to utilize it to provide the best treatment for his patients that the dentist becomes a "doctor" in the true meaning of the word.

George S. Schuster

Contributors

EDITOR:

George S. Schuster, D.D.S., M.S., Ph.D.
Professor and Coordinator, Oral Biology/Microbiology
School of Dentistry
Associate Professor of Cell and Molecular Biology
School of Medicine
Medical College of Georgia
Augusta, Georgia

CONTRIBUTING AUTHORS:

Memory P. F. Elvin-Lewis, Ph.D.
Professor of Microbiology in Biomedicine
Head: Section of Microbiology
Washington University, School of Dental Medicine
St. Louis, Missouri

Benjamin F. Hammond, D.D.S., Ph.D.
Professor and Chairman, Department of Microbiology
University of Pennsylvania
School of Dental Medicine
Philadelphia, Pennsylvania

Jeremy M. Hardie, B.D.S., L.D.S., Ph.D., Dip. Bact.
Department of Oral Microbiology
The London Hospital Medical College
Dental School
Turner Street
London, England

Chris H. Miller, B.A., M.S., Ph.D.
Professor and Chairman
Department of Oral Microbiology
Indiana University School of Dentistry
Professor
Department of Microbiology and Immunology
Indiana University School of Medicine
Indianapolis, Indiana

John A. Molinari, Ph.D.
Chairman and Professor
Department of Microbiology and Biochemistry
University of Detroit School of Dentistry
Detroit, Michigan

Mark R. Patters, D.D.S., Ph.D.
Assistant Professor
Department of Periodontology
University of Connecticut
School of Dental Medicine
Farmington, Connecticut

Charles F. Schachtele, Ph.D.
Professor, School of Dentistry and
Department of Microbiology, Medical School
University of Minnesota
Minneapolis, Minnesota

George S. Schuster, D.D.S., Ph.D.
Professor and Coordinator, Oral Biology/Microbiology
School of Dentistry
Associate Professor of Cell and Molecular Biology
School of Medicine
Medical College of Georgia
Augusta, Georgia

Keith R. Volkmann, Ph.D., D.M.D.
Associate Professor, Oral Biology/Microbiology
School of Dentistry
Medical College of Georgia
Augusta, Georgia

Contents

PART 1

MICROBIOLOGICAL CLASSIFICATION AND TECHNIQUES

chapter 1

Microbial Taxonomy

John A. Molinari

INTRODUCTION

Microbiology is a branch of the biological sciences that is concerned with the study of life that is ordinarily too small to be seen with the unaided human eye. Microorganisms included in the field of Microbiology, in order of decreasing size, are the algae, fungi (yeasts and molds), protozoa, bacteria, rickettsiae, chlamydiae, viruses, and viroids. Those that are known to cause infectious diseases in animals are the pathogenic fungi, protozoa, bacteria, rickettsiae, chlamydiae, and viruses. The macroscopic metazoa and microscopic protozoa that are parasites or pathogens are usually grouped in the branch of Biology known as Parasitology.

TAXONOMY

The present concepts of evolution seem to indicate that microbes were derived from primitive ancestors of the Plant and Animal Kingdoms and are, in fact, in a position somewhere between them. This led Haeckel in 1866 to propose that the acellular or unicellular microbes, because of their apparent relative simplicity, should be placed in a separate kingdom designated as Protista (= first of all).

As techniques and the necessary apparatus (chiefly the electron microscope) became available, the cellular organization of microbes was revealed in more detail. It became evident that protozoa, fungi, and most algae could be described as eucaryotic (= true nucleus) because, like the cells of plants and animals, their distinctive nucleus, which was enclosed with a nuclear membrane, contained multiple chromosomes and an apparatus that equally divides their chromosomes during cell division. In contrast, the bacteria and the blue-green algae belonged to a group of cells that was termed as procaryotic. The nucleus or genophore of these cells consisted of a single, circular, naked chromosome not separated from the cytoplasm by a nuclear membrane. Major features that differentiate eucaryotes from procaryotes are presented in table 1/1.

In the eighth edition of *Bergey's Manual of Determinative Bacteriology*, bacteria that are phototrophic and those that are indifferent to light are placed in a Kindgom: Procaryotae, that is distinct from the Plant and Animal Kingdoms. This Kingdom is then divided into two Divisions. Division I includes the Phototrophic procaryotes (or "photobacteria"). The photobacteria are then divided into three Classes: Class I, the blue-green photobacteria; Class II, red photobacteria; and Class III, the green photobacteria. Division II includes the procaryotes that are indifferent to light.

In this text we have adopted the system of classification of bacteria of the eighth edition of *Bergey's Manual of Determinative Bacteriology* because it is the product of over 40 years of evolution and is more widely accepted than any other system.

The utilization of this comprehensive reference, however, does not suggest that the treatment is complete, as important omissions of dentally relevant microorganisms are evident. These are primarily due to the rapid development of sophisticated procedures for culture and isolation of strict

Table 1/1

Comparison of procaryotic and eucaryotic cells[a]

	Procaryotic	Eucaryotic
Cell wall	Complex with glycopeptide	Not as complex, no glycopeptide
Cell membrane	No sterols	Sterols
Mesosomes	Present	None
Nucleus	DNA; no membrane	DNA complexed with histones; membrane
Cell division	Binary fission; budding	Mitosis; meiosis
Ribosomes	70S	80S
Chromosomes	Single	Multiple
Mitochondria	None	Present
Chloroplasts	None	Present
Chromatophores	Present in some organisms	None

[a] From J. A. Molinari and M. J. Phillip: Microbiology and Sterilization. In *Review of Dental Assisting*, edited by B. A. Ladley and S. A. Wilson. C. V. Mosby, St. Louis, 1980.

anaerobes from clinical specimens. A prime example is *Capnocytophaga ochraceus*, a gram negative gliding rod, which appears in *Bergey's* as *Bacteroides ochraceus*.

It is beyond the scope of this text to catalogue each of the microbial characteristics employed in *Bergey's* system of classification. Briefly, organization of bacteria, rickettsias, and mycoplasmas is divided into 19 parts based on morphological appearance, gram reaction, requirement for oxygen, sporulation, and physiological, biochemical, and metabolic patterns.

With pathogenic bacteria and other pathogenic microorganisms, the range of hosts, conditions required to produce an infection, the characteristics of the disease produced, tissue responses, and immune responses are important characteristics used in identification and classification. The immunochemical characterization is also important in bacterial classification. In accordance with current practices, the weight placed on the various characteristics greatly influences the classification of bacteria. For instance, if all characteristics were given equal weight, considerable changes would be made in bacterial classification. Other factors currently being utilized are DNA base composition and cell wall composition.

The practical goal of microbial taxonomy is to identify microorganisms belonging to a species. In plants and animals, the species is composed of individuals that closely resemble each other in most respects and whose sexual forms produce fertile offspring that resemble each other in their most important features. With bacteria, reproduction is normally asexual and the number of discernible and distinctive characteristics is limited, particularly when compared to those of plant and animal species. The species of the procaryotes are named with a Latin binomial for genus and species. The genus name is capitalized and the species name is uncapitalized. Such binomials are underlined in writing and italicized in print, to signify that the names are in a foreign language.

A selected portion of the genera and species of bacteria of medical and dental significance is shown in table 1/2.

EUMYCETES (TRUE FUNGI)

The true fungi may be defined as nonphotosynthetic thallophytes that grow typically in filaments and reproduce by sporulation, *i.e.*, each unit plant produces a large number of spores, whereas most of the sporulating bacteria produce only one spore per cell and can multiply indefinitely without sporulation. Most fungi have well defined sexual modes of sporulation, involving nuclear fusion and reduction in chromosome number, but they form spores asexually most of the time (fig. 1/1).

On germination, the spore enlarges and puts forth one or more processes called germ tubes, which elongate at the distal end to become filaments, called hyphae. In many cases, each hypha lays down cross walls (septa) to form a chain of cells. The cell walls are typically well defined, relatively thick, and extraordinarily resistant chemically, resembling the chitin of the outer coat of crustaceans and insects. As the hyphae grow, they eventually branch and form a tangled mat of filaments called the mycelium, examples of which are familiar to everyone as the growth of molds. A part of the mycelium penetrates the substrate to absorb nourishment and is called a vegetative mycelium; another part extends into the atmosphere and is called an aerial mycelium. When an aerial mycelium begins to bear spores, it is a reproductive mycelium.

A considerable group of fungi, the yeasts, are quite primitive and do not form true filaments but grow instead as single spheroid cells. Yeasts reproduce asexually by putting forth spheroid buds, called blastospores, which break off, enlarge, and reproduce like the parent. One group of yeasts can

Table 1/2
Outline of the Principal Bacterial Genera of Dental and Medical Importance

---

Kingdom: Procaryotae

Single cells or cells in a simple association that do not have a nuclear membrane and are generally but not always enclosed by a rigid cell wall. One or more of these microorganisms inhabits almost every moist environment.

Division II. *The Bacteria.* Division consists of procaryotic microorganisms that are unicellular or in simple association and they usually divide by binary fission or by budding. Some are motile, others are not; some form endospores, others do not. With the exception of the *Mollicutes* the cells are enclosed in relatively rigid cell walls. The cells may be aerobic or anaerobic, or facultative.

Spirochetes

Order 1. *Spirochaetales.* Gram negative, unicellular, slender helical bacteria that are nonsporulating, motile, variable aerobic, facultatively anaerobic or anaerobic. They are either free-living, commensal, or parasitic and some are pathogenic.

Family I. *Spirochaetaceae.* Free-living spirochetes found in sewage, polluted water, and in fresh and salt waters. Anaerobic or facultatively anaerobic. The family contains five genera.

Genus III. *Treponema* (a turning thread). Gram negative, motile, unicellular, helical rods. Fermentative metabolism. Strictly anaerobic. Some have not been cultivated. Found in the oral cavity, intestinal tract, and genital regions of man and other animals. The genus contains 11 recognized species. The more important pathogenic species are *Treponema pallidum* (syphilis), *Treponema pertenue* (yaws) and *Treponema carateum* (pinta or carate). Oral residents of man and other animals include *Treponema macrodentium*, *Treponema denticola*, *Treponema orale*, *Treponema scoliodontum*, and *Treponema vincentii*.

Genus IV. *Borrelia* (after A. Borrel). Gram negative, helical cells that are generally parasitic, living on mucous membranes. Some species are pathogenic for man and other animals and birds, causing such diseases as avian borreliosis and relapsing fever. Nineteen recognized species, with the type species being *Borrelia anserina*.

Genus V. *Leptospira* (a fine coil). Gram negative, flexous, helical, motile cells that have one or both ends bent. The genus is represented by a single type species, *Leptospira interrogans*. Some strains are pathogenic (leptospirosis) whereas others are free-living saprophytes.

Spiral and Curved Bacteria

Family I. *Spirillaceae.* Gram negative, rigid, helical cells that are motile by flagella. Variably aerobic and anaerobic. Do not ferment carbohydrates. Some are inhabitants of fresh and salt water, others are saprophytes or parasites, and some are pathogenic.

Genus I. *Spirillum* (a small spiral). Cellular description as for family. Nineteen recognized species. *Spirillum voluntans* is the type species. *Spirillum minor* is a cause of one type of rat-bite fever in man.

Genus II. *Campylobacter* (a curved rod). Gram-negative, nonsporulating, spirally curved rods that do not ferment or oxidize carbohydrates. Several recognized species with *Campylobacter fetus* being the type species. The various species are found in the oral cavity, intestinal tract, and reproductive organs of man and other animals. Some species are pathogenic for cattle and sheep, causing abortion and human infections.

Gram Negative Aerobic Rods and Cocci

Family I. *Pseudomonadaceae.* Gram negative curved or straight aerobic rods that are motile. Type genus, *Pseudomonas.*

Genus I. *Pseudomonas* (false monad). Description as above. Strictly aerobic with respiratory metabolism. Type species is *Pseudomonas aeruginosa*. The genus is divided into four sections with 10 species in Section I, 5 species in Section II, 10 species in Section III, and 3 species in Section IV. Generally the species are found in the environment in soil and water, with some being pathogenic for mammals and plants. *P. aeruginosa* is isolated from a wide variety of human infections and is occasionally a plant pathogen. *Pseudomonas fluorescens* is associated with the spoilage of foods; *Pseudomonas pseudomallei* is a cause of melioidosis. *Pseudomonas mallei* causes glanders and farcy in horses. *Pseudomonas salanacearum* is an important plant pathogen.

Genera of Uncertain Affiliation

Genus *Brucella* (after Sir David Bruce). Gram negative, nonmotile, nonsporulating, coccobacilli (short rods) that are strictly aerobic and are mammalian parasites and pathogens. *Brucella melitensis* is the type species. Six recognized species. *B. melitensis* is pathogenic for goats, sheep, cattle, and man. *Brucella abortus* is pathogenic for cattle and man. *Brucella suis* is pathogenic for swine, hares, reindeers, and man. *Brucella neotoma* is found in rats. *Brucella ovis* infects sheep, and *Brucella canis* infects dogs.

Genus *Bordetella* (after Jules Bordet). Gram negative, variably motile minute coccobacilli that are strictly aerobic. The members of the genus are parasites and pathogens of mammals. Three recognized species with *Bordetella pertussis* as the type species. *B. pertussis* causes whooping cough in man, while *Bordetella parapertussis* produces a whooping cough-like disease in man. *Bordetella bronchiseptica* causes a bronchopneumonia in dogs and other mammals.

Genus *Francisella* (after Edward Francis). Gram negative, nonmotile, nonsporulating rods and cocci that are extremely pleomorphic. Two species are recognized with *Francisella tularensis* as the type species. *F. tularensis* is found in natural waters and in species of wild animals in North America, Europe, Russia, Turkey, and Japan where it is the cause of tularemia. *Francisella novicida* can induce a tularemia-like disease in white mice, guinea pigs, and hamsters, but it does not affect man.

Gram Negative Facultatively Anaerobic Rods

Family I. *Enterobacteriaceae*. Gram negative, motile and nonmotile, facultatively anaerobic rods that have both a respiratory and fermentative metabolism. The type genus is *Escherichia*.

Genus I. *Escherichia* (after Theodor Escherich). Cells are as described above. The genus contains one species, *Escherichia coli*, which has several hundred antigenic specificities whose different combinations allow for several thousand serotypes.

Genus II. *Edwardsiella* (after P. R. Edwards). Motile, gram negative rods. Contains one species, *Edwardsiella tarda*, which is found in water, intestinal tract of snakes, human intestinal tract, blood, and urine.

Genus III. *Citrobacter* (citrate using rod). Motile, gram negative rods that can use citrate as the sole carbon source. The genus contains two recognized species, *Citrobacter freundii* and *Citrobacter intermedius*. The species are found in water and food and in the feces, urine, and intestinal tract of healthy people.

Genus IV. *Salmonella* (after D. E. Salmon). Gram negative, usually motile rods that can use citrate as a source of carbon. The species of this genus have been named at different times by the disease they produce or by the animal from which they were isolated, by the geographic location at which they were first isolated, or by antigenic formula as established by the Kaufmann-White scheme which designates by numbers and letters the different O, K and H antigens of a given strain. By this scheme the *Salmonella* are divided into some 65 groups and more than 1500 serotypes.

Genus V. *Shigella* (after K. Shiga). Gram negative nonmotile rods that cannot utilize citrate as a sole carbon source. Ferments carbohydrates with the production of acid but no gas. Four recognized species with *Shigella dysenteriae* as the type species. All species inhabit the intestinal tracts of man and higher monkeys and all species produce dysentery in man.

Genus VI. *Klebsiella* (after Edwin Klebs). Gram negative, nonmotile capsulated rods that can use citrate and glucose as the sole carbon source. Three recognized species. *Klebsiella pneumoniae* is widely distributed in the environment and is an inhabitant of the normal intestinal tract of man and animals and may be associated with infections of the intestinal and respiratory tracts. *Klebsiella ozaenae* is found in chronic diseases of the respiratory tract and ozena. *Klebsiella rhinoscleromatis* is found in rhinoscleroma.

Genus VII. *Enterobacter* (intestinal small rod). Gram negative motile rods that can utilize citrate and acetate as the sole carbon sources. Two species recognized. *Enterobacter cloacae* is found in the feces of man and other animals and in the environment in sewage, soil and water; found in pathological material from animals. *Enterobacter aerogenes* is found in sewage, soil, water, dairy products, and human and animal species.

Genus VIII. *Hafnia* (old name for Copenhagen). Gram negative, motile, encapsulated rods that can use citrate and acetate as sole sources of carbon. The genus is represented by *Hafnia alvei*, which is found in human and animal feces, dairy products, sewage, soil, and water.

Genus IX. *Serratia* (after Serafuno Serrati). Gram negative, motile, capsulated rods that form pink, red, or magenta pigments. The genus contains one species, *Serratia marcescens*, which is widely distributed in food, soil, and water.

Genus X. *Proteus* (a god who is able to transform himself into many forms). Gram negative, pleomorphic, motile, not encapsulated, straight rods that form involution forms, coccoids, filaments, and spheroplasts. The genus has five recognized species. The species are found variously in human, chicken, and animal feces, sewage and soil, decomposing protein, urine, and human clinical specimens.

Genus XI. *Yersinia* (after A. J. E. Yersin). Gram negative, not encapsulated, variously motile ovoid cells or rods. The genus is divided into three recognized species with *Yersinia pestis* as the type species. *Y. pestis* is the cause of plague in humans and rodents. *Yersinia pseudotuberculosis* causes a form of pseudotuberculosis in animals, generally in the mesenteric lymph nodes. *Yersinia enterocolitica*, while not pathogenic, is widely distributed in sick and healthy men and animals and in dairy products.

Family II. *Vibrionaceae*. Gram negative, motile, short rods that have a respiratory and fermentative metabolism and are facultatively anaerobic. Inhabit fresh and salt water and the intestinal tracts of animals. Some species are pathogenic for man and fish.

Genus I. *Vibrio* (that which vibrates). Gram negative, motile, nonsporulating rod that is facultatively anaerobic and has a respiratory metabolism. It is found in fresh and salt water and the intestinal tract of man and animals. Some species are pathogenic for man and fish. Five recognized species, with *Vibrio cholerae* as the type species. *V. cholerae* is present in the intestines of normal and diseased man and animals, and classic cholera is related to certain strains of *V. cholerae*. Other species are found in water and fish and other marine animals. Some are found in brine and cured meat.

Genus II. *Aeromonas* (gas-producing monad). Gram negative, motile, rod-shaped cells that are both respiratory and fermentative. The genus has three recognized species, with *Aeromonas hydrophila* as the type species. The various species infect frogs and salmon, and *A. hydrophila* infects humans.

Genus III. *Plesiomonas* (neighbor monad). Gram negative, motile, rod-shaped cells that have a respiratory and fermentative metabolism and are facultative anaerobes. The genus is represented by one species, *Plesiomonas shigelloides* which inhabits the gastrointestinal tracts of man and animals and cause an infectious gastroenteritis in humans.

Genera of Uncertain Affiliation

Genus *Chromobacterium* (a colored rod). Gram negative, motile, nonencapsulated rods that have respiratory or fermentative metabolism and are strict aerobes or facultative anaerobes. They produce a violet pigment. A common inhabitant of fresh water and soils. The genus has two recognized species. *Chromobacterium violaceum* is found in soils and fresh water and causes serious pyogenic or septicemic infections of man and other mammals. *Chromobacterium lividum* has a similar distribution but is not pathogenic for man or other mammals.

Genus *Flavobacterium* (a yellow bacterium). Gram negative, nonsporulating, motile cells that are pigmented, with hues ranging from yellow to brown and are fastidious in their nutritive requirements. Twelve species, of which *Flavobacterium breve* is pathogenic for laboratory animals and *Flavobacterium meningosepticum* is pathogenic for man. Species are commonly isolated from fresh and salt waters.

Genus *Haemophilus* (the blood lover). Gram negative, nonmotile, nonsporulating, parasitic rod-shaped or coccobacillary cells that are facultatively anaerobic and require growth factors present in blood. Some 14 species, with *Haemophilus influenzae* as type species. Species are found in the upper respiratory tract of man and other animals, and in the oral cavity of man, where they cause a variety of infections. *Haemophilus ducreyi* is associated with soft chancre. *Haemophilus vaginalis* is found in the human genital tract but it is not pathogenic for laboratory animals.

Genus *Pasteurella* (after Louis Pasteur). Gram negative, nonmotile, nonsporulating coccoid or rod-shaped cells that are facultatively anaerobic and have a fermentative metabolism. The genus contains four genera without an acceptable type species. The species are widely distributed parasites of many mammals, including man, and birds, and principally cause diseases in domesticated animals.

Genus *Actinobaccilus* (ray baccilus or rod). Gram negative, nonmotile, nonsporulating cells that are spherical, oval or rod-shaped and have a fermentative metabolism. *Actinobacillus lignieresii* is the type species. *A. lignieresii* is pathogenic for cattle and sheep and only slightly for man and the dog. *Actinobacillus equuli* is pathogenic for horses and pigs. Evidence had also been accumulating to assign a role for *Actinobacillus actinomycetemcomitans* in the development of juvenile periodontitis.

Genus *Cardiobacterium* (bacterium of the heart). Gram negative, nonmotile, nonsporulating, pleomorphic rods that have a fermentative metabolism and are facultatively anaerobic. The genus has one species *Cardiobacterium hominis*, which is also the type species. A normal inhabitant of the human nose and throat and causes endocarditis in man.

Genus *Streptobacillus* (a twisted or curved small rod). Gram negative, nonmotile, nonsporulating rods that spontaneously convert to L phase. The cells are facultatively anaerobic and have a fermentative metabolism. The genus contains one species, *Streptobacillus moniliformis*, which is the type species. Its activities range from parasitic to pathogenic for rats and other mammals, including man. A cause of rat-bite fever and arthritis.

Genus *Calymmatobacterium* (the sheathed rodlet). Gram negative, nonmotile, nonsporulating, encapsulated rods. The genus contains one species *Calymmatobacterium granulomatis*, which is the type species. The organism causes granuloma inguinale in man but is not pathogenic for laboratory animals.

Gram Negative Anaerobic Bacteria

Family I. *Bacteroidaceae*. Gram negative, variably pleomorphic, variably motile, obligately anaerobic rods that are present in the cavities of man and other animals and the intestinal tracts of insects. Some species are pathogenic for man and animals.

Genus I. *Bacteroides* (rod-like). Gram negative, nonsporulating, nonmotile, obligately anaerobic rods that ferment sugars to produce organic acids. The genus contains 20 or more species of which *Bacteroides fragilis* is the type species. The various species are found in the oral cavity, upper respiratory tract, genital tract, appendix, lacrymal gland, intestinal tract and feces of man; the rumen of cattle and wild animals; the intestines of poultry, turkeys, and termites; and the infected hoofs of sheep and goats.

Genus II. *Fusobacterium* (a small spindle-shaped rod). Gram negative, nonsporulating, variably motile rods which metabolize carbohydrates to produce organic acids and are obligately anaerobic. The genus contains 16 recognized species, of which *Fusobacterium nucleatum* is the type species. The species are common residents of the cavities of man and other animals. Some are pathogenic and they appear in various human infections.

Genus III. *Leptotrichia* (fine hair). Gram negative, nonmotile, anaerobic, straight or curved rods that produce acid but not gas from carbohydrates. One recognized species in the genus, *Leptotrichia buccalis*, which is also the type species. An inhabitant of the oral cavity of man.

Genus IV. *Eikenella* (rod-like). Gram negative, nonsporulating, nonmotile, facultatively anaerobic rods that reduce nitrates. One recognized, species, *Eikenella corrodens*, is more frequently isolated from clinical specimens than the obligate anaerobe, *Bacteroides corrodens*. Like *B. corrodens*, *E. corrodens* is a component of the normal oral flora and has been cited as the primary agent in certain human infections.

Genera of Uncertain Affiliation

Genus *Selenomonas* (moon monad). Gram negative, motile, nonsporulating, anaerobic, curved or helical rods. The genus contains two species of which *Selenomonas sputigena* is the type species and an inhabitant of the human oral cavity. The other species *Selenomonas ruminantium* is an inhabitant of the rumen of cattle, sheep, and elk.

Gram Negative Cocci and Coccobacilli

Family I. *Neisseriaceae*. Gram negative, nonmotile, spherical bacteria that are aerobic and have complex growth requirements. Heterotrophic, utilizing organic nitrogen and carbohydrates. Cells occur in pairs or masses with adjacent sides flattened, or as rod shapes in pairs or chains. Obligate parasites of the mucous membrane of man. The family consists of *Neisseria*, *Branhamella*, *Moraxella*, and *Acinetobacter*.

    Genus I. *Neisseria* (after A. Neisser). Aerobic or facultatively anaerobes that occur in pairs with interfaces flattened. The genus consists of six recognized species of which *Neisseria gonorrhoeae* (gonococcus) and *Neisseria meningitidis* (meningococcus) are most important medically.

    Genus II. *Branhamella* (after Sara Branham). Gram negative, nonsporulating, nonmotile cocci occurring in pairs with adjacent sides flattened. The genus contains one species, *Branhamella catarrhalis*, which is a parasite of the mucous membranes of mammals; a potential pathogen.

    Genus III. *Moraxella* (after V. Morax). Gram negative short rods that occur in pairs and short chains. Carries out an oxidate metabolism. Five species, of which *Moraxella lacunata* causes conjunctivitis and *Moraxella bovis* causes "pink-eye" (epizootic keratoconjunctivitis) in cattle.

    Genus IV. *Actinetobacter* (nonmotile rod). Gram negative, nonmotile, nonsporulating, short and plump rods. Contains one species, *Acinetobacter calcoaceticus* which is an inhabitant of healthy and diseased man and other animals. Probably an opportunistic pathogen in debilitated individuals.

Gram Negative Anaerobic Cocci

Family I. *Veillonellaceae*. Gram negative, nonmotile, anaerobic cocci that have complex nutritional requirements. A common inhabitant of the intestinal tract of man, ruminants, rodents, and pigs, and a predominant species in the human oral cavity. The family is composed of three genera of which *Veillonella* is the type genus.

    Genus I. *Veillonella* (after A. Veillon). Gram negative, nonmotile, nonsporulating, anaerobic cocci that are unable to ferment carbohydrates and have complex nutritional requirements. Two recognized species in the genus with *Veillonella parvula* as the type species. An abundant inhabitant of the human, rat, and hamster mouth, respiratory and intestinal tracts.

Gram Positive Cocci

Family I. *Micrococcaceae*. Gram positive spheroidal cells that form regular or irregular clusters or packets. Motile or nonmotile. Chemoorganotrophs. The family consists of *Micrococcus*, *Staphylococcus*, and *Planococcus*.

    Genus II. *Staphylococcus* ("grape-like coccus"). Nonmotile cocci that tend to form irregular clusters. Respiratory or fermentative metabolism. Facultative anaerobes that prefer aerobic conditions. The genus consists of *Staphylococcus aureus*, a potential pathogen that is an obligate parasite of the respiratory and intestinal tracts of warm-blooded animals; *Staphylococcus epidermidis*, primarily an inhabitant of skin and mucous membranes of warm-blooded mammals as commensals or parasites; and *Staphylococcus saprophyticus*, a nonpathogen found in the environment, dairy products, and urine.

Family II. *Streptococcaceae*. Gram positive spherical or ovoid cells that tend to form chains. Usually nonmotile and nonsporulating. Facultatively anaerobic with a fermentative metabolism, and complex nutritional requirements. The family consists of five genera: *Streptococcus*, *Leuconostoc*, *Pediococcus*, *Aerococcus*, and *Gemella*.

    Genus I. *Streptococcus* (pliant coccus). Gram positive cells typically in pairs or chains. Fermentative metabolism and facultatively anaerobic, with complex nutritional requirements. Twenty one species are recognized, divided into a hemolytic pyogenic group, subdivided by immunological criteria (*e.g.*, *Streptococcus pyogenes*); a viridians group (turns blood green), of which *Streptococcus salivarius*, *Streptococcus mitis*, and *Streptococcus sanguis* constitute a major part of the oral microbiota; an enterococcus group represented by *Streptococcus faecalis* that contains primarily intestinal parasites but some are also found in the mouth; and a lactic group of primarily plant parasites also used for the manufacture of dairy products (*e.g.*, *Streptococcus lactis*). Not included in these four groups are some 80 types of *Streptococcus pneumoniae* (the pneumococcus), primarily an obligate parasite of the nasopharynx and an important pathogen of the respiratory tract, causing pneumonia.

Family III. *Peptococcaceae*. Gram positive cocci that occur in pairs, tetrads, irregular masses, and cubic packets or in chains. Nonsporulating and nonmotile, with complex nutritional requirements. Inhabitants of the oral cavity and the intestinal and respiratory tracts of man and other animals and the human female urogenital tract.

    Genus I. *Peptococcus*. Consists of six species of spherical bacteria (type species, *Peptococcus niger*) that do not require carbohydrates but obtain energy from protein decomposition products. Inhabitants of the human female urogenital tract, the human oral cavity, the human intestinal and respiratory tract, tonsils, skin and infected areas, but pathogenicity uncertain.

Genus II. *Peptostreptococcus.* Gram positive, nonmotile, nonsporulating spherical or ovoid cells. Anaerobic and generally ferment carbohydrates to form organic acids. Inhabitants of the normal and infected oral cavity and female genital tract and often found in septic wounds, gangrene, osteomyelitis, and appendicitis. There are five recognized species with *Peptostreptococcus anaerobius* as the type species.

Endospore-forming Rods

Family I. *Bacillaceae.* Gram positive, motile or nonmotile, aerobic, facultative, or anaerobic, sporulating rods with one genus having spherical cells.

Genus I. *Bacillus* (a rodlet). Gram positive, sporulating, motile, rod-shaped cells that are aerobes or facultative anaerobes. Some 48 species in the genus with *Bacillus subtilis* being the type species. *Bacillus anthracis* causes anthrax in animals and humans.

Genus III. *Clostridium* (a small spindle). Generally gram positive, occasionally nonmotile, sporulating, generally strictly anaerobic rods. Inhabitants of marine and fresh water sediments, soil, and the intestinal tract of man and other animals and animal products. The genus contains more than 60 species with *Clostridium butyricum* being the type species. Various species infect wounds and cause gas gangrene, tetanus, and botulism.

Gram Positive, Asporogenous Rod-shaped Bacteria

Family I. *Lactobacillaceae.* Gram positive, nonmotile, anaerobic or facultative straight or curved rods with complex nutritional requirements. Metabolize carbohydrates to produce lactate. Widely distributed in plant and animal products. A common organism in the oral cavity, vagina, and the intestinal tract of man and other animals.

Genus I. *Lactobacillus* (milk-rodlet). Gram positive rods that vary from long and slender to short coccobacilli that are generally nonmotile. Metabolize sugars to terminally produce lactate. The genus has 25 recognized species with *Lactobacillus delbrueckii* as the type species. The species are widely distributed in dairy products, grain, meat products, water, sewage, pickled fruit and vegetables, beer, wine, and silage. Particularly common in the oral cavity, intestinal tract, and the vagina of humans and other animals.

Genera of Uncertain Affiliation

Genus *Listeria* (after Lord Lister). Gram positive, motile, nonsporulating, small coccoid rods that are found on vegetation, silage, and the intestinal tracts of man and other animals. The genus has four recognized species with *Listeria monocytogenes* as the type species. Diseases produced include abortion, local abscesses, endocarditis, septicemia, encephalitis, and meningitis. Pathogenicity variable among the species.

Genus *Erysipelothrix* (erysipelas thread). Gram positive, nonsporulating, nonmotile, aerobic, rod-shaped organisms that form filaments. Parasites of birds, mammals, and fish. One species, *Erysipelothrix rhusiopathiae* which is the type species. Causes swine erysipelas and is occasionally pathogenic for man.

Actinomycetes and Related Organism

Coryneform Group of Bacteria. Pleomorphic, mostly nonmotile rods that are frequently banded with metachromatic granules. Generally gram positive. Includes the genera *Corynebacterium, Arthrobacter, Microbacterium, Cellulomonas,* and *Kurthia.*

Genus I. *Corynebacterium* (club bacterium). The cells frequently show club-shaped swelling and "snapping division" that produces palisade arrangement of cells. The genus has been divided into three sections: I—Human and animal parasites and pathogens. II—Plant pathogenic corynebacteria. III—Nonpathogenic corynebacteria. Section I is divided into nine recognized species with *Corynebacterium diphtheriae,* the cause of diphtheria, as the type species.

Order I. Actinomycetales. Gram positive, acid-fast bacteria that form branching filaments that fragment to coccoid, elongate, or diphtheroid elements. Some forms reproduce spores on aerial hyphae.

Family I. *Actinomycetaceae.* Gram positive, non-acid-fast bacteria that form filaments, that fragment in diphtheroid-shaped or coccoid cells.

Genus I. *Actinomyces* (ray fungus). Gram positive, non-acid-fast, nonmotile, nonsporulating bacteria that occur as filaments that fragment into diphtheroids. Mostly anaerobic but some are facultative anaerobes. Five species are recognized, with *Actinomyces bovis* as the type species. All species are found in the oral cavity of man and other animals.

Genus II. *Arachnia* (filamentous microcolonies). Similar to, but distinct from, the genus *Actinomyces*. Represented by a single species, *Arachnia propionica,* which is pathogenic for man and mice, causing a disease similar to actinomycosis.

Genus IV. *Bacterionema* (thread-shaped long rod). Gram positive, nonsporulating nonmotile, pleomorphic filaments and bacilli. Facultative anaerobe that ferments carbohydrates. Represented by a single species, *Bacterionema matruchotii,* that is found in the oral cavity of primates and man in calculus and dental plaque.

Genus V. *Rothia* (after G. D. Roth). Gram positive, non-acid-fast, nonsporulating, nonmotile bacteria that can

Table 1/2—*continued*

occur singly or as a mixture of coccoid, diphtheroid, or branched filaments. Represented by the species, *Rothia dentocariosa*, a normal inhabitant of the oral cavity.

Family II. *Mycobacteriaceae*. Cells composed of curved or straight rods that also branch or form filaments. Gram positive, nonmotile, nonsporulating. Aerobic. Slow or rapid growth. Found in the soil, water, also in warm-blooded, and cold-blooded animals. Contains one genus, *Mycobacterium*.

　　Genus I. *Mycobacterium* (fungus rodlet). Cells as described above with a high lipid content. Composed of 30 recognized species, with *Mycobacterium tuberculosis*, the cause of tuberculosis, as the type species. Many of the other species are pathogenic. *Mycobacterium leprae*, the cause of leprosy is another important species.

Family VI. *Nocardiaceae*. Gram positive, variably acid-fast. Nonsporulating, obligate aerobes. Cells vary among filaments, coccoids, and bacillary fragments. Reproductive spores are produced on differentiated hyphae.

　　Genus I. *Nocardia* (after E. Nocard). Cells similar to those described above. The genus consists of some 31 recognized species with *Nocardia farcinica* as the type species. Common inhabitant of soils and humans and other animals. Some species cause nocardiosis, which resembles actinomycosis.

Family VII. *Streptomycetaceae*. Resemble fungi, with vegetative hyphae that produce branched mycelia that do not fragment easily. Forms aerial spores. Gram positive, aerobic. Four genera.

　　Genus I. *Streptomyces* (pliant or bent fungus). Forms slender coenocytic hyphae and aerial mycelia that bear reproductive spores. Many strains are sensitive to antibacterial agents. There are more than 400 recognized species that are widely distributed in the environment. Many of these species and strains produce antibacterial, antifungal, antiviral, antialgal, antiprotozoal, or even antitumor antibiotics.

The Rickettsias

Order I. *Rickettsiales*. Gram negative, nonmotile, pleomorphic, rod-shaped, coccoid, small microorganisms that can multiply only in the cells of a suitable host. Procaryotic microorganisms not related to viruses.

Family I. *Rickettsiaceae*. Small pleomorphic organisms that are intracellular parasites that, with one exception, have not been cultured in cell-free media. Parasites of man and other animals that are transmitted to and from such insect vectors as mites, ticks, fleas, and lice.

　　Tribe I. *Rickettsieae*. Small, pleomorphic, intracellular microorganisms that are obligate parasites and pathogens.

　　Genus I. *Rickettsia* (after H. T. Ricketts). Gram negative, short rods that have not been cultivated without the presence of living host cells. Growth occurs in the cytoplasm of such cells. Man may be either the reservoir or incidental host of *Rickettsia* species. Small rodents and other vertebrates also serve as reservoirs and disseminate rickettsia. Arthropods are main reservoirs and regulate the transmission to and from the susceptible vertebrates. There are 10 recognized species and the type species is *Rickettsia prowazekii*. The various strains of the genus *Rickettsia* can be divided into biotypes that cause either typhus, spotted fever, or scrub typhus.

　　Genus II. *Rochalimaea* (after H. da RochaLima). Similar to the genus *Rickettsia*, and they depend on vertebrates and arthropods for survival. The genus contains one species, *Rochalimaea quintana*, which is also the type species. The organism is the cause of trench fever, which is transmitted to the primary human host by the human louse.

　　Genus III. *Coxiella* (after H. R. Cox). Resembles the genus *Rickettsia* but is more resistant. The genus contains one species, *Coxiella burnetii*, which is the type species. *C. burnetii*, the cause of Q fever is widely distributed throughout the world in domestic animals and their ectoparasites, as well as the ectoparasites of rodents and marsupials. While such vectors transmit the disease it is also an aerosol infection.

Family II. *Bartonellaceae*. Gram negative, pleomorphic, rod-shaped coccoid, and disc-shaped cells that are parasites of human and vertebrate erythrocytes but which can be cultivated on nonliving media.

　　Genus I. *Bartonella* (after A. L. Barton). Gram negative but stain poorly. Found in the host in fixed tissue cells and erythrocytes but can be grown in cell-free media. The genus has one species, *Bartonella bacilliformis*, which is the type species. It is the cause of human bartonellosis, which occurs as either an anemia (Oroya fever), or as cutaneous eruptions (verruga peruana).

Order II. *Chlamydiales*. Gram negative, coccoid microorganisms that require an intracellular mode of reproduction involving an infectious phase (elementary body) and a noninfectious form (initial body).

Family I. *Chlamydiaceae*. Coccoid organisms that have a developmental cycle within the cytoplasm of the host. Cause various diseases.

　　Genus I. *Chlamydia* (a cloak). Gram negative, nonmotile, obligate intracellular parasites that undergo a developmental cycle in the cytoplasm of the host's cells. Greatly dependent on the host cells for metabolic activity. Two recognized species, with *Chlamydia trachomatis* as the type species. *C. trachomatis* causes trachoma, inclusion conjunctivitis, lymphogranuloma venereum, urethritis, and proctitis. The other species, *Chlamydia psittaci*, causes psittacosis, ornithosis, pneumonitis in several domestic animals; polyarthritis in cattle, sheep and pigs; abortion in cattle and sheep; enteritis in cattle; conjunctivitis in cattle and sheep; intestinal infections in cattle and sheep; and encephalomyelitis in cattle.

Table 1/2—*continued*

The Mycoplasmas

Class *Mollicutes*. Procaryotic organisms that lack a true cell wall and are incapable of synthesizing certain cell wall precursors. Cells are gram negative and consist of small, highly pleomorphic coccoids or filaments that are small and sometimes ultramicroscopic. All recognized species are capable of growth in cell-free media. These organisms may be either saprophytic, parasitic, or pathogenic. Pathogenic species cause diseases in both animals and plants.

Order I. *Mycoplasmatales*. Description of the order similar to the class. Only one order, *Mycoplasmatales* in the Class *Mollicutes*. Two families are in the order *Mycoplasmatales*.

Family I. *Mycoplasmataceae*. Description similar to class and order. Require sterols.

Genus I. *Mycoplasma* (fungus form). Gram negative, extremely pleomorphic cells with alternate means of replication. Lack a true cell wall. Form very small colonies (up to 600 μm) on solid media. Generally they have a fermentative metabolism and all species require sterols for growth. They range from aerobes to facultative anaerobes. They may be either parasites or pathogens for a wide range of mammals and birds. The principal diseases are contagious pleuropneumonia of cattle and goats, pink-eye in cattle, chronic respiratory diseases in poultry, infectious synovitis in chickens and turkeys, "rolling disease" in mice, atrophic rhinitis, pneumonia in pigs, primary atypical pneumonia in man, mastitis in cattle, and purulent polyarthritis in rats. More than 36 recognized species with *Mycoplasma mycoides* as the type species.

also form spores asexually. With nuclear fusion and reduction of chromosome number, the cell enlarges to form a spore sac (ascus) containing from one to eight spores, which are termed ascospores. An intermediate yeast, genus *Candida*, forms a pseudomycelium consisting of chains of elongated buds. Quite a few pathogenic fungi can grow either in a yeast-like or mold-like filamentous form depending on cultural conditions. *In vivo*, the yeastlike forms predominate. Such fungi are said to be false yeasts.

Unlike bacteria, most fungi are large enough and exhibit sufficient differentiation of structure to permit classification along standard botanical lines with little resort to physiological and biochemical characteristics. They are classified by the type of colony produced (yeast types, resembling bacterial colonies, or mold type); by the presence or absence of mycelia; by the character of the mycelium (septate or not); by the size, structure, and color of the spores; and most important of all, by characteristic mechanisms of sexual and asexual spore formation. On these bases, eumycetes are divided into four classes:

I. Phycomycetes (literally, "seaweed fungus"). A diverse, widely distributed group but of negligible medical importance.

II. Ascomycetes ("sac fungi"). A diverse and widely distributed group; a few genera occasionally infect man and animals.

III. Basidiomycetes. Except for the species that form powerful poisons, they are not medically important.

IV. Fungi Imperfecti (imperfect fungi). Hyphae septate; no sexual stage known; asexual spores formed in various typical ways as conidia (see Ascomycetes) or directly within, upon, or from the thallus (= mycelium or body of the fungus) as thallospores; practically all of the fungi pathogenic for man fall in this class; many of these grow yeast-like *in vivo* and under appropriate cultural conditions, and mold-like under other cultural conditions.

CLASSIFICATION AND NOMENCLATURE OF VIRUSES

It is generally agreed that four characteristics distinguish a virus. 1) It contains either DNA or RNA but not both, in contrast to other microorganisms and higher forms. 2) It lacks enzymes to convert substrates into high energy compounds needed to drive biosynthetic reactions, and also lacks the enzymes requisite for biosynthesis. 3) It cannot grow and then divide by binary fission. 4) Its reproduction consists essentially of the replication of its nucleic acid genetic material by the metabolic mechanisms of the infected host cell. The incidental production of a proteinaceous coat (capsid) serves primarily to stabilize the nucleic acid component and protect it from nucleases during passage of the virus to a fresh host cell.

In biological terms, a virus is a rudimentary subcellular genetic entity, capable of gaining entrance into a limited range of living cells and capable of reproduction only within such cells. Intracellularly, after conversion into a noninfective form, its genetic information specifically directs biosynthetic pathways of the host cell to replication of the viral genome and its associated capsid. This process does not necessarily impair the infected cell seriously— in some systems the cell survives and liberates new virus indefinitely; in others, the cell and its progeny maintain a persistent infection without the appearance of extracellular virus.

A completely satisfactory definition of viruses is hardly possible at present, let alone a description

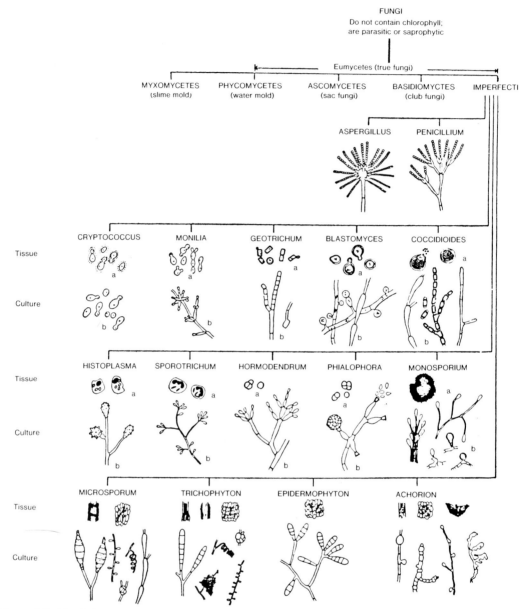

Figure 1/1. Morphological types of the pathogenic fungi as they occur in tissue (*a*) and in culture (*b*). (Adapted from chart prepared by N. E. Conant: In *Musser's Internal Medicine*, Ed. 5, edited by M. G. Wohl. Lea & Febiger, Philadelphia, 1951.)

of their natural relationships to each other and to more familiar microorganisms. The criteria of filterability and size ceased long ago to be definitive, with the discovery of free-living organisms smaller than many viruses. The property of obligate intracellular parasitism is relevant but is not peculiar to viruses, being characteristic of occasional protozoa and bacteria. The property of producing disease is of methodological value only, since many viruses are maintained in their hosts for long periods without producing discernible pathological change.

The modern classification of viruses relates largely to the physicochemical properties of the virus particle. The principal components involved are nucleic acids and proteins, although larger virions may contain carbohydrates and lipids. Like other organisms, the basis for viral nomenclature is varied and often arbitrary. Many names are based on clinical, pathological, or epidemiological features, *e.g.*, Eastern Equine Encephalomyelitis virus. Others are descriptive, being based on some outstanding characteristic of the virus, *e.g.*, Orbivirus group (L. *orbis* = ring), derived from their large doughnut-shaped capsomeres. Some names are ac-

Table 1/3
Current classification of RNA-containing viruses of vertebrates[a]

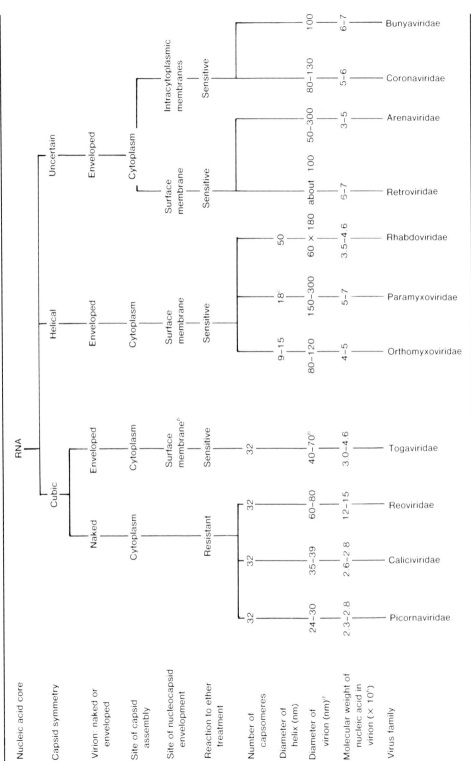

[a] From J. L. Melnick: Taxonomy of Viruses. In *Manual of Clinical Microbiology*, Ed. 3. American Society for Microbiology, Washington, D.C., 1980.

[b] All of the properties shown for Togaviridae apply to the genera *Alphavirus* and *Rubivirus*; however, for the genera *Pestivirus* and *Flavivirus*, envelopment takes place at intracytoplasmic membranes, the number of capsomeres is not clearly established, and the virions are somewhat smaller.

[c] All of the properties shown for Paramyxoviridae apply to the genera *Paramyxovirus* and *Morbillivirus*; however, for members of the genus *Pneumovirus*, the diameter of the helix is 12 to 15 nm.

[d] Diameter, or diameter × length.

Table 1/4
Current classification of DNA-containing viruses of vertebrates[a]

	Poxviridae	Iridoviridae	Herpesviridae	Adenoviridae	Papovaviridae	Parvoviridae
Nucleic acid core	DNA					
Capsid symmetry	Complex	Cubic				
Virion: naked or enveloped	Complex coats	Enveloped		Naked		
Site of capsid assembly[b]	Cytoplasm	Cytoplasm	Nucleus	Nucleus		
Site of nucleocapsid envelopment		Cytoplasmic membrane	Nuclear membrane			
Reaction to ether (or other lipid solvents)	Resistant	Sensitive	Sensitive	Resistant		
Number of capsomeres		1500	162	252	72	32
Diameter of virion (nm)[c]	230 × 300	130–300	100[d]	70–90	45–55	18–26
Molecular weight of nucleic acid (× 10⁶)	160	100–250	92–102	20–30	3.0–5.0	1.5–2.2
Virus family	Poxviridae	Iridoviridae	Herpesviridae	Adenoviridae	Papovaviridae	Parvoviridae

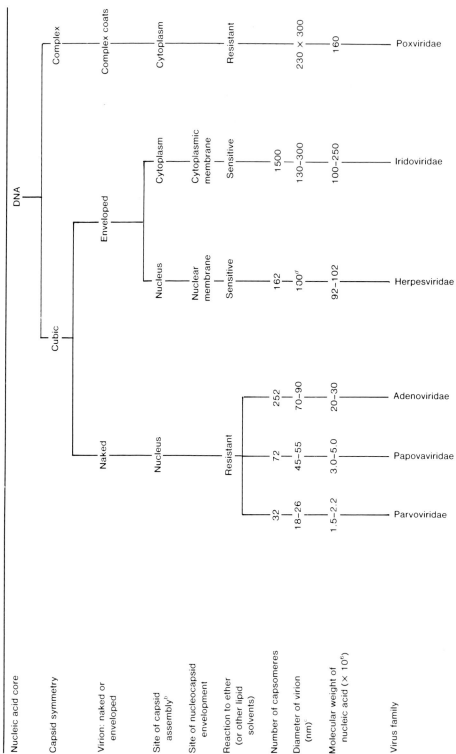

[a] From J. L. Melnick: Taxonomy of Viruses. In *Manual of Clinical Microbiology*, Ed. 3. American Society for Microbiology, Washington, D.C., 1980.
[b] For the DNA viruses whose capsid assembly takes place in the nucleus, a phase of replication occurs in the cytoplasm, as evidenced by the detection of viral messenger RNA associated with polyribosomes.
[c] Diameter, or diameter × length.
[d] The naked virus is 100 nm in diameter; however, the enveloped virions range up to 150 nm in diameter.

ronyms, *e.g.*, *reo*virus from *re*spiratory-*e*nteric-*o*r-phan, while others reflect the name of the individual who first described the virus, *e.g.*, Rous sarcoma virus. Finally, some describe the region where the virus was located or predominates, *e.g.*, Colorado tick fever virus.

Virus classification is based on common, genetically stable properties which include nucleic acid type, strandedness, and molecular weight; virus shape; capsomere number; site of production of maturation; and presence or absence of an outer envelope. These and other major characteristics are summarized for the major families of RNA- (table 1/3) and DNA- (table 1/4) viruses.

ADDITIONAL READING

BUCHANAN, R. E., AND GIBBONS, N. E. (Eds.) 1974 *Bergey's Manual of Determinative Bacteriology*. Williams & Wilkins, Baltimore.

DEMELLO, F. J., AND LEONARD, M. S. 1979 *Eikenella corrodens*: A New Pathogen. Oral Surg, **47,** 401.

FENNER, F. 1974 The classification of Viruses; Why, When and How. Aust J Exp Biol Med Sci, **52,** 223.

MANDEL, M. 1969 New Approaches to Bacterial Taxonomy: Perspective and Prospects. Annu Rev Microbiol, **23,** 239.

MELNICK, J. L. 1980 Taxonomy of Viruses. In *Manual of Clinical Microbiology*, edited by E. H. Lennette, A. Balows, W. J. Hausler, and J. P. Truant. American Society for Microbiology, Washington, D.C.

MOLINARI, J. A., AND PHILLIP, M. J. 1980 Microbiology and Sterilization. In *Review of Dental Assisting*, edited by B. A. Ladley and S. A. Wilson. C. V. Mosby, St. Louis.

RAVIN, A. W. 1960 The Origins of Bacterial Species. Genetic Recombination and Factors Limiting It between Bacterial Populations. Bacteriol Rev, **24,** 201.

SKERMAN, V. V. D. 1959 *A Guide to the Identification of the Genera of Bacteria*. Williams & Wilkins, Baltimore.

SOCIETY OF GENERAL MICROBIOLOGY. 1959 Symposium: The Principles of Microbial Classification. J. Gen Microbiol, **12,** 314.

chapter 2

Isolation and Systematic Examination of Pathogenic Microorganisms

Chris H. Miller

INTRODUCTION

Isolation and identification of pathogenic microorganisms from man is of primary importance in determining the diagnosis and in recommending therapy for infectious diseases. In addition, the techniques used are important in determining the types and numbers of microorganisms present at various body sites under various conditions (*e.g.*, in research studies determining the "anti-caries" effects of an antimicrobial agent, effects on both caries-inducing and less pathogenic oral microorganisms must be measured). During the isolation and identification of microorganisms from the human body, consideration must be given to many procedures each of which can influence the final results: specimen collection; transport and initial processing; selection, inoculation and incubation of growth media; identification of the isolated microorganisms. The specific procedures depend upon the type of specimen, the suspected types of microorganisms present in the specimen and the specific types of results desired. Of particular procedural importance in all phases of microbial isolation, identification and manipulation is the use of aseptic technique—procedures which prevent or reduce unwanted microbial contamination.

COLLECTION OF SPECIMENS

Sampling Sites

The site of specimen collection is usually dictated by the pathogenesis of the disease. Specimens which are usually free of indigenous microorganisms are needle or surgical biopsy tissues, blood, spinal fluid, and exudates or other unnatural accumulations of fluid within various internal body cavities. Contaminating indigenous microorganisms are usually found in specimens associated with mucous membranes and skin. It is necessary to avoid as much as possible contamination of a clinical specimen by normal body flora. This is a constant problem when sampling oral sites. The types of oral lesions or conditions from which microbial specimens are obtained include: periodontal lesions including pericoronitis, acute necrotizing ulcerative gingivitis and periodontitis; lesions of the oral tissues such as might occur in syphilis, oral gonorrhea, denture stomatitis, candidiasis, herpes and other fungal and viral infections; abscesses with suppuration; postoperative infections from extractions or soft tissue surgery; sinus drainage through the oroantral fistula from perforations of the maxillary sinus; salivary gland infections; biopsy tissues; infected root canals.

Sampling Methods

When collecting fluids or biopsy tissue by needle aspiration through the skin or a mucous membrane, the surface must be disinfected with an antiseptic to reduce or prevent both entry into the tissues and contamination of the specimen by normal body flora. Blood, spinal fluid, midstream urine, bronchial washings, sputum, saliva, and feces are best collected directly into sterile containers which are transported to the laboratory. Tissue specimens and dental plaque are collected under aseptic technique and commonly placed into small containers of stabilizing or transport fluid to preserve microbial viability. Swabbing of specific lesions or other sites should involve as little contamination as possible from adjacent sites. For example, a sample of purulent drainage from an excised oral abscess or opened tooth pulp must not be contaminated with saliva. Since plain cotton swabs may contain antibacterial fatty acids, it is best to use sterile swabs made of calcium alginate or Dacron or Fortrel polysters. Commercially available swabs include those which are packaged in a receptacle containing a transport fluid.

In instances where the likelihood for the presence of strictly anaerobic bacteria is great, samples may be collected under anaerobic conditions. Such instances are common with oral infections. The sample may be collected as usual and then immediately placed into a prereduced fluid which has low oxygen tension and a low oxidation-reduction potential. Such fluids are commercially available. A stream of oxygen-free gas also may be used when opening the prereduced fluid container to avoid entrance of air. Other devices have been described for use during the sampling of anaerobic organisms such as might be found in periodontal pockets. The samples are taken through cannulas modified so the site can be continually flushed with oxygen-free gas while the sample is taken. Such samples are then placed in a prereduced medium from which oxygen has been excluded and they may be dispersed and cultured in an anaerobic environment.

TRANSPORT OF SPECIMEN

Transport of clinical or research specimens to the microbiology laboratory for analysis should occur as soon as possible to prevent overgrowth of contaminating microorganisms and death of potential pathogens. When specimens are collected within a hospital or research setting, a common time limit between collection and delivery to the laboratory is 2 hours. Specimens collected in the dental office should be taken to the laboratory immediately. If the specimens must be mailed then they should be placed in a transport medium in a preferably unbreakable tube sealed with waterproof tape, wrapped with absorbent material, placed in a secondary container sealed with waterproof tape, and finally placed in a sealed, properly labeled shipping container. Shipping with dry ice may also help preserve the specimen.

Each clinical specimen must be fully described so that the laboratory will be able to select the proper procedures for analysis. This description should include the type of specimen, site of collection, attempts taken to avoid contamination, patient symptoms or suspected diagnosis, suspected types of microorganisms present, and need for antibiotic sensitivity testing on the predominant or unusual isolates.

INITIAL PROCESSING OF SPECIMENS

Some specimens such as feces and dental plaque must be diluted before culturing so that workable numbers of microorganisms can be obtained. In addition, dental plaque samples must first be dispersed by techniques of controlled sonic oscillation, or vortexing with glass beads to facilitate the separation of the many types of bacterial cells present in this adherent mass. Precautions again must be taken during dispersion and dilution procedures to preserve the strictly anaerobic microorganisms.

Frequently, general types of information on the microbial content of a raw specimen can be obtained by performing various types of bacterial staining and microscopic procedures (*e.g.*, gram stain, capsular stain, dark-field examination). A great deal of research is being conducted on the rapid identification of microorganisms including methods analyzing for specific microbial products directly in raw specimens. Advancements in this field will be of particular importance to the dentist and physician because the sooner the microorganisms can be identified the sooner the diagnosis can be made and appropriate therapy instituted. Until such techniques have been proven, the more time-consuming standard procedures of microbial culturing prior to identification must suffice.

BACTERIA

The characterization and classification of a bacterium require that it be separated from all other microorganisms and that it be maintained in pure culture. Since bacterial identification involves working with a population of like cells rather than with a single cell (due to the small size), a pure culture is commonly defined as an isolated colony of over a million bacterial cells which are direct offspring of a single cell or colony-forming unit (CFU).

Methods of Isolation

Specimens from the human mouth and other body sites contain mixed cultures, and characterization of the different bacteria present requires that each type be separated from the others. The isolation of a pure culture of bacteria can be accomplished with a suitable agar-containing medium by either the streaking method or the pour plate method. Samples are placed on or in a suitable nutrient broth which is made semisolid by the addition of agar. Agar is a polysaccharide from seaweed which is nontoxic and not affected by bacteria. When placed in an aqueous nutrient broth and boiled prior to steam sterilization, the agar liquefies (at about 100 C). When the medium is cooled to near 40 C, the agar solidifies and will not melt again until temperatures of 100 C are reached.

Streak Plate Method. A suitably diluted specimen containing a mixture of bacterial types or species is spread or "streaked" on the surface of a suitable solidified agar medium in a sterile Petri dish. Spreading or streaking is accomplished by the use of a sterilized bacteriological inoculating loop or by a sterilized bent glass rod. As the loop or rod passes over the surface of the agar, individual or small groups of bacterial cells are deposited, and after appropriate incubation each develops into an isolated colony if the sample was diluted sufficiently and spread properly (fig. 2/1). Each isolated colony,

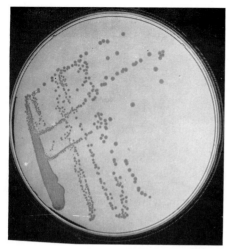

Figure 2/1. Open view of Petri dish containing nutrient agar upon which a bacterial inoculum has been spread sufficiently by means of an inoculating loop to give distinct and separate colonies.

now usually visible to the naked eye, can be counted (if determining numbers of CFU in the original specimen) and subcultured for further tests leading to identification.

Pour Plate Method. This is an alternative to the streak plate method. Sterile, melted agar medium is cooled to about 48 C and the properly diluted specimen is added and gently mixed. The medium is poured into a Petri dish and allowed to cool and solidify. After appropriate incubation, visible, isolated colonies develop throughout the agar.

Aerobic and Anaerobic Culturing

Bacteria have varying requirements for oxygen and carbon dioxide and those from the human body may be aerobic, facultatively anaerobic, microaerophilic, or anaerobic as defined in a later chapter. Plating and culturing of anaerobic bacteria may be carried out in an anaerobic environment using anaerobic chambers or glove boxes in which the air has been replaced with an oxygen-free gas mixture (*e.g.*, 85% N_2, 10% H_2, 5% CO_2). Growth media also may be inoculated under a stream of oxygen-free gas and the vessels sealed or placed in an anaerobic holding jar until ready for incubation. Cultures in sealed anaerobic tubes are incubated in the usual fashion. Unsealed cultures may be incubated in temperature-adjusted anaerobic chambers and glove boxes or they may be placed in sealed, reduced-oxygen jars and placed in a regular incubator. Oxygen can be removed from a closed container by a catalytic process in which hydrogen reacts with the oxygen in the presence of a platinized asbestos catalyst to form water. Commercially prepared units are available whereby water is added to an exact mixture of chemicals and placed in jars which contain the catalyst. The oxygen is removed and also carbon dioxide is produced yielding an anaerobic environment. The media used to culture strict anaerobes should also contain reducing agents (*e.g.*, dithiothreitol, thioglycollate) to lower the oxidation-reduction potential. Reduced media also may be prepared and stored under oxygen-free conditions prior to inoculation.

Bacterial Growth Media

Media used for the isolation of bacteria by the streak or pour plate methods can be divided into two types: nonselective, and selective. In general, both types contain basic growth nutrients in the form of protein digests, extracts of yeasts or plant and animal tissues, salts and frequently blood and sugars. The nonselective media (*e.g.*, blood agar) support growth of many pathogenic and nonpathogenic bacteria commonly encountered. Selective media contain either inhibitors for undesired bacteria, or growth promoters for desired bacteria, or both. Rogosa's medium, selective for the aciduric lactobacilli, contains acetate and other salts to suppress most oral bacteria and enrichments for lactobacilli. Crystal violet and potassium tellurite are used to select for certain oral streptococci (*e.g.*, Mitis-Salivarius medium) and facilitate the isolation of *Streptococcus mitis*, *Streptococcus salivarius*, and other streptococci. In other selective media, dyes, bile, antibiotics, and high salt content are typical inhibitors.

In most microbial analyses of mixed culture specimens a combination of nonselective and selective media are used for primary isolation. Use of only a nonselective medium may result in the masking or interspecies inhibition of important bacteria. Such bacteria may be present in the sample at lower concentration and, thus, would appear only on plates which have a large total number of colonies making isolation and/or enumeration difficult or impossible. The use of appropriate selective media will permit isolation of bacteria masked or inhibited on nonselective media. On the other hand, use of selective media for enumeration of specific bacteria in a given specimen must be done with caution, since this type of medium can select against as well as for the desired bacterium.

Not all pathogenic bacteria can be cultured *in vitro* and some have few, if any, animal hosts. Fully pathogenic *Treponema pallidum* apparently has not been cultured *in vitro* but can be maintained by serial transfer in rabbit testes. *Mycobacterium leprae* has not been cultured *in vitro* and has only one apparent animal host, the armadillo. Nevertheless, animal inoculation is an important means for isolating and, in a few instances, in maintaining pathogenic bacteria. In addition, microscopic studies coupled with microbial isolation and identification suggest that microorganisms are present in the mouth and alimentary canal of man which have never been cultured or identified.

Maintenance of Pure Cultures

While awaiting identification or further study, pure cultures of bacteria must be maintained in such a way as to preserve their viability without significantly changing their properties. Lyophilization is widely used to preserve bacteria. Suspensions in sterile protein solution are quick-frozen in dry ice and alcohol, their water removed under a high vacuum and the tubes sealed and stored under refrigeration. Lyophilized bacteria survive for a long time but they die slowly so that after prolonged storage the surviving population may be selected for some particular characteristic. When lyophilization is not available, pure cultures may be stored at 4 C in sealed tubes of agar-media or frozen in broth media to which a 10% final concentration of sterile glycerin has been added.

Enumeration of Bacteria

It is frequently necessary to determine the concentration of the bacteria present in clinical specimens or laboratory cultures. For example, the microbiological diagnosis of a urinary tract infection is commonly based upon demonstrating that the urine specimen contains more than 100,000 organisms per ml. Recovery of 10,000 to 100,000 per ml with three or more bacterial species represented usually denotes contamination of the urine during collection rather than infection. Enumeration of the different types of bacteria in dental or crevicular plaque or saliva samples has been used to determine the predominant bacteria present during different stages of periodontal disease and dental caries. This approach is also used to measure shifts in the proportions of pathogenic oral bacteria during the testing of various preventive or treatment regimes for caries and periodontal diseases. Additionally, bacterial enumeration is important in the quality control of drinking water and milk, since certified milk is limited to 10,000 bacteria per ml and drinking water to 1 coliform per 100 ml in the United States. Counting bacteria is also important in the determination of growth requirements, measurement of virulence, or in standardization of reference cultures and whole-cell vaccines.

The most useful counting procedures are the direct count and the viable count. A direct count, usually carried out in a counting chamber under the microscope, indicates the total number of cells, whether living or dead. The viable count gives the number of bacterial cells that will grow under given culturing conditions. For a viable count, measured amounts of various sample dilutions are plated by the streak or pour plate method and the colonies which develop after incubation are counted. Each colony theoretically represents a single cell originally deposited on or in the agar medium. In reality, a single colony may be derived from 1 to 25 or more cells (a CFU) due to cell aggregation or natural associations (e.g., chains of streptococci) in the inoculum.

Systematic Examination of Bacteria

Once a bacterium is isolated and established as a pure culture, it is necessary to determine enough of its properties to identify and classify it. In general the systematic examination involves determining colony characteristics, cell morphology, staining reactions, biochemical properties, and occasionally its antigenic properties, virulence in animals, susceptibility to specific bacteriophages, cell wall chemistry, and DNA chemistry (e.g., guanine and cytocine content, hybridization characteristics). In identifying bacteria it must be kept in mind that most bacteria experience mutations, as well as many physiological variations according to age, the type of culture medium, time and temperature of incubation, and other environmental factors. The establishment and the reliability of bacterial characteristics are dependent upon the control and standardization of such factors.

Colony Characteristics. Colony morphology is an important characteristic of bacteria and is one of the first properties of a freshly isolated strain to be observed. It is commonly determined by examination of colonies by the unaided eye or with a stereoscopic binocular dissecting microscope (fig. 2/2).

The most important colony characteristics of bacteria and typical terms used to describe them are:

1. *Size:* diameter in mm.
2. *Form:* punctiform, circular, filamentous, irregular, rhizoid, spindle
3. *Elevation:* flat, raised, convex, pulvinate, umbonate, umbilicate
4. *Margin* (edge of colony): entire, undulant, lobate, erose, filamentous, curled
5. *Color:* white, yellow, black, buff, orange, etc.
6. *Surface:* glistening, dull, other
7. *Density:* opaque, translucent, transparent, other
8. *Consistency:* butyrous, viscid, membranous, brittle, adherent
9. *Changes in medium:* hemolysis, discoloration.

Cellular Morphology. Cellular characteristics, important in defining a bacterial species, are microscopically observed on stained bacterial cells fixed by heat to glass slides. Staining is usually accomplished by gram stain, acid-fast stain, metachromatic stain, or by special stains to demonstrate some specific part of a cell, such as capsules or

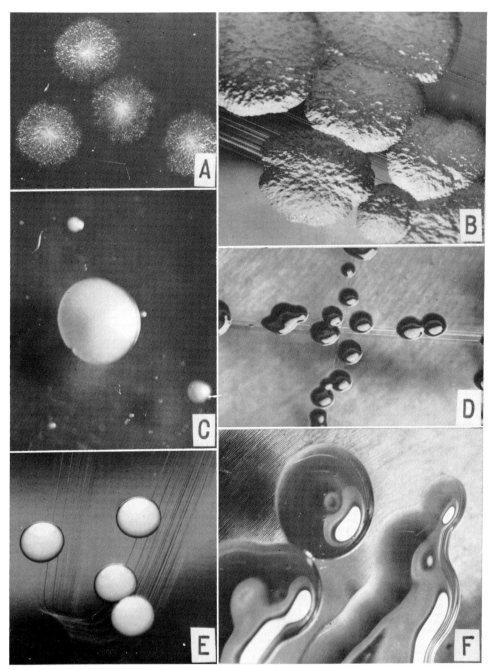

Figure 2/2. Various colonial types of microorganisms. *(A)* Rough filamentous colonies of *Leptotrichia* species. *(B)* Rough colonial forms of *Escherichia coli* grown on beef heart infusion agar. *(C)* The largest colony is that of an oral yeast species, showing a creamy smooth surface, an entire margin, and a heaped-up contour. The medium-sized smooth colonies are those of oral *Lactobacillus* species. The smaller pinpoints are those of oral streptococcal species. *(D)* Mucoid colonies of *E. coli* growing on eosin-methylene blue agar. *(E)* Flattened, smooth colonies of *Staphylococcus epidermidis* growing on beef heart infusion agar. *(F)* Mucoid colonies of *Klebsiella pneumoniae* growing on beef heart infusion agar. *(A,* from B. G. Bibby.)

flagella. Dark-field or phase-contrast microscopy can be used to observe living, unstained bacteria. Electron microscopy, utilizing electrons rather than light, can be used to reveal much of the finer details of bacteria, but it is not always used for bacterial identification. Cellular characteristics used in describing bacteria are size, descriptions of overall shape (sphere, rod, filament, curved, or spiral), arrangement in aggregates or chains, presence and arrangement of spores, staining affinities, presence or absence of capsules, and the presence or absence of flagella (motile or nonmotile).

Biochemical Properties. After determination of colony and cellular morphologies from nonselective and selective growth media along with the gram stain reaction, many isolates can be placed in a "suspected" bacterial group (*e.g.*, streptococci, gram negative bacilli, gram positive bacilli). Further identification of the isolates to genus and species levels usually requires characterization of their biochemical properties and sometimes their immunochemical characteristics. Of the numerous tests available, only select ones are important in differentiating organisms within a "suspected" group. The common types of biochemical tests used include those which measure oxygen requirements, nutritional requirements, sensitivity to specific growth inhibitors or lysing agents, production of specific enzymes, adherence in the presence of certain nutrients, actions on proteins and production of specific metabolic end products. The biochemical nature of the isolates is sometimes reflected in its immunological properties. Antibodies produced by the body in response to a given bacterium are used to detect and identify homologous bacteria. Immunological techniques, in more recent years, have been greatly expanded by the conjugation of antibodies with fluorescent dyes, such as fluorescein. This procedure is a valuable and sensitive tool for identifying bacteria and other microorganisms in a variety of specimens and even in tissues.

As the systematic examination continues, the reactions of the isolate are compared to the known reactions of previously characterized reference bacteria until identification is confirmed. Some bacteria can be identified by only a few characteristics, while others require extensive testing. Some isolates will simply not fit into any known species classification because of changes in their properties or because they have not been previously identified.

RICKETTSIAE AND CHLAMYDIAE

Rickettsiae and chlamydiae are obligate intracellular parasites like viruses, but their structure and chemical composition suggest that they are specialized forms of gram negative bacteria. The rickettsiae, which cause such diseases as typhus, Rocky Mountain spotted fever, and Q fever, reproduce by transverse binary fission only within a host cell, and most (exception: Q fever agent) are transmitted to man through the bite of an infected arthropod. Chlamydiae, which cause diseases such as psittacosis, trachoma, inclusion conjunctivitis, and nongonoccal urethritis, also reproduce by binary fission with host cells. However, unlike rickettsia, they develop into a specialized form for survival when released from the host cell and do not require vectors for transmission.

Both rickettsiae and chlamydiae can be cultured in the yolk sac of embryonated chicken eggs or in specific types of tissue cultures (*e.g.*, mouse lymphoblasts for the scrub typhus rickettsiae and mouse fibroblasts for chlamydiae). Bacterial contamination is suppressed by use of appropriate antibiotics. The systematic examination of these specialized forms of bacteria is mainly based on the clinical and epidemiological features of the diseases produced in animals and man, demonstration of tissue forms of the organisms, immunological properties, and/or effects of physical and chemical agents on growth.

VIRUSES

Viruses, like rickettsiae and chlamydiae, are obligate intracellular parasites and require living cells for growth and reproduction. The isolation and identification of viruses are more difficult than bacteria because of their small size, obligate parasitism, and greater lability. Viral specimens include nasal washings, nasal or pharyngeal swabs, throat washings or swabs, mouth swabs, vesicular fluid and scrapings, exudates, urine, stools and rectal swabs, blood, spinal fluid, or biopsy specimens. Before propagating the specimen, as many bacteria as possible should be removed by centrifugation, filtration through a membrane filter, or by the addition of antibacterial agents (*e.g.*, antibiotics). Viruses are commonly propagated in the host system, cell culture, by animal inoculation, or in embryonated eggs. Characteristics that are commonly looked for in tissue cultures are cell destruction and cell alterations (cytopathic effects). In properly inoculated animals, observations are made of the signs of the disease that develops or of the immunological response. Growth of a virus in an embryonated egg frequently will produce lesions that can be detected by visual examination. Also, viruses may be isolated from the membranes, sac fluids, or homogenates of the embryos. Purification of viruses (*e.g.*, filtration, partition, differential centrifugation) is required before they are examined systematically.

After purification, virus particles are examined for their form, stability, infectivity, host cell specificity, and animal interaction. The viral nucleic acid of the particle is examined for type and form, molecular weight, and molar base ratio. Viral proteins are examined for enzyme activity, antigenic nature, and hemagglutinating ability. Viral lipids, if present, are examined for composition and relation to infectivity. Particle stability is examined in relation to pH, temperature, presence of various ions, and response to lipid solvents. Particle form is described according to size, capsid shape, capsomere number, presence or absence of envelope or accessory structures. Host interactions are described according to sites of synthesis, assembly, maturation, and mode of release.

FUNGI

Fungi are "plant-like" organisms that grow as single cells, the yeasts, or as multicellular filamentous forms, the molds and mushrooms. Most fungi are saprophytic but some can produce serious disease in man. Molds reproduce by spores which germinate into long filaments called hyphae. The hyphae grow and branch forming a mat called a mycelium. Yeasts commonly divide by budding or by fission. Some pathogenic fungi are dimorphic existing as yeasts or molds while others have only one form or the other.

Fungi have relatively simple nutritional requirements and are not sensitive to antibiotics that inhibit bacteria. These characteristics allow for the development of selective media for isolation of fungi which do not support the growth of bacteria (e.g., Sabouraud dextrose agar and Littman oxgall agar). Cornmeal agar is often used to stimulate sporulation and the development of fungal characteristics. Temperature, humidity, age, nutrition, and strain variation affect fungal morphology during in vitro culture.

The systematic examination of pathogenic fungi often requires the demonstration of tissue and lesion forms as well as their examination in culture. In culture, colonial morphology, pigmentation, and cellular characteristics are important in identifying and describing species and strains. Spores, formed by aerial mycelia, vary with the species in size, shape, and arrangement, and are properties useful in identification. Other characteristics required for more detailed identification are biological, biochemical, and immunological, including the development of hypersensitivity in fungal infections.

ADDITIONAL READING

Aranki, A., Syed, S. A., Kenney, E. B., and Freter, R. 1969 Isolation of Anaerobic Bacteria from Human Gingiva and Mouse Caecum by Means of a Simplified Glove Box Procedure. Appl Microbiol, 17, 568.

Blair, J. E., Lennette, E. H., and Truant, J. P. 1974 Manual of Clinical Microbiology, Ed. 2. American Society for Microbiology, Bethesda, Md.

Buchanan, R. E., and Gibbons, N. E. (Eds.) 1974 Bergey's Manual of Determinative Bacteriology, Ed. 8. Williams & Wilkins, Baltimore.

Cowen, S. T., and Steel, K. J. 1974 Manual for the Identification of Medical Bacteria. Cambridge University Press, Great Britain.

Freeman, B. 1979 Textbook of Microbiology, W. B. Saunders, Philadelphia.

Koneman, E. W., Allen, S. D., Dowell, V. R., Jr., and Sommers, H. M. 1979 Color Atlas and Textbook of Diagnostic Microbiology. J. B. Lippincott, Philadelphia.

Manganiello, A. D., Socransky, S. S., Smith, C., Propas, D., Oran, V., and Dogon, I. L. 1977 Attempts to Increase Viable Count Recovery of Human Supragingival Dental Plaque. J Periodont Res, 12, 107.

Rogosa, M., Mitchell, J. A., and Wiseman, R. F. 1951 A Selective Medium for the Isolation and Enumeration of Oral Lactobacilli. J Dent Res, 30, 682.

2 CELLULAR AND MOLECULAR MICROBIOLOGY

chapter 3

Bacterial Structure and Function

Benjamin Hammond

INTRODUCTION

Bacteria are procaryotic cells and therefore have a distinctive pattern of cellular organization. In general, the internal structure of procaryotic cells is simpler than that of eucaryotic cells since procaryotes lack a membrane-bound nucleus, an extensive endoplasmic reticulum, mitochondria, and structures associated with mitosis. As would be expected, however, there are a number of structures common to all cells as dictated by certain universally required biological functions—transmission of genetic material and reproduction (nucleus), protein synthesis (ribosomes), and osmotic regulation (cytoplasmic membrane). There is a central network of chromatin material (nuclear body or nucleus) containing a single molecule of DNA unlinked to protein. The molecule is very thin (25 Å in *Escherichia coli*) but has an extraordinary total length (~ 1 mm) sufficient to specify all the major genetic information of the cell. The total amount of genetic material in the procaryotic bacterial cell is about 600 times less than found in a typical eucaryotic cell (5×10^{-15}g per bacterium vs. 3×10^{-12}g per mammalian cell). In the amorphous cytoplasm surrounding the nucleus there are numerous 70S ribosomes in which protein synthesis occurs. There are also a number of cytoplasmic inclusions (often referred to as reserve energy storage granules) which may be present in some bacteria under appropriate cultural conditions. Other cytoplasmic structures are limited to only a few bacteria—*e.g.*, endospores—and play an important role in the survival and maintenance of these organisms in their environment.

The external or surface structure of the bacterial cell is much more complex with a rigid cell wall surrounding the underlying cytoplasmic membrane. There are additional components of this cell envelope which may include filamentous appendages known as flagella and pili, external surface layers (capsules or slime layers) and other specific surface macromolecules. The details of the structure-function relationships of these surface components have been worked out in rather great detail making it possible to relate function to chemical architecture. Schematic representations of prototype bacterial cells are seen in figure 3/1.

This chapter will introduce bacterial structure with an emphasis on structure function relationships as they relate to oral bacteria.

BACTERIAL MORPHOLOGY AND SIZE

Morphology

There are two principal morphological forms of bacteria: cocci or spheres (modified Latin diminutive of the Greek word *kokkus*, berry); and rod-shaped organisms or bacilli (from the Latin word *baculus*, rod). Many different variants of these two forms are known (fig. 3/2). Cocci may occur as pairs (diplococci), in chains (streptococci) in clusters (staphylococci) or in tetrads (sarcina). Similarly, bacilli may be quite short (cocobacilli), have tapered ends (fusiform bacilli), grow as long threads

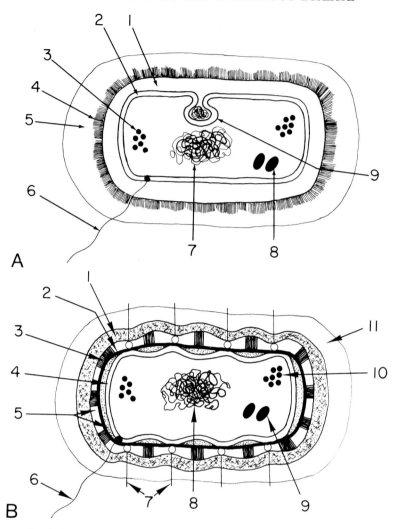

Figure 3/1. Diagram of typical bacterial cells showing most of the structures seen in the cells. (*A*) Gram positive cell: *1*, cell wall peptidoglycan; *2*, cytoplasmic membrane; *3*, ribosomes; *4*, surface proteins; *5*, capsule; *6*, flagellum; *7*, chromosome; *8*, inclusion; and *9*, mesosome. (*B*) Gram negative cell: *1*, outer membrane; *2*, peptidoglycan; *3*, lipoprotein; *4*, cytoplasmic membrane; *5*, periplasmic space; *6*, flagellum; *7*, pili; *8*, chromosome; *9*, inclusion; *10*, ribosomes; and *11*, capsule.

(filamentous forms) or in a curved or "S" configuration as vibrios or spirilla. The spiral forms may be considered as rod-shaped organisms twisted into a helix of variable rigidity. If the helix is flexible the organism is referred to as a spirochete (*Treponema*, *Leptospira*, and *Borrelia*); if the helix is rigid the organism is probably a member of the genus *Spirillum*. The grouping of bacteria is dependent upon two factors: 1) the geometry of successive planes of cell division and 2) the ease with which daughter cells pull apart after division. If the successive planes of division are perpendicular, tetrads will occur; if parallel, the cells will occur singly, in pairs, or in chains depending on their tendency to pull apart. The post-divisional separation of cells (pulling apart) may be determined by a number of

factors including specific enzymes that dissolve cellular material at the point of contact between two daughter cells, flagellar activity in motile cells and the production of certain adherent macromolecules.

The shape of individual cells is genetically determined and characteristic for the various genera and species of bacteria. It is generally agreed that the primary regulator of bacterial shape is the rigid cell wall component (the peptodoglycan or murein) since removal of the wall or prevention of wall synthesis results in cells, even rod-shaped cells, acquiring a balloon or spherical configuration (see "Cell Wall" section below). Other factors, however, have been implicated in this complex and quite variable process. Some of these factors include: 1) differential rate controls of envelope assembly and

2) asymmetric architecture in certain parts of the bacterial cell envelope.

Size

The small size of bacteria is one of the earliest and most important properties of the group (see table 3/1). Their dimensions place them at the upper levels of the size of collodial matter (0.01 to 0.5 μm). In many respects the behavior of bacterial cells is analogous to the behavior of colloids (Brownian movement, light scattering via the Tyndall effect, migration in an electric field). Another important aspect of the small size of bacteria involves their surface/volume relationships. The growth of most organisms, large or small, depends, in part, on the amount of available surface area since it is at the surface that the transfer of metabolites into the cell and the elimination of waste products occur. The generalization is often made that the larger the surface area per unit volume the greater the cell's metabolic rate. *E. coli* with a surface/volume (S/V) ratio of six can catabolize up to 10,000 times its weight of lactose in 1 hour, whereas it has been estimated that a 70-kg man would need 28 years or 250,000 hours to catabolize a comparable weight of lactose. This generalization, however, is valid only up to a point, *i.e.*, there is a lower limit of S/V beyond which viable cells cannot exist. This lower limit reflects a critical amount of space needed to accommodate the metabolic machinery (enzyme proteins, cofactors, organic substances, etc.) and the genetic apparatus of a biologically functional cell.

The *Mycoplasma* or pleuropneumonia-like organisms (PPLO) (diameter of 0.25 μm) are often referred to as the "theoretically minimum cell" with a volume of approximately 0.01 μm^3. The cells consist of a cytoplasmic membrane, ribosomes and a nuclear body. The small amount of DNA is just sufficient to code for all the products needed for self-reproduction at the expense of nutrients in an artifical medium. The cells, therefore, appear to be at, or very close to, the molecular limit of cellular function. The S/V ratio for these cells is approxi-

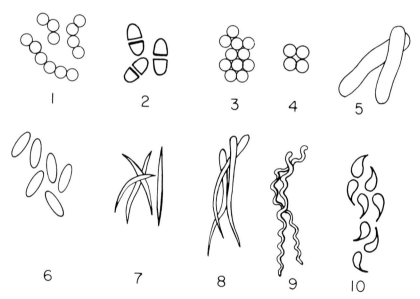

Figure 3/2. Morphological forms of bacteria: *1*, streptococci; *2*, diplococci; *3*, staphylococci; *4*, sarcina; *5*, bacilli; *6*, coccobacilli; *7*, fusiform bacilli; *8*, filamentous bacilli; *9*, spirochetes; and *10*, vibrios.

Table 3/1
Sizes of various microorganisms

Cell Type/Structural Unit	Biological Group	Volume (V) (μm^3)	Surface (S) (μm^2)	S/V (μm)
Eucaryotic cells	Unicellular algae	6.5×10^{13}	7.8×10^9	1.2×10^4
	Yeast (*Saccharomyces cerevisiae*)	110	110	1
Procaryotic cells	*Escherichia coli*	0.52	3.1	6
	Lactobacillus casei	1.6	7.85	5
	Mycoplasma sp.	0.00818	0.196	23.9
Viruses	*E. coli* phage	2.5×10^4	0.02	80

mately 20 although their metabolic rate is considerably less than the rate for *E. coli*. The smallest viable reproductive units of mycoplasmas range from 125 to 250 nm in diameter. An examination of table 3/1 will also show that viruses also have very high S/V ratios and yet their metabolic rate is negligible or nonexistent.

SURFACE STRUCTURES OF BACTERIA

There is no one simple description of the bacterial surface since the variation among the different genera and species regarding surface architecture is enormous. Moreover, as a result of the large surface area provided by cultures of bacterial cells there are continuous opportunities for chemical and physical modifications of surface structure due to environmental stresses. There are also a number of well known genetic mutations that produce major changes in bacterial cell surfaces so that within a single population it is possible to see several subpopulations with different surface structures and properties. The following section describes some of the major surface structures of bacteria but it must be remembered that not all cells have every structure and that considerable variation in the chemical and physical properties of each structure are commonly observed.

Capsules

Most bacteria produce a hydrophilic, gel-like structure of low optical density variously termed microcapsule, capsule, or slime layer and usually located just outside the cell wall. It is most easily demonstrated by negative staining (India ink suspension) where the capsular layer appears as a clear zone between the opaque background and the more refractile cell body. Most capsules are relatively simple polysaccharides composed of repeating units of two or three sugars that may or may not be present in the cell wall. Other bacteria are known to produce capsules of different chemical compositions—*e.g.*, *Bacillus anthracis* forms a capsule of poly-D-glutamic acid linked by a γ peptide bond, while the outer layer of the tubercle bacillus (*Mycobacterium tuberculosis*) is composed of protein, polysaccharide, and mycolic acid. Capsular materials are usually antigenic and can be detected on cells by exposure to specific antibody and the resultant increase in refractility gives the appearance of capsular swelling ("quellung reaction") (fig. 3/3). The specificity of the quellung reaction very often is used in the identification of certain pathogenic bacteria, *e.g.*, the pneumococcus where over 80 different capsular serotypes have been demonstrated. Many oral bacteria are also known to produce extracellular polysaccharides (dextrans and levans of *Streptococcus mutans* and *Streptococcus salivarius*) which may give the appearance of capsular material but are more often found in the medium rather than as well defined surface layers. Other oral bacteria, *e.g.*, *Lactobacillus casei*, *Neisseria* species, and many other gram negative bac-

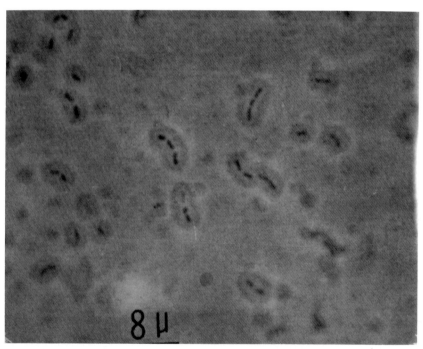

Figure 3/3. The specific capsular swelling reaction ("quellung") of *Lactobacillus casei* cells (strain L324M) exposed to specific antibody to the capsular material.

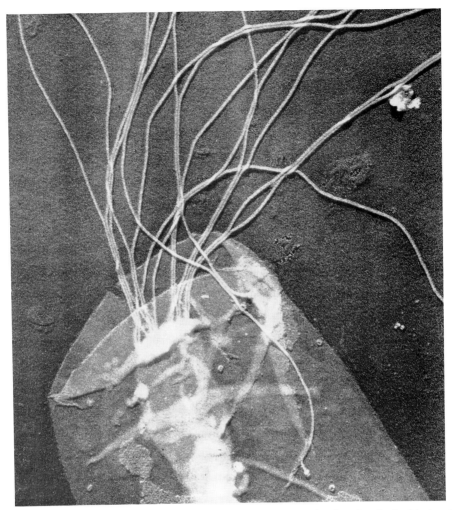

Figure 3/4. *Spirillum serpens* cell autolyzed and digested by trypsin, showing flagella attached to basal granules inside the cell. (From M. R. J. Salton: The Anatomy of the Bacterial Surface. *Bacteriological Reviews*, **25**, 77, 1961.)

teria, produce well defined capsules with some possible significance in the survival and maintenance of these and other species in the oral milieu. The polysaccharide capsule of *L. casei* is known to prevent phage adsorption and possibly serve as a reserve nutrient supply under conditions of nutrient limitation.

Ordinarily the biological significance of capsules in bacteria is limited to a consideration of their antiphagocytic properties. Since capsules are hydrophilic polysaccharides and since the surfaces of phagocytic cells are generally hydrophilic in nature the engulfment or phagocytic process is usually prevented. Thus, there is a positive association between capsule formation and the virulence of some bacteria because capsules interfere with one of the host's first lines of defense, phagocytosis. In a more restricted sense the capsule is more often thought of as a product of metabolism rather than as a structure *per se*. Capsular size, for example,

usually depends on the rate of formation and secretion of capsular material (*e.g.*, microcapsule). In other instances capsules may not be detectable at all unless there is a specific nutrient in the growth medium indicating in part, the nonessentiality of capsule formation to the biological economy of the cell.

Surface Appendages

Flagella. Bacterial cells often have one or more filamentous appendages termed flagella (L. *flagellum*, whip). The flagellum (fig. 3/4) is a long (3 to 12 μm) thin (12 to 25 nm) structure that originates in the cell membrane basal body and terminates outside the cell. Because of their narrow diameter flagella are not seen in the ordinary light microscope unless coated with stains containing a precipitating agent (tannic acid). In living cells the structure is coded in the form of a cylindrical helix but appears in dried preparations as regular sinusoidal curves (or more appropriately as flattened helices) whose wave length is characteristic for the species. The location and number of flagella are relatively constant for a species. Bacteria with a single polar flagellum are *monotrichous*; those with two or more polar flagella are *lophotrichous*; those with a random arrangement of flagella all over their surface are called *peritrichous*. On this basis the common bacteria are separated into two orders, Eubacteriales (peritrichous flagella) and Pseudomondales (polar flagellation).

Purified flagella (obtained by differential centrifugation) consist of a globular protein, flagellin (approximate molecular weight of 40,000), whose chemical composition appears to be the same in different genera of bacteria although differences in primary structure are known and account for serologic differences. The protein is antigenically different from the rest of the cell body and these differences form the basis for the serological identification of many flagellated gram negative bacteria. For example, the combination of flagellar antigens (H or *hauch*—German for breeze, whiff) and somatic antigens (O or *ohne hauch*—without flagella) provides the basis for serological typing of salmonellae in the Kauffman White schema.

The primary function of flagellae is to provide bacteria with a mechanism for motility. There are a few exceptions such as spirochetal motility due to alternate contractions of the axial filament which is attached to each end of the cell, and the gliding movement of certain nonflagellated *Capnocyto-*

phaga and *Mycoplasma* on solid surfaces due to cell binding and pili. However, in the main, bacterial motility is a direct function of flagellar activity. Motility occurs when there is a rotation of the rigid helically coiled flagellum after a tongue is created in the basal body. At the base of the flagellum within the cytoplasmic membrane there are two sets of rings surrounding the flagella cylinder: an inner set which rotates and an outer set which serves as bearings to minimize friction. As the inner set of rings rotates the flagellum to which it is attached also moves, ultimately acting as a propeller for the bacterial cell. The energy for the rotation is thought to be derived from oxidative phosphorylation in the membrane.

Fimbriae or Pili. Bacterial cells, both gram positive and gram negative, often have as many as several hundred filamentous appendages called fimbria, or more recently, pili, that are thinner, shorter, and less rigid than flagellae. They are 75 to 100 nm in diameter and up to 2 μm in length (fig. 3/5). Like flagella, they also arise in the cytoplasmic membrane and are composed of a serologically distinct protein (pilin). They can be easily removed from bacterial cells without affecting vitality and they reform rapidly. Based on the known functions there are two varieties of pili: a sex pilus which was once thought to be a tube through which DNA was transferred during the process of conjugation between two bacterial cells; and a somatic pilus which has adhesive properties that aid in the adherence of bacterial cells to mucosal and other cell surfaces

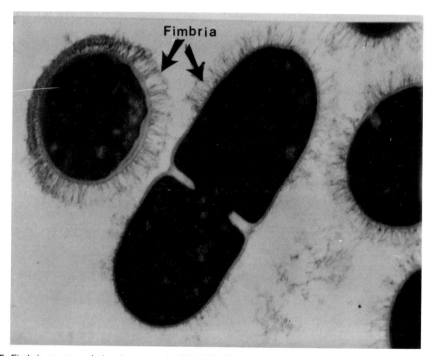

Figure 3/5. Fimbria on an oral streptococcus (×60,000). (Courtesy of Dr. Chern Lai, University of Pennsylvania.)

as a first step in bacterial colonization of the host. Recent evidence suggests that the real function of the sex pilus is to serve as a recognition device between mating cell types followed by the formation of some kind of cytoplasmic bridge between cell envelopes. The significance of the somatic pili in adherence and colonization was first established by oral microbiologists who demonstrated most convincingly that the selective localization of certain oral bacteria depended on the presence of these fibrillar coatings. Studies of numerous other investigators have established the universality of the phenomenon; adherence mechanisms, mediated by pili or other "adhesins" play a fundamental role in the natural ecology of pathogenic and nonpathogenic bacteria. The colonization of *Actinomyces viscosus*, one of the first organisms shown to produce periodontal disease and root surface caries in gnotobiotic (so-called "germ-free") animals is dependent on pili. Avirulent mutants of *A. viscosus* lack pili and are unable to colonize the oral cavity (fig. 3/6). Pili have also been implicated recently in the gliding motion of nonflagellated bacteria on solid surfaces ("surface translocation").

Bacterial Cell Walls. One of the most important characteristics of procaryotic cells (bacteria

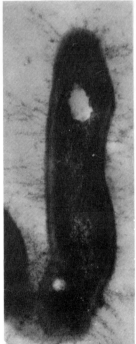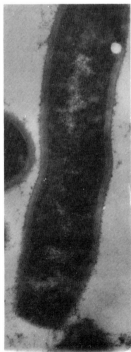

Figure 3/6. Electron micrographs of *Actinomyces viscosus* strains T14V (virulent) and T14AV (avirulent) ($\times$52,650). Note the presence of numerous fimbrial like projections on virulent cells (*left*) and the absence of such projections on avirulent cells (*right*). (Courtesy of Dr. Dale Birdsell and Dr. Werner Fischlschweiger, University of Florida.)

and blue green algae) is the presence of a rigid cell wall containing the unique peptidoglycan (PG or murein) moiety. All bacteria except the mycoplasma and certain halophilic bacteria have rigid cell walls with some variation of the peptidoglycan serving as the basic structural unit of the wall. The significance of the PG is best illustrated in the number of functions it serves:

1. It is responsible for the strength and rigidity of the wall. The walls of some bacteria are able to withstand up to $400,000 \times g$ without rupture or distortion of shape.

2. The inertness of the wall to a variety of chemical agents derives from the resistance of PG to such agents. Equally important is the concept that those agents which affect the integrity or synthesis of the wall are almost always bactericidal in nature. Any compromise of wall structure, function, or synthesis usually leads to cell death.

3. Associated with its strength and rigidity the PG is essentially (although not exclusively) responsible for the shape of the cell. If the PG layer is digested by lysozyme or if its synthesis is blocked by an antibiotic, the cell loses its characteristic shape and becomes a spherical body. (The cell will lyse unless it is placed in a hypertonic medium (*e.g.*, 20% sucrose).) Thus, a rigid rod-shaped bacillus in hypertonic medium will become a flexible spherical body if the wall is lost. (Since the free energy of a system tends towards a minimum a flexible body will assume the smallest possible surface area, and the smallest possible surface area for any given volume is a sphere.) The wall-less forms are called protoplasts or spheroplasts. The difference between them and their significance will be discussed later.

It is possible to isolate and purify cell wall preparations of various bacteria by cell rupture, enzymatic treatment and differential centrifugation. The isolated PG is now known to be a single, giant, bag-shaped macromolecule which may account for 10 to 40% of the cell dry weight. The PG consists of three parts (see fig. 3/7): (a) a backbone chain made up of repeating units of two amino sugars (*N*-acetylglucosamine and muramic acid) joined by a β-1,4-linkage; (b) a set of identical tetrapeptide units joined at the CO end of muramic acid and with an alternating D/L configuration of amino acids and a diamino acid in position 3; and (c) a set of identical cross bridges to hook the backbone chains together.

The basic PG unit is essentially the same for all bacteria but there are variations in the number and nature of the cross bridges, and the diamino acid in position 3 of the tetrapeptide unit. Some of the taxonomic and other implications of these differences in wall structure will be discussed in the sections on gram positive and gram negative cell walls.

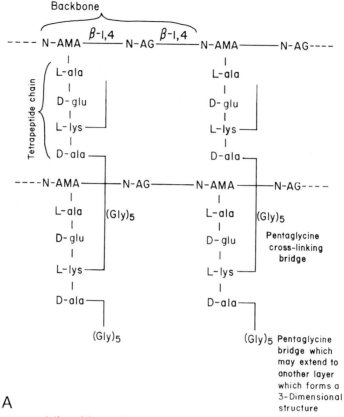

Figure 3/7. Schematic representation of the peptidoglycans of bacteria. The major components are: the polysaccharide backbone chains containing muramic acid (*N-AMA*) and *N*-acetylglucosamine (*N-AG*); the tetrapeptide units containing various amino acids including L/D-alanine, D-glutamic acid, L-lysine or diaminopimelic acid (*DAP*); and cross bridges linking the tetrapeptide units. (*A*) Peptidoglycan structure of gram positive bacteria; (*B*) the extent of cross-bridging in gram positive bacteria; (*C*) peptidoglycan structure of gram negative bacteria; and (*D*) the extent of cross-bridging in gram negative bacteria. Asterisk (*) is simple peptide bond between two amino acids of the tetrapeptides (D-ALA and DAP).

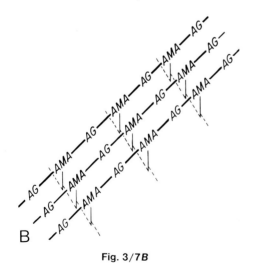

Fig. 3/7B

There are certain similarities in the bacterial PG and the rigid cell walls of the few eucaryotic cell walls. The β-1,4-linkage provides a strong and thermodynamically stable polysaccharide chain; it is also found in cellulose (β-1,4-glucose) of algal cell walls, in chitin (poly-β-1,4-N-acetylglucosamine) of fungal cell walls and in the xylans (β-1,4-xylose) of certain woody plant cells. These similarities explain, in part, the strength and resistance to rupture of these rigid cell walls. There are other chemical explanations on the toughness of the PG including the alternation of D- and L-amino acids in the tetrapeptide (greater strength of structure than L- or D-homopolymers) and the extensive amount of hydrogen bonding between peptide groups. Where there is an extensive amount of cross bridging to produce a mesh-like structure of interlacing strands of disaccharide chains the PG assumes an even greater structural strength. The overall picture of PG is one of a giant, bag-shaped, covalently linked molecule with marked ability to protect the cytoplasmic membrane and other parts of the cell from many physical and chemical forces in the external environment of the cell.

Gram Stain

Bacteria can be differentiated into two large groups by a stain developed in the early 1880s by

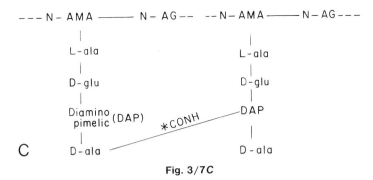

Fig. 3/7C

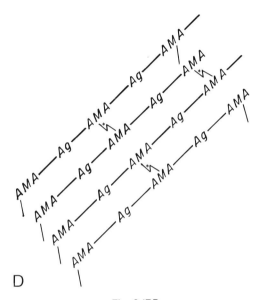

Fig. 3/7D

the Danish bacteriologist Christian Gram. The procedure consists of four basic steps:

1. Primary staining with a slightly alkaline solution of a triphenyl methane dye, such as crystal violet.

2. Mordanting with aqueous iodine solution to form a water-insoluble complex in both cell wall and cell cytoplasm.

3. Differential decolorizing with an organic solvent, usually ethanol. This step is critical, for all bacteria are decolorized by this treatment if exposed long enough. On brief exposure, however, many kinds of bacteria retain much of the iodine complex. These are designated gram positive. The kinds of bacteria that decolorize completely are designated gram negative. Some bacteria (diphtheroids, *Neisseria*) retain varying amounts of the dye-iodine complex and are termed gram variable.

4. Counterstaining with a dye of contrasting color and chemical character, usually aqueous safranin or basic fuchsin (red). This step is necessary to make gram negative bacteria visible. It has no effect on gram positive except for a darkening of the normal purple color.

The mechanism of the gram stain appears to be critically related to the intactness of the cell wall and to the permeability properties of the intact cell envelope. Gram positive bacteria stain gram negative on autolysis, or on loss of osmotic integrity, as occurs in old or dying cells. A unique bacterial cell wall component does not appear to explain the reaction since no specific gram positive substrate has been isolated. Whatever the precise mechanism, two facts are clearly established:

1. The difference in their reactions to the gram stain is but one manifestation of fundamental differences between gram positive and gram negative bacteria—differences in susceptibility to various chemical and physical agents, metabolic potential, chemical composition and structure. These differences in turn are reflected in pathogenic potential (nature of toxins produced, role of antibody in defense, etc.). A summary of these differences is presented in table 3/2.

2. The cell wall structures of gram positive and gram negative cells are clearly different with respect to chemical composition, ultrastructure, physical properties and serologic properties.

Some of the chemical and structural differences between the two kinds of cell wall follow.

Gram Positive Walls

From the standpoints of chemical components, size, and major physicochemical properties the PG dominates the structure of virtually all gram positive walls. Most of the thickness of the wall and the dry weight of isolated wall preparations are due to the PG, and the susceptibility to the various chemical and physical agents reflects the importance of PG as the primary structural unit in gram positive walls. Early ultrastructural and chemical studies showed that the thickness of the PG layer was due to the fact that there were numerous disaccharide chains joined together by extensive cross bridges between the tetrapeptide units giving an enormously intertwined mesh-like structure of considerable strength. There is considerable diversity in terms of some of the individual components of the PG in gram positive bacteria such as the amino acids in tetrapeptides, the nature of the cross

Table 3/2
Some differences between gram positive and gram negative bacteria

Property	Gram Positive	Gram Negative
Cell wall thickness	Greater	Less
Amino acids in cell wall	Few	Numerous kinds
Lipids in cell wall	None or low	Present
Bactericidal action of saliva	Resistant	Susceptible
Digestion by gastric/pancreatic juices	Resistant	Susceptible
Lysozyme lysis	Susceptible	Less susceptible
Inhibition by penicillin	Susceptible	Usually resistant
Inhibition by sulfonamides	Usually susceptible	Usually resistant
Inhibition by streptomycin	Usually resistant	Usually susceptible
Inhibition by basic dyes (crystal violet)	Susceptible	Usually resistant
Lysis by anionic detergents	Very susceptible	Much less susceptible
Autolysis	Less common	More commonly noted
Isoelectric range	pH 2–3	pH 4–5
Nutritonal requirements	Complex generally, none autotrophic	Relatively simpler, many autotrophic
Nature of toxins produced	Exotoxins	Endotoxins
Lysis by antibody + complement	Resistant	Some susceptible

bridges, etc., but two factors are constant: the high total amount of PG (40 to 90% of dry weight) in the wall and the extensive cross-bridging between chains.

The high percentage of PG in the cell wall of gram positive bacteria increases the availability of the β-1,4-linkage of the backbone chains to lysozyme, a naturally occurring substance found in tears and salivary secretions. This enzyme is able to cleave the β-1,4-linkage between the two amino sugars, muramic acid and N-acetylglucosamine breaking the chain, destroying the integrity of the PG structure and ultimately causing cell lysis. Resistance to lysozyme, although more common among the gram negative bacteria, because of the outer membrane cover, also occurs in some gram positive bacteria as well. Many gram positive oral bacteria appear to be resistant to lysozyme, a fact that would explain their high numbers in a milieu such as saliva where lysozyme is known to be present. The basis for this resistance is probably related to modification of PG structure (O-acetylation of muramic acid) or the inability of lysozyme to gain access to the wall PG (steric interference of surface macromolecules or structures). The lethal effect of penicillins on growing populations of bacteria is similarly related to an effect on PG structure, i.e., penicillins block the terminal step of PG synthesis in which the peptide chains are cross-linked.

In addition to PG there are other components of the gram positive wall. The teichoic acids (from the Greek, teichos, wall) are water-soluble polymers of ribitol or glycerol linked covalently to PG via phosphodiester linkages (usually at the C_6 hydroxyl of N-acetylmuramic acid residues). Membrane teichoic acids (lipoteichoic acids, LTA) usually contain only glycerophosphate polymers and terminate in the membrane glycolipid. These polymers, both wall and membrane teichoic acids, are major surface antigens of gram positive cells and are probably important in a number of other surface related phenomena such as adherence and regulation of ion passage through the PG layer. The membrane teichoic acids (LTA) are amphipathic molecules (both polar and nonpolar ends) that can interact with a variety of other biologically active molecular species such as lipids in erythrocyte membranes to produce hemagglutination, or divalent cations, particularly in the regulation of intracellular Mg^{2+}. In many respects, LTA is analogous to the lipopolysaccharide of the gram negative cell wall (see below).

Other wall associated substances of gram positive cells include: antigenic polysaccharides (e.g., group and type-specific streptococcal polysaccharides); teichoic acid polymers covalently attached to the PG and generally formed under conditions of phosphate limitation; and antigenic proteins which are not identical with pili or flagella but which may be associated with adherence. The M protein of group A streptococci is an illustration of such a wall-associated protein. In general, it has been said that the gram positive wall is devoid of proteins because the procedures used in wall isolation often employ proteolytic enzymes (trypsin, etc.) which would destroy ordinary D- or L-homopolymers. However, the tetrapeptides composed of the alternating D- and L-amino acids are resistant to these proteolytic enzymes.

Gram Negative Walls

The gram negative cell wall is considerably more complex than its gram positive counterpart in terms of structural heterogeneity, chemical composition and functional activities. Also, the wall PG is intimately connected with other surface layers of the cell and with membrane-associated functions. Because of the structural complexity of the wall in gram negative bacteria the term "cell envelope" may be preferable to "cell wall" when applied to these bacteria.

The unique three-layered envelope consists of an outer membrane overlaying a thin PG layer which, in turn, is separated from the underlying cytoplasmic membrane by a periplasmic space (fig. 3/8). The outer membrane (6 to 8 nm thick) consists of two layers of protein separated by a layer of phospholipids. This outer membrane structure plays a vital role in the biology of the cell since it contains receptors for antibodies, bacterial viruses, and bacteriocins (see Chapter 4) and performs a number of permeability-related functions consistent with the designation, membrane. The outer membrane serves as a barrier to the passage of many antibiotics (notably, some of the penicillins), detergents, and other chemicals (dyes, bile salts). Part of the barrier effect is due to the presence of outer membrane matrix proteins such as porins which selectively inhibit permeation of molecules with a molecular weight greater than 800. Porins also serve as receptor sites for viruses and bacteriocins.

Another major component of the outer membrane is the lipopolysaccharides (LPS or endotoxins) which are unique to gram negative bacteria including spirochetes. LPS consists of three regions: a lipid portion, termed lipid A; a core polysaccharide common to most LPS molecules and an O-specific polysaccharide side chain. The O-specific side chains may be visualized as projections from the surface of the outer membrane which could prevent the harmful interaction of antibody and complement with the outer membrane. The structures of the different O residues exhibit considerable variation based on the differences in the nature and arrangement of the individual sugars, thereby making it possible to classify different organisms or strains of an organism on the basis of these somatic antigens. When the O antigen is lost by mutation the normally "smooth" colony formation changes to "rough." There appears to be a selective advantage associated with the presence of the O side chains since they tend to make the bacterium resistant to many host defenses (phagocytosis, complement, antibody interaction, etc.). The polysaccharide portions of the LPS are responsible for the antigenic properties of the molecule while lipid A, a glycophospholipid, is responsible for the toxicity of the molecule.

There are a number of similarities between this characteristic molecule of gram negative cells and the lipoteichoic acids of gram positive cells. Both are amphipathic surface macromolecules and both share a number of common biological properties (immunogenicity, hypersensitivity, bone-resorbing capacity, erythrocyte stimulation, Shwartzman re-

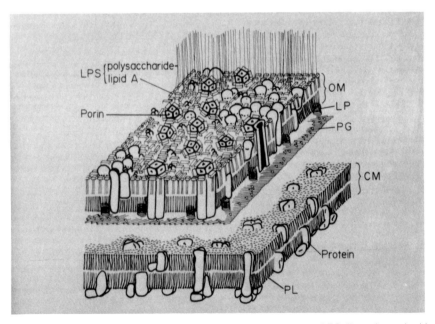

Figure 3/8. An interpretive diagram of the gram negative envelope structure. *LPS*, lipopolysaccharide; *OM*, outer membrane; *LP*; lipoprotein; *PG*, peptidoglycan; *CM*, cytoplasmic membrane; *PL*, phospholipid. (Modified from J. M. DiRienzo et al.: *Annual Review of Biochemistry*, 47, 481, 1978, and presented in *Zinsser Microbiology*, Ed. 17, edited by W. Joklik, H. P. Willett, and D. B. Amos. Appleton-Century-Crofts, New York, 19.)

action). They differ in that only LPS is pyrogenic, mutagenic, and lethal to mice. Of considerable interest in dental medicine are the recent reports that have shown the potential significance of LPS preparations obtained from oral bacteria associated with periodontal disease. Known periodontopathic bacteria, especially those associated with juvenile periodontitis (*Actinobacillus actinomycetemcomitans*) produce potent endotoxins with marked ability to cause *in vivo* bone resorption and other inflammatory changes due to cell systems known to be involved with the disease process (complement activation, release of lysosomal enzymes from inflammatory cells, platelet aggregation).

Some of the major differences in gram positive and gram negative cell walls are summarized in table 3/3. The one additional kind of bacterial cell wall requiring attention is the cell wall of the acid-fast bacteria (members of the genus *Mycobacterium*, including the tubercle bacillus *Mycobacterium tuberculosis* and some species of *Nocardia*). They are called acid-fast because once they are stained with carbolfuchsin they resist decolorization with acid-alcohol. This staining property is correlated with the presence of cell wall bound mycolic acids, a group of large α-branched, β-hydroxy-fatty acids (C_{30} to C_{90} chain lengths). The wall of *M. tuberculosis* contains roughly equal amounts of lipid, peptidoglycan, and arabinogalactan (a polymer of arabinose and galactose). The arabinogalactan is bound to the PG at muramic acid and the mycolic acid via the C_5 hydroxyl group of arabinose. The lipids in the cell wall and elsewhere in the envelope of the tubercle bacillus have a profound effect on the surface properties of this organism and its pathogenic potential (see Chapter 23).

Protoplasts and Spheroplasts

As indicated earlier, protoplasts (usually gram positive in origin) and spheroplasts (usually gram negative in origin) arise when the structural integrity of the cell walls is compromised. Protoplasts are devoid of cell wall whereas incomplete removal of the wall (usually occurring in gram negative bacteria because of the intimate association between the wall and the membranes) results in spheroplasts. Protoplasts and spheroplasts can be produced by exposing sensitive vegetative cells to antibiotics (*e.g.*, penicillin) that inhibit cell wall formation or to an enzyme (*e.g.*, lysozyme) which disrupts the wall. Both protoplasts and spheroplasts are osmotically fragile and their cytoplasmic membranes easily ruptured, but they can be maintained in a hypertonic solution if they are protected from mechanical shock. Many protoplasts and spheroplasts cannot divide normally or reform cell walls. Those resulting from the action of penicillin can often grow, divide, and resume formation of cell walls if the antibiotic is removed. The mycoplasmas previously discussed lack the ability to form cell walls but they are capable of growth and cell division. Another group of procaryotic wall-less cells (or cells with impaired cell walls) are the L-forms. L-Forms are bacterial mutants of gram positive or gram negative parents in which peptidoglycan synthesis has been severely deranged but they have developed compensatory changes in the mem-

Table 3/3
Differences in gram positive and gram negative cell walls

	Gram Positive	Gram Negative
PEPTIDOGLYCAN	Thick layer	Thin layer
Disaccharide chain	Numerous, intertwined mesh in 3 dimensions	Few chains and in a 2 dimensional monolayer
Cross bridges	Extensive (up to 100% in *Staphylococcus aureus*)	Minimal (30% in *Escherichia coli*)
	Combinations of one or more amino acids or a single amino acid, *e.g.*, glycine	Simple peptide bonds often
Tetrapeptide amino acids	Alternating L- and D-forms with a diamino acid in position 3 (L-lysine usually but also DAP,[a] ornithine, DAB[b])	Same except L-lysine is usually substituted for by DAP
OTHER		
Teichoic acids	Yes	No
Endotoxin (LPS)	No	Yes
Amino acids	Few in number	Numerous
Membrane lipids	No (but lipoteichoic acids)	Yes (outer membrane)
Surface antigens	Yes (polysaccharides, teichoic acids, protein appendages)	Yes (of many kinds but usually do not cross react with gram positive antigens)

[a] DAP, diaminopimelic acid.
[b] DAB, 2,4-diaminobutyric acid.

Table 3/4
Characteristics of procaryotic bacteria without cell walls or with defective cell walls

Microorganism	Origin	Osmotic Fragility	Cell Division	Cell Wall Status
Mycoplasma	Mycoplasma	±	+ (slow)	Absent
Protoplasts	Known gram positive bacterium	+ +	− to ±	Absent
Spheroplasts	Known gram negative bacterium	+ +	− to ±	Part of wall remains
L-Forms	Known gram positive or gram negative bacterium	±	+ (slow)	Absent or part of wall may remain

brane that allows them to grow and divide. Although most L-forms are osmotically fragile, some can grow at the osmolality of serum. Their role in human infectious disease is unclear even though they have been cultured from cases of pyelonephritis and oral aphthous ulcers. What is clear and disturbing about them is the threat that they pose in view of their resistance to most wall inhibitory antibiotics. Some of the characteristics of protoplasts, spheroplasts, L-forms and mycoplasma are summarized in table 3/4.

CYTOPLASMIC STRUCTURES

Cytoplasmic Membrane

Internal to the cell walls of all bacteria is a cytoplasmic membrane, the principal osmotic barrier of the cell. It is composed of a phospholipid bilayer into which membrane proteins are intercalated ("unit membrane"). The polar regions of the phospholipids are found in the outer surfaces of the bilayer while the hydrophobic fatty acid chains extend into the center of the membrane (see also fig. 3/8). The membrane makes up 10% of the dry weight of the cell and 20% of the total protein of the cell. As is true for all procaryotic cells, bacteria and their cell membranes do not contain or synthesize sterols. (Some *Mycoplasma* species are able to incorporate exogenous sterols from the medium into their surface layer but still lack the ability to synthesize sterols.) Membranes may be observed with both light and electron microscopy by placing bacterial cells in hypertonic solutions which results in plasmolysis, *i.e.*, shrinkage of the membrane and cytoplasm from the cell as a result of the osmotic membrane.

The osmotic barrier function of the membrane is also indicated by the ability of bacteria to transport selectively many organic and inorganic nutrients into the cell. The membrane proteins responsible for this specific transport across the membrane are known as permeases. The activity of these enzyme-like proteins is rapid (more rapid than passive diffusion), and exhibits considerable substrate specificity (discrimination between enantiomorphs of optically active compounds—*e.g.*, D- vs. L-amino acid). It is therefore possible to effect the intracellular accumulation of a specific compound against a concentration gradient of that substance.

The membrane is also a major metabolic center for the cell since many of the enzymes involved in biosynthesis, electron transport, DNA replication, and membrane permeability are found here. Many of the biosynthetic reactions involved in cell wall assembly occur in/on the membrane as do the energy yielding reactions associated with electron transport and coupling mechanisms employed in active transport of substrate molecules. The assembly of extracellular polysaccharide units that form capsules and other extracellular polymers (dextrans, levans, etc.) occurs in the membrane when a phosphorylated lipid carrier molecule translocates these units to the exterior surface where they are covalently bound to the growing extracellular polymer.

Mesosomes

The cytoplasmic membranes of some bacteria, particularly gram positive cells, may be invaginated to form internal structures called mesosomes (fig. 3/1A, item 9). They are connected to the membrane and do not occur as free membrane-bound organelles in the cytoplasm (*e.g.*, mitochondria) (fig. 3/9). The only known exceptions to this rule among the procaryotes are the thylakoids found in some photosynthetic bacteria in which these chloroplast-like, membrane-bound organelles are distinct and separate from the membrane. Mesosomes appear to be associated with cell wall synthesis, segregation of nucleic acid during cell division and secretion of enzymes; they also increase the surface area of the membrane and its transport systems.

Ribosomes

The cytoplasm of bacterial cells is filled with a large number of small (18 nm in diameter), dense, roughly spherical particles termed ribosomes whose primary function is the synthesis of proteins. They contain RNA (60 to 70%) and protein (30 to 40%) and make up about 40% of the cell dry weight and

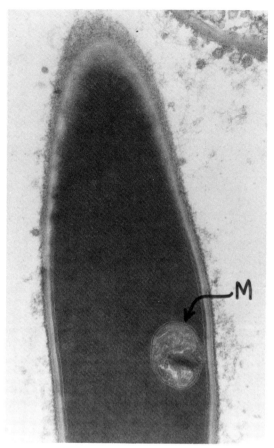

Figure 3/9. A transmission electron micrograph of the oral bacterium *Bacterionema matruchotii* (strain 100) showing mesosome (*M*) and its attachment to the cell membrane (×68,000). (Courtesy of C. Lai.)

fortunately, some of these antibiotics (chloramphenicol, tetracycline, streptomycin) also inhibit the 70S ribosomes found in eucaryotic mitochondria and chloroplasts making it clear that the concept of selective toxicity is not absolute regarding these antibiotics.

Nucleus (Nuclear Region, Nucleoid)

One of the primary reasons that bacteria are grouped with procaryotic cells is that they have a "primitive nucleus," a repository for the DNA that serves as genetic material but not enclosed by a nuclear membrane. Since there does not appear to be a clear line of structural distinction between nucleus and cytoplasm the term "nuclear region" is often used. This term is, however, a misnomer since it is possible to isolate discrete masses of biologically active DNA by gentle lysis of cells indicating that one is dealing with a structural entity rather than some indefinite space. Moreover, the physical and cytological demonstration of the material are complementary to and consistent with genetic data. It is difficult to demonstrate the nucleus in ordinary staining reactions because the presence of large amounts of RNA throughout the cytoplasm obscures the nucleus. One or more chromatin bodies (chromosomes) can be demonstrated and they serve as the functional equivalents of the eucaryotic nucleus. Bacterial DNA appears as a fibrillar network which often runs parallel to the cell axis. The bacterial chromosome usually exists as a single circular DNA molecule from 100 to 1400 μm long. The fibrillar appearance arises from the considerable amount of folding of this extremely long DNA molecule. (see fig. 3/1, *A* and *B*).

Although the bacterial nucleus serves as the principal repository for DNA and carries all the genetic information ordinarily associated with the growth, metabolism and survival of the cell, there are other repositories for DNA termed plasmids. Many bacteria harbor these extrachromosomal, circular DNA molecules, capable of autonomous replication and carrying the determinants for several phenotypic characters (*e.g.*, drug resistance, pilus formation, bacteriocin formation, enzyme synthesis, etc.). The amount of DNA in a plasmid is from 0.1 to 5% of that found in chromosomal DNA, supporting the view that plasmids may be lost from the cell without any real impairment of cell viability. Several oral bacteria have been reported to contain plasmids but their role in oral disease and oral microbial ecology has not yet been established. Plasmids for which there is no known phenotypic property are called cryptic plasmids.

80 to 90% of the cellular RNA. When grouped together by attachment to a single strand of messenger RNA, they are called polysomes or polyribosomes. The RNA of bacterial cells consists of ribosomal RNA (rRNA), transfer RNA (tRNA), and messenger RNA (mRNA). Twenty to 30 individual proteins are also present in the ribosomes. There are from 1 to 4 kinds of tRNA for each of the 20 amino acids. There are also many kinds of mRNA, each acting as the template for synthesis of individual proteins. *E. coli* is estimated to contain between 2,000 and 3,000 different proteins and approximately 1,000 different kinds of mRNA.

All of the ribosomes of bacteria are of the 70S variety (based on their sedimentation rate in an ultracentrifuge; S=Svedberg units) and are therefore different from the 80S ribosomes characteristic of eucaryotic cells. This difference in ribosome structure forms the basis of selective toxicity of several antibiotics known to inhibit protein synthesis, *i.e.*, it is possible selectively to prevent protein synthesis in a procaryotic bacterial cell without substantially affecting the eucaryotic host cell. Un-

Cellular Inclusions

Most if not all bacteria are capable of forming some kind of cytoplasmic inclusion if the appropriate cultural or environmental conditions are present. Until recently the full significance of these inclusions in the overall biological economy of the cell was not recognized. A few general facts about their synthesis have been known for a long time: 1) Most are high molecular weight polymers (no osmotic energy is required to keep them inside the cell); 2) most inclusions are formed under conditions of unbalanced growth (carbohydrate excess, nitrogen limitation, phosphate excess); and 3) not all inclusions are formed by any one organism at any one time. However, very little information was available about the catabolism of these inclusions and their possible significance in cellular physiology. Most of these inclusions are found in various oral bacteria and their roles in oral microbial ecology have been investigated in some detail.

Glycogen. A large number of bacteria during the later phases of growth when the synthesis of nucleic acids and proteins is decreased, *i.e.*, nitrogen limitation and in the presence of residual carbohydrate (*e.g.*, glucose), accumulate large amounts of an α-1,4-linked glucose polymer (glycogen). This material is produced by a large number of plaque-forming bacteria including most oral streptococci, *Lactobacillus casei*, diphtheroids, *Veillonella*, and other plaque-related bacteria. In several of these cases it has been shown that this intracellular polysaccharide (IPS) amounts to 50 to 60% of the cell dry weight and is used as a reserve storage material that can be stoichiometrically converted to lactic acid in the absence of exogenous carbohydrate (fig. 3/10). This possibility could account for the sustained production of acid by human dental plaque in the absence of dietary carbohydrate. The hypothesis was given additional support when it was found that IPS-producing bacteria were more numerous in plaques and carious lesions from caries-active persons than from similar materials taken from caries-inactive individuals. However, studies using IPS-defective mutant strains were less clear in demonstrating a positive correlation between IPS production and cariogenicity—some mutants produced fewer carious lesions; some mutants produced higher caries scores than uninfected controls. Other roles for glycogen catabolism in oral ecology have included a possibly enhanced survival since (glycogen-producing cells of *Streptococcus mitis* have a much higher viability upon prolonged storage than non-glycogen-producing cells). Also, IPS catabolism provides the cell with utilizable energy for enzyme induction (β-galatosidase induction was much faster in IPS positive cells than in IPS negative cells under otherwise identical conditions).

Poly-β-hydroxybutyrate (PβHB). Poly-β-OH-butyric acid is a polymer of the C_4 fatty acid. Whereas glycogen-type polymers are found in both eucaryotic and procaryotic cells, PβHB is uniquely found in procaryotes such as species of *Pseudomo-*

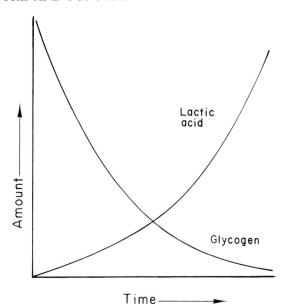

Figure 3/10. Catabolism of intracellular glycogen to lactic acid by washed cells of *Lactobacillus casei* (strain 32-1I). Note that there is an almost stoichiometric conversion of glycogen to lactic acid when there is no exogenous substrate.

nas, Bacillus, and *Spirillum.* Procaryotes use this material as a reserve storage material in contrast to the neutral fat stored by eucaryotes. Catabolism of PβHB occurs after the material is activated by a Ca^{2+}-requiring enzyme and the final products include acetoacetate and β-OH-butyrate. In the presence of CoA the synthesis of PβHB may be recycled with the formation of acetoacetyl CoA. Accumulations of PβHB range from 7 to 40% of the cell dry weight.

Volutin Granules (Babès-Ernst or Metachromatic Granules). Volutin granules are acid-insoluble polymetaphosphates and characteristically seen in *Cornyebacterium diphtheriae* and *L. casei.* They are called "metachromatic" because they appear red when stained with a blue dye. The granules are formed under starvation conditions and appear to function as intracellular phosphate reserves that can be mobilized as a phosphorus source for nucleic acids. The degradation of polymetaphosphate has also been considered as a possible source for ATP although this function has not yet been proved.

BACTERIAL SPORES AND SPORE FORMATION

The ability of some bacteria to produce the highly refractive and highly resistant internal structures known as endospores represents an extraordinary example of differentiation. The process leads to the production of a new type of cell, structurally, antigenically, and physiologically different from the parent cell (sporangium) from which it is formed and ultimately released. A considerable amount of work has been done to define in mechanistic terms the nature of sporulation not just because it presents a series of fascinating problems related to cellular differentiation but also because of certain medical and public health implications. Although spore formation is uncommon among most pathogenic bacteria the two genera, *Bacillus* (aerobic) and *Clostridium* (anaerobic) in which it occurs are highly important. *Bacillus anthracis* is the etiologic agent of anthrax and its spores are the single most important factor in disease prevention and transmission of the infectious agent. Members of the genus *Clostridium* are responsible for tetanus (*Clostridium tetani*) and botulism (*Clostridium botulinum*), and once again it is the spores of both organisms that play a critical role in the dissemination of the disease. Most sterilization procedures also use spore destruction as one of the major criteria for sterilizing efficiency (see Chapter 7).

Spores are formed by an invagination of the double layer of cell membrane within which is enclosed part of the host cell genome and a small amount of cytoplasm (forespore). The process usually begins at the end of exponential growth under conditions in which there is a limiting supply of C, N, or P and the entire process (completion of sporulation) requires 6 to 8 hours. Spore integument forms between the double membranes, and the cytoplasm condenses to complete the inner core, which is enclosed by a thin membrane (spore wall). Surrounding the spore wall is a laminated cortex, which is, in turn, surrounded by two rather impervious coats that account for some of the resistance of spores to heat, drying or chemicals. The spore wall and cortex contain different types of peptidoglycan. The coats are composed of keratin-like protein which provides resistance to chemicals and ultraviolet and ionizing radiation. Resistance to heat is associated with a calcium salt of dipicolinic acid in the core (fig. 3/11) and also the extreme state of dehydration.

Spores have very little metabolic activity. Selective synthesis and uptake of metabolites result in a cell containing the minimal constituents necessary for resumption of growth at a later time. Spores may remain in a "dormant" state for long periods of time and serve as a source of contamination when activation into the vegetative state occurs (germination). Some spores germinate spontaneously in a nutritionally favorable medium while

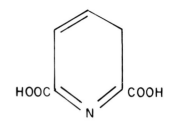

Figure 3/11. Dipicolinic acid (pyridine 2,6-dicarboxylic acid).

others are activated by some sort of trauma (mechanical disturbance of spore coat, fatty acids, low pH, or an SH-compound) in which the integrity of the impermeable surface layers is broken. Spore germination involves the following five events: 1) uptake of water, 2) hydrolysis of the cortical peptidoglycan with change in refractility, 3) dilution of the core condensate, 4) loss of calcium dipicolinate, and 5) formation of the vegetative cell wall from the inner spore membrane.

ADDITIONAL READING

BRINTON, C. C., JR. 1967. Contributions of Pili to the Specificity of the Bacterial Surface, and a Unitary Hypothesis of Conjugal Infectious Heredity. In *The Specificity of Cell Surfaces*, pp. 37–70, edited by B. Davis and L. Warren. Prentice-Hall, Englewood Cliffs, N.J.

GIBBONS, R. J., AND VAN HOUTE, J. 1975. Bacterial Adherence in Oral Microbial Ecology. Annu Rev Microbiol, **29**, 19.

HAMILTON, I. R. 1976. Intracellular Polysaccharide Synthesis by Cariogenic Microorganisms. In *Microbial Aspects of Dental Caries* (H. M. Stiles, W. J. Loesche, and T. C. O'Brien, eds.), Microbiol Abstr Spec Suppl **3**, 683–701.

LAMANNA, C., MALLETTE, M. F., AND ZIMMERMAN, L. N. 1973. *Basic Bacteriology*, Ed. 4. Williams & Wilkins, Baltimore.

LEIVE, L. (ED.) 1973. *Bacterial Membranes and Walls*. Marcel Dekker, New York.

LIN, E. C. C. 1970. The Genetics of Bacterial Transport Systems. Annu Rev Genetics, **4**, 225.

MEYNELL, G. G. 1973. *Bacterial Plasmids*. The M.I.T. Press, Cambridge, Mass.

SHIVELY, J. M. 1974. Inclusion Bodies of Procaryotes. Annu Rev Microbiol, **28**, 167.

STANIER, R. Y., ADELBERG, E. A., AND INGRAHAM, J. L. 1976. *The Microbial World*, Ed. 4. Prentice-Hall, Englewood Cliffs, N.J.

WATSON, J. D. 1976. *The Molecular Biology of the Gene*, Ed. 3. W. A. Benjamin Inc. Menlo Park, Calif.

WICKEN, A. J., AND KNOX, K. W. 1977. Biological Properties of Lipoteichoic Acids. In *Microbiology-1977*, pp. 360–365, edited by D. Schlessinger. American Society for Microbiology, Washington, D.C.

chapter 4

Bacterial Genetics

Benjamin Hammond

INTRODUCTION

An orderly mechanism of inheritance in bacteria has always been implied by the fact that they "breed true." If the distribution of genetic material at bacterial cell division were not uniform, progeny identical with the parent bacteria would occur only by chance. In general, the morphologic and physiologic identity of most bacteria is maintained from one generation to the next. This constancy in properties is the basis upon which routine identification of unknown organisms in nature is made. Similarly, the control of infectious diseases would be greatly compromised if the genetic stability of microorganisms was not so common. Antigenic variation would nullify the benefits of vaccines and variation in drug susceptibility would create chemotherapeutic nightmares. Indeed, one of the early considerations about the efficacy of the proposed caries vaccines was the possibility of "antigenic drift" in the serotypes of *Streptococcus mutans*. Thus, genetic stability in microorganisms is not absolute and gene mutations do occur. The natural antibiotic resistance in bacteria is well known and has caused serious problems. Moreover, we know that the evolution of microorganisms is predicated on change and the ability to change.

One of the more positive aspects of these genetic changes in microorganisms, especially the bacteria, is that it has provided the molecular biologist with a powerful tool to study various aspects of cell biology in a rapid and easily reproducible way. The significance of a property (A) can be determined by using mutant pairs (A^+ and $A-$) of otherwise identical organisms, many of which have doubling times (generation times) of less than 30 minutes. Thus, many generations of a population can be studied in a very short time to determine the significance of a single property.

Typical genetic processes and molecular mechanisms operate in procaryotic microorganisms even though their organization is simplified when compared to the eucaryotic mammalian cell. The basic structure of DNA and mechanisms for replication, transcription, and translation of genetic information should be familiar to most students. However, a brief summary of genetic structures and mechanisms as they relate to bacteria will be presented. Additional information will be provided concerning recent work on the genetics of oral bacteria and how the application of basic genetics is clearly relevant and necessary in dental medicine.

THE BACTERIAL CHROMOSOME

As indicated in the section on bacterial structure, the chromosome of all bacteria thus far reported is a single, circular DNA molecule. The molecular weight of the *Escherichia coli* chromosome is 3×10^9 and contains about 5×10^6 base pairs: The bacterial chromosome does not have histones attached to it, but small polyamines may serve similar functions (stabilize the DNA molecule and increase resistance to strand separation). As is true for eucaryotes, bacterial DNA is a polymer of the deoxyribonucleotides of adenine (A), guanine (G), thymine (T), and cytosine (C), connected by phosphodiester linkages to form a chain. The DNA molecule takes the form of two adjacent chains arranged in a double helix and stabilized by hydrogen bonds between pairs of bases on the two side chains. Pairing occurs between adenine and thymine and between guanine and cytosine (see fig. 4/1).

DNA replication in the bacterial chromosome occurs in a semiconservative fashion so that progeny chromosomes consist of one chain from the parent molecule and one newly formed chain. The latter chain is the result of enzymatic polymerization of a sequence of nucleotides arranged on a template consisting of one strand of a parental DNA molecule.

The genetic information encoded in the order of the nucleotides and divided into hereditary units known as genes is transcribed into mRNA, then translated into proteins by reactions typical of this process. Bacterial mRNA is polygenic, *i.e.*, it con-

BACTERIAL GENETICS

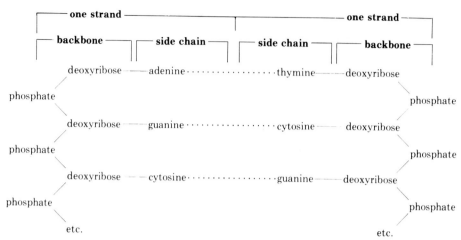

Figure 4/1. Schematic representation of double strand deoxyribonucleic acid. The molecule consists of two polynucleotide strands wound vertically around a longitudinal axis held together by hydrogen bonds (····) between adjacent purine-pyridine pairs. The code for a particular protein consists of a DNA made up of the necessary number and variety of base triplet sequences which code for an amino acid arranged in the order in which the respective amino acids occur in the protein. A single gene has been estimated to contain about 1,000 base pairs and a bacterial chromosome about 10,000,000 base pairs. Assuming an average of 300–400 amino acids per protein whose synthesis is determined by a gene and that three base pairs control the incorporation of a single amino acid into protein, the bacterium must possess of the order of 10,000 different proteins. *Escherichia coli* has been estimated to contain about 3,000 to 4,000 proteins. (Reproduced with permission from C. Lamanna and M. F. Malette. 1973 *Basic Bacteriology*, Ed. 4, p. 591. Williams & Wilkins, Baltimore.)

tains information from more than one gene. The information contained in such a molecule generally specifies proteins whose functions are related, *e.g.*, the enzymes for a specific pathway.

MUTATION

Any alteration in the nucleotide sequence of the gene changes the structure and therefore the function of the protein under the control of that sequence. Such an alteration in protein structure and function resulting from changes in the DNA is called a mutation. Changes in nucleotide sequence can occur in many ways including: 1) base-pair substitution (one base pair is substituted for another base pair as the result of an error during replication) and 2) breakage of the sugar-phosphate backbone of DNA with subsequent deletion, inversion or insertion of old/new segments (see fig. 4/1).

The expression of the mutation (phenotypic change) can occur for any property of the cell (cell nutrition, morphology, drug susceptibility, etc.). Besides producing recognizable changes in structure or function, mutations may be lethal to the cell, produce no visible effects, or perhaps go unrecognized until the organisms are placed under conditions of a selective or permissive environment, *e.g.*, absence of a metabolite or at an abnormal temperature. Mutations may be spontaneous or

caused by mutagens which specifically alter DNA structure. In all instances, however, it should be remembered that mutations are random events and occur irrespective of environmental factors and pressures. Resistance to an antibiotic among bacterial cells in a culture occurs in the complete absence of the antibiotic and at the same rate as would have occurred if the antibiotic was present.

Spontaneous mutations, occurring with a frequency of 10^{-7} to 10^{-10} per organism per cell division, are those that occur in the absence of a known mutagen. The most likely mechanism for spontaneous point mutations is thought to be a rare tautomeric shift of electrons in one of the four bases resulting in a change of H bonding patterns, *e.g.*, thymine in the enol form (rather than the normal keto state) will form a hydrogen bond with guanine instead of adenine and change the base sequence and triplet code. Other postulated mechanisms include 1) production of mutagens from normal metabolites, 2) loss of a segment of DNA, or 3) alteration in activity or synthesis of enzymes involved in DNA synthesis.

A more specific explanation for spontaneous mutation reflects recent advances in our understanding of gene structure. There are genetic elements termed *insertion sequences* and *transposons* which are capable of moving about from one region of the genome (chromosome, plasmid) to another region of the same or different genome. The insertion of these "mobile genes" into different areas of the chromsome or plasmid DNA modify gene function because the coding sequences are interrupted. Insertion sequences (IS) are small pieces of DNA (800–1400 base pairs), whereas the transposons (Tn) are larger and contain additional genes unrelated to insertion functions, *e.g.*, antibiotic resistance genes. The potential for rapid and extensive alterations in genetic functions of bacteria by these elements is enormous, since they do not depend on DNA homology and may jump from one genome (chromosome, plasmid, bacteriophage DNA to another).

Mutagens and Induced Mutations

There are a number of agents and techniques that increase the errors a cell makes in DNA replication. Many of these errors lead to cell death (lethal mutations) but proper selection methods can permit isolation of other nonlethal mutants. Agents that increase the overall incidence of mutations are termed mutagens. None of these agents is able to produce specific or directed mutational events, rather to increase the overall or total number of mutations.

Several kinds of mutagenic agents are known:

1. Agents which Cause Base-pairing Errors during Replication. For example, 5-bromouracil (5-BU), a structural analogue of thymine, is incorporated into DNA in place of thymine and 5-BU tautomerizes to the enol form more frequently than thymine. Similarly, 2-amino purine (2-AP), is incorporated in place of adenine and it (2-AP) pairs with cytosine rather than thymine. Thus, G-C pairs replace A-T pairs.

2. Agents which Alter Chemical Structure of DNA, Promoting Replication Errors. Nitrous acid (HONO) deaminates adenine and cytosine to hypoxanthine and uracil, both of which have different hydrogen bonding possibilities than the original bases:

$$\text{Adenine} \xrightarrow{\text{HONO}} \text{hypoxanthine}-$$

H bonds with cytosine not thymine

$$\text{Cytosine} \xrightarrow{\text{HONO}} \text{uracil}$$

H bonds with adenine not guanine

HONO deaminates guanine as well but the deamination product (xanthine) does not have different H bonding properties.

3. Alkylating Agents. Agents which substitute aliphatic hydrocarbon radicals at various positions on the DNA bases may cause pairing errors or the hydrolytic removal of the purine (depurination and gap formation). These alkylating agents, ethylme-

thanesulfonate (EMS) or nitrogen mustards are extremely potent and require caution in their use.

4. Intercalating Agents. Certain compounds such as the acridine dyes (proflavine, acridine orange, etc.) are able to be intercalated between the stacked base pairs of DNA in such a way as to cause insertion or deletion of one or a few base pairs during replication. Such an insertion or deletion in the DNA will cause a shift in the "reading frame"— *i.e.*, the message encoded in an RNA must be read as a series of triplets in uninterrupted order. Addition or loss of a base will change the sequence of the three bases in the altered and subsequent triplets.

5. Radiations (Ultraviolet Light, X-rays). The mechanism of UV-induced radiation has been attributed to the production of covalent bonds between neighboring pyrimidines in DNA. The dimers cause gaps to appear in the complimentary strands during replication. Some of these gaps may be repaired by photoactive enzymes that excise the dimers and allow subsequent replacement of bases by DNA polymerases using information on the complimentary strand.

In a number of cases the genetic damage due to mutation may be circumvented by two other processes: suppression and complementation.

Suppression

Loss of activity by a protein as a result of a mutation may be partially or completely removed by a second mutation at a different site. The second mutation, called a suppressor mutation, may occur in the same gene as the primary mutation (intragenic suppression) or in a different gene (extragenic suppression). Intragenic suppression may cause the substitution of an amino acid which compensates for the first change. Extragenic suppression involves suppression of mutations by mechanisms involving alterations of tRNA in the anticodon portion of the molecule, a three nucleotide sequence of tRNA that pairs with a compatible sequence, the codon, in the mRNA molecule. The change in the anticodon permits it to read a mutated codon resulting from an alteration in DNA structure. However, since the change is limited to the anticodon loop of tRNA, it is still able to bind the correct amino acid and insert it into the correct place in the polypeptide chain. The primary mutation occurred in the gene that specified the codon, resulting in an incorrect codon, while the second mutation occurred where the tRNA is specified and permitted the tRNA to read the altered codon. Another possible mechanism of suppression involves opening an alternate pathway for production of the product which cannot be synthesized due to a primary mutation, or production of a product which replaces that of the mutated gene.

Results of Mutation

Since genes regulate protein structure, which determines the structural and metabolic properties of the cell, mutations cause changes in various cell properties. Loss of certain functions is not critical as in the cases where an alternate pathway is possible or where the synthesis of a polymer (e.g., capsule) will not affect the viability of the cell. However, some gene products are indispensible, for the cell dies if they are lost through mutation (lethal mutations). Another form is the conditional lethal mutation, which is expressed under one set of environmental conditions but not another. Conditions where the lethal mutation is expressed are called nonpermissive, while those where they are not expressed are called permissive. One of the more common mutations is that affecting temperature sensitivity, where protein structure is altered so that it is nonfunctional at one temperature but functional at another. If this change occurs and affects an indispensible protein, the cell dies when it is placed at nonpermissive temperatures.

GENE TRANSFER

In eucaryotic cells new gene combinations arise by gamete fusion. Diploid cells are formed and recombinant chromosomes result from the transfer of genetic material from one cell to the other. A similar process may occur in bacteria, whereby a recombinant chromosome is formed from genetic material of two different parental cells. For this to occur in bacteria, the genetic material from one parent must be transferred to the other. Transfer may occur by transformation, conjugation or transduction, resulting in part of the donor cell genetic material being transferred to the recipient making the latter a partial diploid. The original genome of the recipient is called an endogenote, while the donor DNA is called the exogenote. In transformation, a single-stranded piece of donor DNA replaces a strand of endogenote; in transduction a small fragment of donor DNA is transferred to the recipient by a bacterial virus, a bacteriophage; in conjugation the donor DNA is transferred between cells which are in direct contact. If the exogenote has a base sequence homologous to a segment of the endogenote, pairing occurs and a recombinant chromosome is formed, a step that is called integration. If integration does not occur, the exogenote may be segregated upon subsequent cell division, it may replicate independently, or it may be degraded. Recombination occurs by breakage of the parental DNA followed by reunion of the broken ends with the donor DNA, producing a chromosome with the exogenote incorporated into it.

Several generalizations can therefore be made about all these mechanisms of gene transfer.

1. The transfers are always unidirectional—from DNA donor to DNA recipient. There is not a genetic exchange in the sense that both partners receive part of the genetic material, only one partner is the recipient.

2. The transfer of genetic material is usually incomplete. Except in a very few instances only part of the donor DNA is transferred so that *meromixis* (from the Greek roots meaning *partial mixing*) is used to describe the bacterial process of genetic transfer. Similarly, the term merozygote is substituted for zygote to indicate a recipient (partial zygote) without the complete complement of the donor's haploid genome.

3. Not all organisms are capable of all the genetic transfer mechanisms described below. In some instances specific cultural or environmental conditions prevent transfer (e.g., "competency" in transformation) whereas in other instances the presence of a specific surface structure (sex pilus in conjugation) appears to be a prerequisite. Thus, the mechanism of gene transfer is dependent in large measure on the individual properties of the bacterium in question.

4. The successful completion of gene transfer (incorporation and integration of the donor DNA into recipient DNA) requires some positive level of DNA homology. DNAs with low homology—*i.e.*, very few similar nucleotide sequence, do not hybridize. It is therefore possible to make some conclusions about evolutionary relationships between bacteria on the basis of their ability to "mate" successfully.

Some of the various mechanisms of gene transfer in bacteria are described below and summarized in table 4/1.

Transformation

The transfer of extracted soluble DNA from one bacterium to a recipient cell of different genotype was the first mechanism of gene transfer to be described and perhaps the first major discovery in the field of molecular genetics since it led to the first direct evidence that DNA was the ultimate genetic determinant. When DNA of a heat-killed, encapsulated strain of one type of pneumococcus (*Streptococcus pneumoniae*) was mixed with a live nonencapsulated pneumococcus of a different type it was found that the live cells now had the genetically stable ability to form capsules of the same type as the killed pneumococci.

Live nonencapsulated cells (originally derived from type II cells) + DNA of heat-killed, type I (encapsulated cells) → type I encapsulated cells

Subsequently transformation was observed in several bacterial genera with numerous kinds of genetic properties including: antigen production, en-

Table 4/1
Summary of genetic transfer mechanisms

Genetic Process	Representative Organisms	State of DNA as Transfer Agent	Direction of Transfer	Frequency	Amount of Transfer	Other
Transformation	*Streptococcus pneumoniae, Haemophilus influenzae, Bacillus species, Neisseria species, oral streptococci (Streptococcus sanguis, Streptococcus mitior)*	"Naked" DNA	DNA donor → DNA recipient	10^{-3} up to 25%	Few genes (1/200 of chromosome)	1. "Competency" of cell surfaces 2. Environment plays a major role in transfer process 3. Historically, the first mechanism of gene transfer reported in bacteria
Transduction	*Salmonella* species, *Escherichia coli; Shigella*	Bacteriophage carrier	Phage donor → Phage recipient	10^{-5}–10^{-6}	Small linkage groups	1. Two kinds of transduction: restrictive and generalized 2. Nature of infective phage (lytic/lysogenic)
Lysogenic conversion	*Corynebacterium diphtheriae* and other exotoxin-producing bacteria	Phage/prophage	Lysogenic → Nonlysogenic	100%	1 or 2 genes	
Conjugation	*E. coli, Shigella Salmonella, Proteus, Bacillus, Streptococcus mutans, Bacteroides* species, *Streptococcus faecalis*	DNA via cytoplasmic bridge	HFr → F⁻ (F⁺ → F⁻)	10^{-3} 10^{-6}–10^{-7}	Large linkage group	1. Requirement for fertility factor (F) 2. Cell to cell contact required 3. Oriented transfer of linkage group (origin → end)

zyme synthesis, drug resistance, colony morphology, fermentation reactions, etc. For transformation to occur the recipient cell must be competent, a physiological state wherein the recipient has the ability to take up donor DNA which must be double-stranded and have a molecular weight greater than 5×10^5. Competency is determined by the cell's ability to form protein receptors at the cell surface for DNA. These receptors are nonspecific since DNA from heterologous species, which do not transform, can compete successfully for these receptor sites. In transformation the double-stranded donor DNA binds to competent cells, and after certain alterations by membrane bound endonuclease activity the DNA traverses the cell membrane. Only one strand of donor DNA functions in this entry, while the other is usually degraded; therefore, only single-stranded DNA enters the cell. The DNA pairs with the homologous region of the endogenote, recombination occurs and a portion of the endogenote is replaced by the transforming DNA. As is true for most genetic transfers, recombination does not occur unless the exo- and endogenotes have considerable homology in their base pair sequences of DNA.

Transformation studies on oral bacteria have been used to study a number of problems in oral microbial ecology and oral disease. The possibility that genetic transfer could contribute to the enhanced fermentability of sorbitol by oral streptococci has been studied. It was shown that this trait (sorbitol fermentation) was gained by sorbitol nonfermenting strains of *Streptococcus sanguis* by exposing them to naked DNA from sorbitol fermenting strains of *S. sanguis* and *Streptococcus mitior*. Other studies with oral bacteria have shown several other transformable traits including 1) antibiotic resistance, 2) colonial morphology, and 3) resistance to chlorhexidine (an antimicrobial agent). Other related studies show that adherence, a critical ecological determinant for colonization and pathogenicity by many oral bacteria, can also be mediated by transformable properties between cells.

Conjugation

Conjugation, or transfer of DNA from one cell to another following their direct contact, occurs in bacteria. Such transfer requires the presence of extrachromosomal DNA (episomes) which replicate autonomously or are integrated into the bacterial chromosome and replicate as part of the chromosome. The episome necessary for conjugation is capable of promoting gene transfer to other cells and is called the F (fertility) factor. This factor consists of a relatively large piece of double-stranded DNA. It specifies many proteins including products required for its own replication and structural proteins of the specialized F (sex) pili that are necessary for the recognition and aggregation of male and female cells. Male cells are those which have F factor, while females lack it (F⁻). If the F factor is only in the cytoplasm the cell is designated F⁺, whereas if it is integrated in the bacterial chromosome, the cells are designated HFr (high frequency of recombination). F⁺ cells can transfer the F factor with high efficiency to F⁻ cells but usually without any chromosomal markers. In doing so, an F⁻ cell becomes F⁺. HFr cells do transfer part of a cell's chromosome at a relatively high frequency but usually do not transmit the F factor. This failure to transfer F results from the fact that the HFr chromosome is transferred into the F⁻ cell in a linear fashion with F at the end of the chromosome. Therefore, F is the last part of the chromosome to become integrated (oriented direction of transfer). Since the whole chromosome is rarely transferred due to breakage at various times during transfer, F is rarely transferred. The DNA is thought to be transferred through a cytoplasmic bridge into the recipient (F⁻) cell and subsequently is known to be integrated into F⁻ cells giving the partial diploid (merozygote) referred to earlier.

F factor may either come out of the chromosome of HFr cells by itself or bring with it a piece of bacterial DNA. If the latter occurs, the genetic information attached to the F factor will be transferred to a new recipient along with the F factor. (This process has been termed sexduction or F duction and the F factors now called F'. Since these hybrid F' factors are transmitted to F⁻ cells with high efficiency they are of potential significance—depending on the specific gene locus adjacent to the F locus, *e.g.*, antibiotic resistance.

Conjugation requires cell-to-cell contact. The affinity of male and female microbial cells relates to a male-borne structure, the F pilus (see Chapter 3), which promotes contact. With cellular contact, a break occurs in the DNA carrying the F factor, converting it to a form that can be transferred. Transfer is initiated by replication of DNA in the male cell. One of the daughter DNA molecules passes to the female while the other remains with the male. This method of transfer ensures the gentic integrity and the post-mating viability of the male cell and also provides for the zygotic condition of the female cell.

Conjugation has been demonstrated in a variety of microorganisms. As in transformation a variety of characteristics can be transferred but integration of donor DNA does not occur unless there is sufficient homology to permit pairing.

Transduction

Transduction is the transfer of DNA from one bacterial cell to another by means of a bacterial virus (bacteriophage) (see fig. 4/2). Transduction

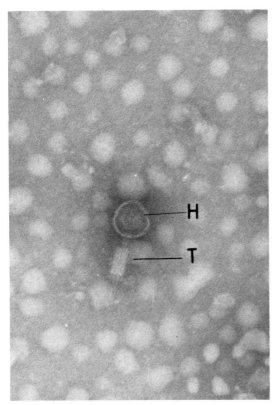

Figure 4/2. An electron micrograph of a bacteriophage against *Actinobacillus actinomycetemcomitans*, a well known periodontal pathogen associated with juvenile periodontitis. Note the head (*H*), tail (*T*) and contractile fibers. The preparation was negatively stained with 1% phosphotungstic acid. (Courtesy of Dr. R. H. Stevens and Dr. Chern Lai, University of Pennsylvania School of Dental Medicine.)

where any chromosomal marker can be transferred is termed generalized transduction. Where only certain genes are capable of being transferred by a phage, the process is called restricted transduction. The ability of a phage to mediate transduction of one or the other type depends upon the relationship of the phage to host DNA.

Host-Bacteriophage Relationships. Bacteriophages infect by attaching to bacterial cells into which they inject their DNA. If the phage is virulent, it goes through a vegetative cycle in which the phage replicates to produce new virus particles which are released by lysis of the host cell. A temperate phage, on the other hand, may follow alternate pathways after infection. It may go through a lytic cycle, or a repressor may be produced which prevents the lytic cycle. In the latter instance, phage DNA enters into a nonvirulent relationship with the host cell and is incorporated into the host chromosome. Such a relationship is called lysogeny or the lysogenic state, and the phage DNA in this state is called the prophage. With

lysogeny the host cell acquires new properties. First, it is immune to infection by a homologous phage. Second, any genetic characteristics accompanying the phage DNA are imparted to the cell and may be expressed.

During assembly of phage particles in a host cell prior to release by lysis, host DNA may be packaged into the phage coat, forming a generalized transducing particle. The packaging is random with regard to which host DNA is packaged; it occurs at a low frequency, and the amount of DNA is equivalent to the size of the genome normally carried by the phage. In generalized transduction the transducing particles contain no detectable phage DNA, but when a generalized transducing phage infects a new host, the bacterial DNA it is carrying is transferred to the new host. On the other hand, production of phages for restricted transduction depends on formation of the lysogenic state. The integration of phage DNA is not irreversible, but it can be induced to come out of the host chromosome and initiate a lytic cycle. Induction is caused by ultraviolet light, changes in environment, or sometimes occurs "spontaneously." If this occurs and if the prophage carries a portion of host DNA with it, there may be production of specialized transducing particles. However, the amount of host DNA is limited since the total amount of DNA in a phage is limited. The reason that specialized transducing particles carry only specific genes is that the phage DNA integrates into a host at a very few specific sites, and thus the host genes it can take with it are only those adjacent to it. In this process a portion of the phage DNA is excluded, the amount depending on how much host DNA is present (analogous to F duction).

Abortive Transduction and Lysogenic Conversion. In many instances the exogenote pairs with the endogenote and recombination occurs, producing a recombinant type organism. In others, the exogenote may persist and function but not replicate so that when cell division occurs only one cell in the population contains the exogenote. In some cases a given suspension of phage will produce 10 times more abortive transductions than the normal ones. Since abortive transduction results when recombination does not occur between the exogenote and the endogenote it follows that procedures which stimulate recombination (exposure to UV light) will convert abortive transductions to normal transductions.

Certain properties of bacterial cells are controlled solely by phage genes and are manifested in lysogenic or phage-infected cells, *e.g.*, *Corynebacterium diphtheriae* produces toxin only if it is infected with a particular strain of phage (*β*); phage-free cells do not produce toxin. This process in which a new property is acquired as the result of phage infection is termed lysogenic conversion. Several other examples of lysogenic conversion are well known: 1) antigenic changes in the cell surface of *Salmonella* strains; 2) toxin formation by major bacterial pathogens (*Streptococcus pyogenes* and its erythrogenic toxin, leukocidin of *Staphylococcus aureus* and the highly potent toxin of *Clostridium botulinum*; and 3) some virulence-associated property of *Vibrio cholerae* (El Tor biotype). In all of these cases a lysogenic phage is necessary for the expression of a property that is never expressed in the absence of phage infections.

Plasmids and Episomes

One of the primary differences between eucaryotes and procaryotes is the absence in procaryotes of membrane-bounded organelles containing DNA (mitochondria, chloroplasts). These autonomously replicating centers were thought to be analogous in many respects to the bacterial chromosome. With the discovery of the F factor it became clear that some bacteria do occasionally harbor extrachromosomal packets of DNA on a temporary basis. Unlike mitochondria and chloroplasts these extranuclear bacterial elements 1) do not have membrane coverings, 2) lack the machinery for transcription and translation of organellar protein synthesis, and 3) are not essential to life. Two types of extrachromosomal DNA are known for bacteria: plasmids and episomes. Plasmids are autonomous genetic elements not capable of integration into the chromosome, while episomes can exist autonomously or can be integrated into the chromosome. Some elements are plasmids in one species and episomes in others. (F is an episome in *E. coli* but a plasmid in *Proteus mirabilis* indicating that episomes are host-specific.) Both may be eliminated from the cell by treatment with various ("curing") agents including acridine dyes, UV light and heat. This criterion of elimination is further evidence that plasmids and episomes are dispensable, autonomous elements not coding for essential gene functions.

Extrachromosomal genetic elements have been divided into large and small factors. Large factors, composed of 100 to 200 genes, include F (fertility factor—see above), antibiotic resistance factors and a few bacteriocinogens (see below). Small factors (only about 15 genes) include most bacteriocinogens and a number of cryptic plasmids (plasmids with no known gene function). Both kinds of factors can be recognized by standard genetic and physical techniques. Genetically, a plasmid is revealed if a gene function(s) can be shown *not* to be linked to the chromosome *re* autonomous replication. The autonomous replication of such an extranuclear element is assumed if the factor is transferred at conjugation independent of the chromosome or by

"curing" experiments with acridine dyes in which case the plasmid function is irreversibly eliminated. Physical detection of plasmids is based on differences in the physicochemical properties of plasmid and chromosomal DNAs: 1) Plasmid DNAs are often less dense and show up as "satellite bands" on ultracentrifugation in a density gradient and 2) if the densities are similar, plasmid DNA can be differentiated from chromosomal DNAs by the intercalation of various acridine dyes which increase the density of plasmid DNA but not chromosomal DNAs. This latter method (dye-buoyant density) is based on the fact that plasmid DNA is a supercoiled, closed, circular molecule and much more likely to take up the dye molecules than the linear fragments of chromosomal DNA.

Replication of large factors is usually synchronous with the bacterial chromosome. Mutations that prevent replication of the bacterial chromosome may also prevent replication of large plasmids. Replication of small plasmids is not synchronous with replication of the bacterial chromosome and the replication rate of these small plasmids may differ widely from the chromosome under certain conditions giving rise to numerous copies of the plasmid within a single cell. Many of the large plasmids are transmissible to other cells by formation of their own conjugation apparatus whereas the small plasmids do not usually code for enough proteins to ensure self replication and self-transfer. Several cryptic plasmids have been detected among bacteria associated with oral disease. Particular attention has been directed toward *Streptococcus mutans* and other lactic acid bacteria regarding the acquisition of pathogenic potential as a result of a plasmid-mediated gene transfer. A small plasmid from *S. mutans* LM7 was recently cloned in *E. coli* cells and shown to be associated with the production of a protein of unknown function, but no association with cariogenicity of *S. mutans* was demonstrated. Attempts to demonstrate a positive correlation between glycogen formation and the small plasmids in *Lactobacillus casei* were also unsuccessful. Conjugal transfer of a plasmid from a streptococcus (group F) to strains of *L. casei* has recently been demonstrated although the biological significance of this transfer (antibiotic resistance) in a context of oral health is also not clear. The original idea behind many of these investigations was to determine the extent to which genetic transfer between oral bacteria could explain the observed variations of clinical isolates. Since most of the plasmids are cryptic the original question remains unanswered. Many possibilities seem quite reasonable in view of the known role of plasmids as critical determinants of pathogenicity in other infectious diseases such as enterotoxin production in pathogenic strains of *E. coli*, pili formation and adherence of the gonococcus, sucrose fermentation, antibiotic resistance and bacteriocin formation.

Related studies also have demonstrated that certain *S. mutans* genes, those that code for glycosyltransferases or GTF, can be cloned in *E. coli* cells. Glycosyl transferases are enzymes that catalyze the synthesis from sucrose of adherent glucose polymers that *S. mutans* needs to colonize teeth prior to initiating the caries process. If GTF were used in a vaccine, specific antibodies would be induced which are capable in interacting with GTF produced by *S. mutans*. These would presumably inhibit the enzyme's biological activity and therefore reduce the likelihood of this bacterium colonizing teeth. The advantages of using GTF clones in *E. coli* are: 1) the absence of competing sucrose-degrading enzymes normally present in *S. mutans*, and 2) the absence of cross-reacting substances in *E. coli* that could interfere with the safety of a GTF vaccine. (Antisera to whole *S. mutans* cells contain antibodies that could react with human myocardial tissue.)

ANTIBIOTIC RESISTANCE

Resistance Involving Extrachromosomal Factors

One of the most important clinical implications of gene transfer is the ability of plasmids to transfer resistance to a number of antibiotics and chemicals in mixed populations of bacteria. Thus, a single bacterium can develop multiple resistance to several antibiotics as a result of one plasmid transfer and, subsequently, can transfer this multiple resistance to yet another bacterium, often of another genus or species. When multiple resistant strains of *Shigella* were mixed with antibiotic-sensitive strains of *E. coli* the multiple resistance was transferred to the sensitive organisms. The plasmids responsible for this type of multiple resistance to antibiotics and other antibacterial agents are termed R factors. The R factor consists of two parts: one part, the resistance transfer factor, (RTF) carries the genes for replication and the conjugative transmission of the plasmid and the other part consists of one or more sequentially linked resistance determinants (genes for enzymes that inactivate or otherwise modify the antibiotics in question). These two components may exist as separate, autonomously replicating elements in which case the resistance determinants appear to be incapable of undergoing transfer unless mobilized by an RTF. In many respects R factors are analogous to the F factor in that both code for surface pili and other factors associated with their conjugative transmission, *e.g.*, R and F pili, and both may exist as autonomously replicating units in the cytoplasm or they may be integrated into the chromosome, *i.e.*,

they are in the strict sense episomes although they are usually designated as plasmids.

Resistance Involving Chromosomal Mutation

It is to be remembered that resistance due to R factors and plasmids is clearly different from resistance arising from spontaneous chromosomal mutations. First, there are enormous differences in the *occurrence* of chromosomal mutations responsible for drug resistance as compared to the en bloc conjugative transfer of resistance genes in plasmids. The likelihood of simultaneous chromosomal mutations to resistance to 4 or 5 antibiotics is infinitesimally small since the probability is the algebraic sum of the mutation frequencies for the universal drugs, *i.e.*,

Mutation rate to antibiotic X is 10^{-5}
Mutation rate to antibiotic Y is 10^{-6}
Mutation rate to antibiotic Z is 10^{-7}

Therefore, the likelihood of a simultaneous mutation to resistance to X, Y, and Z antibiotics is 10^{-18}.

Furthermore, chromosomal mutations obviously do not require conjugation or some other means of genetic transfer. There are also differences in the mechanisms of resistance associated with R factors as opposed to chromosomal mutations. Plasmid genes encode enzymes that chemically inactivate the antibacterial agent (e.g., chloramphenicol transacetylase), whereas chromosomal resistance genes usually modify the cellular target of the drug (e.g., cell wall, ribosome).

Penicillinase Plasmids

Many bacteria produce a β-lactamase (a penicillinase) that hydrolyzes the β-lactam ring of the penicillin molecule (Chapter 8) resulting in high levels of resistance to penicillin. The gene for this enzyme along with others is located on a plasmid and is responsible for almost all cases of penicillin resistance in clinical isolates. The one penicillinase plasmid that has been studied most intensively is the one found in *Staphylococcus aureus*; an important human pathogen that causes skin and wound infections. Unlike the enterobacteria, *S. aureus* is unable to conjugate and its plasmids are transferred by transduction. There is considerable epidemiologic evidence in human studies that *S. aureus* transduction occurs naturally and may be responsible for the widespread resistance so frequently observed in clinical isolates of this organism. Certainly, lysogeny is well documented in clinical isolates of staphylococci.

Bacteriocins

Many bacteria produce low molecular weight, heat stable bactericidal proteins called *bacteriocins*.

Most bacteriocins kill only those bacteria closely related taxonomically to the producing organism, i.e., S. mutans bacteriocin-producer strains affect other closely related streptococcal strains, not E. coli. Also, since bacteriocin-producing strains are resistant to their own bacteriocins, it is possible to use bacteriocins for "typing" (see below). The genetic determinants for bacteriocins are carried on plasmids (bacteriocinogens) but may under certain circumstances be integrated into the bacterial chromosome. These proteins are very toxic at low doses. Their actions are very specific but differ among the various types of bacteriocins. They may, for example, stop nucleic acid synthesis, cause cell lysis, or inhibit respiration. The colicins are the most widely studied bacteriocins. One inhibits ATP formation in E. coli while another causes breaks in DNA. Streptococcus mutans strains produce bacteriocins (mutacins) which have proved useful in grouping or classifying strains of S. mutans and in epidemiological studies. Their possible role in the natural environment is not known but the susceptibility of bacteriocins to proteolytic enzymes could compromise their activity in a salivary milieu.

ADDITIONAL READING

ELWELL, L. P., AND SHIPLEY, P. L. 1980 Plasmid-mediated Factors Associated with Virulence of Bacteria to Animals. Annu Rev Microbiol, 34, 465.

GOTS, J. S., AND BENSON, C. E. 1974 Biochemical Genetics of Bacteria. Annu Rev Genet, 8, 77.

HAMADA, S., AND SLADE, H. D. 1980. Biology, Immunology and Cariogenicity of Streptococcus mutans. Microbiol Rev 44, 331.

HAYES, W. 1968 The Genetics of Bacteria and Their Viruses, Ed. 2. Blackwell, Oxford, England.

KELSTRUP, J., RICHMOND, S., WEST, C., AND GIBBONS, R. J. 1971 Fingerprinting Human Oral Streptococci by Bacteriocin Production and Sensitivity. Arch Oral Biol, 15, 1109.

RILEY, M., AND ANILONIS, A. 1978 Evolution of the Bacterial Genome. Annu Rev Microbiol, 35, 519.

STILES, H. M., LOESCHE, W. J., AND O'BRIEN, T. C. (Eds.) 1976 Microbial Aspects of Dental Caries; Vol III. Biochemical and Genetic Determinants of Virulence Microbiol. Abstr Spec Suppl.

WATSON, J. D. 1976 Molecular Biology of the Gene, Ed. 3. W. A. Benjamin Inc., Menlo Park, Calif.

chapter 5

Metabolism of Bacteria

Benjamin Hammond

INTRODUCTION

Unity, Diversity and Oral Bacteria

The growth and maintenance of bacteria are the results of an extraordinary series of chemical and physical reactions that occur within the cell. Two general groups of reactions may be identified: 1) synthesis of cellular constituents (*anabolism*) which requires energy and 2) the opposite process of *catabolism* (the decomposition or breakdown) of cellular components which is accompanied by the release of energy and the accumulation of breakdown products. Anabolic reactions are essentially similar in all cells, eucaryotic as well as procaryotic—*i.e.*, the synthesis of proteins, nucleic acids, lipids and polysaccharides are governed by a few common-denominator reactions characteristic of all biological systems. Indeed, the concept of unity in biochemistry derived from studies based on bacterial metabolism. Catabolic reactions in bacteria while sharing a number of biochemical pathways with other cell systems exhibit an extraordinary diversity as well. Thus, unity amid diversity is one of the hallmarks of bacterial metabolism and is fundamental to the taxonomy, classification and physiology of bacteria. The catabolic mechanisms of bacteria range from the oxidation of inorganic compounds such as ammonia, nitrites, sulfides, ferrous salts or hydrogen to the oxidation of carbohydrates, hydrocarbons and many other compounds for energy sources. This metabolic versatility is especially important in the human oral cavity since variations in diet and other environmentally induced changes provide an enormous number of metabolizable substrates and possibilities for bacterial action.

This chapter will be concerned with some of the catabolic reactions of bacteria with emphasis on the metabolism of oral bacteria. It does not purport to be a detailed analysis or even a survey of bacterial metabolism; a more comprehensive coverage will be found in the supplemental readings listed at the end of this chapter.

ENERGY LIBERATION AND STORAGE

The essential task of metabolism is to carry out thermodynamically possible chemical reactions that do not occur directly under the conditions of life, notably at neutrality and at temperatures from 10 to 45 C, or for which no direct path is known. We know, for example, that glucose can be oxidized directly to carbon dioxide and water:

$$C_6H_{12}O_2 + 6O_2 \rightarrow 6CO_2 + 6H_2O \qquad \Delta G = 688,000 \text{ calories}[1]$$

This reaction occurs only at temperatures destructive to life, and the available chemical energy escapes as heat. Consider also the reactions by which glucose is converted to lactic acid:

$$C_6H_{12}O_6 \rightarrow 2CH_3\text{—}CHOH\text{—}COOH \qquad \Delta G = 55,000 \text{ calories}$$

However, no way is known to accomplish this conversion directly. Such a conversion is possible in many biological systems except that it involves a series of intermediate reactions each of which involves only a modest exchange of energy. The process (called glycolysis) entails at least eleven steps, some receiving energy, others liberating energy. The free energy available from this conversion still totals −55,000 calories. Much of this energy is captured and stored by the cell in the form of high energy phosphate bonds of adenosine triphosphate (ATP).

There are three methods by which the energy released as a result of catabolic reactions can be trapped as ATP: 1) substrate level phosphorylation,

---

[1] The symbol ΔG denotes the so-called free energy change, *i.e.*, the energy available for work from the reaction of 1 gram molecule of reactant. A negative sign means that the starting materials release free energy and that the reaction should theoretically proceed spontaneously. A positive sign would mean that the reaction would go in the direction indicated only if energy were supplied. The ΔG under physiological conditions have not been determined exactly. Revision of the values used here, however, would not change the outcome of the reactions described.

2) oxidative phosphorylation, and 3) the most complex of all, photosynthesis.

Substrate Level Phosphorylation

Substrate level phosphorylation is a term used to describe the process in which the energy released through oxidation is localized in a high energy phosphate bond of the oxidized substrate. In this process organic compounds serve as both electron donors (being oxidized) and electron acceptors (becoming reduced). For example:

$$\text{3-Phospho-} \atop \text{glyceraldehyde} + P_i \xrightarrow[]{\text{NAD} \quad \text{NADH}} \text{1,3-Diphospho-} \atop \text{glyceric acid}$$

The best known examples of substrate level phosphorylations occur in the fermentations. In fermentations the substrate (usually a carbohydrate) gives rise to a mixture of end products, some of which are more oxidized and some of which are more reduced, i.e., there is a balance in the oxidation and reduction levels of the products. Other fermentable compounds include organic acids, amino acids, purines, and pyrimidines. All fermentations occur under anaerobic conditions and result in the incomplete oxidation of the substrate. Pasteur referred to fermentation as "la vie sans l'air" and recognized its importance in the metabolism of many bacteria. Many bacteria are strict anaerobes (see Chapter 6 for a discussion of the mechanisms of strict anaerobiosis); others are facultative anaerobes and are able to grow in the presence or absence of air. Many of these facultative organisms in the presence of air are able to convert their mode of ATP generation to respiration (see below). However, one group of very important oral bacteria (the lactic acid bacteria—streptococci and lactobacilli) are exceptions since they continue to ferment even in the presence of air. The inefficiency of this method of energy generation is in sharp contrast to other ATP generative processes.

Oxidative Phosphorylation (Electron Transport)

In this process it is possible to get complete oxidation of a substrate with a much greater release of energy for growth and maintenance of the cells. Unlike fermentation and substrate level phosphorylation the final electron acceptor is oxygen and the process is often referred to as respiration. Electrons are passed sequentially from one electron carrier to the next in an electron transport chain.

$$\text{Organic substrate} \rightarrow \text{NAD} \rightarrow \text{flavoprotein} \xrightarrow{\text{quinone}}$$
$$\text{cytochrome } b,\ c,\ a \rightarrow O_2$$
Redox potential: 0.32 v   0.20 $\rightarrow\rightarrow$ + 0.01 $\rightarrow$ 0.022   +
0.81

The mechanism of ATP generation by the trans-

port of electrons is not completely clear but the current explanation that has received the greatest amount of support is called the chemiosmotic hypothesis. This explanation suggests that the electron transport system is oriented in the cell membrane in such a way as to cause the outward flow of protons which cannot reenter the membrane except at specific membrane sites where ATP areas are found. As a consequence a proton gradient (Δ pH) is created across the membrane. This gradient derives the following reaction resulting in the generation of ATP.

$$\text{ADP} + P_i + H^+ \xrightarrow{\text{ATPase}} \text{ATP} + H_2O$$

In any event, the breakdown of one mole of glucose by this respiratory mechanism (i.e., oxidative phosphorylation involving electron transport) yields about 12 times more energy than the fermentative (anaerobic) breakdown to organic end products such as lactic acid. Some of the comparative differences between fermentation and respiration are shown in the following table:

	Fermentation	Respiration
Electron donor	Organic compound	Organic compound
Final electron acceptor	Organic compound	O_2
Energy liberation from 1 mole of glucose	55 kcal	688 kcal
Method of ATP generation	Substrate phosphorylation	Electron transport (oxidative phosphorylation)
Oxygen requirement	Oxygen absent	Oxygen required

Photosynthesis

Photosynthesis is the third method of ATP generation and uses light as the energy source. This process is rarely, if ever, found in bacteria of medical importance but it is critically important in a context of ecology. Many photosynthetic bacteria occupy a wide range of habitats and are able to fix nitrogen and regulate the supply of dissolved oxygen in lakes where there is a high amount of nitrate and phosphate. The photosynthetic process is not unlike oxidative phosphorylation since ATP is once again formed by the passage of electrons through special electron transport chains. This photophosphorylative process begins when light is absorbed by a chlorophyll molecule. The excited chlorophyll molecule emits an electron which is accepted by an iron-containing electron acceptor called ferredoxin and then is passed through a series of cytochrome pigments where 2 moles of ATP are formed from ADP for each pair of electrons passed.

Overview

Cells are not capable of utilizing energy liberated in reactions outside themselves. Energy must be made available by a catabolic reaction within the cell and retained in one of its products, which is the energy-transferring link to the next reaction in the metabolic chain. In most cases only a fraction of the energy produced is captured and the rest is lost as heat. In a catabolic process, substrate is converted into products of lower energy content and the energy released is captured in various compounds. It can then be used to "prime" additional catabolic reaction and drive synthetic functions. Since carbohydrate occupies an important position in metabolism, the various relationships are best summarized by a consideration of its utilization.

In a context of oral ecology, however, it is important to point out that many of the organisms found in the human gingival crevice (*Bacteroides gingivalis/asaccharolyticus*, *Vibrio* species and other gram negative anaerobes) are asaccharolytic and are unable to utilize carbohydrates including many of the common dietary sugars (sucrose, fructose, maltose or glucose). These organisms obtain their energy from other sources, *e.g.*, amino acid fermentations, hydrogen, etc. Thus, while the centrality of carbohydrate metabolism is well established for all of the cariogenic lactic acid bacteria, carbohydrates are much less important for many other oral microorganisms.

CARBOHYDRATE METABOLISM

The discussion of carbohydrate metabolism will be divided into six parts: the first five related to carbohydrate breakdown, the sixth part a discussion of the carbohydrate metabolism of dental plaque and oral bacteria. Carbohydrate utilization may occur in the following phases: 1) cleavage of hexoses and pentoses into three-carbon and two-carbon compounds, principally pyruvate or lactate and acetate or ethanol (plus carbon dioxide); 2) cleavage of pyruvate to carbon dioxide and a two-carbon fragment ("active acetyl") and conversion of other two-carbon compounds to "active acetyl"; 3) oxidation of the acetyl residue to carbon dioxide and water via the tricarboxylic acid cycle; 4) transfer of hydrogen from NADH and NADPH (formed in the preceding reactions) to oxygen via the cytochrome system; and 5) utilization and synthesis of polysaccharides. The various reactions in carbohydrate metabolism are presented from the viewpoint of dissimilation, but since many of the intermediate steps are reversible, they may serve as well for the synthesis of carbohydrates. Many of the intermediate compounds may be diverted by interconnecting reactions into amino acid, nucleic acid, and fatty acid metabolism.

Embden-Meyerhof Pathway (Glycolysis)

The primary cleavage of sugars is best exemplified by the fermentation of glucose to lactic acid via the classical Embden-Meyerhof pathway. A condensed summary of the essential stages of this fermentation is shown in table 5/1. Other hexoses, such as fructose, galactose, and mannose, enter this pathway at the hexose monophosphate stage through phosphorylations and (where necessary) isomerizations.

The conversion of the glucose molecule in two lactates in the Embden-Meyerhof pathway releases 55,000 calories of free energy, of which about 40% (21,000 calories) is captured in the high energy phosphate groups of two ATPs, where it is available for cellular processes that require energy. When compared to the complete oxidation of glucose, which captures about $\frac{2}{3}$ of 688,000 calories of free energy, lactic fermentation is clearly not an efficient means of obtaining cellular energy. Nevertheless, homofermentative lactobacilli and streptococci rely almost entirely on lactate fermentation, even in the presence of oxygen. Heterofermentative organisms proceed by an alternative route, sometimes called the pentose-phosphate pathway, and produce considerable products other than lactate.

An alternative route for the primary splitting of hexoses via five-carbon compounds is used in part by some organisms, and wholly by others that lack aldolase. This process may be summarized as follows: glucose-6-phosphate is partially dehydrogenated via $NADP^+$ to form 6-phosphogluconate, which is further dehydrogenated via $NADP^+$ to keto-6-phosphogluconate, which is decarboxylated to form a ketopentose, ribulose-5-phosphate. The latter is the connecting link to the metabolism of pentoses, since it is reversibly isomerized enzymatically to ribose-5-phosphate, a common denominator in pentose dissimilation. This reaction provides pentose phosphate for nucleic acid synthesis. In dissimilation, pentose phosphate is split into glyceraldehyde-3-phosphate, which follows the path to lactate indicated in table 5/1 and a two-carbon fragment, "active glycolaldehyde," which accepts hydrogen from NADPH to form ethanol, or is rearranged to form acetate.

A third method of bacterial dissimilation of glucose down to pyruvate is known as the *Entner-Doudoroff* pathway. This pathway is found in certain groups of procaryotic cells (notably the pseudomonads) and is unlike the Embden-Meyerhof and pentose phosphate routes which are found in both eucaryotes and procaryotes. Glucose 6-phosphate is the first intermediate in this pathway (see fig. 5/

Table 5/1
Lactic fermentation of glucose (Embden-Meyerhof pathway)

Glucose	
+ ATP ↓ Hexokinase, Mg^{++}	High energy phosphate transfer, practically irreversible
Glucose 6-phosphate + ADP	
↑↓ Phosphohexose isomerase	Isomerization
Fructose 6-phosphate	
+ ATP ↓ Phosphofructokinase	High energy phosphate transfer, practically irreversible
Fructose 1,6-diphosphate + ADP	
↑↓ Aldolase	Reversible aldol condensation
Glyceraldehyde-3-phosphate + dihydroxyacetone phosphate	
+ 2 NAD$^+$ Triosephosphate isomerase	Isomerization
+ 2 H$_3$PO$_4$ Triosephosphate dehydrogenase	Dehydrogenation + phosphorylation → high energy phosphate; mechanism obscure
Two 1,3-diphosphoglycerate + 2 NADH	
+ 2 ADP ↑↓ Phosphoglycerate kinase	High energy phosphate transfer regenerates ATP
Two 3-phosphoglycerate + 2 ATP	
↑↓ Phosphoglyceromutase	Phosphate transfer
Two 2-phosphoglycerate	
↑↓ Enolase, Mg^{++}	Dehydration and creation of high energy phosphate
Two phospho-enol-pyruvate + H$_2$O	
+ 2 ADP ↑↓ Pyruvate kinase	High energy phosphate transfer regenerates ATP
Two pyruvate + 2 ATP	
+ 2 NADH ↑↓ Lactic dehydrogenase	Regeneration of NAD$^+$
Two lactate + 2 NAD$^+$	

Glucose + 2 phosphate + 2 ADP →
          2 lactate + 2 H$^+$ + 2 ATP   Net reaction. ΔG = −34,000 calories

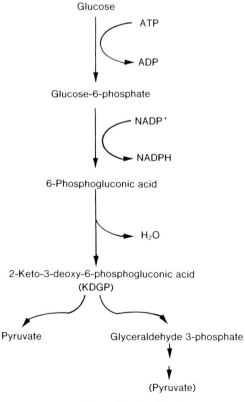

Figure 5/1. Entner-Doudoroff pathway.

1) and is oxidized to 6-phosphogluconic acid. The unique or "signature" intermediate in the pathway is 2-keto-3-deoxy-6-phosphogluconic acid (KDPG) and it is formed by the dehydration of the 6-P-gluconic acid. KDPG is cleaved to 1 mole of pyruvate and 1 mole of glyceraldehyde-3-phosphate which is subsequently metabolized via glycolysis to a second mole of pyruvate. The net yield of 1 mole of glucose through this pathway is 1 mole of ATP and 2 moles of NADH.

Further Metabolism of Pyruvate and Two-Carbon Fragments

The focal reaction of the next stage in biological oxidation is the formation of "active acetyl" directly from two-carbon fragments or from pyruvate by oxidative decarboxylation. Acetyl-CoA is the normal end-product of this phase of the metabolism of pyruvate and two-carbon fragments. The various reactions coupled to these transformations yield three high energy phosphates per molecule of pyruvate.

Depending on available cellular enzymes, acetyl is also converted to compounds such as acetate, ethanol, and butanol, either by transfer from acetyl-CoA, acetyl lipoate, or a presumed acetaldehyde-carboxylase intermediate. Acetyl is a connecting link to fatty acid metabolism. Pyruvate is converted by other mechanisms to propionate, propanol, or acetone; or to acetate and formate. Some bacteria convert formate by hydrogenlyase to carbon dioxide and hydrogen. The direct path from pyruvate, however, leads to the oxidation of acetyl via the "tricarboxylic acid cycle." Pyruvate, through the reversible condensation of its methyl group with carbon dioxide, forms oxalacetate ($COOH—CH_2—CO—COOH$), a key compound that initiates the cycle.

Tricarboxylic Acid Cycle

Active acetyl, in the form of acetyl-CoA, is condensed through its methyl group with the carbonyl group of oxalacetate to form citrate. This initiates a remarkable series of reactions which convert acetyl into carbon dioxide and reduced hydrogen acceptors, and regenerate oxalacetate. The essential stages of the cycle are shown in table 5/2. Because they are incompletely understood, the energy-capturing reactions are omitted. A part of this capture occurs during the subsequent oxidation of the reduced hydrogen acceptors in the cytochrome pathway.

The tricarboxylic acid cycle is an essential part of aerobic metabolism in animal tissues but it seldom operates in its entirety in a microorganism.

Intermediate reactions can be carried out by various bacteria which utilize an incomplete or modified version of the cycle. Since its reactions are reversible, the cycle serves synthetic as well as catabolic purposes. It is also a metabolic crossroads that serves as a bridge between carbohydrate and protein metabolism; through acetyl-CoA it connects with fatty acid synthesis.

Terminal Path to Oxygen

Hydrogen is accepted by NAD^+, $NADP^+$, or another acceptor at four stages in the tricarboxylic acid cycle and in various other reactions involved in carbohydrate metabolism. In aerobic metabolism, hydrogen is eventually transferred to oxygen by a series of reactions apparently coupled so that 3 high energy phosphates are created, making a total of 12 for the 4 acceptors in the tricarboxylic acid cycle.

In animal tissues, carbohydrate appears to be completely utilizable by the tricarboxylic acid cycle. Bacteria form a metabolic spectrum beginning with obligate aerobes such as *Neisseria* species. Intermediate in the spectrum are staphylococci, typhoid, dysentery, and colon bacilli, which possess cytochromes but are able to grow and multiply anaerobically. At the other end of the spectrum there are

Table 5/2
Tricarboxylic acid cycle

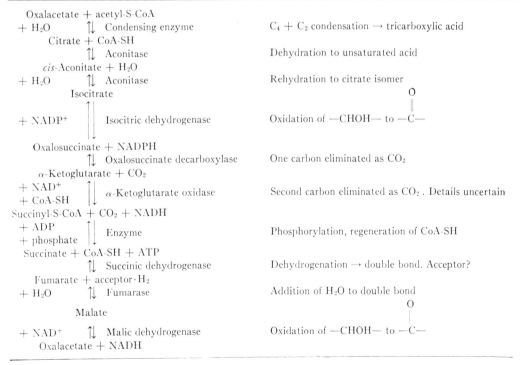

Oxalacetate + acetyl-S-CoA + H_2O ⇅ Condensing enzyme Citrate + CoA-SH	$C_4 + C_2$ condensation → tricarboxylic acid
⇅ Aconitase *cis*-Aconitate + H_2O	Dehydration to unsaturated acid
+ H_2O ⇅ Aconitase Isocitrate	Rehydration to citrate isomer
+ $NADP^+$ Isocitric dehydrogenase	Oxidation of —CHOH— to $—\overset{O}{\overset{\|}{C}}—$
Oxalosuccinate + NADPH ⇅ Oxalosuccinate decarboxylase α-Ketoglutarate + CO_2	One carbon eliminated as CO_2
+ NAD^+ α-Ketoglutarate oxidase + CoA-SH Succinyl-S-CoA + CO_2 + NADH	Second carbon eliminated as CO_2. Details uncertain
+ ADP Enzyme + phosphate Succinate + CoA-SH + ATP	Phosphorylation, regeneration of CoA-SH
⇅ Succinic dehydrogenase Fumarate + acceptor·H_2	Dehydrogenation → double bond. Acceptor?
+ H_2O ⇅ Fumarase Malate	Addition of H_2O to double bond
+ NAD^+ ⇅ Malic dehydrogenase Oxalacetate + NADH	Oxidation of —CHOH— to $—\overset{O}{\overset{\|}{C}}—$

$CH_3CO\text{-}S\text{-}CoA + 3H_2O + 4\text{ Acceptor} \rightarrow$
$2CO_2 + CoA\text{-}SH + 4\text{ Acceptor·}H_2$

Net reaction

the fermentative streptococci, pneumococci, and lactobacilli and the obligate anaerobes of the genus *Clostridium*, which lack cytochromes and are able to utilize only a small fraction of the free energy potentially available from nutrient.

Utilization and Synthesis of Polysaccharides

Many bacteria produce enzymes that release utilizable monosaccharides from nonutilizable polysaccharides. The intracellular formation of polysaccharides and their utilization as stores of energy have not played as prominent a role in bacterial metabolism as in animal and plant metabolism, although, as will be seen subsequently, production and degradation of intracellular polysaccharides seem to be important in the metabolism of plaque bacteria. Many of these bacteria accumulate polysaccharides during growth on sugars that are consumed during sugar deprivation. When grown on glucose, 60 percent of the cultivable organisms from human carious material produced enough glycogen to stain deeply with iodine. Such carbohydrates may permit the bacteria to form extracellular acid in the absence of exogenous carbohydrate (see Chapter 3).

Of interest for the general problem of biochemical polymerization is the enzymatic synthesis of bacterial polysaccharides during dissimilation of disaccharides. *Streptococcus mutans* is capable of converting sucrose to water-soluble and -insoluble glucans. The soluble glucans contain glucose primarily in α-1,6-linkages while insoluble glucans possess a high degree of branching involving α-1,3-linkages (fig. 5/2). These polysaccharides are synthesized by enzymes, glucosyltransferases, which for the most part are extracellular or bound to the cell surface. This extracellular synthesis transfers glucose units from sucrose to an acceptor which usually is the growing dextran-like polymer. The enzyme conserves the energy of the link ($\Delta G=6600$ calories) between the C1 of glucose and C2 of fructose present in sucrose and it is used to create the new bond in the polymer. The reaction may be summarized as follows:

$$n\text{Sucrose} + \text{acceptor} \xrightarrow{\text{glucosyl-transferase}} (\text{glucose})_n + {}_n\text{fructose}$$

By similar reactions *Streptococcus salivarius* utilizes fructosyltransferase to make levan (fructose polymer) and glucose from sucrose. The monosaccharides released can be utilized by the organism as energy sources. In addition, sucrose can be hydrolyzed by extracellular and intracellular invertase activity to glucose and fructose, which is then metabolized mainly to lactic acid through the Embden-Meyerhof pathway. Apparently these latter reactions are quite important, and only a few percent of glucosyl moieties of sucrose find their way to glucan, particularly if the amount of sucrose is limited. This will be discussed more thoroughly in the context of dental caries production (Chapter 16).

The glucan formed by *Streptococcus mutans* in the presence of sucrose contributes importantly to the mucinous consistency of the dental plaque and cohesion of its bacterial cells, and to its tenacious adherence to the enamel surface.

The synthesis of plant, animal, fungal, and bacterial polysaccharides involves uridine triphosphate (UTP). Starting with glucose-6-phosphate, this reaction is exemplified by the synthesis of type 3 pneumococcus capsular polysaccharide, a polymer of glucose and glucuronic acid (see below).

$$\text{Glucose 6-phosphate} \xrightarrow{\text{phosphoglucomutase}} \text{glucose 1-phosphate}$$

$$\text{Glucose 1-phosphate} + \text{UTP} \xrightarrow{\text{uridyl transferase}} \text{uridine diphosphoglucose (UDPG)} + \text{pyrophosphate}$$

$$\text{UDPG} + 2 \text{ NAD} \xrightarrow{\text{UDPG dehydrogenase}} \text{uridine diphosphoglucuronic acid (UDPGA)} + 2 \text{ NADH}$$

$$\text{UDPG} + \text{UDPGA} \xrightarrow[\text{enzyme}]{\text{Type 3 pneumococcal}} (\text{glucose-glucuronic acid})n + \text{inorganic phosphate}$$

Through the action of enzymes on other uridine diphosphate (UDP) sugars and uronic acids, a variety of polysaccharides have been synthesized, including bacterial cell wall polysaccharides. The capsular polysaccharides have great significance because they protect the bacterial cell against phagocytosis.

CARBOHYDRATE METABOLISM OF DENTAL PLAQUE

The metabolism of carbohydrates by dental plaque is extraordinarily complex since it depends upon the interactions of a number of constantly changing variables. The bacterial composition of

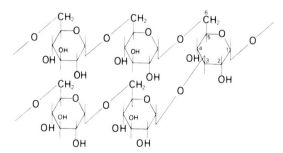

Figure 5/2. Chemical structure of a bacterial glucan molecule showing α-1,6-linkage and branching at C_3 in an α-1,3-linkage. Straight lines represent hydrogens.

plaque is the major variable and exhibits all the variation one would expect of a complex ecosystem. There are well over 100 different bacterial species isolable from various plaques representing a remarkable spectrum of biochemical possibilities. The expression and realization of these biochemical possibilities is, in turn, influenced and, in part, controlled by numerous environmental/ecologic factors (diet, salivary components, bacterial interactions). Moreover, the intraoral location of the plaque, the time of day, oral hygiene, age of the patient are also factors that contribute to the heterogeneity of plaque. Thus, plaque is not an entity but a heterogenous series of bacterial communities attached to the tooth; the composition and biochemical activities of these communities vary from mouth to mouth, from tooth to tooth, even from one surface of the tooth to another surface of the same tooth. Changes in the bacterial composition of various plaques are especially important and are associated with specific pathogenic mechanisms and ecologic niches, e.g., some cariogenic, supragingival plaques contain a large percentage of lactic acid-forming streptococci whereas a subgingival plaque associated with a form of periodontal disease may contain few, if any, streptococci but have a majority of gram negative anaerobes. The end product of the streptococcal plaque may be lactic acid whereas the major end product of the gram negative plaque may be butyric acid, e.g., a metabolic product of certain *Bacteroides* species.

Most of the recent research on plaque metabolism has concentrated on the metabolism of carbohydrates by supragingival plaque in an attempt to relate the biochemical activities of plaque samples and pure cultures of plaque bacteria to various aspects of human dental caries. It has been known since 1897 in the pioneering work of W. D. Miller and subsequently by G. V. Black in 1899 that carious lesions on tooth surface were always preceded by the accumulation of adherent bacterial plaques. The isolation of lactic-acid-forming bacteria from such plaques by numerous investigators over the years led to the notion that the carious dissolution of the enamel was due to the decalcification caused by accumulations of lactic acid in plaque. In the presence of a fermentable carbohydrate in the diet, certain bacteria would catabolize the carbohydrate via glycolysis to lactic acid and the critical pH necessary to initiate the carious lesion or "white spot." The homofermentative nature of plaque was assumed since *in vitro* pure culture studies of known cariogenic bacteria (*Streptococcus mutans, Lactobacillus casei*) demonstrated that lactic acid was the sole (over 95%) end product of glucose breakdown by these organisms.

It is surprising that this belief has persisted up until recently since early work by Muntz in 1943 had shown that lactate was not the sole metabolic end product of plaque carbohydrate metabolism. More recent work by Gilmour and associates showed that plaque and materia alba incubated with glucose resulted in the formation of acetate, propionate and lactate. Furthermore, the concentrations of acetate and propionate were similar to or greater than that of lactate. Subsequent *in vivo* work showed that the addition of sucrose or glucose to *in situ* plaque resulted in the formation of butyrate as well as acetate, propionate and lactate (both D(−) and L(+) forms). Moreover, and more complicating, it was also shown that the proportions of these acids vary with respect to time after exposure to the sugar—e.g., lactate was high immediately following sugar ingestion but declined with time. The decline in lactate (a nonvolatile acid) concentration was paralleled by an increase in volatile acids (acetate, propionate) and ethanol.

Other studies done on pure cultures of cariogenic streptococci, including S. *mutans* have provided a possible explanation for the heterofermentative character of plaques dominated by these classically designated homofermenters. The primary reason for the variation in fermentation patterns of these oral streptococci is associated with the regulation of two enzymes: lactic dehydrogenase (LDH) and pyruvate formate lyase (PFL). LDH has an absolute requirement for an activator, fructose 1,6-diphosphate (FDP) in order to function (see "Regulation of Enzyme Activity" in Chapter 6). Under conditions of glucose/sucrose excess the cellular concentration of FDP was high while that of phosphoenolpyruvate (PEP) was low; under conditions of sugar limitation the reverse was true. The high level of FDP in glucose/sucrose rich cells explains why lactate is the main end product; and the low level of FDP in glucose/sucrose-limited cells explains why there is a decrease in lactate. Pyruvate breakdown under carbohydrate limitation now proceeds via PFL to formate, acetate, and ethanol (see fig. 5/3).

The regulation of PFL is under the control of glyceraldehyde-3-phosphate (GAP). Unlike FDP, a positive effector (activator) for LDH, GAP is a negative effector for the enzyme PFL. Under glucose/sucrose-limiting conditions the cellular concentrations of both FDP and GAP are low, thereby inhibiting LDH and releasing the negative inhibition of PFL with the resulting formation of formate, acetate, and ethanol. Conversely, when cells are grown with excess glucose the concentrations of FDP and GAP are high and since PFL is inhibited by GAP only, LDH is activated and lactate is the sole end product. Under most conditions the organisms in plaque are limited with respect to a carbohydrate source and therefore carry on a heterofermentative metabolism *except* when there is a

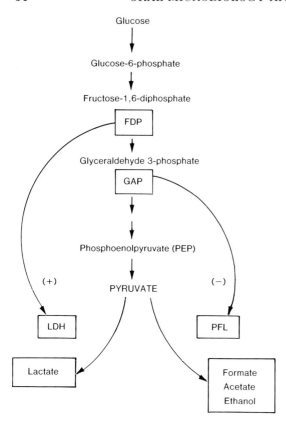

Glucose excess ⇌ Glucose limitation

Figure 5/3. Pathways of carbohydrate metabolism of *Streptococcus mutans* under conditions of glucose excess and glucose limitation. Lactic dehydrogenase (LDH) showing activation (+) by fructose 1,6-diphosphate (FDP); pyruvate formate lyase (PFL) showing negative effect (−) of glyceraldehyde-3-phosphate (GAP). (Adapted from T. Yamada and J. C. Carlsson: The Role of Pyruvate-Formate-Lyase in glucose Metabolism of *Streptococcus mutans.* In Microbiology Abstracts, Spec. Suppl., **3**, 809, 1976.)

dietary intake of carbohydrate (*e.g.,* candy ingestion) allowing the positive activation of LDH by FDP and the negative effect of GPA on PFL.

Other Aspects of Plaque Carbohydrate Metabolism

The endogenous carbohydrate metabolism of plaque bacteria has been discussed previously (see Chapter 3) in a context of cariogenic potential and structure-function relationships of oral bacteria (glycogen granules). There are, however, two other aspects which merit discussion:

1. Acid Utilization and Nature of the Dietary Carbohydrate Source. One of the factors thought to modify the cariogenic potential of dental plaque is the ability of several plaque bacteria to utilize acids, particularly lactic acid. These include species of *Veillonella* (formerly *Micrococcus lactilyticus*),

Neisseria, and *Bacterionema matruchotii.* Both aerobic and anaerobic mechanisms for acid utilization have been described, but because the micro environment of most plaques is largely anaerobic, more interest has been shown in the anaerobic mechanism. Some of these mechanisms are summarized below:

Aerobic:
    Neisseria species
    B. matruchotii

Lactate $\xrightarrow{+O_2}$ acetate + CO_2

Anaerobic
    Veillonella species

Lactate $\xrightarrow{-O_2}$ propionate + acetate + CO_2 + H_2

Many *Veillonella* strains lack the enzyme hexokinase and are therefore unable to utilize sugars via the glycolytic pathway. Their ability to utilize lactate represents an attractive ecologic possibility by which these numerically important members of the plaque microflora could convert lactate into weaker acids (propionate and acetate). Several suggestions have been made that the ratio of *Veillonella* to acidogenic bacteria might be related to cariogenic potential. "Germ-free" animal experiments have provided indirect support for this hypothesis since diassociations of *Veillonella* with known acidogenic and cariogenic streptococcal strains resulted in caries reductions as compared to animals inoculated with the streptococci alone.

Changes in dietary carbohydrate are also known to change plaque metabolism. Not only does the amount of lactic acid vary but the rate of acid formation and the fermentative pathway are also known to depend on the nature of the carbohydrate substrate. More lactic acid is produced and the pH drop more rapid by plaque incubated with sucrose or glucose than with lactose or starch. Practical advantage is taken of the fact that sugar alcohols, although sweet in taste, are not metabolized in the same way as sugars, *i.e.,* sorbitol and mannitol are used as sweetening agents in certain chewing gums and foods because they are metabolized to weak acids and ethanol. Another sugar alcohol with great sweetening power, xylitol, has the added advantage of not being fermented by most plaque microflora including. *S. mutans.* Xylitol was once considered to be an ideal sugar substitute because of this property but others, possibly toxic, complications in animals have recently compromised its use for widespread use and human consumption.

2. Inhibitors of Carbohydrate Metabolism in Plaque. A variety of inhibitors of plaque metabolism are known to occur in the oral milieu (salivary lysozyme, lactoferrin, lactoperoxidase, etc.) and various attempts have been made to exploit these inhibitors to prevent or restrict plaque formation and the parallel biochemical activities of the plaque microflora. The major inhibitor receiving the largest amount of attention has been fluoride in its several forms. It is clear that fluoride inhibits microbial growth and metabolism in dental plaque and in saliva and the principal mechanism of action on oral microorganisms is inhibition of acid formation via glycolysis. Inhibition of the glycolytic pathway is due to the inhibition of enolase activity. Enolase converts 2-phosphoglycerate to PEP. Not only is the glycolytic pathway blocked but the cellular transport mechanism (PEP phosphotransferase sytem) is also inhibited. The inhibition of the transport system is crucially important in the caries process since the marked cariogenicity of certain bacteria, *e.g.*, *S. mutans* depends upon the rapid entry of glucose into the cell allowing for an equally rapid production of acid. The PEP phosphotransferase system of *S. mutans* is known to be remarkably effective in glucose uptake and transport—and the glycolytic rate for this streptococcus is considerably more active than for other oral bacteria, *e.g.*, *Actinomyces viscosus*. The third metabolic function inhibited by fluoride is the synthesis of glycogen since the supply of glucose 6-phosphate is markedly diminished or absent as a result of the glycolytic shut down. It is interesting to note that endogenous glycogen breakdown by whole cells continues at an appreciable rate even in the presence of fluoride-once again reflecting the critical importance of glucose transport into the cell. (Catabolism of glycogen does not require phosphorylation of glucose to glucose 6-phosphate as part of the entry process).

PROTEIN METABOLISM

Bacteria are unable to ingest intact proteins, but many species produce proteinases and peptidases

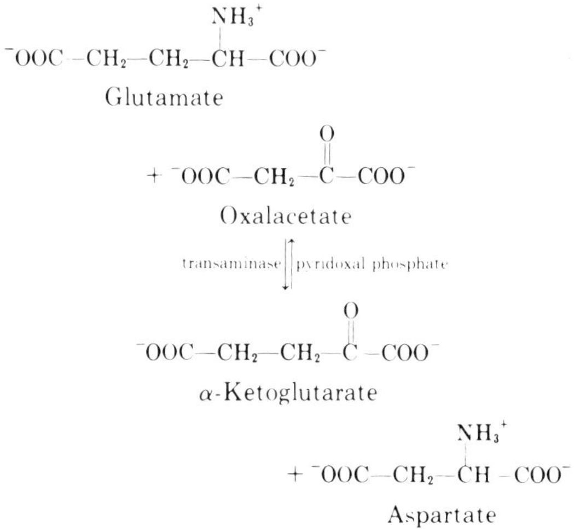

$$NH_3^+$$
$$^-OOC-CH_2-CH_2-CH-COO^-$$

Glutamate

$$+ \ ^-OOC-CH_2-\overset{O}{\underset{\|}{C}}-COO^-$$

Oxalacetate

transaminase ‖ pyridoxal phosphate

$$^-OOC-CH_2-CH_2-\overset{O}{\underset{\|}{C}}-COO^-$$

α-Ketoglutarate

$$NH_3^+$$
$$+ \ ^-OOC-CH_2-CH-COO^-$$

Aspartate

Figure 5/4. Transamination illustrated by the reaction between glutamate and oxalacetate.

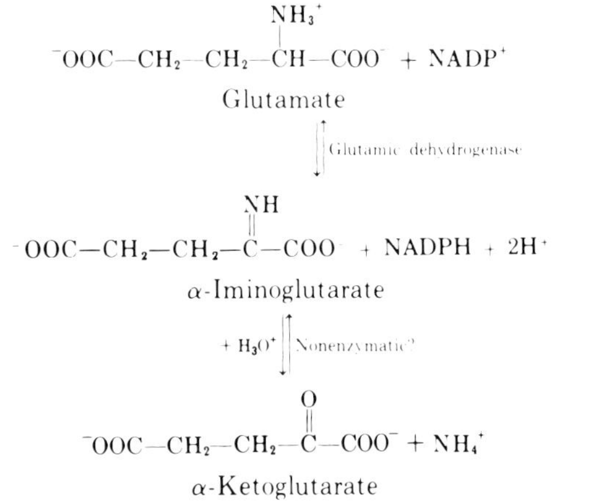

$$NH_3^+$$
$$^-OOC-CH_2-CH_2-CH-COO^- \ + \ NADP^+$$

Glutamate

Glutamic dehydrogenase

$$NH$$
$$^-OOC-CH_2-CH_2-\overset{NH}{\underset{\|}{C}}-COO^- \ + \ NADPH + 2H^+$$

α-Iminoglutarate

$$+ \ H_3O^+$$ Nonenzymatic?

$$^-OOC-CH_2-CH_2-\overset{O}{\underset{\|}{C}}-COO^- \ + \ NH_4^+$$

α-Ketoglutarate

Figure 5/5. Oxidative deamination illustrated with glutamate.

that hydrolyze proteins successively to peptides and amino acids, which the cell can assimilate. Proteolytic bacteria generally cannot initiate growth on intact protein but require at least traces of amino acids or ammonia to get started. Amino acids are utilized as such for the synthesis of proteins or they may be metabolized in several ways to produce intermediates such as pyruvate, α-ketoglutarate, and oxalacetate, which interconnect with the pathways of carbohydrate metabolism.

Probably the most general reaction of this type is transamination between an amino acid and a keto acid (fig. 5/4). Since keto acids are available from carbohydrate metabolism or other reactions, transamination is an important source of the corresponding amino acids.

Another common reaction of amino acids is oxidative deamination (fig. 5/5). The reverse reaction, reductive amination of keto acids by ammonia, may be a source of amino acids from carbohydrate metabolism.

Decarboxylation of amino acids to their corresponding amines is a common reaction. However, bacterial decarboxylases are formed most actively at about pH 5; their activity at neutrality has been doubted. Nevertheless, amines have been detected in the contents of the gingival sulcus.

Amino acids are derived through various biosynthetic pathways from a variety of precursors. For example, α-ketoglutarate gives rise to glutamate, which can then form glutamine. It can also form proline by another pathway or, through a series of reactions, go through ornithine or citrulline to arginine. Similarly, oxalacetic acid can, by transamination, form aspartic acid, which can then form a whole group of other amino acids. Protein is synthesized by successive coupling of amino acids by peptide bonds in a definite sequence determined by DNA.

LIPID METABOLISM

Bacterial lipids occupy intermediate positions in metabolism. They are made of building blocks from a variety of chemical classes, *e.g.*, phospholipids are derivatives of glycerol phosphate. Amines and amino acids can be attached to phosphate, while hydroxyl groups of other glycerol carbons are linked to fatty acids or hydrocarbons. Glycerol can be metabolized by ways of its connection with carbohydrate metabolism. Fatty acid synthesis can be converted to carbohydrate metabolism. Also, some amino acids can be transformed to fatty acids. Relatively few bacterial species are effective in attacking lipids, but most synthesize them to a significant degree. They may be utilized when the medium is low in oxidizable substrates. Internal storage may provide available lipids. For a more complete discussion of lipid metabolism, the reader is referred to Lamanna, Mallette, and Zimmerman (1973).

NUCLEIC ACID METABOLISM

Nucleic acids make up an unusually high proportion of bacterial protoplasm, so much of the bacterial cellular activity relates to nucleic acid biosynthesis and catabolism. In some bacterial species RNA seems to serve as a reserve food material.

The structural units of nucleic acids are the purines, adenine and guanine; the pyrimidines, cytidine, thymine, and uracil; and phosphates of the pentoses, D-ribose and D-deoxyribose. These substances derive from intermediates of amino acid and carbohydrate metabolism by a lengthy series of enzymatic reactions too detailed to present here (see Lamanna, Mallette, and Zimmerman (1973)). Transglycosidation converts the purines, pyrimidines, and pentose phosphates to the corresponding ribosides (nucleosides) and inorganic phosphate. Nucleosides are phosphorylated with the aid of ATP to form nucleotides and nucleotide pyrophosphates (ATP is a nucleotide pyrophosphate), which are polymerized enzymatically to the nucleic acids. Nucleic acids can be returned to the metabolic pools whence they came by the successive actions of nucleases, nucleotidases, and nucleosidases.

ADDITIONAL READING

BOWDEN, G. H. W., ELWOOD, D. C., AND HAMILTON, I. R. 1979 Microbial Ecology of the Oral Cavity. Adv Microb Ecol, **3,** 135.

HAMADA, S., AND SLADE, H. D. 1980 Biology, Immunology and Cariogenicity of *Streptococcus mutans*. Microbiol Rev, **44,** 331.

LAMANNA, C., MALETTE, M. F., AND ZIMMERMAN, L. N. 1973 *Basic Bacteriology*, Ed. 4, Ch. 12, 13, and 14. Williams & Wilkins, Baltimore.

MANDELSTAM, J. AND McQUILLEN, K. (Eds.) 1973 *Biochemistry of Bacterial Growth*, Ed. 2. Wiley, New York.

SANAWAL, B. D. 1970 Allosteric Controls of Amphibolic Pathways in Bacteria. Bacteriol Rev, **34,** 20.

STANIER, R. Y., ADELBERG, E. A., AND INGRAHAM, J. L. 1976 *The Microbial World*, Ed. 4, Ch. 6, 7, and 8. Prentice-Hall, Englewood Cliffs, N. J.

VOLK, W. A. 1982 *Essentials of Medical Microbiology*, Ch. 5. J. B. Lippincott, Philadelphia.

YAMADA, T., AND CARLSSON, J. C. 1976 The Role of Pyruvate-Formate Lyase in Glucose Metabolism of *Streptococcus mutans*; Microbial Aspects of Dental Caries. Microbiol Abstr Spec Suppl **3,** 809.

chapter 6

Physiology

Benjamin Hammond

INTRODUCTION

Bacterial growth consists essentially of the balanced synthesis of cytoplasmic components and cell walls from materials available in the immediate environment. After synthesis, the components are assembled to reproduce the original units. Following sufficient production and assembling of components, multiplication of the cells (cell division) normally occurs.

Bacterial growth requires that proper concentrations of essential nutrients be available to the cells in a suitable environment. Bacterial synthesis also requires the availability of a continuous source of energy, usually obtained from a series of coupled oxidation-reduction reactions. So far as nutritional and energy requirements are concerned, bacteria fit somewhere between two extremes. At one extreme are the autotrophic or lithotrophic bacteria, which are generally not pathogenic for man. They require only simple nutrients such as inorganic salts and CO_2, and they obtain their energy from light (photosynthetic autotrophs) or by the oxidation of inorganic substances (chemosynthetic autotrophs) such as sulfur, iron, nitrite, or ammonia. At the other end of the spectrum are the heterotrophic or organotrophic bacteria, which include the common pathogens. These bacteria use organic compounds, such as glucose, as an energy source and convert a portion of their energy source to the other organic compounds they require.

PHYSICAL AND INORGANIC REQUIREMENTS

Temperature

Most bacteria grow variably over a temperature range of 30 degrees or more but grow best at an optimum temperature which has a relatively narrow range. This is a relatively stable characteristic that is widely used as a criterion in taxonomy. Bacteria can be divided into three groups, depending on their temperature ranges of growth. Psychrophils grow over a range of 0 to 30 C, with an optimum near or only slightly below 29 C. Such bacteria do grow and multiply at 0 C, making them important in relation to food or biologicals stored at refrigerator temperature. Growth of the mesophils, which include common pathogens in mammalian bodies, occurs at 10 to 45 C. Most bacteria that are human pathogens grow best at or near 37 C. Thermophils grow over a range from 25 to 75 C, with an optimum of 50 to 55 C.

Hydrogen Ion Concentration

Bacterial growth extends over a hydrogen ion range of 3 to 4 pH units, with optimal growth usually occurring within a span of less than 1 unit. Most pathogenic bacteria grow best between pH 7.2 and 7.6. While acid-forming bacteria such as *Acetobacter* and *Lactobacillus* species produce and tolerate acids to pH 3 or even below, few such bacteria are human pathogens. Some bacteria (*e.g.*, the cholera vibrio and *Escherichia coli*) tolerate an alkalinity of pH 8 to 9.

Oxidation-Reduction Potential

Bacteria can be divided into groups according to requirements for oxygen. Obligate anaerobes grow only in the absence of oxygen or in a highly reduced medium. Facultative bacteria grow either in the absence of oxygen (reduced state) or in the presence of oxygen (oxidized state). Obligate aerobes require oxygen, although some species can grow at a very low oxygen tension. Microaerophilic bacteria require a reduced oxygen tension, for growth is suppressed at a high oxygen tension. The oxidation-reduction potential (E_h) of a medium is critical for initiating the growth of a given bacterial species. The E_h, expressed in volts or millivolts, may be positive (+ volts), indicating an oxidized state, or negative (− volts), indicating a reduced state. A typical aerobic culture broth has an E_h of +0.3 volts. Facultative or obligate anaerobes require a negative E_h for growth. The reduced state required by anaerobes can be attained by culturing them in closed containers from which oxygen has been removed catalytically or by the chemical actions of chromous sulfate or pyrogallol. An anaerobic or reduced state can also be accomplished even in a medium exposed to the atmosphere by the addition of an oxidation-reduction buffer such as sodium thioglycolate (0.1%) or glutathione (glutamyl-cyteinyl-glycine) which will poise the oxidation-reduction potential at the proper reduced level.

Aerobic bacteria require oxygen for growth. However, oxygen dissolved in culture media is rapidly utilized by such bacteria, and since atmospheric oxygen diffuses slowly across an air-medium interface, an oxygen insufficiency soon results in such cultures. Growth in aerobic cultures can be increased by forced aeration.

Oxygen Toxicity and Strict Anaerobes

As indicated in the preceding paragraph, obligate or strict anaerobes grow only in the absence of oxygen. More than this, oxygen is actually toxic to these cells. The toxicity of oxygen results from the formation of two toxic substances produced by the oxidations of flavoproteins and other enzymes by oxygen: hydrogen peroxide (H_2O_2) and the extremely toxic free radical,[1] superoxide (O_2^-). Aerobic and aerotolerant organisms produce an enzyme superoxide dismutase which catalyzes the following reaction:

$$O_2^- + O_2^- + 2H^+ \xrightarrow[\text{dismutase}]{\text{superoxide}} O_2 + H_2O_2$$

These organisms also have one or more mechanisms for disposal of H_2O_2. The enzyme catalase decomposes H_2O_2 into oxygen and water:

$$H_2O_2 \xrightarrow{\text{catalase}} 2H_2O + O_2$$

and is found in most organisms able to grow in the presence of oxygen. One notable exception to this rule is the lactic acid bacteria that lack catalase but have a peroxidase system that reduces H_2O_2 to water at the expense of oxidizable organic substrates, e.g.,

$$NADH + H^+ + O_2 \xrightarrow[\text{oxidase}]{\text{NADH}} NAD^+ + H_2O_2$$

$$NADH + H + H_2O_2 \xrightarrow[\text{peroxidase}]{} NAD^+ + 2H_2O$$

Net reaction: $2NADH + 2H^+ + O_2 \rightarrow 2\,NAD + 2H_2O$

The absence of catalase, peroxidase, and superoxide dismutase from almost all obligate anaerobes provides an explanation (albeit not absolute) for the toxicity of oxygen to these organisms. Since the large majority of the oral microflora are anaerobic it is not difficult to understand why H_2O_2 was used for years in reducing oral infection and sepsis.

---

[1] A free radical is a compound with an unpaired electron. Superoxide having gained an extra electron carries a negative charge.

Carbon Dioxide

All bacteria seem to require some CO_2, to initiate and even to continue growth. Many bacteria, particularly when first isolated, require a level of CO_2 greater than that found in the atmosphere (and culture medium) to initiate growth. Others find atmospheric CO_2 (about 0.03%) sufficient. Once growth has begun, bacterial cultures may furnish sufficient CO_2 to meet most growth requirements. In practice, in bacterial culturing, an increased CO_2 tension is provided by placing the cultures in a closed environment to which CO_2 is added. It is of interest that many oral bacteria have an absolute requirement for increased levels of CO_2 in order to grow and metabolize. Two such organisms have been associated with the etiology of one form of periodontal disease, *Actinobacillus actinomycetemcomitans* and *Capnocytophaga* species. They are found in the gingival crevices of patients with localized juvenile periodontitis and are obligate capnophiles (capno=CO_2; philes=loving).

Inorganic Ions

The inorganic ions required by bacteria for growth are usually supplied by water or by the ingredients that are used to make up the medium. Among these inorganic ions, Mg^{2+}, K^+, NH_4^+, SO_4^{2-}, and PO_4^{3-} are required by practically all bacteria. Co^{2+} is essential to vitamin B_{12}. When there is no organic sulfur or nitrogen, SO_4^{2-} and NH_4^+ or NO_3^- may be used for growth by some bacteria. Phosphates are related to the transport of energy in bacteria. K^+ is essential to protein synthesis. Mg^{2+} is an essential cofactor for many enzymes and for ribosomal activity. $Fe^{3+(2+)}$ is considered an essential trace ion because it is required by heme protein, by the oxidative enzymes of aerobic bacteria; even anaerobic bacteria have iron-containing enzymes. Ca^{2+} is important to spore formation and to enzyme secretion from gram positive bacterial cells. Zn^{2+} and Mn^{2+} are important constituents of enzymes. Na^+ and Cl^- are not required by most bacteria and, in fact, with some exceptions, may be inhibitory as their concentration increases.

ORGANIC REQUIREMENTS OF BACTERIA

The heterotrophic pathogenic bacteria require sources of carbon in organic forms. They also require growth factors, vitamins, as well as trace amounts of fats, lipids, and other organic compounds, depending on the peculiar requirements of a given bacterial species.

Carbon Requirements

Apparently, elemental carbon is not utilized by bacteria. However, all bacteria, including autotrophic and heterotrophic forms, require some CO_2

for the initiation of growth and for cell division as described above. In addition to the CO_2 requirements, heterotrophic bacteria must have an organic source of carbon which is usually supplied by a wide variety of mono- and disaccharides, with glucose being the most common source; amino acids can serve alternatively in many cases. A few bacteria and fungi (but not yeast) can utilize starch as a source of carbon. Cellulose is also utilized by some bacteria, particularly those associated with the gut tract of herbivorous animals and termites.

Nitrogen Requirements

Heterotrophic bacteria usually require a complex source of nitrogen, including amino acids, peptones, and peptides, and specific nitrogenous growth factors. At present these are primarily supplied by digests and infusions, and extracts of plants, animal tissues, or in some cases, yeasts, singly or in combination. Blood or serum is often used as a source of accessory growth factors for streptococci or *Haemophilus* species. Serum albumin is protective since it has an affinity for small molecules that may inhibit bacterial growth.

The vitamin requirement of bacteria varies widely, but in some species it is extensive. For example, some streptococci and lactobacilli require as many as 9 B vitamins, 17 amino acids, as well as purines, and pyrimidines.

ACQUISITION OF NUTRIENTS BY BACTERIA

The acquisition of food in the proper chemical state from the immediate environment is a particular problem for bacteria since they are surrounded by a cytoplasmic membrane which controls the entry into the cell of both small and large molecules. Small molecules are mostly transported across this membrane by specific transport mechanisms. However, the transport systems are unable to take larger components across the plasma membrane. In order for bacteria to acquire the components of insoluble foods and large molecules, they elaborate and release exoenzymes into the immediate environment to break them down so that their constituents can be transported across the plasma barrier. Microbial exoenzymes may be found that will break down almost any naturally occurring substance. Macromolecular substances most commonly attacked by the exoenzymes of pathogenic bacteria are proteins, polysaccharides, mucopolysaccharides, and lipids. The hydrolytic enzymes of gram positive bacteria are released from the periplasmic space, located between the inner cytoplasmic membrane and the peptidoglycan layer, and most readily diffuse through the cell wall. In gram negative bacteria, in addition to the exoenzymes that are released into the microbial environment, some are retained on the surface of the cell just exterior to the plasma membrane, due to their inability to pass through the outer membrane.

GROWTH AND MULTIPLICATION OF BACTERIA IN A CLOSED SYSTEM

For the purposes of the present discussion, growth means the progressive increase of the cells' protoplasm, as by the synthesis of cell components, and by inhibition of water and electrolytes that eventuates in cellular division. Multiplication, then, may be regarded as a necessary response to the pressure of growth. Indeed, if multiplication is prevented without other injury to the cell, as it can be by certain antibiotics, the cell grows, becomes grossly distorted, and eventually perishes.

When a few quiescent bacteria are introduced into an environment that meets their requirements for growth and multiplication, they first pass through a period of adjustment, commonly called the lag phase, during which there is no multiplication or increase in number (up to point *a* in fig. 6/1). The physiology of this phase of adaptation is not completely understood. *A priori,* there seems to be no reason that the cell should not grow and multiply promptly. Actually, growth of cells commences and becomes exponential after a much shorter phase of adjustment (dry weight per milliliter) than shown in figure 6/1. Growth is evidenced also by a rapid increase in individual cell weight (dry weight per cell count) and by an even more

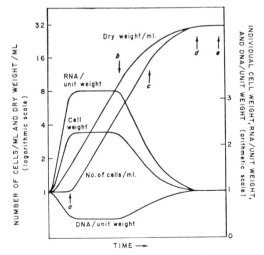

Figure 6/1. Diagram correlating typical changes in cell size, number, and chemical composition during bacterial growth in broth inoculated with a culture in early stationary phase (*e*). Initial values of all variables equalized as one arbitrary unit. (From D. Herbert: *Microbial Reaction to Environment*, p. 395. Cambridge University Press, New York, 1961.)

rapid rise in RNA per unit weight, presumably reflecting intensive protein synthesis. Because each cell is larger and metabolically more active, there are corresponding increases in the rates per cell of oxygen consumption, carbon dioxide production, and heat evolution. In sum, cellular growth runs ahead of cellular division. However, as many as four nuclei (chromatinic bodies) per cell may accumulate because of nuclear division without cellular division. Although DNA per unit weight declines steadily and reaches a minimum at the end of the lag phase, DNA per nucleus remains nearly constant.

It is not at all certain what influences stimulate cellular division. Most theories have been based on the consideration that the cell should outgrow its ability to nourish itself, which is limited by the proportion of its surface to its volume.

It is quite understandable that at some critical size the rate at which nutrients could be transported into the cell would become insufficient for maintenance of the enclosed volume of protoplasm, and division into smaller cells would become necessary. Alternatively, the need could be met from without by providing a greater concentration of nutrients, which would, up to a point, increase their rate of transport into the cell. Richer media should, therefore, support a population of larger cells, but in general the reverse seems to occur.

Whatever may be the various factors that determine the lag in multiplication, it terminates after a period of a few hours in a transition period when the physiological activity per cell, RNA per unit weight, and individual cell weight are greatest, DNA per unit weight is least, and cellular division begins (a in fig. 6/1). The population now enters what is termed the exponential or logarithmic phase of multiplication (a to c), since the logarithm of the number of cells now increases linearly with time. Physiologically, the cells have reached a steady state in relation to their environment. Total bacterial mass increases exponentially, but individual cell weight, RNA per unit weight, and DNA per unit weight remain constant. Cellular division occurs regularly at a definite time interval called the mean generation time, which is characteristic for each species under given conditions. For a wide variety of oral bacteria in optimal media at body temperature, it falls between 20 and 90 minutes. An extreme example is the tubercle bacillus, which may not divide more than once a day, even under favorable conditions. Nuclear division typically occurs during the middle third of the interval between cell divisions. If the medium is regularly removed and replaced by a fresh sample of the same medium at the same temperature, the cells will continue to grow and multiply at the exponential rate indefinitely. Approximately these circumstances proba-

bly prevail in the mouth, for, except for the addition of extra nutriment at mealtimes and a period of stagnation at night, the culture medium is being renewed constantly, although at a variable rate.

If the medium is not renewed, the period of exponential multiplication commonly lasts from 3 to 24 hours to yield a total growth of 10^8 to 10^{10} cells per ml. The larger the original inoculum, the more limited the nutrients, and the faster the inherent rate of multiplication of the organism, the shorter is the period of exponential multiplication, and vice versa. The cells next enter a second transitional phase during which first the growth rate (fig. 6/1, b) and then the multiplication rate (c) decline. Concurrently, RNA synthesis and individual cell weight decrease. Finally (d), RNA per unit weight, DNA per unit weight, and cell size return to values characteristic of resting cells. Growth and multiplication cease and the cells enter the stationary phase (e). The total number of cells now remains constant for a considerable period, after which the "phase of decline" sets in, with progressive death and, in many cases, autolysis of the cells. Bacteria in the stationary phase are so-called resting cells. Although they have ceased to multiply, such cells retain their ability to carry on metabolic processes. It follows that microorganisms in general can continue to function in pathological processes long after they have passed the peak of their growth and multiplication.

The growth of bacteria may be limited by suboptimal concentrations of essential nutrients (fig. 6/2), but even though all are provided in excess, the total number of cells per unit volume cannot exceed a maximal value, called the M concentration, which is characteristic for each organism and medium. The first explanation of this limitation that occurs to one is that the medium has been "staled" by the accumulation of toxic metabolic end products of the organism. This explanation is certainly applicable to some cases. For example, the presence of utilizable carbohydrate greatly stimulates the growth of a microorganism (fig. 6/3), but it also limits growth owing to the acidification of the medium. The situation is different in sugar-free broths in a number of instances. If the majority of the cells is removed from such a broth culture in the stationary phase and the supernatant fluid reincubated, the typical multiplication cycle is repeated by the remaining cells. Obviously, such a medium had not become "staled" by the first growth. It has been noted also that when equal amounts of two nonantagonistic species with the same M concentrations are inoculated together, each reaches only ½ its usual final concentration. This has given rise to the concept that growth is limited by the "available biological space," which although descriptive, does not explain the phenomenon. Since the volume of

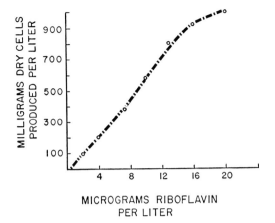

Figure 6/2. Limitation of total growth of a bacterium (*Lactobacillus casei*) by insufficient supply of an essential nutrient (riboflavin) in an otherwise complete medium. Below 16 μg per liter, growth is directly proportional to the concentration of riboflavin and is limited by exhaustion of the supply. Above 20 μg per liter, additional riboflavin has less and less effect and total growth approaches the limiting M concentration for this organism in this medium. This form of curve is generally applicable to microbiological assay, whether the limited essential nutrient is a vitamin, amino acid, carbohydrate, mineral, or other substance. (Compiled from the data of E. E. Snell: Nutritional Requirements of the Lactic Acid Bacteria. *Wallerstein Laboratories Communications*, **11, 81**, 1948.)

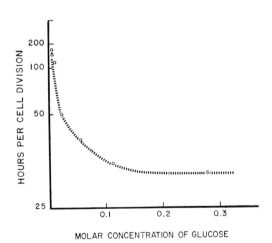

MOLAR CONCENTRATION OF GLUCOSE

Figure 6/3. Effect of changing the concentration of a nutrient (glucose) on the rate of division of a bacterium (*Mycobacterium tuberculosis* in Dubos' medium). In 0.005 M glucose (1 g per liter), there was only one division per week; in 0.3 M glucose (50 g per liter) one in 30 hours; further increase of the concentration of glucose would have little effect. (Compiled from the data of W. Schaeffer: Recherches sur la croissance du *Mycobacterium tuberculosis* en culture homogène. *Annales de l'Institut Pasteur*, **74**, 458, 1948.)

a typical bacterial cell is of the order of 10^{-12} ml, even in a dense culture containing 10^{10} cells per ml, the total cellular volume would not exceed 1% of the total volume of the medium. If the cells in such a culture are killed by heating but not removed, the spatial constraint no longer exists, for a fresh inoculum will go through the usual multiplication cycle. Evidently, we have to deal with an obscure antibiotic effect that occurs even between presumably identical living cells.

The duration of the stationary phase depends in part on the inherent tendency of the given organism to autolyze and in part upon the nature of the medium. In general, the presence of fermentable carbohydrate is unfavorable for survival, since it leads to a bactericidal degree of acidification of the medium. If this is avoided, cultures of the gram negative bacilli of the "enteric" group, for example, survive for months if refrigerated. Special requirements may be important, but if these are met, survival will be prolonged.

The typical growth and multiplication cycle described for bacteria is by no means peculiar to them or even to microorganisms in general. Rather, it describes the course of events to be expected whenever a few self-reproducing units are introduced into a favorable environment.

BACTERIAL GROWTH ON SOLID MEDIA

In the early days of bacteriology, due to the lack of adequate media, it was difficult to obtain a pure culture or even attempt to enumerate bacteria. With the introduction of agar, a suitable solid culture medium was devised by adding 1.5 to 2.0% agar to an otherwise adequate fluid medium to produce a "solid medium." Solid media are used to isolate bacteria in a pure culture by the streaked or poured techniques. Culturing on solid media is a means of enumerating viable bacteria. It is also used to induce bacteria to form colonies, whose morphology, size, color, and surface texture are used to identify and classify bacteria.

Due to the lack of suitable techniques, the growth characteristics of bacteria on solid media, particularly those related to population dynamics, have not been ascertained as thoroughly as they have in fluid media. It is assumed that if a bacterial cell is cultured on adequate solid medium, it goes through phases of growth similar to those of the same bacterial cell growing in liquid medium. Under such circumstances nonmotile bacteria form colonies that are usually limited to a total of 10^{10} cells. Motile bacteria may spread over the surface of solid media, forming a relatively thick film that contains many more cells than ever form in the largest colony.

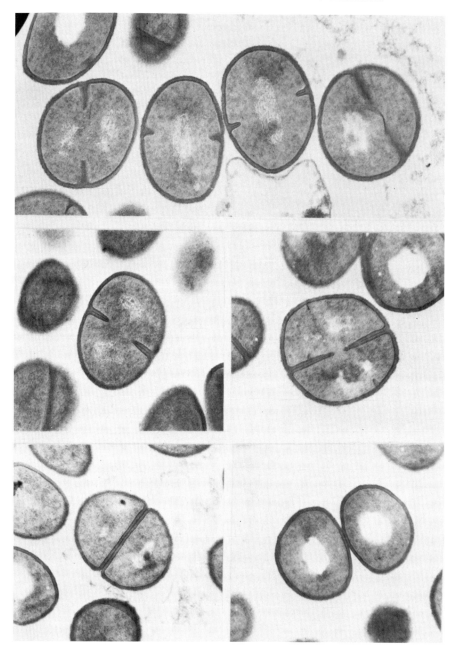

Figure 6/4. Successive stages of cross-wall formation and division in log phase growth of a strain of *Staphylococcus aureus.* (Courtesy Dr. R. M. Cole (R. M. Cole, A. N. Chatterjee, R. W. Gilpin, and F. E. Young: Ultrastructure of Teichoic Acid-Deficient and Other Mutants of Staphylococci. *Annals of the New York Academy of Science,* **236,** 22, 1974).)

GROWTH AND DIVISION OF SINGLE BACTERIAL CELLS

Most data about growth and division of bacterial cells have been obtained as averages of large unsynchronized bacterial populations, or, at best, by a population that is roughly synchronized for only a few generations. With the advent of the electron microscope and the attainment of longer periods of synchronized bacterial growth, considerable information has been obtained about the sequences and events that are involved with the reproduction cycle of individual bacterial cells.

Cell Division

The genetic information for the sequence of events required to duplicate bacterial cells is found in the DNA of the bacterial chromosomes. The number of chromosomes in a bacterial cell is partially related to its physiological state at a given time. Bacterial cell division begins with the initiation of DNA replication, followed by its complete duplication.

When replication of the DNA is complete, the duplicate chromosomes separate from each other, resulting in a type of nuclear division. Separation of the duplicate chromosomes relates to a function of the cytoplasmic membrane. In gram positive bacteria, the chromosomes are attached to an extension of the cytoplasmic membrane, called a mesosome. When the chromosome has been replicated, the mesosome splits and the two parts separate, each carrying one of the chromosomes with it. The separation of the mesosomes is accomplished by the formation of new cell membrane in the area between the separated mesosomes. In gram negative bacteria the mesosomes are not formed or they are not so prominent in chromosome separation. In these bacteria the chromosomes seem to attach directly to the cell membrane.

When the duplicate bacterial chromosomes have been separated from each other, the formation and separation of the two daughter cells are accomplished by the synthesis of a transverse equatorial septum, by plasma membrane growth, and by cell wall synthesis. Initiation of septum formation is dependent on the completion of chromosome replication and the elapse of a period to allow for protein synthesis. The place and time of the formation of the septum is essential for the proper division of the materials in the mother cell (fig. 6/4). Cell wall formation follows septum formation. In gram positive bacteria, the cell wall forms equatorially and by diffuse intercalation. In cell wall formation, the mesosome moves toward the center of the cell, followed by the developing cell wall septum. After the transverse cell wall septum is completed, the cells separate by a process mediated by hydrolases.

MICROBIAL REGULATORY PROCESSES

In their independent existence in a widely fluctuating environment, the cells of microorganisms must be able to maintain an individual biological steady state (homeostasis) in order to metabolize, grow, and reproduce. The growth and survival of microorganisms depend on a variety of mechanisms, which include the structure and composition of their cell walls and the regulation of the intake and outgo of metabolites, as well as their concentration in microbial cells, and osmotic and specific transport activities of their plasma or cytoplasmic membranes. In addition, microorganisms, particularly bacteria, possess a number of intracellular regulatory mechanisms which allow them to adapt to a wide variety of environments. These regulatory mechanisms relate to the factors involved in the synthesis and activities of enzymes as well as the control of the synthesis of nucleic acid and protein.

Metabolic Uptake

Relatively early in the development of bacteriology, it was evident that permeability and osmotic barriers existed in bacterial cells. An enzyme that was present and active in the bacterial cytoplasm of an intact cell did not attack its specific substrate if the substrate was outside of the cytoplasmic membrane. It was also evident that cytoplasmic membranes took some active part in the transport of substances across such barriers. Bacterial cells exposed to a dilute concentration of amino acids accumulated a higher concentration of these amino acids inside the cell than existed outside the cell, indicating some form of active transport across the membrane.

The plasma membrane has at least three main functions in regard to metabolism and growth (and cell division) of bacterial cells. For metabolism, growth, and cell division to occur in bacteria, their membrane must either transport or at least allow essential nutrients to come into the cell. It must also transport or permit passage of the waste products from the cell to the environment. As importantly, it must not allow essential metabolites to diffuse or be transported from the cell. The membranes which carry out these essential functions are thought to be made up of two layers of lipid molecules, surrounded on each side by layers of protein. While the general arrangement is similar in different plasma membranes, they may differ in their overall structure, they may differ in different areas of a membrane, and they may differ in a given area at different times.

Characteristics of the Transport System

The transport systems of bacterial plasma membranes have a specificity similar to that of enzymes. Transport systems also resemble enzymes in their stereospecificity, by requiring protein synthesis, and by their formation's being influenced by induction, repression, and nutrition. Also, they usually do not follow diffusion kinetics. They do not resemble enzymes in that the material being transported does not undergo enzymatic conversion. Specificity of a transport system seems to relate to the protein portion of the membrane. A given transport system can accept and transport only a limited number of different substances that have closely similar chemical structures. The rate of transfer of a substance is initially related to its concentration. As the concentration increases, the rate of transport reaches a steady state, indicating a limited number of adsorption sites. A given transport system may be at least partially involved in the transportation of substances both in and out of bacterial cells. Tranportation across the plasma membrane against a concentration gradient requires energy. In such instances active transport can be halted by chemical substances which interfere with energy metabolism. Plasma membrane transport occurs in three stages. In the first stage, the substance being transported combines with a specific chemical group or molecule on the exterior of the membrane. The substance is then transported across the membrane. In the final step, the substance is released inside the cell, and the transport system returns to its original state. Energy is supplied to the transport system at one of the steps in the transportation cycle.

Active transport systems require energy for transport of materials across the bacterial plasma membrane. However, some transport systems do not utilize energy and are passive transport systems, shuttling back and forth across the cell membrane in a manner somewhat analogous to the gravity flow of liquids. Some sugars enter cells in this manner when they are present in high concentration in the immediate environment of a bacterial cell. The term "facilitated diffusion" is also applied to passive transport.

The variety of transport functions may be exemplified by the growth of E. coli in the presence of β-galactoside. This results in the formation of β-galactosidase by the cells, as well as the mechanism for transport of β-galactoside into the cells. The transport of the substrate is not against a concentration gradient, and hence it does not require energy. On the other hand, E. coli can actively transport nonhydrolyzable analogues of β-galactoside against a concentration gradient if it is supplied energy. The same transport system is evidently used by both β-galactoside and its analog whether or not energy is required for their transfer. When a substance is utilized inside the cell more rapidly than it is transported, systems capable of active transport sometimes become uncoupled from their energy source and they function as facilitated or passive transport systems that shuttle back and forth without utilizing energy. Actually, a few transport systems, particularly those found in yeast, are capable only of facilitated transport. In contrast, the transport of sugars across cytoplasmic membranes of bacteria is mostly by active transport, which requires energy.

The rate at which a substance that has been taken into a cell by transport exits from a cell is in proportion to its intracellular concentration. This indicates that such substances could exit from the cell by passing through pores in the membranes, by dissolving in the membrane, or by a transport system that has little affinity for the substance being transported.

Metabolite Transport

There are numbers of substances that have been shown to be specifically transported across cytoplasmic membranes. These include amino acids which are transported by constitutive transport systems that have relatively broad specificity and rapidity of action. Various oligopeptides and compounds covalently attached to them are transported across cytoplasmic membranes. Even inhibitors are transported by systems that ordinarily transport metabolites. Most phosphorylated compounds are not transported, but glucose phosphate is transported intact across cytoplasmic membranes. Several sugars are transported by specific transport systems. Others are transported by a phosphotransferase system. For example, in the course of entering the cell, glucose is phosphorylated to glucose phosphate in the cytoplasmic membrane as the first step in its metabolism. Thus, the compound released into cytoplasm is different from the one that entered the cytoplasmic membrane.

Microorganisms may have a specific enzyme for a substrate but may have lost its specific transport system. Even without a transport system they are able to metabolize the substrate, but very slowly. This suggests that the substrate may enter the cell in small amounts by the transport systems of other compounds, by diffusion through pores in the membranes, or by dissolving in the membrane.

The exact mechanism of active transport across cytoplasmic membranes is unknown. Proteins that firmly bind compounds that are transportable across cytoplasmic membranes have been released from the cells of E. coli. Specific binding proteins have been released also from the periplasmic space of the cell membrane by osmotic shock. Such binding proteins may well be a part of the transport system of the membrane.

Enzyme Regulation

In a preceding section of this chapter we have indicated how bacterial cells cope with their environment and maintain a biologically steady state by the regulatory activities of their cytoplasmic membranes. In addition, bacterial cells have several equally important mechanisms for intracellular regulation of their metabolic activities which allow them to live in and adapt to many different environments.

Few, if any, bacterial enzymes are produced at a steady rate in all environments. The enzymes of bacteria vary widely, as to both their presence and their concentration. The production of an enzyme in a given environment depends on the corresponding metabolites' being present in the medium in which they are grown. Regulation of metabolism by enzyme regulation may be at the level of enzyme activity or enzyme synthesis.

Regulation of Enzyme Activity. Regulation at the level of enzyme activity is very rapid and there is no significant time lag required for the effects of such regulatory action to occur. Generally the enzymes which are subject to control at the activity level are those which occupy strategic points, particularly branch points, in the sequence of reactions of metabolism, so that changing their activity immediately affects the entire pathway beyond that enzyme. The enzymes involved are called allosteric (other shape) enzymes since they can change their configuration, and the type of regulation in which they are involved is called end-product or feedback inhibition, since their activity is subject to regulation by the end-product of that pathway or branch. Allosteric enzymes can be inhibited (or activated) by substances which are structurally dissimilar to their substrate. This can occur because these enzymes have two different kinds of combining sites, a site for the substrate and a site for the inhibitor or activator. The enzyme molecule is flexible, so its shape can be changed by combination with the substrate or the inhibitor. This ability to change shape influences the shape of the catalytic site. If this site is occupied by substrate, or if the other site is occupied by an activator, the enzyme is stabilized in the active configuration. An inhibitor complexing at the inhibitor site favors the inactive form of the enzyme. There are multiple sites of each type on an enzyme, so they act in the concert to promote a given configuration, and when one site of a type is complexed, that configuration is promoted at other sites.

Regulation of Enzyme Synthesis. Besides regulation at the level of enzyme activity, bacterial metabolism may be controlled at the level of enzyme synthesis. Regulation of enzyme synthesis generally involves regulation at the genetic level. Some substrates and metabolites can effect enzyme synthesis by acting as inducers, which increase enzyme synthesis, while others act to repress the rate of synthesis. Enzymes which are always present whether or not substrate is present, are constitutive, while those present only when substrate is available are said to be inducible. The mechanism of enzyme regulation was discovered while examining the β-galactosidase system in *E. coli*. During this study a gene product was discovered which inhibits synthesis of this enzyme. It was called a repressor, and subsequently shown to be a tetrameric protein product of a specific gene called a regulatory (R) gene. The general mechanism for this type of regulation indicates that inducible enzymes are those for which the cell continually synthesizes repressor. When substrate is present it acts

to induce enzyme synthesis by combining with the repressor and inactivating it. The repressor normally binds to a receptor site on the DNA, the operator locus, and shuts off enzyme synthesis. If the repressor is inactivated it no longer can bind to the operator locus. The operator locus controls the expression of adjacent structural genes, and if repressor does not bind, the structural genes, in this case for the enzyme(s) of lactose metabolism, are expressed and enzyme(s) produced. An operator and the genes it controls is called an operon and they act as a unit of coordinated expression. For example, the operon for lactose metabolism contains an operator, the enzyme β-galactosidase which breaks down lactose, and a permease that transports β-galactoside into the cell. There is also a third enzyme, a galactoside transacetylase, whose specific role in lactose metabolism has not been defined. These genes are linked and form a linear array. As described previously, the primary structure of polypeptide chains is encoded in structural genes and transcribed into mRNA as a linear molecule, so regulation of the operon is regulation of the production of this messenger.

In addition to the regions described above, another region known as a promoter is present on the DNA, located next to the operator but distal to the structural genes. This is the binding site for RNA polymerase and its relation to the operator adds to the regulation of transcription by the operator and repressor.

Repressors are freely diffusible, so a regulator gene does not have to be adjacent to the genes it regulates. The operon is an efficient control system for metabolic regulation since all enzymes must function as a unit. They must be present in equivalent amounts and turned on or off at equal rates. Even though enzyme synthesis begins rapidly after induction, several generations must occur before the effects are seen in a culture. This lag occurs because there must be time for the enzyme to reach an adequate level to be effective. Similarly, when repression occurs the enzyme already present must disappear through dilution and turnover before the effects are seen in the population, or even the individual organism. To reiterate briefly, the method of regulation is as follows: RNA polymerase attaches to DNA at the promoter site and the information in the genes of the operon is transcribed sequentially. The operator regulates the production of polygenic mRNA, so the genes are transcribed as a unit. If the operator has repressor bound, transcription is inhibited, but if repressor is inactivated, the mRNA can be formed and subsequently translated into enzymes.

If end product of a specific pathway is present, it can regulate enzyme synthesis by repression. This is the reverse of induction in that inducers cause an increase, while end products cause a decrease in synthesis. The mechanisms whereby end products suppress enzyme synthesis are not well understood. Some features may be similar to induction, but the exact mechanism and relation to induction are not well defined.

Functions of Bacterial Regulatory Mechanisms

Induction, repression, and inhibition are most important mechanisms in bacterial metabolism and biosynthesis. These mechanisms allow bacteria to control their intracellular activities sufficiently so that they can adapt to a given environment. Induction relates to the regulation and economy of bacterial enzyme production in that it allows an enzyme to be produced only if the substrate is available for it to act upon. If the enzymes of a given bacterial cell were constitutive and they were produced at a steady rate regardless of their need in a particular environment, then most of the biosynthetic and metabolic economy of such cells would be so misdirected that the cell could no longer grow, for it could not obtain the energy and metabolites that it required.

Feedback inhibition and repression are also important mechanisms that allow bacterial cells to control their endogenous metabolic and biosynthetic activities in relation to the availability of exogenous metabolites. Repression is concerned mostly with control of the synthesis of the macromolecules of the cell that are the metabolic building blocks. End-product inhibition is related to the control of the economy of metabolite synthesis. The loss of only feedback inhibition by mutation (not by repression) results in the cell's producing excessive amounts of the end product and excreting it. Feedback inhibition allows bacteria to produce their metabolic building blocks in such amounts that their excretion does not occur, even under widely varying temperature or pH.

The regulatory mechanisms allow bacteria to economize their synthetic and metabolic activities if a required product is present in the environment. Thus, if small molecules are supplied in an enrichment medium, the bacterial cell will no longer produce them because they can be obtained more easily from the environment. This will allow the cell to redirect its metabolic efforts and to grow at a more rapid rate.

Another important factor that often confronts bacterial cells is the exhaustion of one or more nutrients in the environment. When this occurs the production of the enzymes for the metabolic pathway would cease and they would no longer be present in the cell. If the metabolite is restored to the environment, the various regulatory mechanisms of the cell permit preferential formation of the requisite enzymes for that metabolic pathway, allowing the metabolic recovery of the cell.

ADDITIONAL READING

ALEXANDER, M. 1971 *Microbial Ecology.* Wiley, New York

ATKINSON, D. E. 1969. Regulation of Enzyme Function. Annu Rev Microbiol, **23,** 47.

CALVO, J. M., AND FIND, G. R. 1971 Regulation of Biosynthetic Pathways in Bacteria and Fungi. Annu Rev Biochem, **40,** 943

GUIRARD, B. M., AND SNELL, E. E. 1962 Nutritional Requirements of Microorganisms. In *The Bacteria,* Vol. IV, edited by E. C. Gunsalus and R. Y. Stanier. Academic Press, New York.

HELMSTETTER, C. E. 1969 Methods for Studying Microbial Division Cycle. In *Methods in Microbiology,* Vol. I, edited by J. R. Norris and D. W. Ribbons. Academic Press, London.

HUGHES, E. C., AND WIMPENNY, J. W. T. 1969 Oxygen Metabolism by Microorganisms. Adv Microb Physiol, **3,** 197.

INGRAHAM, J. L. 1962 Temperature Relationships. In *The Bacteria,* Vol. IV, edited by I. C. Gunsalus and R. Y. Stanier. Academic Press, New York.

JOKLIK, W. K., WILLETT, H. P., AND AMOS, D. B. (Eds.) 1980 *Zinsser Microbiology,* Ed. 17, pp. 66, 79. Appleton-Century-Crofts, New York.

KOSHLAND, D. E. 1970 The Molecular Basis for Enzyme Regulation. In *The Enzymes,* Ed. 3, Vol. 1, p. 342, edited by P. D. Boyer. Academic Press, New York.

MALLETTE, M. F. 1969. Evaluation of Growth by Physical and Chemical Means. In *Methods in Microbiology,* Vol. I, edited by J. R. Norris and D. W. Ribbons. Academic Press, London.

PAIGEN, K., AND WILLIAMS, B. 1970. Catabolic Repression and Other Control Mechanisms in Carbohydrate Utilization. Adv Microb Physiol, **4,** 252.

ROGERS, J. J. 1970 Bacterial Growth and the Cell Envelope. Bacteriol Rev, **34,** 194.

SETLOW, P., AND KORNBERG, A. 1970 Biochemical Studies of Bacterial Sporulation and Germination. J Biol Chem, **245,** 3637.

chapter 7

Sterilization and Disinfection

John A. Molinari

INTRODUCTION

Since the oral cavity normally contains a diversity of potentially pathogenic microorganisms, disinfection and sterilization in dental practice are both important and difficult to accomplish. This becomes very apparent when one considers the types of diseases that can be transmitted between patients and personnel. A few of these "occupational" infections are summarized in table 7/1. Many of the agents find favorable growth environments in various areas of the mouth, and may be spread by either direct contact with a lesion or microorganisms, indirect contact via contaminated instruments or office equipment, inhalation of aerosols induced by handpieces and ultrasonic cleaners, and routine scrubbing of instruments (fig. 7/1).

Since diseases such as hepatitis B and tuberculosis may have long incubation periods, it is difficult to trace suspected outbreaks back to their source; thus, it is the responsibility of dental professionals to make certain they are doing their utmost to provide "safe" oral procedures for their patients. Utilization of proper sterilization, disinfection and clinical aseptic procedures minimize the infectious risk that certain patients present to the attending personnel. Control of the hazards of cross-infection and post-treatment infection is thereby facilitated by the use of appropriate chemical disinfectants and physical methods of sterilization.

In this chapter procedures and agents will be considered which attempt to prevent the spread of infectious disease during and following dental treatment.

TERMINOLOGY

Sterilization is defined as the destruction or removal of all forms of life, with particular reference to microorganisms. The practical criterion of sterility is the absence of microbial growth in suitable media. Other criteria are loss of motility and inhibition of metabolism and particular enzymes. The limiting requirement is the sterilization of bacterial and fungal spores. Agents capable of sterilizing are steam under pressure, high temperature, including an open flame, filters, ethylene oxide and radiation.

Germicide means literally "a killer of germs" and is not readily susceptible to ambiguity. *Antiseptic* indicates an agent that inhibits growth as long as there is contact between agent and microorganism. By custom, the term antiseptic is reserved for agents that can be applied to the body.

Disinfection properly refers only to the inhibition or destruction of pathogens. By custom, the term *disinfectant* is reserved for agents applied to inanimate objects. *Bacteriostatic agents* act by inhibiting the growth of microorganisms without killing them, and their effects are reversible. If any organism is held in a state of suspended animation long enough, it dies, so the distinction between bacteriostatic and bactericidal disappears. At any rate, *bactericidal agents* kill microorganisms by an action that is not reversible.

There are other qualifications to disinfection. *Complete disinfection*, in effect, means sterilization, for it is defined as the killing of all spores and vegetative forms of microorganisms. *Concomitant* or *concurrent disinfection* signifies the killing of pathogens (and any other incidental microorganisms in the vicinity) in the discharges from a sick patient during the course of a disease. *Terminal disinfection* is the destroying of microorganisms in the discharges after a patient has recovered from a disease or has died.

There is also another group of substances known as *sanitizers*, which includes the detergents. These are agents or processes involving agents which are used to maintain the microbial flora of food-handling equipment at a safe public health level.

Asepsis, in contrast to antisepsis, denotes the avoidance of pathogenic microorganisms. In practice, it refers to those techniques that aim to exclude all microorganisms. Modern surgery is antiseptic in its attempts to disinfect the site of the operation and the hands of the surgeon. It is aseptic in the use of sterile instruments, sutures and dressings, and the wearing of sterile masks, caps, gowns and

Table 7/1
Representative occupational diseases in dentistry

Disease	Etiologic Agent	Incubation Period
Bacterial		
Staphylococcal infections	Staphylococcus aureus	4–10 days
Tuberculosis	Mycobacterium tuberculosis	Up to 6 months
Streptococcal infections	Streptococcus pyogenes	1–3 days
Gonorrhea	Neisseria gonorrheae	1–7 days
Syphilis	Treponema pallidum	2–12 weeks
Viral		
Recurrent herpetic lesion	Herpes simplex, types 1 and 2	Up to 2 weeks
Hepatitis A	Hepatitis A virus	2–7 weeks
Hepatitis B	Hepatitis B virus	6 weeks–5 months
Infectious mononucleosis	Epstein-Barr virus	4–7 weeks
Hand-foot and mouth disease	Primarily Coxsackievirus A16	2 days–> 3 weeks
Herpangina	Coxsackieviruses Group A	5 days

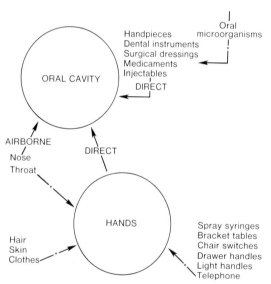

Figure 7/1. Representative vehicles of microbial cross-contamination in dental practice. (Adapted from J. J. Crawford: *Disinfection, Sterilization and Preservation,* edited by S. S. Block, Lea & Febiger, Philadelphia, 1977.)

rubber gloves. Bacteriological laboratory techniques are aseptic. They minimize contamination by flaming wire transfer loops and other instruments, flaming the mouths of containers when opened, exposing open Petri plates and other containers for the shortest time possible, and working under as dust-free conditions as possible.

While each of the above defined terms may be distinguished from one another on the basis of clinical and antimicrobial application, the expression *cold sterilization* represents an often abused aspect of office asepsis. This concept refers to disinfection of instruments at room temperature by immersion in a chemical solution. Since the solutions routinely utilized cannot guarantee destruction of all microbial forms, cold sterilization is actually a misnomer, and should not be confused with acceptable methods of sterilization.

The goal of antimicrobial sterilization and disinfection is to reduce the spread of infectious agents. This necessitates an understanding of *cross-infections,* that is, the passage of microorganisms from one person to another. The potential for cross-infection in the dental office exists for direct or indirect transmission, as well as via aerosols routinely created during clinical procedures.

FACTORS AFFECTING THE DEATH RATE OF MICROORGANISMS

Time and Concentration of Organisms. The concentration of microorganisms affects the rate at which they are killed. Microorganisms, when exposed to a sterilizing agent, die at a progressively decreasing rate that is proportional to the number of survivors. Whatever the agent, the graph of logarithms of number of survivors against time falls in a straight line over most of its course (fig. 7/2). The greater the total number at the outset, the longer it takes to reach complete sterility.

Time and Concentration of Agent. The concentration of the agent affects the rate at which microorganisms are killed. The time required for sterilization by a chemical decreases as its concentration increases and vice versa. For many chemicals doubling the concentration halves the time required. For some popular antiseptics such as phenols and alcohol, their efficacy changes extremely rapidly with changes in concentration (fig. 7/3).

Time and Temperature. Temperature affects the rate at which microorganisms are killed. Two effects of temperature must be distinguished: the increase in activity of a chemical with rising temperature, and killing by heat alone. The rate of sterilization behaves like a chemical reaction; that is, it doubles or trebles for every 10 C rise in temperature.

The susceptibility of microorganisms to heat has been expressed as thermal death time or thermal death point (more accurately, thermal death temperature). Thermal death time is defined as the time it takes to kill microorganisms at a given temperature. The thermal death point of bacteria is defined as the lowest temperature that sterilizes a 24-hour culture in broth at pH 7 in 10 minutes.

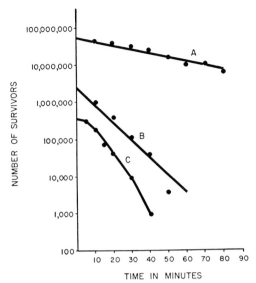

Figure 7/2. Effect of size of inoculum on the death rate of bacteria. Three experiments with *Escherichia coli* in 0.005 N sodium hydroxide at 30 C. In all cases, the death rate was logarithmic over most of the course. Starting with 55,000,000 cells per ml (*A*), however, only 2.5% of survivors died per minute, whereas starting with 2,500,-000 (*B*) or 350,000 (*C*), the rate was 10% per minute. A similar although less pronounced effect of numbers was observed with heat at 55 C at neutrality. Even though the death rate is approximately the same in (*B*) and (*C*), 70 minutes would have been required to reduce the survivors in (*B*) to 1,000, whereas (*C*) reached this figure in 40 minutes. Theoretically, (*A*) would have required 7 hours. (*C*) illustrates also the lag that often occurs at the beginning and the acceleration of killing at the end, when the numbers are very small. Frequently, however, the death rate at the end is much slower, owing to a fraction of more resistant cells in the original population. (Data for compilation of graph from I. H. Watkins and C. E. A. Winslow: Factors Determining the Rate of Mortality of Bacteria Exposed to Alkalinity and Heat. *Journal of Bacteriology*, **24**, 243, 1932.)

Effect of Organic Matter.

Since the chemicals considered in the present discussion act for the most part by chemical combination with microbial protoplasm, they combine also with the constituents of tissue, especially with proteins. This reduces the efficacy of the chemicals.

Hydrogen ion concentration affects the killing of microorganisms. Acids and acidic substances are more easily sterilized than are neutral or alkaline substances. Organic acids produced in fermentations often protect fluids and solid food and the gastrointestinal tract from the activities of undesirable, contaminating microorganisms.

EVALUATION OF STERILIZING AGENTS

Laboratory Measurement of Antimicrobial Action.

Sterilization *in vitro* is determined either by exposure of organisms to an agent in liquid medium with subsequent tests for viability, or by direct application of the agent to cultures on agar plates. The former is exemplified by the determination of the *phenol coefficient*. A standard inoculum of a standard strain of *Staphylococcus aureus* or *Salmonella typhi* is added to a series of dilutions of phenol in a standard broth at 20 C and to a series of dilutions of the substance under comparison. After 5, 10, and 15 minutes, a standard sample of each mixture is transferred to fresh broth, containing, if necessary, a neutralizer of the agent being tested. After incubation, it is noted in which subcultures growth occurred and, accordingly, which dilutions of the substances had killed all organisms in 10 minutes but not in 5.

If the test for viability is carried out by animal inoculation, it can be applied to viruses, rickettsiae, and protozoa that cannot be cultivated. This procedure has been much used for the assay of antibiotics, using known amounts of the pure substance

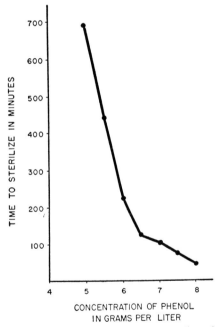

Figure 7/3. Effect of changing concentration of phenol on time required to sterilize paratyphoid bacilli in a concentration of 6,000,000 per ml in aqueous phenol at 20 C. The data fit closely the curve, $C_5 t = 6.65$, which means that doubling the concentration reduces the time required 45-fold ($= 2^{5.5}$) and vice versa. By extrapolation, a concentration of 1% (10 g per liter) would have sterilized in 14 minutes, and 2%, in 20 seconds. Note, however, that concentrations of phenol as low as 0.25% may be used to protect solutions from contamination. (From H. E. Watson: A Note on the Variation of the Rate of Disinfection with Change in the Concentration of the Disinfectant. *Journal of Hygiene (Cambridge)*, **8**, 536, 1908.)

instead of phenol in the reference series. When done in this way, the test resembles the agar plate method, in which a test organism is seeded in a pour plate or streaked uniformly on the surface and a sample of the agent is applied either directly, or in hollow cylinders, or in impregnated thick disks of filter paper. After incubation, growth develops everywhere except in the vicinity of the agent (fig. 7/4). The area of the clear zones is proportional to the amount of the agent applied.

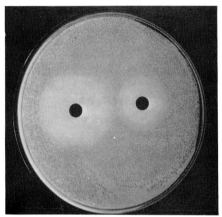

Figure 7/4. The plate method for determining sensitivity of microorganisms to antibiotics. A poured plate is prepared on the test organism(s), the disks impregnated with a given concentration of antibiotic(s) are placed on the surface, and the plate is incubated. The area of clear zone about the disks is proportional to the amount of agent applied and to the sensitivity of the microorganism.

Evaluation in Use. Some physical and chemical methods have been found useful in general sanitation and for the sterilization of inanimate objects. The success of a chemical against a defined infection can be measured satisfactorily, *e.g.*, the use of silver nitrate to prevent gonococcal ophthalmia neonatorum. It is all-purpose antiseptics that defy exact evaluation.

PHYSICAL METHODS OF STERILIZATION

Certain routine procedures must be employed to sterilize instruments, mirrors, burs, metal bands and other intraoral materials. The importance of this approach was affirmed in March of 1974 by the House of Delegates, American Association of Dental Schools. At that time, they passed the following resolution:

Resolved, that the Association adopt the following statements: Disinfection of dental instruments with chemical agents is unacceptable in preventing the transmission of infectious disease. Therefore, the Association strongly recommends the use of autoclaving, dry heat, and gaseous sterilization, which are acceptable and effective methods of preventing the transmission of disease-causing agents.

The following section will consider the most appropriate physical methods of sterilization: steam autoclaving, dry heat and chemical vapor, as well as other physical modes which are useful as sterilizing systems. Effective conditions and wrapping requirements for the major physical modes are given in table 7/2.

Table 7/2
Major methods of sterilization[a]

Method	Temperature	Pressure	Cycle Time	Pakaging Material Requirements	Acceptable Materials	Unacceptable Materials
Steam autoclave	121 C 134 C	15 psi 30 psi	15–20 min 3–5 min	Must allow steam to penetrate	Paper, plastic, surgical muslin	Closed metal and glass containers
Dry heat oven	160 C 170 C		2 hr 1 hr	Must not insulate items from heat; must not be destroyed by temperature used	Paper bags, muslin, aluminum foil, aluminum trays, pans	Plastic bags
Unsaturated chemical vapor	131 C	20 psi	30 min	Vapors must be allowed to precipitate on contents; vapors must not react with packaging material; plastics should not contact sides of sterilizer	Perforated metal trays, paper	Metal trays, sealed glass jars
Ethylene oxide	Room temperature (25 C)		10–16 hr (Depends on material)	Gas must be allowed to penetrate	Paper, plastic bags	Sealed metal or glass containers

[a] Adapted from J. A. Molinari and J. York: *Detroit Dental Bulletin*, **49**, 5, 1980; and R. J. Whitacre *et al.*: *Dental Asepsis*, Stoma Press, Seattle, 1979.

Moist Heat

Boiling. Moist heat is the most widely utilized means for sterilizing heat stable items. The application of this method may occur in several forms: boiling, steam at atmospheric pressure and steam under pressure. As applied at 100 C or higher, heat is effective by denaturation of proteins. Microbial destruction is accomplished by immersion of articles in boiling water for 10 to 20 minutes. All vegetative cells and most spores are destroyed in this way but a fraction of tetanus, gas gangrene, and botulinum spores are likely to survive. Hepatitis viruses require a longer exposure interval (30 minutes) for inactivation, however, boiling water is not recommended for routine destruction of these viruses. In addition, because of the unrealistically prolonged time required for ultimate destruction of all spores, 100 C water is not considered a sterilizing process. This method however, has certain advantageous features as a disinfection mode: it is rapid, economical, does not require any elaborate equipment, has effective penetration capability, and is harmless to a wide range of dental materials. Serious disadvantages are the dulling of the edges of cutting instruments and corrosion of carbon steel instruments. The use of stainless steel instruments will alleviate the latter problem, while the dulling effects can be reduced, but not eliminated, by addition of sodium carbonate to the water. This chemical, and similar mild alkaline detergents, remove protein deposits (tissue, blood, pus) from instruments and form an emulsion on the instrument surfaces which accelerates disinfection.

Steam Sterilization. Complete sterilization is achieved by the use of moist heat at higher temperatures in the form of saturated steam under pressure in air-tight vessels such as autoclaves and pressure cookers (fig. 7/5). At the appropriate conditions, autoclaving represents the most efficient sterilization process. Steam may also be employed as free-flowing at atmospheric conditions, although at 1 atmosphere pressure its efficacy is in reality only analogous to that of boiling water.

Most commonly, a temperature of 121 C (249.8 F) is applied for 15 to 20 minutes. This temperature corresponds to 15 pounds pressure of steam at sea level. Direct exposure to saturated steam at 121 C for 10 minutes normally destroys all forms of life. In practice, additional time must be allowed for the temperature to reach this point in the center of thick packages of dressings or large containers of liquids. With few exceptions, a maximal period of 30 minutes suffices. Higher temperatures for shorter periods of time are employed in equipment modified for office use.

As efficient as autoclaving can be in instrument sterilization, this procedure is effective only when suitable conditions are present in the pressured

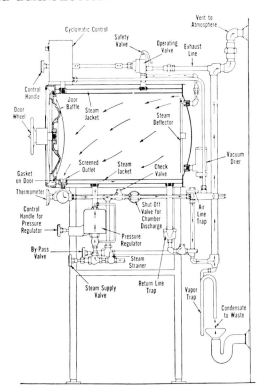

Figure 7/5. The structural details of a steam autoclave with automatic controls. (From American Sterilizer Company.)

chamber. Areas of preparation and operation which pose the most problems for steam sterilization are: faulty preparation of materials for sterilization (packaging which does not allow for penetration of steam), improper loading of instrument chamber, improper functioning of sterilizer (failure to reach temperature and/or pressure), presence of air in the chamber (may delay microbial destruction up to 10 times longer), and excess water in the steam (can serve as passageway for microorganisms to get through wet instrument packages).

Unsaturated Chemical Vapor. Chemical vapor sterilization in dental practices and clinics is considered an acceptable method of sterilization by the Council on Dental Therapeutics and its use has increased substantially in recent years. This system depends on heat, water and chemical synergism for its efficacy; a mixture of alcohols, formaldehyde, ketone, acetone and water is employed. As shown in table 7/2, the temperature and pressure required with chemical vapor sterilizers are greater than those for the autoclave. The principle of operation has similarities with steam sterilizers, but also some important distinctions. The solution of premixed chemicals added to the jacket reservoir must be purchased from the manufacturer, since the ratio of each in the preparation is critical. After the apparatus is preheated, clean, dry, loosely wrapped instruments are placed in the chamber. The package wraps must be loose to allow the chemical vapors to condense on the instrument surfaces during the cycle. Thick, tightly wrapped items will require longer exposure because of the inability of the unsaturated chemical vapors to penetrate as well as saturated steam under pressure. Metal instruments must be dry prior to sterilization, or chemicals will accumulate in the wetted surfaces and corrosion will occur.

The major advantages of chemical vapor sterilization are: a short cycle time which is analogous to that for the autoclave, no rusting of instruments and burs in contrast to steam sterilization, the removal of dry instruments at the end of the cycle, and automatic, preset cycle timing. The presence of only about 8 to 9% water vapor in the chemical solution is significantly below the 15% minimum for rusting and dulling, and this property prevents destruction of dental items such as endodontic files, orthodontic pliers, wires and bands, burs and carbon steel instruments. Thus a wide range of items can be routinely sterilized. A requirement for adequate ventilation can constitute a problem for practioners that use this type of apparatus, however. Chemical vapors, particularly formaldehyde, can be released when the chamber door is opened at the end of the cycle, and these leave a temporary unpleasant odor in the area. Although numerous toxicity studies by the manufacturer indicate little chance of eye irritation from these residual vapors, dental personnel may occasionally report some discomfort if the sterilizer is in an area with poor air circulation. To counteract this detrimental aspect, newer models are equipped with a special filter which further reduces the amount of vapor left in the chamber at the end of the cycle.

Dry Heat

The destruction of all forms of microbial life in the absence of moisture requires very different conditions than those discussed previously. As proteins dry, their resistance to denaturation increases. Thus, at a given temperature dry heat sterilizes much less efficiently than moist heat, and as shown in table 7/2 higher temperatures are required for a properly functioning hot air oven.

Destruction of microorganisms by dry heat is accomplished either by incineration or placement of items in a hot air oven. Obviously, direct flaming constitutes the most drastic application of dry heat, yet it is also one of the simplest procedures. No special apparatus is necessary and 100% effectiveness is guaranteed. Disposal of infectious materials and organic wastes is safely accomplished using large incinerators. The practical application of this method in clinical areas, however, is limited at best. Aside from the flaming of wire loops in the micro-

biology laboratory prior to the sterile inoculation of cultures, other metallic items are unable to maintain their integrity with repeated flaming.

The proper use of a dry heat oven is recognized as an effective means of sterilization in dental practices. Since dry air is not as efficient a heat conductor as moist heat at the same temperature, a much higher temperature is required for sterilization. The usual recommended practice is to hold the temperature at 160 C for 2 hours. A 1-hour exposure at 170 C will also be effective. These conditions are suitable for sterilizing glassware and metal instruments that rust or dull in the presence of water vapor. Many dental practitioners prefer the use of dry heat sterilizers in their offices because of the preservation of sharp, cutting edges on their surgical instruments. In addition, many types of oils and powders with high heat resistance may be sterilized at 160 to 170 C. However, these high temperatures will destroy many rubber and plastic based materials, melt the solder of most impression trays, and weaken some fabrics, as well as discolor other fabrics and paper materials.

One of the most common problems with the employment of a dry heat sterilizer, is the failure of clinical personnel to properly time the sterilization interval with large instrument packages. Since the penetration of dry heat into the center of the pack is slow and dependent on both the size of packages and the type of wrapping material, one must be certain that a proper temperature is attained in the chamber (preheating) before setting the timer. Thick wraps such as muslin and larger than normal packages can significantly increase the interval required for assured sterility. Some individuals also view the prolonged exposure times for dry heat as a disadvantage. The argument is made that if only one sterilizer is available, the 1- to 2-hour period plus cooling time disrupts a smooth flow of instrument recirculation. These aspects may be compared with those inherent for autoclaving and chemical vapor in table 7/3.

Pasteurization

The principal use for pasteurization is in the food-processing industries (milk and other dairy products, fruit juices, wine and beer). Its purpose is to disinfect and to postpone spoilage. As defined for the treatment of milk, pasteurization consists of holding the fluid at 143 F (61.7 C) for 30 minutes in tanks or at 160 F (71.1 C) for 15 seconds by continuous flow through heat exchangers. The infectious agents that cause milk-borne diseases such as tuberculosis, brucellosis, salmonellosis, Q fever and diphtheria are destroyed under these conditions, and in fact, the killing of *Mycobacterium tuberculosis* and *Mycobacterium bovis* was classically used to test the efficiency of the pasteurization process.

Table 7/3
Features of sterilization methods

Method	Advantages	Disadvantages
Autoclaving	1.Short cycle time 2.Good penetration 3.Wide range of materials can be processed without destruction	1.Corrosion of unprotected carbon steel instruments 2.Dulling of unprotected cutting edges 3.Packages may remain wet at end of cycle 4.May destroy heat-sensitive materials
Dry heat	1.Effective and safe for sterilization of metal instruments and mirrors 2.Does not dull cutting edges 3.Does not rust or corrode	1.Long cycle required for sterilization 2.Poor penetration 3.May discolor and char fabric 4.Destroys heat-labile items
Unsaturated chemical vapor	1.Short cycle time 2.Does not rust or corrode metal instruments including carbon steel 3.Does not dull cutting edges 4.Suitable for orthodontic stainless wires	1.Instruments must be completely dried before processing 2.Will destroy heat-sensitive plastics 3.Chemical odor in poorly ventilated areas
Ethylene oxide	1.High capacity for penetration 2.Does not damage heat-labile materials (including rubber & handpieces) 3.Evaporates without leaving a residue 4.Suitable for materials that cannot be exposed to moisture	1.Slow—requires very long cycle times 2.Retained in liquids and rubber materials for prolonged intervals 3.Causes tissue irritation if not well aerated 4.Requires special "spark-shield"—explosive in presence of flame or sparks

Microbial spores are not inactivated however, and some nonpathogens like *Streptococcus lactis* can also survive.

Radiant Energy

Lethal levels of energy may be transmitted to microorganisms by ultraviolet light, which is absorbed in their DNA over a considerable range of wavelengths from 220 to 290 nm. Bactericidal efficiency is proportional to the adsorption. Killing of microorganisms by ultraviolet light involves inducing lethal mutations or sufficient chemical modification of DNA so as to interfere with subsequent replication. Ultraviolet light may act indirectly on DNA, by production of H_2O_2 or organic peroxides in fluids which contain oxygen and organic compounds. Modern germicidal lamps are usually of the mercury vapor type, because they can be designed to have most of their output at 254 nm, the resonance radiation of mercury. Unfortunately the poor penetration capability of the energy rays constitutes a serious factor limiting their use. Ultraviolet light is so readily absorbed by glass, liquids and a variety of organic substances that it is effective only on surfaces or thin layers of material. It should also be noted that so-called sun lamps have little bactericidal power since their major output is in the "tanning" wavelengths longer than 300 nm.

High energy electromagnetic waves (X-rays and γ-rays) and particulate radiations (cathode, α-, and β-rays; fast protons, neutrons, and deuterons; heavy atomic particles from nuclear fission) have been tested extensively as sterilizing agents. They are called ionizing radiations because they ionize molecules in their path which absorb them. Their lethal action may occur directly on such vital molecules as enzymes and nucleic acids, particularly DNA, but for the most part they act indirectly by splitting water into hydroxyl radicals and hydrogen atoms, both of which are highly reactive and interfere with vital cellular activities.

The practical effectiveness of ionizing radiations in sterilization is limited because it depends on random hits of molecules; therefore, complete killing of bacterial cells requires many times the dosage that reduces the population partially. The sensitivity of bacteria to ionizing radiation varies with the growth phase, being least during the lag phase, greatest during the logarithmic phase, and gradually decreasing in the latter to the sensitivity of "resting" bacteria. Freezing decreases sensitivity and so does drying.

The vegetative forms of bacteria are most susceptible to ionizing radiation, but there is little difference between gram positive and gram negative species. Bacterial spores are quite resistant, those of *Clostridium botulinum* most of all. A major medical industrial application of electromagnetic waves is found in the sterilization of heat-sensitive plastic hypodermic syringes and sutures.

Ionizing radiation has also been studied as a means of sterilization, pasteurization, disinfection, or disinfestation, or all four, particularly with regard to food preservation. Studies have been made of the preservation of foods by ionizing radiation, and irradiated bacon was the first food found acceptable for human consumption by the Food and Drug Administration in 1963. In general, the sterilization of foods with ionizing radiation has not been proven acceptable to the Food and Drug Administration. The high level of irradiation required to achieve sterility in foods also causes sufficient changes to make them unacceptable or potentially dangerous as foods.

Ultrasonic Vibration

Cells of all kinds can be disrupted by intense sonic and ultrasonic vibrations generated by magnetostriction oscillators or piezoelectric crystals. This technique is widely used as a laboratory tool for the release of cell contents, such as nuclei, mitochondria, antigens and enzymes, with minimal damage, but it is not a practical means of sterilization. Bacteria and viruses are more resistant to it than are mammalian cells. Ultrasonics have been used with some success to cleanse but not sterilize dental and surgical instruments, by removing blood, pus and other tissue debris from grooves and other areas which are difficult to clean. The effective scrubbing capabilities of ultrasonic cleaners make them a valuable piece of equipment in dental offices as a preparatory step to instrument sterilization.

Filtration

In microbiology, filtration is used to free liquids and gases from suspended particles, either inanimate or animate. The Seitz, sintered glass and membrane filters are in common use in microbiology.

Seitz filter pads are made of a mixture of asbestos and cellulose, supported by a woven base and held in place by a suitable holder. Numerous types of filter pad holders are available for either pressure or vacuum filtration, but such filters should not be subjected to a change in pressure of more than 5 pounds per square inch. Seitz filters and holders may be sterilized by autoclaving.

Sintered glass filters are available in several grades. The pores of such filters are not uniform, however, necessitating the determination and certification of the average pore diameter of each filter. Sintered glass disks are either fused into glass funnels or fitted into funnels by means of rubber cones.

Membrane filters are composed mostly of cellulose esters, usually cellulose acetate or triacetate, but not cellulose nitrate. Pore size usually ranges from 0.22 to 10 μm, but filters can be produced with a pore size as small as 0.05 μm. Each square centimeter of a membrane filter with an average pore size of 0.45 $\pm$ 0.02 μm contains millions of pores, the volume of the open spaces being about 80% and the solid material being about 20% of the total volume. A membrane filter with a 0.45 μm pore size will prevent the passage of almost all nonviral microorganisms. Membrane filters have a flow rate at least 40 times faster than other types of filters with similar pore size. Clogging occurs with stable gels and with liquid-borne particles which are approximately pore size. Liquid-borne particles larger than pore size and air-borne particles cause negligible clogging because they do not penetrate into the pore structure.

Membrane filters are widely used to prepare cell-free solutions, particularly those that will not withstand heat. They are also used for the separation of bacteria and viruses; for the clarification of solutions by removing cells; for microbial isolation and cultivation—bacteria collected on a membrane filter can be cultivated by placing the filter in contact with nutrients; for analysis of airborne microorganisms and biological specimens; for contamination control and microbial analysis of food, meats, soft drinks and dairy products; for investigation of antibiotics, antiseptics and disinfectants; for water and sewage control; and for soil microbiology.

Freezing

Depending on the species, the composition of the suspending fluid, the rate of temperature reduction or increase, and the temperature at which microorganisms are stored, freezing both kills and preserves viable microorganisms. Freezing of bacterial cells usually does not occur until they are supercooled to -10 to -15 C. Water then freezes inside the cells or it moves out of the cells, dehydrating them in either instance. When a microbial suspension is cooled, considerable ice crystal formation occurs inside the cell. The formation and movements of internal ice crystals disrupts the cell by cytoplasmic and membrane damage. The rate of thawing also affects the survival of frozen microbial cells. Slow thawing is more harmful than rapid thawing.

As the microbial cells become dehydrated during cooling, their salts tend to concentrate in pockets sufficiently to crystalize when the temperature is lowered to their eutectic point, which is about -20 C for NaCl. Local concentration and crystallization of intracellular salts damages the cytoplasm, cell wall and membrane.

When present in the suspending medium, nonelectrolytes such as glycerol, sucrose, or dimethyl sulfoxide partially protect bacteria from damage during freezing by preventing electrolytes from concentrating locally in cells. Impermeable, high molecular weight substances are also protective by some unknown method.

While most metabolic activities of bacteria cease below the freezing point of water, microorganisms are best preserved at the lowest temperature possible. Untoward reactions occur at a temperature as low as −130 C, but the temperatures commonly used are those of solid carbon dioxide (−78 C) and liquid nitrogen (−180 C).

Cold can also be used to destroy microorganisms and to obtain their component parts by alternate freezing and thawing, which decreases but does not eliminate the viable organisms in a microbial suspension.

Drying

The preservation of microorganisms by drying from the frozen state has been previously discussed. The spontaneous drying of water or saline suspensions of bacteria on glass usually kills them, while viruses are more resistant. The smaller particles of salivary spray expelled during coughing, sneezing, many dental procedures or simply talking, dry within seconds, encasing their bacterial contents in a protective mucinous coat. In this way, viable hemolytic streptococci survive indoors for at least several weeks. Staphylococci in dried pus survive for at least several months. On the other hand, pneumococci, meningococci and *Haemophilus influenzae* do not survive for more than a few days under such conditions. Air-dried spores may remain viable for years.

CHEMICAL AGENTS

Antiseptics and disinfectants are the most widely used of all drugs in public health practice, in hospital practice, sanitation and in the household. These agents are used extensively in dental practices and hospitals despite the demonstrated limited effectiveness of certain substances. They continue to be used for treatment of local infections and infections of the urinary tract. Many are applied to the skin of the patient, to the hands of the surgeon, and to the operating room for use in controlling the microbial content of the human environment.

Ideal Properties

When chemical disinfectants and antiseptics are considered for use, their clinical application and limitations should be first compared with the desirable properties for an *ideal* agent. The latter may be summarized as follows:

Ideal Antiseptics. An ideal antiseptic should be germicidally potent and lethal in low concentrations. An antiseptic may be either rapid- or slow-acting and have either a broad or narrow antimicrobial spectrum. It should be stable and not inactivated by body cells, body fluids, or exudates of infections. It should neither corrode instruments nor cause the disintegration of cloth, rubber, or other materials. A low surface tension is desirable for penetration when applied topically, but it should not be absorbed by tissues sufficiently to cause systemic toxicity. An ideal antiseptic should have a good therapeutic index, *i.e.*, it should be effective against microorganisms at a concentration which will not irritate tissue or interfere with healing and tissue repair. It should also not induce hypersensitivity.

Ideal Disinfectants. A disinfectant should always have the widest possible antibacterial spectrum and should always have a rapidly lethal action on all vegetative forms and spores of bacteria and fungi, on protozoa and on viruses. In addition to being lethal to microorganisms in the presence of organic matter such as blood, sputum and feces, it should be compatible with soaps, detergents and other chemicals encountered in use. It should also be inexpensive.

Modes of Action

Most chemicals that act as antiseptics and/or disinfectants function as cytoplasmic poisons. This lack of specificity generally limits the application of the agents to inanimate objects and the outer surfaces of the body. Any part or all of three major portions of cells may be affected: cell wall, protoplasm (particularly enzymes) and nuclear material. The resultant microbial destruction is accomplished by one of a limited number of reactions or by a combination of them; these effects with representative chemical substances are summarized in table 7/4.

Surface-active Substances (Detergents)

Surface-active substances are those that alter the nature of interfaces to lower surface tension and increase detergency. At the cell membrane, the effect is to alter the osmotic barrier and increase permeability so that the cell cannot maintain its integrity. There may also be surface denaturation of enzymes in the cell membrane.

The surface-active substances are classified as nonionic, anionic, cationic, and amphoteric. Nonionic agents have essentially no antibacterial effect. Anionic substances are soaps and synthetic anionic detergents. Soaps are the salts of the long-chain aliphatic carboxylic acids of animal and plant fats. Most synthetic anionic detergents are alkyl, aryl, or alkyl-aryl sulfates or sulfonates. The alkali content and sodium salt are responsible for the cidal effect

Table 7/4
Antimicrobial mechanisms of chemical agents

Mechanism of Action	Representative substances
Protein denaturation	Alcohols
	Phenols
	Detergents
	Acids
	Organic solvents
Hydrolysis	Acids
	Alkalis
Formation of insoluble or poorly dissociable salts of proteins	Mercuric, cupric and silver ions
Oxidation	Hypochlorite
	Hydrogen peroxide
Halogenation	Iodine
	Iodophors
	Chlorine
Disruptive, increased membrane permeability	Detergents
	Alcohols
	Phenols
Poisoning active groups of enzymes	Mercurials
	Detergents
	Acid dyes
Production of an unfavorable oxidation-reduction potential	Dyes
Inhibition of enzymes containing iron or copper	Cyanide
	Azide
	Hydroxylamine

of soaps on treponemes, streptococci, pneumococci, gonococci, meningococci and influenza viruses. They are not very active against most gram negative bacilli and quite ineffective against staphylococci. Overall, the value of anionic detergents seems to depend as much on their mechanical cleansing power as on their germicidal action.

Cationic surface-active substances (also termed quaternary ammonium salts) are modifications of a basic formula in which the four hydrogen atoms of the ammonium ion have been replaced with alkyl and alkyl-aryl groups. Cationic surface-active agents are germicidal in a much lower concentration than anionic detergents and are bacteriostatic in surprisingly high dilutions. They persist when they are applied to inanimate objects, and form a film on the skin, the inner surface of which is not antibacterial. They likely act on the cell membrane, releasing essential enzymes and metabolites of both gram positive and gram negative bacteria; however, the cationic detergents are much more effective against gram positive bacteria. They have little or no action on bacterial spores, viruses, or fungi. Severe limitations in the use of cationic detergents arise because of their inability to penetrate organic debris on instrument surfaces, and their incompatibility with anionic agents or soaps, calcium, magnesium, and iron of hard waters, and organic matter. They are readily absorbed by porous material

(cotton, rubber, and other materials). Quaternary ammonium solutions also easily become contaminated by gram negative bacteria.

A substantial amount of scientific evidence has proven the ineffectiveness of quaternary ammonium compounds against many pathogenic microorganisms that are transmitted in dental practice. These include the causative agents for hepatitis and tuberculosis. Since dental personnel are exposed to a significant occupational risk of infection for these diseases, it is unfortunate that some practitioners continue to use aqueous quaternary ammonium preparations for the disinfection of dental and surgical instruments. In what amounted to removing any doubt concerning the feasibility of these preparations, the Council on Dental Therapeutics eliminated quaternary ammonium preparations in 1978 from the Acceptance Program as disinfecting agents. Thus, benzalkonium chloride, dibenzalkonium chloride and cetyldimethylethylammonium bromide are no longer recommended for routine use in dentistry.

Heavy Metals

All metallic ions inhibit microorganisms if applied in sufficient concentration, but only a few are useful antiseptics or disinfectants. None is of practical use in killing bacterial spores. Metals inhibit nonsporulating bacteria in very low concentration (1:1,000,000 or less) by what is termed oligodynamic action (Greek, small powerful). This potency in small concentrations means simply that the ions of these elements have such an exceptionally strong affinity for proteins, and especially for sulfhydryl groups, that the bacterial cells or other organic matter readily absorb them out of solution. As with many other chemical antiseptics and disinfectants, the antimicrobial activity of metallic ion substances is sharply reduced by the presence of organic matter.

Mercury Compounds. The mercuric ion, far from being an ideal antiseptic, is both an indiscriminate protein precipitant and an inactivator of sulfhydryl enzymes, the latter action being easily reversible.

Mercury Bichloride. Mercuric chloride, N.F., the oldest of the mercury antiseptics, is used for skin disinfection and disinfecting inanimate objects, including some surgical instruments, but it is ineffective against spores. Water-insoluble mercury compounds are used principally for treatment of skin infections. The organic mercurial antiseptics are, in general, less irritating, less toxic, and more antiseptic than inorganic mercurial salts.

Merbromin, N.F. (Mercurochrome), used widely for application to skin, wounds, and mucous membranes, is not an effective germicide. Some other organic mercurials (*thimerosal*, N.F., *phenylmercuric nitrate*, N.F., and *nitromersol*, N.F.) are used in solutions, ointments, tinctures, jellies, and suppositories. They are not effective against spores, cannot be depended on to disinfect instruments, and are prone to cause allergic sensitization.

Mercury-containing compounds, particularly the soluble salts of mercury, are a common cause of poisoning. In acute poisoning, mercury is corrosive to the alimentary tract and causes irreversible kidney damage. In chronic poisoning, it causes gastric irritation and gingivitis, in addition to nephritis and hepatitis.

Silver Compounds. Simple silver salts (silver nitrate, silver lactate, silver picrate) and colloidal silver preparations are used as antiseptics. *Silver nitrate*, U.S.P., is used as a caustic and in lesser concentrations for local application as an antiseptic or astringent. Silver nitrate was also employed in the management of dental caries. The routine application of 1 or 2% silver nitrate into the eyes of new born infants has practically eliminated gonococcal ophthalmia.

Colloidal silver preparations (mild silver protein, N.F., strong silver protein, silver chloride colloidal, and silver iodide colloidal), although used as antiseptics, have been displaced by antibiotics.

Zinc Compounds. *Zinc sulfate*, U.S.P., *zinc chloride*, U.S.P., and *zinc oxide*, U.S.P., are mild antiseptics, mostly noted for their astringent action. They are used in the treatment of conjunctivitis, skin infections, and as a nasal spray.

Copper Compounds. While many copper salts act as astringents, germicides, and fungicides, the concentration required for bactericidal activity is usually too great to be useful.

Alcohols

Ethyl alcohol and isopropyl alcohol are among the most widely used surface disinfectants and antiseptics. They have been shown to be effective in disinfecting surfaces such as counters and dental light handles. Alcohols are not recommended for use on dental instruments, however, because of a number of serious problems inherent with these chemicals: they are corrosive to metal instruments (especially with ethanol); they do not inactivate any of the hepatitis viruses, nor are they sporicidal; the presence of tissue debris and/or blood on instrument surfaces prevents penetration of the agent; and certain plastics swell in the presence of alcohol. Both of the above alcohols denature proteins and act as lipid solvents. This latter property probably enhances their range of activity because of the destructive effect on many enveloped viruses. Vegetative bacteria are killed by exposure to high concentrations of alcohol (50 to 70% optimum), the

most notable pathogen being *M. tuberculosis*. As a matter of fact, these alcohols constitute the tuberculocidal disinfectants of choice in many instances. The concentration of an alcohol preparation is critical to its antimicrobial effectiveness. When the concentration exceeds 70%, the initial dehydration of microbial proteins allows these cell components to resist the detrimental denaturation effects. Thus, the exposed microorganisms are able to remain viable for longer periods of time.

Ethyl alcohol is relatively nontoxic, colorless, nearly odorless and tasteless, and readily evaporates without residue. During its denaturation of protein, ethanol may precipitate a protective coat around bacteria contained in blood, pus, mucus, and other organic matter. It should not be used on instruments unless they have been thoroughly cleansed. A justifiable antiseptic use of ethyl alcohol is for a 2-minute rinse as part of the presurgical scrub, where it reduces the resident flora of the skin temporarily to $\frac{1}{10}$ its normal number. However, the rarity of infection following the usual superficial wiping of the skin with alcohol in preparation for hypodermic injections is a strong testimonial to the tolerance of the body for its resident flora.

Isopropyl alcohol is somewhat more germicidal than ethanol and has tended to displace the latter since it is free from the legal restrictions of a potential beverage. Isopropanol is also less corrosive to metallic instruments, since it is not oxidized to acetic acid and acetaldehyde as rapidly as ethyl alcohol. Finally, higher alcohols have progressively greater phenol coefficients but no practical value because of their insolubility, odor, and expense.

Halogens

Iodine. Iodine is one of the oldest and still most used antiseptics for application onto skin, mucous membranes, abrasions and other wounds. The high reactivity of this halogen with its substrate provides iodine with potent germicidal effects. It acts by iodination of proteins, and subsequent formation of protein salts by halogenation. Since iodine is insoluble in water, it is routinely prepared as a tincture by dissolving an iodide salt in alcohol. Iodine in this form continues to be one of the most effective antiseptics, as shown by the fact that at different concentrations, tinctures of iodine are toxic for both gram positive and gram negative bacteria, *M. tuberculosis*, spores, fungi and most viruses. However, this chemical suffers from some serious drawbacks, since it is irritating and allergenic, corrodes metals and stains skin and clothing. Hypersensitivity reactions to iodine may range from very mild to servere.

Iodophors. Attempts to utilize the powerful germicidal action of iodine, while reducing its caustic and staining effects, have led to the synthesis of organic iodine compounds and to the devising of preparations in which the iodine is held in dissociable complexes. These compounds, called iodophors, retain a similar broad-spectrum antimicrobial range to iodine tinctures, but have the following added features: less irritating to tissues, significantly less allergenic, not staining skin or clothing and having a prolonged activity after application. Iodophors are prepared by combining iodine with a solubilizing agent or carrier. Two of the most common carriers for iodophors are polyvinylpyrrolidine (PVP) and undecoylium chloride. These agents stabilize the iodine, minimize its toxicity, and slowly release the iodine to the tissues. The carriers themselves are surface-acting substances (usually nonionic) which are water soluble and react with epithelial areas to increase tissue permeability. Thus, the active iodine that is released is better absorbed. Well-known iodophors used in clinical medicine and dentistry include Betadine, Isodine (PVP) and Virac (undecoylium chloride). Many oral surgery clinics and periodontists use iodophors to prepare the oral mucosa for local anesthetic injections and surgical procedures. Iodophors have also been found to be very effective handwashing antiseptics. In addition to removing microbial populations from the skin in large numbers, these cleansers are not generally washed off completely; therefore, a residual antimicrobial effect may remain in the scrubbed areas. Other iodophor preparations such as Wescodyne, Iosan and Kleenodyne serve as disinfectants in hospitals, clinics, food-processing establishments and restaurants.

Chlorine. Chlorine has been used to arrest putrefaction and destroy odors since shortly after its discovery in 1774. Chlorine acts primarily by oxidation, as hypochlorous acid, into which it is quickly converted by water:

$$Cl_2 + H_2O \leftrightarrows HOCl + HCl$$

$$HOCl + NaOH \leftrightarrows NaOCl + H_2O$$

Chlorine is therefore more active in acid solutions. Elemental chlorine is a very potent germicide, killing most bacteria in 15 to 30 seconds at concentrations of 0.10 to 0.25 p.p.m. Chlorine-containing compounds in common use are hypochlorite solutions, and chlorinated lime. Two officially recognized preparations are *sodium hypochlorite solution*, N.F., containing 5% NaOCl, and *diluted sodium hypochlorite solution*, N.F., containing 0.5% NaOCl. The first solution contains too much available chlorine for use on tissue but the second solution can be used for surgical purposes. Sodium hypochlorite is useful as a disinfectant, especially in areas considered to have been contaminated with hepatitis viruses. The Center for Disease Control

has recommended the use of 500 to 5,000 p.p.m. (0.05 to 0.5%) sodium hypochlorite as an effective agent in destroying hepatitis B viruses. Since this chemical is unstable, fresh solutions must be prepared daily. Despite its effectiveness as a disinfectant, this chlorine-releasing preparation has some obvious disadvantages. It is corrosive to metals, irritating to skin and eyes, dissolves necrotic tissue, and disadvantageously dissolves blood clots and delays clotting.

Phenols and Derivatives

The classical antiseptic for surgical procedures was carbolic acid. It was first thought that postoperative infections would be virtually eradicated with widespread use of this phenol. However, due to the severe toxicity reported in individuals exposed to carbolic acid, its application has been significantly diminished. Other phenolic compounds have filled roles as effective disinfectants or antiseptics. These agents act as cytoplasmic poisons penetrating and disrupting microbial cell walls, leading to denaturation of intracellular proteins. The intense penetration capability of phenols is probably the major factor associated with their antimicrobial activity; unfortunately, they can also penetrate intact skin causing local tissue damage and possible systemic complications. Thus, with the exception of the bisphenols, most phenolic derivatives are used primarily as disinfectants.

Phenol. Phenol is bacteriostatic at about 0.2%, lethal to most bacteria at 1.0% and fungicidal at about 1.3%. Its penetrating power on epithelial surfaces can cause necrosis and gangrene. Phenol is now seldom used as a disinfectant or germicide but has slight value as a fungicide. It is still utilized as the standard against which other antimicrobial chemicals are compared.

Resorcinol. Resorcinol, a derivative of phenol, is only about one-third as active. It is used to treat superficial mycotic infections in a 10% ointment.

Hexylresorcinol. This phenolic derivative is widely used as an antiseptic, specifically as an antihelminthic. In addition, some commercial mouth rinses also contain hexylresorcinol in very low concentrations.

Picric Acid. Picric acid (2,4,6-trinitrophenol) is a germicide used as a 1% aqueous solution for the treatment of minor burns and exudative wounds and as a 5% alcoholic solution to treat skin disorders.

Cresols. Cresols, which are alkyl derivatives of phenol, are composed of mixtures of *ortho*-cresol, *meta*-cresol, and *para*-cresol. Cresols are widely used and are superior to phenol as disinfectants. This latter property is illustrated by the greater tuberculocidal activity of such cresols as Lysol. The primary disinfection of many inanimate areas such as floors, counter tops and walls is accomplished through routine use of these agents. Because they retain the capacity to irritate superficial tissues, cresols are not applicable as antiseptics. Concentrations which are nonirritating are ineffective against most bacteria.

Halogenated Phenols. Chlorinated phenols are active germicides. Camphorated p-chlorophenol (1 part p-chlorophenol and 2 parts camphor; also, 1 part p-chlorophenol and 7 parts camphor) has been used in dentistry as a root canal antiseptic. Their spectrum of activity and toxicity are similar to those of phenol; however, the antimicrobial efficacy of the chlorinated phenols appears to be greater due to the halogen substitution.

Bisphenols. This group of phenolic compounds contains two agents possessing properties which make them effective handwash antiseptics. Hexachloraphene and chlorhexidine, by virtue of their dual phenolic ring structure, have a relatively low toxicity and a high bacteriostatic level at low concentrations. While they are somewhat insoluble in water, they are soluble in dilute alkali. Thus, both antiseptics remain effective even when mixed with soaps. Bisphenols are more active against gram positive than gram negative bacteria, and this property makes them suitable as routine handwashing agents. Hexachloraphene and chlorhexidine do not affect many resident skin microorganisms following a single application; instead, they require repeated washings throughout the day to attain maximal effectiveness. Both preparations can accumulate and remain in the skin in an active form for prolonged periods, thereby leaving a residual anti-bacterial effect after each wash. This property, called *substantivity*, fosters the build-up of an "antimicrobial layer" against many common skin contaminants. Since neither hexachloraphene nor chlorhexidine is effective against tubercle bacilli and spores, they are not functional as disinfectants.

A series of clinical reports in the late 1970s indicated that products containing 2 to 3% hexachloraphene could accumulate to toxic levels in the body with extensive use. As a result, pHisoHex has been banned by the Food and Drug Administration from over the counter sales in the United States. Similar adverse findings have not been reported for chlorhexidine, and the chlorhexidine gluconate, Hibiclens, is routinely used in many hospitals, dental clinics and practices.

Oxidants

Oxidizing agents are toxic to microorganisms. The more common oxidants used as antiseptic drugs are hydrogen and metallic peroxides, sodium perborate, potassium and zinc permanganate, and potassium chlorate. Of these, hydrogen peroxide is the most frequently employed as an oxygenating agent in the treatment of oral anaerobic infections, such as acute gingivitis and maxillofacial abscesses.

Hydrogen peroxide in quite small concentrations will inhibit bacteria in culture, but its antiseptic action is brief when applied to tissues, owing to its rapid decomposition by tissue catalase. Zinc peroxide releases its oxygen more slowly than hydrogen peroxide and leaves a residue of zinc oxide, an astringent. The other metallic peroxides, used extensively in the past, are seldom used now.

Dyes

Dyes have been recognized as antiseptics for many years, even though their practical use is very limited. Some are used as antiprotozoal and wound-healing agents. Generally, they are more active against gram positive than gram negative bacteria. Dyes are used in selective culture media and in some diagnostic procedures. Merbromin (Mercurochrome), a combination of mercury and fluorescein, although widely used, has limited value for disinfection of skin, mucous membranes, and wounds. The triphenylmethane rosaniline dyes, a group of basic dyes, of which gentian or crystal violet is the most important, are active against bacteria and some pathogenic fungi. Crystal violet is used as a differential bacterial stain (gram stain).

Glutaraldehydes

Glutaraldehyde ($C_5H_8O_2$) has two aldehyde units, one at each end of the carbon chain. Accepted preparations of glutaraldehydes are sold under the trade names of Cidex-7 (Johnson and Johnson), Sonacide (Ayerst), and Sporicidin (Sporicidin). A 2% solution is used for disinfection, which is activated by addition of a buffer to bring the solution to the desired pH. The maximum effective pH ranges for each are 8.0 to 8.5 (Cidex-7), 2.7 to 3.7 (Sonacide), and 7.0 to 7.4 (Sporicidin). The activated solutions have a positive antimicrobial and economic feature of retaining their maximum disinfectant activity for several weeks (28 to 30 days).

In a 2% solution, glutaraldehydes are effective against all vegetative bacteria, including *M. tuberculosis*, fungi and viruses within 10 to 20 minutes, but require as long as 10 hours to destroy spores. Claims of efficacy against hepatitis viruses have not been conclusively documented. In addition to their wide antimicrobial range, glutaraldehydes also offer other important advantages as disinfectants. They are noncorrosive to stainless steel and do not affect the cutting edges of dental instruments when used properly. Their low surface tension also permits them to penetrate blood and/or pus to reach instrument surfaces and facilitates rinsing. Rubber and plastic items are not degraded during prolonged immersion, and, in fact, these chemicals are very useful in removing blood from suction hoses.

While glutaraldehydes are highly effective as disinfectants, they are not functional as antiseptics. Irritation of hands is common and thus, contact with glutaraldehyde solutions should be as brief as possible. They may also induce hypersensitivity reactions on the skin or oral mucous membranes. For these reasons exposed instruments should be thoroughly rinsed with water or 70% isopropyl alcohol. Finally, nickel-plated impression trays and carbon steel burs will discolor and corrode if immersed in a glutaraldehyde preparation.

Vapors and Gases

Glycol Vapors. In 1941 it was demonstrated that glycol vapors readily kill bacteria in air. Aerosols of propylene or trimethylene glycol, hypochlorite, or substituted phenols were widely tested for sterilization of air. Their use is limited because of difficulty in controlling humidity, distribution of the vapors, and the accumulation of glycol films that have little or no antibacterial activity on room surfaces.

Formaldehyde. Formaldehyde, a gas at room temperature, was formerly used for fumigation. It is too toxic to apply to body tissues and is allergenic, causing eczematoid dermatitis. It is used in solution (formalin), as a tissue specimen fixative and endodontic medicament.

β-Propiolactone. β-Propiolactone, in its vapor phase, has been used to disinfect dental instruments. It is more active than formaldehyde, is a good sporicide, but there is some indication that it may be carcinogenic.

Ethylene Oxide. Ethylene oxide is a highly penetrative, colorless gas at room temperature. This agent is unusually effective against spores, is virucidal, does no damage to materials and evaporates without a residue. These features have led to the acceptance of ethylene oxide as a recognized method of sterilization (see table 7/2), especially for items that can be damaged by moisture and/or heat. Materials such as suction tubing, all handpieces, radiographic film holders and dental prostheses may be sterilized without adverse effect by this means.

Since ethylene oxide is rather toxic, allergenic, slow in action and forms explosive mixtures with air, commercial preparations are mixed with carbon dioxide or an inert gas to form a more stable combination. This preparation functions as an alkylating agent by irreversibly inactivating cellular nucleic acids and proteins. Susceptible chemical groups of these intracellular molecules are the —NH_2, —COOH, —SH and —OH sites. Since the toxic effects are not selective for microbial sub-

strates and the potential remains for explosion, materials must be processed in a special container placed in a well-ventilated area.

The slow penetration of gas throughout the container necessitates a protracted sterilization period followed by another prolonged aeration interval. Usually, 10 to 16 hours are sufficient for sterilization of most nonrubber-based items. For those containing rubber an additional 24 hours may be required to allow for complete dissipation of ethylene oxide from the porous material. Trapped gas can cause painful burns when the improperly aerated item comes into contact with epithelial tissues. Liquids to be sterilized may have to aerate even longer and may not even be able to be treated with ethylene oxide.

STERILIZATION AND INACTIVATION OF VIRUSES

The successful inactivation of a virus by physical or chemical means requires permanent loss of infectivity. Inactivation may result in the complete destruction of the virus, or it may result in loss of infectivity and the retention of immunogenicity. The rate of virus inactivation relates to the concentration of the agent and the length of exposure. Inactivating agents that are nucleotropic are formaldehyde, ethylene oxide, ultraviolet light with a wave length of 260 nm, hydroxylamine, and radioactive elements. Agents that are active against viral proteins (proteotropic agents) are heat, proteolytic enzymes, mild acids, ultraviolet light with a wavelength of 235 nm, compounds containing sulfhydryl bonds, and detergents. Some viral lipotropic agents are enzymes and lipid solvents (alcohols). Agents such as X-radiation and photodynamic sensitization are not very specific in their actions on viruses.

MONITORING OF STERILIZATION

An integral component of office sterilization procedures is monitoring the efficiency of the system. A multitude of factors may diminish the effectiveness of an autoclave, dry heat sterilizer or unsaturated chemical vapor apparatus. Two of the more frequent problems encountered are improper wrapping of instruments preventing adequate penetration to the instrument surface, and defective control gauges which do not reflect actual conditions inside the sterilizer.

One may employ chemically treated tapes that change color or biological controls to check for the proper functioning of an office sterilizer. Materials that change color generally inform the practitioner that sterilizing conditions have been reached, but do not necessarily indicate that sterilization of the chamber contents has been achieved. In addition, certain indicators change color long before sterilization occurs and before appropriate conditions are met. Autoclave tape is probably the worst offender in this regard, as it will change to show the striped markings following very brief exposure to steam. It appears that the major use of specific chemical indicators to monitor sterilization is as a routine check for each load of items processed through the sterilizer. Gross malfunctions can be usually detected very quickly by utilization of indicator labels, strips, and steam pattern cards.

The employment of calibrated biological controls remains the main guarantee of sterilization. These preparations contain bacterial spores which are more resistant to heat than viruses and vegetative bacteria. Since a spore vehicle designed for one sterilization method is not necessarily the proper mode to use for other procedures, manufacturers produce both glass vials containing spores and biological test strips. A dental office with two different types of sterilizers (*i.e.*, an autoclave and a chemical vapor sterilizer) may therefore utilize spore ampules (for the autoclave) and spore strips (for the vapor apparatus) to be certain that the sporicidal assays are providing maximal effectiveness. The organisms most used are calibrated concentrations of either *Bacillus stearothermophilus* or *Bacillus subtilis* spores. These are either suspended in a nutrient medium (ampule form) or impregnated onto a test strip with the broth in an adjacent capsule. A pH indicator in the medium is also present; this changes color when spores germinate, thereby visually demonstrating a failure to sterilize. Since the spore preparations are relatively heat-resistant the proof of their destruction after exposure to the sterilization cycle is used to infer that all microorganisms exposed to the same conditions have been destroyed. The demonstration of sporicidal activity by an office sterilizer thus represents the most sensitive check for efficiency.

ASEPSIS IN DENTAL PRACTICE

The control of microbial flora in dental practice by sterilization and disinfection by either physical or chemical means is difficult to completely accomplish. The main problems in dentistry relate to instruments and equipment, cavity and tooth preparation in restorative dentistry, mucous membranes in oral and periodontal surgery, local anesthesiology and root canals in endodontics.

Instruments and Equipment

Some types of dental instruments and equipment can be effectively sterilized whereas others cannot. In dental practice all means available should be utilized to their maximum extent. Procedures in order of their usual preference by clinicians are steam under pressure, dry heat, unsaturated chem-

ical vapor and ethylene oxide. The application of each of these for sterilizing instruments and other intra-oral items is presented in table 7/5. Earlier sections of this chapter have included pertinent conditions and features of sterilization modes; the following information is meant to serve as adjunct material for further application.

As discussed earlier, saturated steam at 15 pounds pressure in an autoclave is preferred for instruments not unduly affected by moist heat. The length of exposure ranges from 15 to 30 minutes, depending on the bulk of the package. A fundamental assumption requires that all instruments be thoroughly cleansed before sterilizing. Instruments and other dental items should then be properly wrapped so that steam can penetrate through the package and bring the interior temperature to 121 C during the sterilizing period. The effectiveness of any sterilization method is dependent upon the preparation, packaging and storage of the items processed. A summary of appropriate packaging materials for each of the accepted sterilization modes is included in table 7/2.

Oils, waxes, petroleum, zinc oxide, water-insoluble powders, and other substances that are not water soluble cannot be readily sterilized by autoclaving. In some instances they can be sterilized by dry heat or by the use of ethylene oxide. The latter is often used for sterilization at the time of manufacture or at the time of packaging.

Corrosion or rusting of metallic instruments is a major fault of using steam under pressure for sterilization. Even the best autoclaves contain sufficient oxygen to cause corrosion of carbon steel during sterilization. At the temperature of the autoclave, the iron in carbon steel is converted to ferrous hydroxide:

$$Fe + 2H_2O \rightleftharpoons Fe(OH)_2 + H_2$$

In the presence of oxygen and water, ferrous hydroxide is converted to ferric hydroxide:

$$4Fe(OH)_2 + O_2 + 2H_2O \rightleftharpoons 4Fe(OH)_3$$

On drying ferric hydroxide is converted to ferric oxide:

$$2Fe(OH)_3 \rightleftharpoons Fe_2O_3 + 3H_2O$$

A coating of ferric oxide on the surface of an instrument does not protect the unoxidized metal beneath it from attack. An approach has been made with chemicals that vaporize in the autoclave and protect iron or steel from oxidation by hydrolysis. The utilization of a dry heat oven, chemical vapor sterilizer or an ethylene oxide unit prevents the above adverse effect.

Attempts have also been made to disinfect or sterilize small dental instruments, used mostly in

Table 7/5
Suitable methods for sterilizing common dental instruments and items[a,b]

Materials	Steam Autoclave[c]	Dry Heat Oven	Chemical Vapor	Ethylene Oxide
General hand instruments				
Stainless steel	1	1	1	2
Carbon steel	3	1	1	2
Mirrors	2	1	1	2
Burs[d]				
Steel	2	1	1	2
Carbon steel	3	1	1	2
Tungsten-carbide	2	1	2	2
Stones				
Diamond	2	1	1	2
Polishing	1	2	1	2
Sharpening	2	1	2	2
Polishing wheels and disks				
Rubber	2	4	3	2
Garnet and cuttle	4	3	3	2
Rag	1	2	2	2
Rubber dam equipment				
Carbon or carbide steel clamps	3	1	1	2
Stainless steel clamps	1	1	1	2
Punches	3	1	1	2
Plastic frames	3	4	4	2
Metal frames	1	1	1	2
Impression trays				
Aluminum	1	2	1	2
Metal, chromeplated	1	1	1	2
Custom acrylic resin	4	4	4	2
Plastic (discarding is preferred)	4	4	4	2
Fluroide gel trays				
Heat-resistant plastic	1	4	3	2
Nonheat-resistant plastic	4	4	4	2
Orthodontic pliers				
High quality stainless	1	1	1	2
Low quality stainless	4	1	1	2
With plastic parts	4	4	3	1
Endodontic instruments				
Reamers and files, broaches, stainless metal handles	1	1	1	1
Nonstainless, metal handles	4	1	1	1
Stainless with plastic handles	3	3	3	1
Pluggers and condensers	1	1	1	2
Glass slabs	1	2	1	2
Dapen dishes	1	2	1	2
Handpieces[e]				
High speed	3	3	3	2
Low speed straight	3	3	3	2
Prophy-angles	2	2	2	2
Contra-angles	4	4	4	2
X-ray equipment				
Plastic film holders, columating devices	3	4	4	2
Stainless steel surgical instruments	1	1	2	2
Ultrasonic scaling tips	2	4	4	2
Electrosurgical tips and handles	4	4	4	4
Needles				
Disposable (do not reuse)	4	4	4	4
Reusable	2	2	4	4

[a] From "Current Status of Sterilization Instruments, Devices and Methods for the Dental Office, CDMIE. *Journal of the American Dental Association,* **102,** 685, 1981; copyright by the American Dental Association, reprinted with permission.

endodontics, by exposing them to heat-transfer media such as molten metal, table salt, steel balls $\frac{1}{16}$ inch in diameter, or fine glass beads. Most instruments or objects need to be exposed to such media for at least 10 seconds or longer at 218 C to be effective. Larger instruments require longer to heat to the desired temperature than do smaller ones and with all such sterilizers the temperature may vary throughout the sterilizing medium.

The use of chemical disinfectants in destroying microorganisms on instrument surfaces is not considered a sterilizing end by itself. The limitations and problems with different types of agents are well documented, and even the routine 10- to 20-minute use of glutaraldehydes should be thought of as disinfecting. In many instances items may be initially immersed in a chemical agent after a dental procedure to reduce the microbial population until the materials can be scrubbed and sterilized. It thus becomes important to use a chemical that can inactivate viruses and other pathogens, and to avoid those that can cause corrosion of instruments. Since debris such as blood and saliva can retard sterilization, hand-scrubbing of instruments is necessary to accomplish mechanical cleaning.

An alternative or additional measure of cleaning instruments utilizes an ultrasonic bath. This apparatus can achieve instrument cleaning in 5 minutes, and should be operated with the cover on to prevent expulsion of contaminants into the atmosphere. Some disinfectants are suitable for use with the ultrasonic bath and commercially prepared cleaning solutions may be purchased. However, it is important to remember that solutions used for instrument cleaning are not suitable for re-use with items such as dentures and appliances which will be placed in patients' mouths.

Storage

Instruments should be stored in a manner protecting them from environmental contaminants. Ideally, instruments should be kept wrapped until use, however, those stored unwrapped in drawers should be touched only with clean hands or forceps. Basic setups can be packaged together for prophylaxis and operative procedures. Those seldomly used can be packaged together according to type, and taken from the package as needed.

Disinfection of the Operatory

Since it is not possible to provide absolute asepsis for all surfaces and objects during a dental procedure, decontamination attempts should be directed toward those things which are sources of cross-infection. These include light handles, switches, drawer handles, water faucets, X-ray cones, chair buttons, bracket tables, hose ends, unit controls, couplings to the saliva evacuator tip, the tip itself, headrests, and the arms of dental chairs. The most desirable disinfectants for these purposes are tuberculocidal and virucidal. By using the previously discussed desired properties as guidelines, a few of the commonly employed disinfectants used to achieve surface decontamination may be assessed. Thus, disinfectants containing mixtures of phenolic and chlorinated phenolic derivatives are tuberculocidal and destroy most lipophilic viruses. Ethyl alcohol is an effective disinfectant whose properties are enhanced by combining with benzalkonium chloride. This latter approach reinforces the aforementioned Council on Dental Therapeutics recommendation that quaternary ammonium compound solutions are inappropriate by themselves. A very effective method of disinfection employs iodophor solutions. These have been shown effective against hepatitis B, but they require at least 30 minutes of exposure to attain this level of efficacy.

Personal Cleanliness

Considerations in the area of personal cleanliness include the use of gloves, safety glasses, face masks, hair restraints and suitable clothing. Specific implementations for these include:

1. Disposable gloves to protect the operator from contact with blood and salvia, especially when cuts and abrasions are present.
2. Eyeglasses to protect the operator's eyes from blood, saliva and splattering particles.
3. Face masks to prevent respiratory cross-contamination.
4. Restraint of long hair to prevent contamination of the operative field and restriction of vision.
5. No jewelry worn on hands or arms since it may harbor blood, saliva, mercury and other contaminants.
6. Clinic jackets or smocks with short sleeves.

---

[b] *Key:* 1 indicates preferred method with minimum risk of damage; 2 indicates that materials should withstand treatment with minimum risk of damage; 3 indicates that treatment is usually not suitable and may damage materials; manufacturer should be consulted; 4 indicates that materials are likely to be damaged or process may be ineffective.

[c] Chemical protection of certain nonstainless instruments may permit steam autoclaving. A rust-preventive dip (1% sodium nitrite) is recommended before sterilization.

[d] Steel burs may also be sterilized in a hot salt endodontic sterilizer for 15 to 20 seconds at 475 F (246 C), but the process may not be suitable for carbide burs.

[e] Some common latch-type contra-angles cannot withstand repeated heat sterilization; short, heat-sterilizable contra-angle handpieces are now available.

Gloves, protective lenses, and face masks are always indicated in treating patients whose medical history indicates a risk of transmission of hepatitis, tuberculosis, or venereal disease.

Handwashing

A basic procedure related to personal cleanliness executed many times during the day, yet commonly overlooked in its importance, is handwashing. The handwashing procedure for general dentistry is effective in removing transient microorganisms which can be transferred from patient to patient. A liquid antibacterial antiseptic should be used since soaps generally do not kill many bacteria or viruses. Hands should be scrubbed for 20 seconds and rinsed well. It is important to remember that between patients and the handling of items, such as charts and radiographs, the hands should again be washed to prevent cross-contamination.

Overview

Procedures aimed at preventing the spread of infectious disease during dental treatment are constantly being evaluated by the profession and an increasingly inquisitive public. The dilemma faced by dental practitioners was concisely summarized by Crawford (1978):

Discrepancies between "the ideal" and "the real" in dental asepsis provide fertile ground for rash statements of two kinds: "Sterilize everything!" versus "Do nothing, the mouth is a dirty place!" Both are expressions of compulsion, fear or frustration about a seemingly impossible dilemma. They may reflect the sentiment, "Go away; let me alone." Practical reality, of course, dictates that to prevent the possible spread of infectious diseases, dental professionals must be provided with inclusive, up-to-date information that can be utilized to develop an optimal program of asepsis.

When such a program has been implemented by the practitioner and auxiliary staff, the risk of disease transmission is significantly reduced.

ADDITIONAL READING

ACCEPTED DENTAL THERAPEUTICS. Ed. 37. 1979 American Dental Association, Council on Dental Therapeutics.

AMERICAN DENTAL ASSOCIATION COUNCIL ON DENTAL THERAPEUTICS. 1978 Quaternary Ammonium Compounds Not Acceptable for Disinfection of Instruments and Environmental Surfaces. J Am Dent Assoc, **97,** 855.

BLOCK, S. S. (Ed.) 1977 *Disinfection, Sterilization and Preservation.* Lea & Febiger, Philadelphia.

CASTLE, M. 1980 *Hospital Infection Control. Principles and Practice.* John Wiley & Sons, New York.

CENTER FOR DISEASE CONTROL, United States Department of Health, Education and Welfare. 1977 Hepatitis Surveillance, Report 41.

COUNCIL ON DENTAL MATERIALS, INSTRUMENTS AND EQUIPMENT. 1981 Current Status of Sterilization Instruments, Devices and Methods for the Dental Office. J Am Dent Assoc, **102,** 683.

CRAWFORD, J. J. 1977 Sterilization, Disinfection and Asepsis in Dentistry. In *Disinfection, Sterilization and Preservation*, pp. 685–704, edited by S. S. Block. Lea & Febiger, Philadelphia.

CRAWFORD, J. J. 1978 *Clinical Asepsis in Dentistry.* R. A. Kolstad, Publisher, Dallas.

DINEEN, P. 1978 Handwashing Degerming: A Comparison of Povidone-iodine and Chlorhexidine. Clin Pharm Ther, **23,** 63.

ERNST, R. R. 1974 Ethylene Oxide Sterilization Kinetics. Biotechnol Bioeng Symp, **4,** 865.

FIRTELL, D. N., MOORE, D. J., AND PELLEN, G. B., JR. 1972 Sterilization of Impression Materials for Use in the Surgical Operating Room. J Prosthet Dent, **21,** 315.

GILMAN, A. G., GOODMAN, L. S., AND GILMAN, A. 1980 *The Pharmacological Basis of Therapeutics*, Ed. 6. Macmillan, New York.

KIMBROUGH, R. D. 1973 Review of Recent Evidence of Toxic Effects of Hexachlorophene. Pediatrics, **51,** 391.

LILLY, H. A., AND LOWBURY, E. J. L. 1971 Disinfection of the Skin: An Assessment of Some New Preparations. Br Med J, **3,** 674.

MOLINARI, J. A., AND YORK, J. 1980 Asepsis in Dental Medicine. Detroit Dent Bull, **49,** 6.

PETERSON, A. F., ROSENBERG, A., AND ALATARY, S. D. 1978 Comparative Evaluation of Surgical Scrub Preparations. Surg Gynecol Obstet, **146,** 63.

RILEY, R. L. 1971 Air Disinfection in Corridors by Upper Air Irradiation with Ultraviolet Light. Arch Environ Health, **22,** 551.

SYKES, G. 1969 Methods and Equipment for Sterilization of Laboratory Apparatus and Media. In *Methods in Microbiology*, Vol. 1, p. 77, edited by J. R. Norris and D. W. Ribbons. Academic Press, New York.

TABER, D., LAZARAS, J. C., FAUCHER, O. E., AND CALANDRA, J. C. 1971 The Accumulation and Persistence of Antibacterial Agents in Human Skin. J Soc Cosmet Chem, **22,** 369.

VIRAL HEPATITIS TYPE B, TUBERCULOSIS AND DENTAL CARE OF INDOCHINESE REFUGEES. 1980 Morbidity Mortality Weekly Report **29,** 1.

WHITACRE, R. J., ROBINS, S. K., WILLIAMS, B. L., AND CRAWFORD, J. J. 1979 *Dental Asepsis.* Stoma Press, Seattle.

chapter 8

Antimicrobial Chemotherapy

John A. Molinari

INTRODUCTION

The advent of antibiotics for practical therapy of infectious diseases began in 1928 with the observation of Fleming that staphylococci growing on a culture plate were inhibited by a chance contamination with a species of *Penicillium*. This mold produced an antibiotic which Fleming called penicillin. After much investigation penicillin was isolated by Chain and Florey as an impure brown powder, and by 1941 its therapeutic efficacy was well established. After 1941 an extensive systematic search was begun for molds and bacteria that might produce other antibiotics. The results indicated that many types of penicillin were produced by mutant strains and species of *Penicillium notatum* and *Pencillium chrysogenum* as well as other species of *Pencillium*. The search also revealed that many species of the genus *Streptomyces* produced a variety of antibiotics. A few species of the genus *Bacillus* produced antibiotics, but these are not as useful as those produced by species of *Penicillium* and *Streptomyces*, principally because of their toxicity. Some species of *Nocardia* and *Aspergillus* also produce antibiotics. As the search continues, undoubtedly new antibiotics will be discovered, either produced naturally by microorganisms or synthesized by biochemists.

The list of microbial agents causing oral and maxillofacial infections continues to expand as cultural and diagnostic procedures become more sensitive. The dental practitioner is thus required to be familiar with the principles and general approaches to chemotherapy as they relate to the wide range of infections encountered. Many of these infections, such as those involving strict anaerobes, were frequently not diagnosed correctly and often led to long-term complications for both patient and dentist. It is not the purpose of the following chapter to present an exhaustive pharmacological discussion of antibiotics. Excellent texts and references (see Additional Readings) have been recently published which provide the student and practitioner with detailed therapeutic information on virtually every chemical agent. Instead, the intent is to present an overview of the principles of antimicrobial chemotherapy with the emphasis on different mechanisms by which antibiotics interfere with infectious microorganisms. Selected drugs will be discussed as they relate to these mechanisms and their appropriateness for dental medicine.

CHARACTERISTICS OF IDEAL CHEMOTHERAPEUTIC AGENTS

As the search for useful chemotherapeutic agents progressed it became evident that they must have certain properties. It also became evident that an agent could be useful even if it did not possess all the properties of an ideal agent, depending on the circumstances of its clinical use. The characteristics of an ideal agent became a useful guide in the search for antibiotics and in the development of chemosynthetic agents. Therefore, an ideal chemotherapeutic agent:

1. Should have selective activity. It will have true selectivity if it affects some essential biochemical reaction of the microorganism that is not an essential reaction of the host. The agent may have relative selectivity even if the reaction is essential to both pathogen and host. For instance, such an agent would be useful if the pathogen metabolizes or reproduces more rapidly than the host cells, or if the membranes of the pathogen were more permeable to the agent than the host cells.

2. Should have spectrum of activity that includes only the causative pathogen or pathogens involved in a given disease. It should not upset the normal microbiota of the various body areas.

3. Is generally more useful if it is bactericidal rather than bacteriostatic.

4. Should not induce bacterial resistance.

5. Should have no significant toxic effects on the host at its highest useful dose.

6. Should not be allergenic.

7. Should retain its activity in the presence of body fluids and tissues.

8. Should be soluble and stable in water.

9. Is one with which a bactericidal blood level can be rapidly attained and maintained for the time required to effect a cure.

10. Is one that can be administered either systemically or orally.

11. Is one that can be easily disposed of by the body at a rate that will maintain a bactericidal blood level.

12. Should be reasonable in cost.

CLASSIFICATION OF ANTIBIOTICS AND CHEMOTHERAPEUTICS

Antibiotics and chemotherapeutic agents can be classified by their mode of action on microbial cells (table 8/1). Thus, the various agents can be divided into groups that 1) interfere with cell wall synthesis, 2) inhibit or interfere with protein synthesis, 3) affect nucleic acid function, 4) damage plasma membranes, and 5) are metabolite antagonists.

As shown in table 8/1, penicillin, cycloserine, vancomycin, bacitracin, and novobiocin inhibit the synthesis of bacterial cell walls, or more specifically, they interfere with some phase of peptidoglycan synthesis. Antibiotics that inhibit protein synthesis can be subdivided into one group that affects protein synthesis at the level of transcription (actinomycin, rifampin), and another that inhibits microbial protein synthesis at the level of translation. This later group includes streptomycin, neomycin, paromomycin, kanamycin, gentamycin, spectinomycin, chloramphenicol, erythromycin, linomycin, clindamycin and the tetracyclines. While there are a number of inhibitors of nucleic acid function, most are not routinely used because of their deleterious effects on the host. Many nucleic acid inhibitors that are not included in table 8/1, such as the alkylating agents nitrogen mustard and cyclophosphamide, have found an important function in antineoplastic treatment regimens.

The cell or cytoplasmic membrane is also an important regulator of bacterial cell activity, particularly as a selective barrier affecting the transport of compounds both into and out of the cell and in biosynthesis and metabolism. Polymyxin, nystatin, and amphotericin B are examples of antibiotics that attack the cytoplasmic cell membrane directly. These agents are relatively nonspecific, for they are usually not able to distinguish between mammalian and target microbial membranes. This affects their application and will be discussed in a later section.

The sulfonamides and related compounds are classified in a group of antimetabolites that interfere with the enzymes involved in the production and utilization of essential bacterial growth factors (vitamins, amino acids). These essential enzymes combine with antimetabolites that are structurally related to their normal substrate and prevent normal substrate-enzyme reaction.

Table 8/1
Chemotherapeutic agents according to their mode of action

Mode of Action	Antibiotic
Inhibitors of cell wall formation	Penicillin
	Cycloserine
	Vancomycin
	Bacitracin
	Novobiocin (partially)
Inhibitors of protein synthesis:	
A. At the level of transcription	Actinomycin
	Rifampin
B. At the level of translation	Streptomycin
	Neomycin
	Paromomycins
	Kanamycin
	Gentamycins
	Spectinomycin
	Chloramphenicol
	Erythromycin
	Lincomycin
	Clindamycin
	Amikacin
	Tobramycin
	Tetracyclines
Inhibitors of nucleic acid function	Mitomycin
	Nalidixic acid
	Novobiocin
	Griseofulvin
Inhibitors causing cytoplasmic membrane damage	Polymyxin
	Nystatin
	Amphotericin B
Metabolite antagonists	Sulfonamides
	Sulfones
	p-Aminosalicylic acid
	Isoniazid

There does not appear to be any classification scheme for antibiotics which is appropriate in all instances. While each method is plagued by exceptions and footnoted explanations, a few approaches other than the format shown in Table 8/1 must be mentioned. First, antibiotics and chemotherapeutic agents can be classified by their antimicrobial spectrum. This classification, quite useful in clinical practice, divides the agents into 1) those that have primarily a gram positive spectrum, 2) those that have primarily a gram negative spectrum, 3) those that have a broad spectrum, 4) those that have an antifungal spectrum, and 5) those that have an antiviral spectrum. Agents with a gram positive spectrum include penicillin, erythromycin, lincomycin, bacitracin, and vancomycin. Agents with a gram negative spectrum include gentamycin, tobramycin and polymyxin B. Broad spectrum agents, acting on both gram positive and gram negative bacteria include tetracycline, kanamycin, neomycin, cephalosporin, chloramphenicol, and streptomycin. Antifungal agents are nystatin, amphotericin B, and griseofulvin. There are few antiviral agents, but 5-iodo-2′ deoxyuridine, vidarabine and amantadine are clinically useful.

Another method of categorizing antimicrobial agents is by their route of administration. Routes of administration are topical or systemic. Some agents that are applied topically include bacitracin and nystatin. Some agents that can be applied both topically and systemically are polymyxin and neomycin. Among the numerous agents that are applied systemically, griseofulvin, streptomycin, amphotericin B, cephalosporins, tetracycline, clindamycin, erythromycin and penicillins have found application in dental medicine.

A less useful method of classifying antimicrobial agents, at least clinically, is by their source. Sources are 1) fungi or molds, 2) bacteria, 3) the actinomycetes, and 4) synthetic compounds. Antibiotics produced by fungi include the penicillins, griseofulvin, and cephalosporins. Major agents derived from bacteria are polymyxin, colistin and bacitracin. Most antibiotics derived from bacteria are applied locally. The majority of antibiotics in current use are produced by actinomycetes. They include streptomycin, neomycin, kanamycin, vancomycin, clindamycin, nystatin, amphotericin B and erythromycin. Another source of antibiotics and chemotherapeutic agents is by synthesis or semisynthesis. The most notable examples of this type of agent are the semisynthetic penicillins.

The scheme chosen for the present chapter utilizes the categories in table 8/1. As mentioned in the introduction, the extent of discussion for different agents will be influenced by the application of the antibiotics in dental medicine.

Inhibitors of Cell Wall Formation

Penicillins. The basic structure of penicillins consists of a condensation product of the D-isomers of an alanine and a β-dimethyl-cysteine residue, to which is attached an R-C-group (fig. 8/1). From strains of *P. notatum* and *P. chrysogenum* growing in ordinary culture media, many useful types of penicillin have been isolated, designated as G, K, X, O, V, F, and dihydro-F. Penicillin G, O, and V are useful therapeutically. Many additional "biosynthetic" penicillins have been isolated by the addition of certain chemical intermediates, as sources of different R-groups, to species and strains of *Penicillium* growing in standard media. For penicillin to have antibacterial activity, the lactam and thiazolidine rings must be intact. Most forms of bacterial penicillinase inactivate penicillins by breaking the lactam ring, resulting in inactive penicilloic acid. The side chain, or R-group, largely determines stability of the molecule and is responsible for many of the antibacterial and pharmacological features of different penicillins. In 1959, 6-aminopenicillanic acid was obtained in crystalline form without side chain precursors. While it has little or no antibacterial activity, it can be acylated to yield strongly antibacterial semisynthetic penicillins, which have become very important in the treatment of certain penicillin-resistant and gram negative infections. A functional classification of the major penicillins is presented in table 8/2. Structural formulas of the principal penicillins in use are diagramed in figure 8/2.

Penicillin Activity. Penicillins are mainly effective against gram positive bacteria, spriochetes and

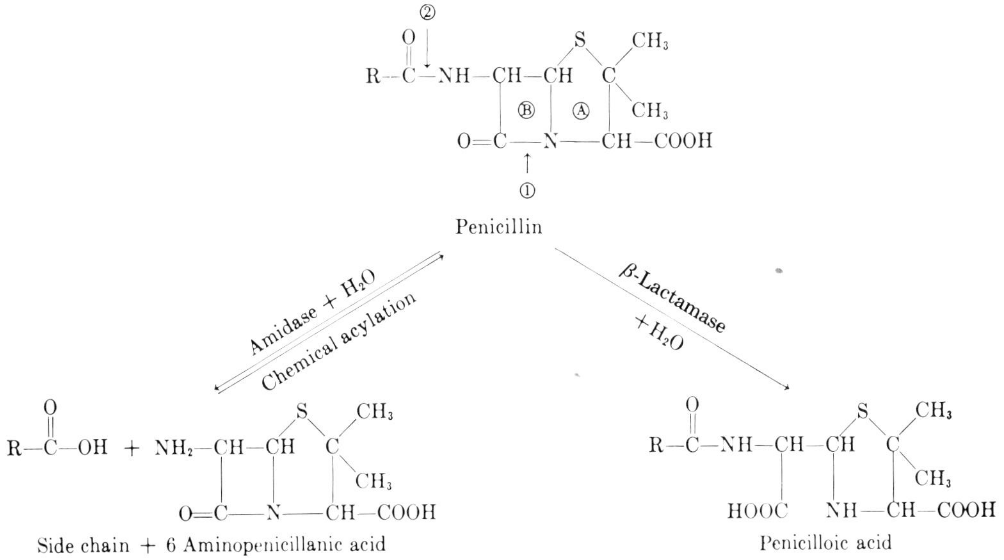

Figure 8/1. Basic structure of penicillins, and some of their important chemical reactions. Ⓐ, thiazolidine ring. Ⓑ, β-lactam ring. ①, site of action of β-lactamase. ②, site of action of amidase.

Table 8/2

Penicillins and the infectious organisms for which they are the antimicrobial agents of choice[a]

Penicillin G

Streptococcus pneumoniae[b]
Streptococcus pyogenes
Viridans streptococci
Anaerobic streptococci
Staphylococcus aureus (nonpenicillinase-producing)
Neisseria meningitidis
Neisseria gonorrhoeae[c]
Bacillus anthracis
Clostridia
Leptotrichia buccalis
Erysipelothrix rhusiopathiae
Pasteurella multocida
Streptobacillus moniliformis
Bacteroides (nonfragilis strains)
Treponema pallidum
Sprillum minor
Leptospira
Fusiform bacteria
Actinomyces israelii

Methicillin, oxacillin, nafcillin, cloxacillin, dicloxacillin

Staphylococcus aureus (penicillinase-producing)

Ampicillin

Streptococcus faecalis (usually with an aminoglycoside)
Proteus mirabilis
Haemophilus influenzae[b]
Actinomyces muris ratti
Listeria monocytogenes
Salmonella other than Salmonella typhi

Carbenicillin

Pseudomonas aeruginosa

---

[a] From C. J. Wilkowske, Special Series on Antimicrobial Agents, Mayo Clinic Proceedings, **52**, 616, 1977.
[b] Penicillin-resistant strains occur in the absence of penicillinase synthesis.
[c] Penicillinase-producing resistant strains occur.

a few gram negative bacteria (table 8/2). However, in high concentrations they are effective against many gram negative microorganisms.

The semisynthetic penicillins include some with broadened antimicrobial spectrum. for example, 6-aminobenzylpenicillin (ampicillin) is much more active than penicillin G against many gram negative bacteria. This is evidently due to its greater ability to penetrate through the gram negative cell wall. Ampicillin, however, is less active than penicillin G against many gram positive microorganisms.

Penicillin Resistance. Penicillin-resistant microorganisms usually develop by the production of the adaptive enzyme, penicillinase. Although pathogenic strains of *Staphylococcus aureus* remain as the major infectious agents possessing this enzyme, other infections have been traced in recent years to penicillinase-producing strains of *Neisseria gonorrhoeae* and *Haemophilus influenzae*. These strains are becoming increasingly prevalent. In addition, penicillin-resistant strains of *Streptococcus pneumoniae* began appearing in South African outbreaks in 1977, and since that time a number of countries including the United States and Canada have reported strains resistant up to 2 μg/ml penicillin. Multiple drug resistance has also become a characteristic feature of these pneumococci.

Penicillinase synthesized by adaptive mutants can occur in either a β-lactamase or an amidase form (fig. 8/1). The first is the most common, resulting in cleavage of the β-lactam ring with subsequent inactivation of the drug. Most *S. aureus* and gram negative bacteria that produce a penicil-

linase do so by releasing a β-lactamase. The amidase type of enzyme destroys the antimicrobial activity of penicillins by cleaving side groups from the parent molecule. The development of semisynthetic penicillins such as methicillin and oxacillin has countered some of the above resistance, as these forms of the drug are penicillinase-resistant. They are poor substrates for β-lactamase and thus are not inactivated in the presence of lactamase-producing strains. Agents such as methicillin, cloxacillin, nafcillin and oxacillin have found significant usage in dental medicine against penicillin G-resistant staphylococcal infections.

Penicillin Toxicity. The penicillins in common usage have very little significant toxicity or pharmacological action *per se* even when used in large dosages. They are toxic when applied directly to the central nervous system in concentrated solution, but not in dilute solution. After parenteral or oral administration, very little penicillin reaches the undiseased central nervous system.

Penicillins, however, seem to be among the worst allergens of the antibiotics in current use. Largely because of the indiscriminate use of penicillins, more than 10% of the population has become seriously hypersensitive to them. Some 25% of all patients treated with penicillins show some form of dermal sensitivity. The less severe symptoms of penicillin sensitivity are epidermal reactions (urticaria, dermatitis), gastrointestinal disturbances (diarrhea is common with ampicillin), pain in muscles or joints, headache, eosinophilia, fever resembling serum sickness, faintness, and malaise. Most

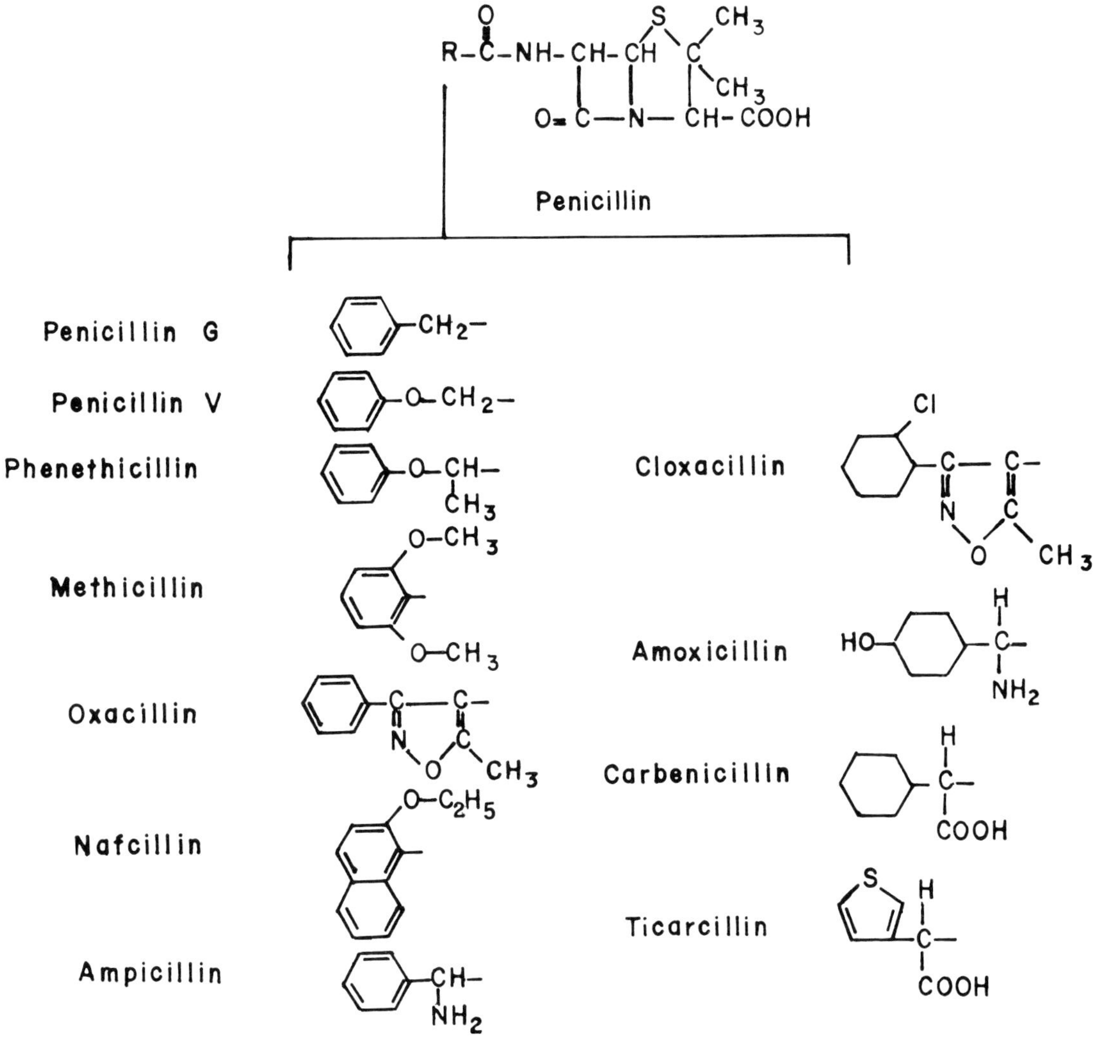

Figure 8/2. Structures of penicillin derivatives.

of these reactions are transient and subside when penicillin is no longer administered. The use of long-lasting or repository types of penicillin complicates the treatment of allergic reactions, for even though such penicillins are withdrawn, they persist in the tissues. The most serious sensitivity reaction is anaphylactic shock. Its occurrence is infrequent and usually, but not always, follows parenteral administration.

Routes of Administration. Penicillins can be administered orally, intramuscularly, or intravenously. The onset of antibacterial action following various routes of penicillin administration relates to the rate of absorption, the tissue level obtained, the resistance to degradation by gastric acids and the degree of protein binding. Two of these factors, extent of absorption after oral administration and acid resistance, are very noteworthy to the practicing dentist and specialist (table 8/3).

Only about one-third of orally administered penicillin G is absorbed, mostly from the duodenum; the other two-thirds is destroyed in the stomach and colon. Some penicillins are resistant to gastric juices and are well absorbed, particularly from an empty stomach. Oral administration also yields a lower blood serum concentration than is obtained by the other routes. The intramuscular administration of penicillin is more effective than the oral route, but the risk of an untoward reaction is greater. Blood serum concentrations obtained by intramuscular injection are intermediate between oral (lowest) and intravenous (highest) administration. Finally, the intravenous injection of penicillins is most dangerous with regard to hypersensitivity, but a high serum concentration can be obtained almost immediately. It is not routinely used except in life-threatening situations.

Metabolism and Excretion. A number of sub-

Table 8/3
Classification of penicillins[a]

Types and Generic Names	Trade Names	Oral Absorption	Acid Resistance[b]
Natural			
Penicillin G	Many	Variable (poor)	+
Phenoxymethyl penicillin (penicillin V)	Many	Good	+ +
Phenoxyethyl penicillin (phenethicillin)	Many	Good	+ + +
Semisynthetic			
Penicillinase-resistant			
Methicillin	Staphcillin	Poor	◯
Oxacillin	Bactocill, Prostaphlin	Good	+ +
Nafcillin	Unipen	Variable	+ +
Cloxacillin	Tegopen	Good	+ + +
Dicloxacillin	Dynapen, Pathocil, Veracillin	Good	
Extended spectrum			
Ampicillin	Many	Good	+ + +
Bacampicillin	Spectrobid	Good	+ + +
Hetacillin	Versapen	Good	+ + +
Amoxicillin	Larotid, Amoxil, Polymox	Excellent	+ + +
Carbenicillin	Geopen, Pyopen	Poor	+ +
Ticarcillin	Ticar	Poor	◯

[a] Modified from C. J. Wilkowske, Special Series on Antimicrobial Agents, *Mayo Clinic Proceedings* 52, 616, 1977.
[b] ◯ = acid sensitive; + = slightly resistant; + + = moderately resistant; + + + = highly resistant.

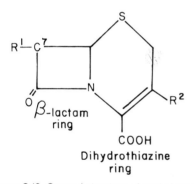

Figure 8/3. General structure of cephalosporins.

stances in the body act on penicillin. Most penicillins are hydrolyzed to some extent by gastric acids. Amidases convert penicillins to the inactive 6-aminopenicillanic acid. Bacterial penicillinase (β-lactamase) converts penicillins to penicilloic acid. Absorbed penicillins that are not hydrolyzed in the body are excreted unchanged. Most penicillin is excreted in urine (60 to 90%), the remainder being excreted in bile, saliva, or in other body fluids.

Dosage of Penicillin. The dosage for intramuscular administration is usually from 300,000 to 1 million units daily. Orally, penicillin is generally administered three to four times daily in 400,000-to 500,000-unit doses.

Cephalosporins. The cephalosporins are semisynthetic derivatives of 7-aminocephalosporanic acid, an antibacterial compound, produced by the fungus *Cephalosporium acremonium.* 7-Aminocephalosporanic acid is the active component of the fungal product cephalosporin C. The nucleus of this latter compound is closely related to penicillin in structure and mechanism of antibacterial action (fig. 8/3). The major difference between the structures of the cephalosporins and penicillins is the presence of a dihydrothiazine ring in place of the penicillins' five-membered thiazolidine ring. The R^1 and R^2 side groups distinguished the various cephalosporins from each other with regard to antimicrobial spectrum, stability and oral absorption. The available forms of cephalosporins are categorized in table 8/4.

Cephalosporin Activity. These drugs usually are reserved for serious infections in hospitalized patients, although in general the cephalosporins are bactericidal against most gram positive cocci and common gram negative bacilli such as *Escherichia coli, Klebsiella pneumoniae, Proteus mirabilis, Salmonella species* and *Shigella species.* A notable exception among the gram positive cocci is the resistance demonstrated by enterococci, specifically *Streptococcus faecalis.* Maxillofacial and periapical abscesses caused by this bacterium are as resistant to cephalosporins as they are to simple penicillins. The above antimicrobial spectrum is remarkably similar for most of the cephalosporins. The main exceptions are cefamandole and cefoxitin which have broad-spectrums.

Table 8/4
Types of cephalosporins[a]

Parenteral Use	Oral Use	Extended Spectrum
Cephalothin	Cephalexin	Cefamandole
Cephapirin	Cephradine	Cefoxitin
Cefazolin		
Cephaloridine	Cephaloglycin	
Cephradine	Cefaclor	

[a] Modified from R. L. Thompson, Special Series on Antimicrobial Agents, *Mayo Clinic Proceedings*, **52**, 625, 1977.

This group of antibiotics is rarely mentioned as the agent of choice for treatment of infections, although cephalosporins are effective against certain orofacial infections that are refractive to penicillins. Serious methacillin-resistant *Staphylococcus aureus* infections serve as examples for the use of an agent like cephalothin, in conjunction with an aminoglycoside such as gentamycin, as an appropriate replacement for ineffective penicillin regimens.

Patients with a history of minor penicillin hypersensitivity have also been transfered onto a cephalosporin, generally without any subsequent incidents. Although there is some immunologic cross-reactivity between penicillins and cephalosporins, scientists and clinicians have found that the latter usually are contraindicated only in patients with anaphylactic or other severe immediate hypersensitivities.

Cephalosporin Resistance. Induced mechanisms of antimicrobial resistance are similar to those demonstrated against the penicillins. β-Lactamases, or more specifically cephalosporinases, are capable of inactivating the drug in a fashion analogous to that for penicillinase. In addition, mutant bacteria can prevent the penetration of most cephalosporins to the active site in the cell wall. These two forms of resistance can be overcome by substituting a less susceptible cephalosporin. One example of this latter practice is the utilization of cefamandole against soft tissue infections caused by β-lactamase-producing gram negative bacilli.

Cephalosporin Toxicity. The development of allergic reactions comprises the major adverse manifestation. These are most commonly maculopapular rashes with anaphylactic responses occurring only occasionally. A positive Coombs test is a frequent problem in individuals receiving larger doses of cephalosporins; fortunately hemolysis generally does not occur in this situation. In the main, similar adverse effects are associated with both cephalosporins and penicillins.

Bacitracin. Bacitracin is an antibiotic produced by strain of *Bacillus subtilis*. It is active against many gram positive bacteria, as well as *Neiserria* species, *Haemophilus influenzae* and *Treponema pallidum*. This agent functions by interfering with dephosphorylation of the carrier lipid formed in the course of subunit transfer to the growing cell wall. Bacitracin frequently induces nephrotoxicity following parenteral administration, so its use is now limited to topical application. The dental practitioner would have little, if any, occasion to use this drug.

Novobiocin. Novobiocin, produced by *Streptomyces niveus*, *Streptomyces griseus*, and *Streptomyces spheroides*, is bactericidal against gram positive bacteria, with an antibacterial spectrum similar to that of penicillin and erythromycin. Novobiocin interferes with the integrity of the cytoplasmic membrane, DNA replication, and cell wall formation. It does not induce formation of spheroplasts and, in fact, is quite active against L-forms and spheroplasts. Still, novobiocin has serious drawbacks in clinical usage. Susceptible bacteria readily develop resistance to it and the drug is allergenic and toxic. These toxic symptoms, principally anemia, leukopenia, pancytopenia, and gastrointestinal irritation, preclude clinical utilization of this antibiotic.

Vancomycin. Vancomycin, produced by *Streptomyces orientalis*, is active against a few gram positive bacteria and spirochetes. It has a complex molecular structure composed of amino acids and sugars, and it acts by interference with the second stage of cell wall formation in preventing the transfer of subunits from the carrier to the growing peptidoglycan component. Vancomycin should only be used in instances when penicillins, cephalosporins and other classes of antibiotics cannot be employed. An application in dentistry would be in the prophylactic administration of intravenous vancomycin to a patient with a history of endocarditis or rheumatic heart disease, who is allergic to penicillin and erythromycin. Vancomycin also is effective in treating endocarditis caused by viridans streptococci in a similar patient. One unexpected use of vancomycin came about recently in investigating the etiology of pseudomembranous colitis. The causative organism, *Clostridium difficile*, is an exotoxin-producing bacillus which is susceptible to orally administered vancomycin. Since the antibiotic is poorly absorbed through the intestinal lining, it remains in the lumen and is thus bactericidal to the *C. difficile* present.

Bacteria seldom develop resistance to vancomycin, and it does not develop cross-resistance with other antibiotics. However, vancomycin is ototoxic, nephrotoxic, allergenic and occasionally causes dermatitis and localized phlebitis. It should also not be administered to patients with impaired renal function.

Inhibitors of Protein Synthesis

Protein Synthesis. Two major processes are essential to protein synthesis. One is transcription, in which a complementary sequence of RNA is formed by RNA polymerase in response to the genetic information present in DNA. In transcription, antibiotics may alter the structure of template DNA or inhibit RNA polymerases. The other process relates to the translation of mRNA, formed in transcription, into protein. Translation of mRNA into the synthesis of a peptide chain occurs in initiation, elongation, and termination stages. This complex activity, resembling an assembly line, occurs in ribosomes that undergo assembly and disassembly while synthesizing protein.

Translation differs between prokaryotes and eukaryotes both in structural features of mRNA and ribosomes, and in the specific steps involving initiation and elongation of polypeptides. These differences allow for inhibition of microbial protein synthetic mechanisms, with a minimum of concurrent disruption of mammalian intracellular functions.

There are a relatively large number of clinically useful chemotherapeutic agents that inhibit some stage of translation. These antibiotics can be categorized primarily into groups according to their reaction with either the 30S or 50S ribosomal subunits of procaryotes. In addition to their inhibitory activity against certain pathogenic microorganisms in disease, many of the following chemotherapeutic agents also have been utilized in delineating individual steps in the process of protein synthesis.

Inhibitors of Transcription

Actinomycin. Actinomycin, produced by several *Streptomyces* species, is an oligopeptide that interferes with protein synthesis in both gram positive and gram negative bacteria and mammalian cells. Its clinical usage has been in the form of the derivative, dactinomycin, a potent antineoplastic chemotherapeutic agent.

Rifampin. Rifampin is a semisynthetic derivative of rifamycin B, the latter being produced by *Streptomyces mediteranei*. Rifampin is effective against numerous gram positive and enteric gram negative bacteria, *Chlamydia* and some viruses, but is best utilized clinically as a potent antitubercular drug. It has the widest range of activity *in vitro* of all the major agents against *Mycobacterium* species. Rifampin's bactericidal effect is directed against DNA-dependent RNA polymerase, impairing RNA synthesis. It has little or no effect on mammalian RNA polymerases, due to their inability to bind the drug. Because of the rapid emergence of bacterial resistance, this antibiotic is not used alone in the treatment of tuberculosis. Instead, rifampin administered concurrently with isoniazid comprises the most effective drug combination for antitubercular therapy. Prophylactic therapy for *Neisseria meningitidis* infection also has been successfully accomplished with oral rifampin used alone.

Side effects vary with use of the drug, the most obvious being development of an orange-pink color to saliva, tears, urine and perspiration. Less frequent adverse reactions include rashes, nausea, vomiting, fever and jaundice.

Inhibitors of Translation

Streptomycin and Other Aminoglycosides. Streptomycin, an aminoglycoside produced by *Streptomyces griseus*, inhibits many gram positive and gram negative bacteria as well as *Mycobacterium tuberculosis*. Although it is toxic to the eighth cranial nerve and vestibular apparatus, it is sometimes used to treat tuberculosis, meningitis caused by *Haemophilus influenzae*, plague, tularemia, and *Salmonella* and *Shigella* infections, usually in combination with other drugs. Orofacial infections and endocarditis caused by enterococci, *i.e.*, *Streptococcus faecalis*, are controlled by intramuscular administration of streptomycin in combination with oral ampicillin. Even so, streptomycin is not a commonly employed antibiotic in dental medicine, due to its toxicity and the rapid development of bacterial resistance.

In vitro, streptomycin has been shown to bind irreversibly to the 30S ribosomal subunit of a sensitive bacterial cell inhibiting protein synthesis at the initiation of the cycle and inducing a misreading of mRNA and phenotypic suppression. The net result of the addition of streptomycin to growing bacteria is a reduction in their negative surface charge resulting in agglutination, a rapid discharge of potassium into the environment, the cessation of protein synthesis, the depression of DNA and RNA synthesis, RNA dissolution, and the resultant death of the cell.

In addition to streptomycin there are a number of other aminoglycoside antibiotics that are mostly produced by *Streptomyces species* and prevent protein synthesis by reacting with the 30S ribosomal subunits. They all contain amino acids and sugars and either a streptamine (streptomycin) or a deoxystreptamine moiety (kanamycin, neomycin). Of this group, neomycin, gentamycin, kanamycin, tobramycin and amikacin are used clinically to suppress gram negative rods like *Pseudomonas aeruginosa* on burns and wounds, and in some types of gastroenteritis. Although a bacterium may develop resistance to one aminoglycoside during such treatment, it will still be sensitive to the other drugs of this group.

Tetracyclines. Tetracyclines, produced by various species of *Streptomyces*, belong to a group of closely related bacteriostatic antibiotics that include tetracycline, chlortetracycline, dimethylchlortetracycline, doxycycline and oxytetracycline. They are termed broad spectrum antibiotics since they act on both gram positive and gram negative bacteria as well as microorganisms that are insensitive to other antibiotics. Bacteria that become insensitive to one tetracycline are insensitive to all others. The clinical value of tetracyclines as drugs of first choice and alternative therapy is summarized in table 8/5. The recognition of appropriate and inappropriate application becomes very important when dental practitioners consider using one of these drugs to treat routine oral infections.

Tetracyclines act by inhibiting protein synthesis. Inhibition is accomplished by preventing the binding of aminoacyl-tRNA to the acceptor site on the 30S ribosome, stopping peptide chain formation. Figure 8/4 shows the basic structure of tetracycline.

Tetracyclines may be administered either orally or parenterally and are absorbed into all tissues except the brain. Tetracyclines do enter the cerebrospinal fluid. Due to their chelating activity, tetracyclines are deposited in forming bones and teeth causing discoloration. They also interfere with the normal growth and development of bones and teeth. Accordingly, their use should be avoided during the last trimester of pregnancy, the neonatal period, and early childhood. Their affinity for calcium chelation also may result in vitamin K deficiency and a prolonged clotting time.

Although tetracyclines have a relatively low systemic toxicity, they can produce untoward effects, and some decomposition products are toxic. In addition, oral administration of tetracyclines can upset the normal microbiota of the mouth, vagina, and intestine. *Candida albicans*, which is not susceptible to the tetracyclines, is ordinarily held in check by the normal bacterial flora. During tetracycline therapy it may grow in abundance causing local and even systemic infection. In addition, staphylococcal enteritis, or pseudomembranous colitis may develop when the normal ecological balance is upset during prolonged tetracycline therapy.

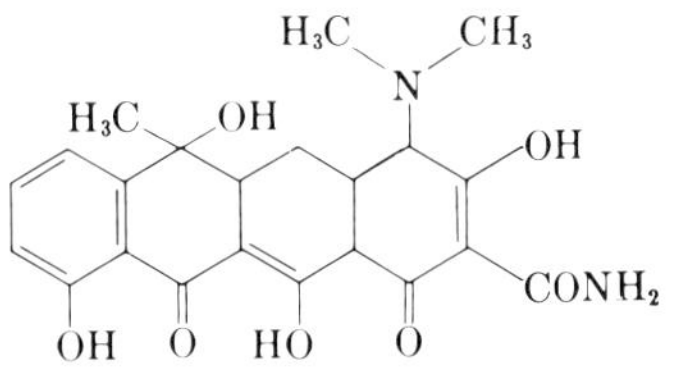

Figure 8/4. Basic structural formula of tetracycline.

Table 8/5
Clinical applications of tetracyclines[a]

Drug of first choice
> *Chlamydia* (*e.g.*, nonspecific urethritis, psittacosis)
> *Rickettsia* (*e.g.*, Rocky Mountain spotted fever, Q fever) (chloramphenicol also effective)
> *Mycoplasma* (erythromycin also effective)
> Brucellosis
> Cholera
> Relapsing fever
> Granuloma inguinale
> Tularemia

Alternative for patient with allergy to penicillin
> Gonococcal disease (spectinomycin, erythromycin also effective)
> Syphilis (erythromycin also effective)
> Tetanus
> *Listeria monocytogenes*
> *Pasteurella multocida*

Alternative for certain other disease states
> Urinary tract infection caused by *Escherichia coli*, *Klebsiella*, *Enterobacter*, *Proteus*, *Pseudomonas*, and enterococci
>   (other drugs preferred)
> Household and similar contacts of patients with meningococcal infection (rifampin first choice)
> Plague (streptomycin first choice)
> Chancroid (sulfas first choice)

Should not be used
> Streptococcal pharyngitis
> Gram positive cocci before sensitivity testing results known; other agents are generally preferred
> Gram negative rods before sensitivity results known; other agents are generally preferred
> *Bacteroides fragilis* and other anaerobic infections

[a] From M. Ginsberg, and I. Tager, *Practical Guide to Antimicrobial Agents.* Williams & Wilkins, 1980.

Chloramphenicol. Closely related to the tetracyclines in its antibiotic spectrum but not in its chemical structure is chloramphenicol, produced either by *Streptomyces venezuelae* or synthetically. Chloramphenicol, a bacteriostatic antibiotic, is active against gram positive and gram negative bacteria, *Rickettsia*, and the *Chlamydia*. Because of its toxicity, the use of chloramphenicol is restricted to the treatment of typhoid fever, salmonellosis, staphylococcal infections resistant to other less toxic antibiotics, anaerobic infections such as *Bacteroides fragilis* sepsis and some other severe, life-threatening infections.

The chief toxic effects are severe blood dyscrasias, optic neuritis, and depression of marrow activity. Less serious symptoms of toxicity are bitter taste, dry mouth, gastritis, diarrhea, and nausea. While it is toxic, chloramphenicol can be administered with reasonable safety to seriously ill patients if proper precautions are observed.

The mode of antibacterial action of chloramphenicol is to prevent protein synthesis by binding exclusively to 50S ribosomal subunits. The antibiotic does not inhibit the initiation of protein synthesis, but interferes with peptide bond formation (transpeptidation). Chloramphenicol does not react with mammalian ribosomes due to the absence of appropriate reacting sites.

Chloramphenicol, erythromycin, lincomycin and clindamycin compete for the same binding sites on 50S ribosomal subunits. Therefore, the simultaneous use of antibiotics affecting these sites is of no more value than if they are used singly. Resistance to such antibiotics generally develops by the bacteria's either becoming impermeable to the drug or by acquiring the ability to degrade the antibiotic to an inactive form.

Macrolide Antibiotics. The macrolide group, which includes erythromycin, oleandomycin and spiramycin also inhibits bacteria by reacting with 50S ribosomal subunits. These antibiotics have an antibacterial spectrum similar to penicillin and are primarily bacteriostatic.

Erythromycin, produced by *Streptomyces erythraeus*, is frequently employed as a therapeutic drug in dental medicine. Many general practitioners and specialists use this macrolide as an alternative to penicillins for common infections. This complex compound is effective both as a drug of first choice and as an alternative mode for individuals with demonstrated penicillin hypersensitivity (table 8/6). Erythromycin prevents protein synthesis by reacting with 50S ribosomal subunits near or at the same site as chloramphenicol. The coupling of the peptide bonds is inhibited, but the ribosome cycle continues without protein synthesis. Resistance to erythromycin is generally controlled with bacterial acquisition of a plasmid that can result in alteration

Table 8/6
Structure and antimicrobial spectrum of erythromycin

STRUCTURE

SPECTRUM OF ACTIVITY
Drug of First Choice
Prophylaxis of elective colonic surgery (with neomycin)
Prophylaxis of household contacts of whooping cough
Eradication of the carrier state of diphtheria
Mycoplasma pneumoniae (tetracyclines also effective)
Legionnaires' disease
Alternative for patient with allergy to penicillin
Prophylaxis of subacute bacterial endocarditis
Prophylaxis of rheumatic fever
Pneumococcal pneumonia (cephalosporins also effective)
Streptococcal pharyngitis (cephalosporins also effective)
Gonococcal disease (spectinomycin, tetracyclines also effective)
Syphilis (tetracycline also effective)

[a] From M. Ginsberg, and I. Tager, *Practical Guide to Antimicrobial Agents.* Williams & Wilkins, 1980.

of the bacterial RNA. This change occurs primarily following exposure to low concentrations of the antibiotic, and diminishes the bacteriostatic effectiveness of the macrolide.

Lincomycin and Clindamycin. Lincomycin, produced by *Streptomyces lincolnensis*, is related structurally to other antibiotics, but it has an antibacterial spectrum similar to erythromycin. The 7-deoxy, 7-chloro derivative of lincomycin, termed clindamycin, is better absorbed than the parent molecule and is more active with fewer adverse reactions. Therefore, clindamycin has replaced lincomycin in clinical usage. Clindamycin is used in dental medicine as a substitute for penicillin in patients allergic to the drug and also in cases of anaerobic infection, especially where *Bacteroides fragilis* is involved. The antibiotic binds to 50S ribosomes interfering with the binding of aminoacyl-tRNA, and resulting in the breakdown of polyribosomes. It does not bind to mammalian rRNA thereby furthering its usefulness. However, since diarrhea can occur which can lead to pseudomembranous colitis, clindamycin is advised only when other antimicrobials are contraindicated.

Inhibitors of Nucleic Acid Function

A number of antibiotics interfere with DNA structure and function, but only a few are clinically useful because their toxic action is not very selective. These antibiotics affect DNA by either cross-linking or intercalation.

Mitomycin. Mitomycin, produced by *Streptomyces* species, has been used principally in the study of bacteriophages, and as an antineoplastic agent. *In vitro*, it blocks DNA synthesis, causing filamentous forms, cessation of growth, and ultimate death. *In vivo* it is converted to an active hydroquinone derivative which cross-links with DNA on each of its complementary strands, preventing their separation, and halting DNA synthesis. Mitomycin has some selectivity, for it will sometimes halt bacterial cell DNA synthesis but allow the synthesis of bacteriophages.

Nalidixic Acid. Nalidixic acid, a synthetic compound, is used clinically against urinary tract infections caused by species of *Escherichia*, *Aerobacter*, and *Proteus*. Because it stops DNA synthesis, it also has been used to study the factors regulating bacterial cell division.

Griseofulvin. Griseofulvin is produced by *Penicillium griseofulvum*. It has few toxic effects, and does not elicit resistance in clinical use. It is useful in treatment of superficial mycotic infections by interference with DNA replication. Griseofulvin is given orally and is assimilated through the intestinal wall into the blood. The drug eventually becomes located in the new epithelial tissues of the skin, nails, and hair, which replace those being sloughed from fungal infection. This antibiotic thus localizes in the specific tissue area infected with dermatophytes.

Inhibitors Causing Cytoplasmic Membrane Damage

There are several antibiotics that affect one or more essential activities of microbial cytoplasmic membranes. Among those that are used clinically are polymyxin, nystatin, and amphotericin B.

Polymyxins. The polymyxins, produced by *Bacillus polymyxa*, are a group of five polypeptides, of which polymyxin B and polymyxin E (colistin) are of clinical value. They act on gram negative bacteria and are used in urinary tract infections and infections caused by resistant *Pseudomonas aeruginosa* and *Shigella* species. The polymyxins are sufficiently nephrotoxic to strictly limit their use. Polymyxins bind specifically to cytoplasmic membranes, break down the osmotic barrier, and cause the leakage of metabolites out of the cell.

Nystatin. Nystatin, produced by *Streptomyces noursei*, is a relatively nontoxic member of the polyene group of antibiotics. It is active against many fungi, particularly *Candida albicans*. This yeast-like fungus is the most common cause of intraoral mycotic infection. Nystatin binds to a sterol-containing site on cytoplasmic membranes of fungi, causing leakage. Nystatin is not active against bacteria, since the cell membranes of bacteria contain no sterol.

Amphotericin B. Amphotericin B, produced by *Streptomyces nodosus*, is also a member of the polyene group of antibiotics. It is active against many pathogenic fungi, but can be nephrotoxic to the patient. Amphotericin B, administered intravenously, reacts with a sterol-containing site on the fungal cytoplasmic membrane, causing it to leak intracellular constituents.

Metabolite Antagonists

Sulfonamides. Even though sulfonamides are not used in dental medicine except in rare instances, their discovery and development as therapeutic agents are important in a historical context. The elucidation of their antimicrobial activity, absorption and toxicity served as the forerunner for investigation of later antibiotics. The following sections are thus presented in detail, despite the limited application of sulfonamides in dental therapeutics.

Domagk, in Germany in 1932, developed Prontosil, an azo dye containing p-aminobenzenesulfonamide, which was inactive *in vitro*. It was *in vivo*, however, for with it he successfully treated experimental streptococcal infection in mice in 1935. In the same year, French investigators found that Prontosil owed its antibacterial activity in the mammalian body to the release of its p-aminobenzenesulfonamide moiety (Sulfanilamide).

Sulfanilamide itself proved to be too toxic for general therapy but its discovery stimulated a successful search for variant compounds that were antibacterial and sufficiently nontoxic for systemic human therapy. This effort resulted in the production of thousands of sulfanilamide derivatives, sulfones, and other related compounds, but only a dozen or so are useful therapeutic agents.

Sulfonamides are effective because they competitively inhibit the synthesis of folic acid. As structural analogues of p-aminobenzoic acid, an essential metabolite which is a precursor of folic acid, sulfonamides interfere with the synthesis of these compounds. In general, the sulfonamides are administered orally and only in exceptional circumstances, intravenously. Most of the sulfonamides are readily absorbed from the gastrointestinal tract, but a few are poorly absorbed. After absorption, they are well distributed to all tissues except the central nervous system.

The sulfonamides are bacteriostatic and their

inhibiting activity can be easily reversed by their dilution or removal or by the addition of p-aminobenzoic acid. Their successful use in vivo requires active phagocytosis. In vitro, they have a wide range of antibacterial activity against gram positive and gram negative bacteria. Clinically useful sulfonamides include sulfadiazine, used in the treatment of meningitis; sulfisoxazole, sulfamethoxazole, and sulfamethoxydiazine, used in the treatment of urinary tract infections; sulfadimethoxine, used in respiratory infections; and phthalylsulfathiazole and succinylsulfathiazole, used before surgery to control the intestinal flora or to treat bacillary dysentery.

Renal damage is the most common complication in sulfonamide therapy. Hypersensitivity, usually manifested as a dermatitis, may develop, particularly if sulfonamides are administered for long periods of time.

Sulfones. A class of sulfonamide derivatives, the sulfones, can be orally administered and are useful in the treatment of leprosy. Such derivatives as sodium sulfoxone, dapsone and sodium glucosulfone are used. Oral sulfone therapy usually effects clinical improvement if given for months or years, but it is not certain that it ever eliminates *Mycobacterium leprae* completely. Toxic manifestations include hemolytic anemia, methemoglobinemia, sulfhemoglobinemia, allergy, and the Jarisch-Herxheimer reaction. Another complication is that the resident bacterial flora of the patient, under long periods of treatment, becomes resistant to sulfonamides in general.

FURTHER CONSIDERATIONS OF ANTIMICROBIAL CHEMOTHERAPY IN DENTAL PRACTICE

The management of infectious diseases with antibiotic therapy is well established in dental medicine. Dental practitioners routinely utilize chemotherapeutic drugs for prophylaxis and treatment of infections. Unfortunately, a tendency has persisted among some to abuse the therapeutic knowledge accumulated in this area. Much of this casual, uninformed approach stems from the observation that many routine cases of dentally-related infection can be controlled with the empirical use of penicillin. The more intelligent management of a patient with an infection requires a complete medical history, an understanding of the etiology of the infection and a comprehension of the application of available antibiotics. These major responsibilities involve some fundamental actions and comprehensions on the part of the general dentist and specialist.

Diagnosis and Antibiotic Sensitivity Testing

A dental clinician is familiar with the discomfort, soft tissue edema, erythema, and dysfunction that classically designate a localized dentoalveolar infection. A more complete diagnosis of the problem can be reached by evaluation of the patient's overall status in regard to onset and sequence of symptoms, the presence of malaise or nausea suggesting intermittent bacteremia or septicemia, the development of palpable lymphadenopathy, the presence of a skin rash or joint pain, and the presence or absence of fever. The dentist also should consider the significance of these localized processes in relation to other factors such as very young or advanced age; preexisting cardiac, liver, or kidney disease; the presence of diabetes mellitus or steroid dependence.

A definitive diagnosis in any infectious process depends upon a microbial culture. Until recently, collection of a specimen for culture was a neglected art not only in dentistry but in other disciplines as well, primarily because "shotgun" therapy with penicillin or broad-spectrum antibiotics was apparently effective. The materials necessary for taking a culture are readily available for both aerobic and anaerobic specimens. The latter provide an oxygen-free environment for the culture material and must be used if one is to obtain the complete picture of bacterial growth within many facial infections. The disposable collection devices with appropriate culture media have a prolonged shelf life and can be obtained along with the necessary descriptive paperwork for identification from a commercial microbiology laboratory. The clinician should submit with this specimen a concise description of the site of infection, the patient's current antibiotic therapy, and the request for aerobic and/or anaerobic bacterial and/or fungal culture with antimicrobial sensitivity patterns. Many hospital and clinical laboratories also request a slide smear preparation from the infection site. The laboratory can then perform a routine stain procedure, such as the gram stain, in order to obtain an idea of the microbial forms present in the lesion at the time of culture. Procedures for obtaining and preparing samples from various types of lesions have been described in Chapter 2. When the laboratory has the specimen and requisite clinical information, microbial identification and determination of antibiotic susceptibility may proceed. The major antibiotic sensitivity procedures employed are summarized in Table 8/7. For many infections, even though antibiotic therapy would have been initiated at the time of sample collection, the practitioner should at least have a tentative identification from the laboratory within 12 to 48 hours. The dentist will then be able to better assess the value of the initial antibiotic prescribed and to modify the regimen if necessary.

Therapeutic Indication and Use

Once it has been established that continued antibiotic therapy is necessary, the proper agent

Table 8/7
Comparison of antimicrobial susceptibility tests [a]

Property	Type of Susceptibility Test			
	Dilution			Agar Disc Diffusion (Bauer-Kirby)
	Broth		Agar	
	Tube	Micro [b]		
Will give minimum inhibitory concentration	+	+	+	−
Can be used to determine lethal action of antimicrobial agent	+	+	−	−
Accurate to within ± 1 dilution	+	+	+	−
Requires relatively little effort (cost)	−	+	+ [c]	+
Information about a large number of microorganisms easily obtainable	−	+	+	+
Contamination easily recognized	−	−	+	+

[a] From G. Youmans, P. Paterson, and H. Sommers, *The Biologic and Clinical Basis of Infectious Diseases*, Ed 2. Saunders, Philadelphia, 1980.
[b] Microdilution performed in microtiter dilution plates.
[c] Will depend on number of isolates.

should be administered in an appropriate dosage for a period of time sufficient to allow destruction and removal of the infectious organisms. The patient should be monitored at frequent intervals to assure that the chosen antibiotics are effective in controlling the symptoms and course of the infection.

Prophylactic Indications

Much has been written concerning appropriate indications for antibiotic prophylaxis in dental medicine. The only definitive instances agreed upon by pharmacologists, microbiologists and clinicians are for those patients with rheumatic heart diseases or other cardiac valvular damage, and individuals with heart prostheses. At the present time there is substantial disagreement regarding chemotherapeutic coverage for circumstances involving those individuals with hip prostheses and for the prevention of post dental surgical infection. Detailed discussions dealing with the beneficial and detrimental aspects of dental and medical prophylaxis may be found by consulting specific references cited at the end of this chapter.

Factors Influencing Antibiotic Use

Superinfection. Antibiotics can suppress the normal microbial flora and may result in the development of superinfections, especially when the resistance of the host is lowered. Examples of such superinfections are oral or systemic candidiasis and staphylococcal pneumonia. Broad-spectrum agents often allow the greatest opportunities for superinfection. Organisms such as *Candida albicans*, that are not affected by routine antibiotics, are no longer held in check by the drug-sensitive resident flora, and may proliferate in a virtually uncontrolled environment. This situation can lead to microbial replacement in normal "ecological niches" with potential pathogens, culminating in an abnormally high presence of drug-insensitive organisms with resultant clinical superinfection.

Nature of Antibiotic and Host Factors. The state of activity of the infecting bacteria influences the effectiveness of antibiotics. For instance, penicillin and other antibiotics affecting cell walls require actively growing cells to be effective. The dosage of an antibiotic also is influenced by the extent of the infection and the tissues involved. For an antibiotic to be effective, a certain concentration of the antibiotic must be obtained in the circulation and in the affected tissues. This concentration is influenced by dosage, absorption, vascularity of the infected tissue, swelling, and the extent of protein binding by the drug.

In choosing an antibiotic the clinician also must consider host factors that may influence the patient's response to treatment. Whether an agent is bactericidal or bacteriostatic must be taken into consideration. Bacteriostatic antibiotics inhibit the replication and growth of the organism but depend upon the defenses of the host to actually eradicate the organism; bactericidal antibiotics interfere with the integrity of the microbial cell itself and directly kill the organism. The effectiveness of bacteriostatic antibiotics thus depends on the ability of the patient to overcome the infecting agent with his own defense mechanisms. When host defenses are altered or compromised, as in pregnant women, the elderly, steroid-dependent individuals, diabetics, patients with advanced liver disease or nutritional compromise, or individuals on prolonged steroid therapy, bacteriostatic antibiotics may prove insufficient and should not be prescribed. Toxic reactions to antibiotics also may be increased by allergies, decreased liver or kidney function, and other debilitating diseases.

Development of Microbial Resistance. The induction of resistant microorganisms to therapeu-

Table 8/8

Mechanisms for development of antimicrobial resistance

Mechanism	Examples of Antibiotics to Which Resistance Is Acquired
Induction of specific drug-Inactivating enzymes	Penicillins
	Chloramphenicol
Prevention of drug entrance into cell	Tetracyclines
	Isoniazid
Decreased affinity of drug due to alteration of receptor site	Erythromycin
	Streptomycin
	Sulfonamides
Loss of enzymes responsible for intracellular drug conversion	Flucytosine (antimycotic)
Alteration in concentration of drug receptor	Sulfonamides

Table 8/9

Representative therapeutic antibiotic combinations

Drug Combination	Clinical Efficacy
Carbenicillin or ticarcillin with tobramycin or gentamycin	Synergistic activity against *Pseudomonas aeruginosa*
Ampicillin with streptomycin	Effective against enterococcal infection (*i.e.*, *Streptococcus faecalis*)
A cephalosporin with an aminoglycoside	Effective against severe *Klebsiella pneumoniae* infections
Isoniazid with Rifampin	Therapeutic and prevents development of resistant *Mycobacterium tuberculosis*

tic drugs remains a constant threat during antibiotic treatment. The most common mechanisms of acquired resistance have been mentioned in previous sections for specific antibiotics. A brief summarization of the induction of drug resistance is presented for completeness in table 8/8.

Complications of Antibiotic Therapy. Local tissue or organ irritation may result from antibiotic therapy. This may occur in the oral cavity in response to oral administration as a stomatitis or glossitis; at the site of an intramuscular injection as an abscess; at the site of absorption in the gastrointestinal tract resulting in nausea, vomiting, and diarrhea; or at the site of elimination as a colitis or perianal lesion.

Antibiotics of value in dental medicine also may cause irritation of organ systems. The principal irritations of this type include neurotoxicity, particularly the eighth cranial nerve; nephrotoxicity; hepatotoxicity; and depression of the hematopoietic system.

In addition, allergic reactions have become increasingly frequent complications of dental-related antibiotic therapy. These reactions may occur locally as a stomatitis or dermatitis, or they may occur as systemic reactions ranging in severity from a mild reaction, such as hives, itching, and urticaria, to anaphylactic shock. Chemotherapeutic agents discussed earlier that are quite allergenic are sulfonamides, penicillin, and amphotericin. Tetracyclines are moderately allergenic, while erythromycin and nystatin are seldom allergenic.

Antibiotic Combinations. Most infections treated by general dentists and specialists are effectively managed by the judicious use of a single appropriate antibiotic. There are instances, however, in which combinations of agents are prescribed. These include acutely ill hospitalized patients with undiagnosed bacterial infections requiring broad antimicrobial coverage; cases of orofacial infection with a mixed bacterial etiology and different antibiotic susceptibility patterns; prevention of the development of resistant mutants against a single antibiotic; and the necessity for an additive or synergistic antimicrobial effect against very adaptable microorganisms. Specific examples of antibiotic combinations are given in Table 8/9.

Despite their effectiveness in certain clinical infections, the use of multiple antibiotic combinations is only recommended in circumstances when the therapeutic efficacy for a single drug is deemed unsatisfactory. In addition to possible antagonism between the agents, resulting in minimal activity, the risks for superinfection are usually greater, as well as the potential for increased toxicity reactions.

ADDITIONAL READING

ACCEPTED DENTAL THERAPEUTICS, 37th ed. 1979 American Dental Association, Council on Dental Therapeutics.

APPLEBAUM, P. C., KOORNHOF, H. J., JACOBS, M. *et al.* 1977 Multiple-Antibiotic Resistance of Pneumococci-South Africa. Morbidity and Mortality Weekly Report, **26,** 285.

ATHAR, M. A., AND WINNER, H. I. 1971 The Development of Resistance by *Candida* species to Polyene Antibiotics *In Vitro*. J Med Microbiol, **4,** 505.

BARTLETT, J. G., CHANG, T. W., GURWITH, M., GORBACH, S. L., AND ONDERDONK, A. B. 1978 Antibiotic-Associated Pseudomembranous Colitis Due to Toxin-Producing *Clostridia*. N Engl J Med, **298,** 531.

BARTLETT, J. G., CHANG, T. W. TAYLOR, N. S. AND ONDERDONK, A. B. 1979 Colitis Induced by *Clostridium difficile*. Rev Infect Dis, **1,** 370.

BARTLETT, J. G., AND O'KEEFE, P. 1979 The bacteriology of Perimandibular Space Infection. J Oral Surg, **37,** 407.

BENNETT, J. E. 1974 Chemotherapy of Systemic Mycoses: Parts I and II. N Engl J Med, **290,** 30, 320.

BENVENISTE, R., AND DAVIES, J. 1973 Mechanism of Antibiotic Resistance in Bacteria. Ann Rev Biochem,

42, 471.

CEFAMANDOLE, AND CEFOXITIN. 1979 Med Lett Drugs Ther, **21,** 13.

FINEGOLD, S. M. 1976 Laboratory Diagnosis of Anaerobic Infections. Mt Sinai H Med, **43,** 776.

GILMAN, A. G., GOODMAN, L. S., AND GILMAN, A. 1980 *The Pharmacological Basis of Therapeutics,* Ed. 6 Macmillan, New York.

GINSBERG, M., AND TAGER, I. 1980 *Practical Guide to Antimicrobial Agents.* Williams & Wilkins, Baltimore.

GOLDBERG, I. H., AND FRIEDMAN, P. A. 1971 Antibiotics and Nucleic Acids. Ann Rev Biochem, **40,** 775.

GREENWOOD, D., AND O'GRADY, F. 1975 Lysis Enhancement: A Novel Form of Interaction Between β-Lactam Antibiotics. J Med Microbiol, **8,** 205.

HANDBOOK OF ANTIMICROBIAL THERAPY. 1980 Medical Letter Inc., New Rochelle.

HEMAN-ACKAH, S. M. 1976 Comparision of Tetracycline Action of *Staphylococcus aureus* and *Escherichia coli* by Microbial Kinetics. Antimicrob Agents Chemother, **10,** 223.

HODGE, W. R., AND SCHNEIDER, L. S. 1972 A New Antibacterial Mode of Action for Sulfonamides. J Phar Sci, **61,** 142.

JACOBS, M. R., KOORNHOF, H. J., ROBINS-BROWNE, R. M., ET AL. 1978 Emergence of Multiple Resistant Pneumococci. N Engl J Med, **299,** 735.

KANNANGARA, D. W., HARAGOPAL, T., AND McQUIRTER, J. L. 1980 Bacteriology and Treatment of Dental Infections. Oral Surg, **50,** 103.

KAPLAN, E. L., ANTHONY, B. F., BISNO, A., ET AL. 1977 Prevention of bacterial endocarditis. American Heart Association Committee Report. Circulation, **56,** 139A.

KOCH, A. L. 1981 Evolution of Antibiotic Resistance Gene Function. Microbiol Rev, **45,** 355.

MONTES, L. F. 1971 Oral Amphotericin B in Superficial Candidiasis. Clin Med, **78,** 14.

NEIDLE, E. A., KROEGER, D. C., AND YAGIELA, J. A. 1980 Pharmacology and Therapeutics for Dentistry, Mosby, St. Louis.

OIKARINEN, V. J., AND MALMSTROM, M. 1972 Penicillin V Concentration in Dental Alveolar Blood after Tooth Extraction. Scand J Dent Res, **80,** 279.

OLSON, R. E., MORELLO, J. A., AND KIEFF, E. D. 1975 Antibiotic Treatment of Oral Anaerobic Infections. J Oral Surg, **33,** 619.

PETZ, L. D. 1978 Immunologic Cross-Reactivity Between Penicillins and Cephalosporins: A Review. J Infect Dis, **137,** 574.

PRATT, W. B. 1977 *Chemotherapy of Infection.* Oxford University Press, New York.

REHAL, J. J., JR. 1978 Antibiotic Combinations: The Clinical Relevance of Synergy and Antagonism. Medicine, **57,** 179.

SABISTON, C. B., JR., AND GOLD, W. A. 1974 Anaerobic bacteria in oral infections. Oral Surg, **38,** 187.

SABISTON, C. B., JR., GRIGSBY, W. R. AND SEGERSTROM, N. 1976 Bacterial Study of Pyogenic Infections of Dental Origin. Oral Surg, **41,** 430.

SCHUEN, N. J., PANZER, J. D., AND ATKINSON, W. H. 1974 A Comparison of Clindamycin and Penicillin V in the Treatment of Oral Infections. J Oral Surg, **32,** 503.

SEVERIN, M. J., AND WILEY, J. L. 1976 Change in Susceptibility of Group B Streptococci to Pennicillin G from 1968 through 1975. Antimicrob Agents Chemother, **10,** 380.

SOMMERS, H. M. 1980 Drug Susceptibility Testing *In Vitro*: Monitoring of Antimicrobial Therapy. In *The Biologic and Clinical Basis of Infectious Diseases*, p. 782, edited by G. P. Youmans, P. Y. Paterson and H. M. Sommers. Saunders, Philadelphia.

THOMPSON, R. L. 1977 The Cephalosporins. Mayo Clin Proc, **52,** 625.

THORNSBERRY, C., GAVAN, T. L. AND GERLACH, E. H. 1977 Cumitech G: *New Developments in Antimicrobial Agent Susceptibility Testing.* Coordinating Ed., J. C. Sherris. American Society for Microbiology, Washington, D.C.

TURNER, J. E. MOORE, D. W., AND SHAW, B. S. 1975 Prevalence and antibiotic susceptibility of organisms isolated from acute soft-tissue abscesses secondary to dental caries. Oral Surg, **39,** 848.

WILKOWSKE, C. J. 1977 The Penicillins. Mayo Clin Proc **52,** 616.

WISOTZKY, J. 1972 Effect of Tetracycline on the Phosphorescence of Teeth. J Dent Res, **51,** 7.

WOODS, R. 1978 Pyogenic Dental Infections: A Ten-Year Review. Aus Dent J, **23,** 107.

PART 4

INFECTION AND RESISTANCE

chapter 9

Host-Parasite Interactions

Chris H. Miller

PARASITISM

Introduction

The association of a microorganism with another living entity is called parasitism. This is a natural outcome of the struggle for existence by living organisms. From the constant interactions of microbes with other life and with the physical and chemical environment, the microbial world has developed into life forms with differing requirements for growth, reproduction and survival. As a result microorganisms demonstrate varying degrees of dependency upon parasitism, and when free-living or parasitic microbes associate with a potential host there are several possible outcomes as shown in table 9/1.

Host-Parasite Associations

The human body is constantly bombarded with microorganisms from the environment with one of several reactions occurring. The intruder may be immediately removed in host secretions or excretions, or destroyed by nonspecific host defense activities after a brief residence. This is the fate of most free-living types of microorganisms that find themselves translocated from the general environment to the human body because they are unsuited for parasitic life in that host.

Other species find specific sites on or within the host suitable for growth and multiplication. The most successful of these parasites are those which exist in harmony with the host and cause no damage. Such associations result in establishment of the indigenous or normal body flora. With some other parasites the growth and multiplication acci-

dently cause damage to the host resulting in a violent reaction called infectious disease. These types of parasites are called pathogens.

In the most unfavorable relationship between host and pathogen, the host dies from being unable to limit the destructive activities of the pathogen. Alternatively, in encounters between a host and pathogen, the host becomes ill and recovers, whereupon the pathogen may be eliminated by the host's adaptive reactions or it may persist in the state of truce that we call the carrier state.

Host Adaptations

In an individual, the state of pathogenicity has evolved into a host-parasite complex owing to adaptations of the host. Generally, pathogens are not maintained solely by transfer from diseased to healthy individuals. It is also a great principle that health prevails only so long as the host adaptations are able to keep the parasite in check. If host adaptations become community-wide over a number of generations, as by hereditary selection, immune responses, and cultural changes, the severity of the disease declines, the carrier state becomes more general, and the parasite may disappear.

Parasite Mutations

A parasite may adjust to an environment by mutation, losing some of its undesirable characteristics. It is not certain how significant this factor has been under natural conditions; although, it has been demonstrated experimentally very often.

Facultative Parasites

A number of microorganisms find themselves equally well adapted to existence when they are

Table 9/1
Possible stages in the development of parasitism

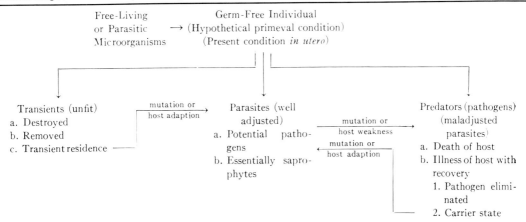

free in the general environment or as harmless parasites within a host. For example, certain species of *Clostridium* are primarily inhabitants of soil or animal and human intestinal tracts and cause no harm as long as they remain there. However, under appropriate conditions they can be potent pathogens, producing tetanus or gas gangrene.

Indigenous Parasites

Few of the indigenous parasites of man are found elsewhere except as parasites of other animals and possibly a few plants. This situation appears to have come about through progressive loss (possibly by mutations of the parasites) of functions that could be carried out by the host, and by elimination of nutritionally facultative parasites from the general environment by the antibiotic activities of other microorganisms. The first of the above-mentioned mechanisms is the most likely for the development of viruses and of such transitional forms as the rickettsiae, which are special types of parasitic bacteria. Similarly, it would be difficult for bacteria such as streptococci and lactobacilli to meet their exceedingly complex nutritional requirements in many environments outside their natural hosts. For example, extensive surveys have shown that *Streptococcus mutans* is worldwide in distribution but is found only in the dentulous mouths of man and some lower animals or on saliva-contaminated environmental surfaces. The meningococcus has relatively simple nutritional requirements, but it can carry on its vital functions only within a narrow range of temperature approximating that of the animal body, and it has a very limited ability to survive in an inactive state. On the other hand, *Escherichia coli* which comprises a large fraction of all sorts of animal feces can synthesize everything it needs from simple media. Its pH and temperature requirements are not critical within a broad range, and it can grow anaerobically as well as aerobically.

These needs can be met in a variety of environments. However, the colon bacillus is not found in soils and waters not recently contaminated with animal feces; it actually disappears quickly from farm soil, presumably owing to the antibiotic activities of the other microbial residents, for it survives and grows if the soil is autoclaved. It is likely that the colon bacillus cannot compete successfully in the open and, as an evolutionary adjustment, has taken refuge in the protected environment of the animal gut.

Microbial Steady State

An individual normally harbors an indigenous parasitic flora characteristic for his species and environment (table 9/2). Environmental saprophytes (free-living organisms) rarely get a foothold. By inherent and adaptive mechanisms, summarized as "resistance," the host holds in check the pathogenic potentialities (virulence) of the parasites. Infectious disease, then, is a combination of the damage to the host's tissues plus the host's adaptive reactions that occur when a parasite gets out of control, owing either to an increase in microbial virulence or to a decrease in the host's resistance.

Probably no microorganisms can be considered nonpathogenic. Under appropriate conditions (*e.g.*, with a compromised host or with excessive contamination) essentially any species may cause varying degrees of damage to the host. In addition, animals reared in a germ-free environment are surprisingly susceptible to generalized invasion by some of the common "nonpathogens," such as lactobacilli and enterococci, in doses that are entirely innocuous for normal germ-bearing animals of the same species which evidently have built up a tolerance. Dosage, then, is another important determinant. All of these relationships between parasite and host may be summarized in an equation which symbolizes the relative nature of health and disease.

Table 9/2
The biological steady state and infectious disease

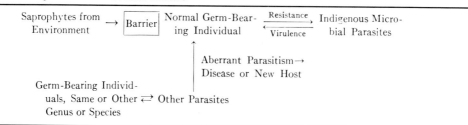

$$\text{Disease or Health} = \frac{\text{Virulence of Parasite} \times \text{Dosage}}{\text{Resistance of Host}}$$

Aberrant Parasitism

If a parasite wanders from its usual habitat into one it is not accustomed to, it may behave as a predator (Table 9/1). This is termed aberrant parasitism. The parasite may simply stray from one part of its host to another to produce disease (such as a bacterial endocarditis caused from a bacteremia with an oral organism) or the parasite may be transfered from a symptomless carrier to an uninfected individual of the same species. The result has been seen most dramatically whenever a virgin population has been infected. Thus, the introduction of measles into the South Sea Islands decimated the native populations. Of epidemiological interest, because of the possible development of new host species, is the transfer of a parasite from its regular host species to a new one, commonly with the production of severe disease. Representative examples can be found among all forms of microorganisms. For example, the rickettsiae are primarily harmless parasites of the intestinal cells of various arthropods, but many of them cause serious disease when transferred to man by the bites of these insects. The initial wandering of a parasite from a well-adjusted association to a foreign host tends to be a biological dead end, since effective mechanisms for transmission within the new host group usually do not exist.

Host Benefits

The universal occurrence of parasitism naturally has raised the question whether the parasitic biota has become indispensable to its host. Although many instances of useful function by parasites appear possible, it is difficult to actually demonstrate the beneficial aspects of the indigenous flora. Man probably derives most of his vitamin K from his intestinal bacteria and some individuals can supplement the supply of B-vitamins by absorption from the same source. The successful rearing of germ-free animals provided a proper diet demonstrates, however, that the microbial functions are dispensable even though they may play a useful role under natural conditions. It also is possible that small numbers of organisms which enter the bloodstream through small breaks in the mucous membranes of the body openings could induce an immunogenic response. If the antigens from such organisms are closely related to those of given pathogens (*e.g.*, common antigens among *Streptococcus mitis*, *Streptococcus sanguis* and the pathogen *Streptococcus pneumoniae*) cross-reacting antibodies may provide some degree of protection against the invading pathogen. This may prevent potential pathogens from establishing in the oral cavity in significant numbers if there are cross-reacting antigens. Secretory-IgA also is produced against some indigenous species. Indigenous species also may antagonize the colonization or growth of some invading pathogens expressing the "first come-first served" adage. For example, it is very difficult to establish a new strain of *S. mutans* in the mouth which is already colonized with an indigenous strain of that organism. The indigenous strain has a selective advantage for specific colonization sites. In addition, the suppression of the indigenous bacterial flora with antibiotics can result in the proliferation of potentially harmful organisms resistant to the antibiotics, as sometimes occurs in candidasis or colitis. Thus, the normal indigenous flora apparently assists in keeping some potentially dangerous organisms in check. Since it is not appropriate to rear normal humans in a germ-free state, the potential benefits to man of his indigenous flora will have to be inferred from the indirect types of evidence available.

HEALTH VERSUS DISEASE

The concepts, health and disease, are reciprocal. Each is conventionally defined by the absence of the other. However, no independent absolute standard of either health or disease is possible. Therefore, we can only evaluate the degree to which the individual adapts to and functions effectively in his relation to his natural environment. The degree to which these adaptations are effective is a measure of the well being of the individual. The average behavior of a species in a given environment describes the reference standard of its normal health.

Such "average" or "normal" is of course not necessarily the optimum.

When microorganisms first associate with a host, the host is said to be *contaminated*. If the microorganisms establish themselves and grow and multiply for a period of time, the host is said to be *infected*. If the infection causes damage, the host is said to have an *infectious disease*. Thus, an infectious disease is an impairment of host function by an infecting microorganism. With a few exceptions, infectious diseases are caused by obligate parasites. Yet, only a minor fraction of the obligate parasites carried by every form of life is involved in the production of overt disease. Conversely, a variety of potentially pathogenic microorganisms can be isolated at any time from healthy individuals. Generally, infectious disease is an infrequent by-product of the parasitization. The fact that parasitization is universal, whereas overt disease is exceptional, means that the host-parasite relationship tends to be an equilibrium. Thus, consideration of those factors which maintain or disturb this equilibrium are important to the understanding of health versus disease.

DETERMINANTS OF HEALTH AND DISEASE

Introduction

We can group determinants that set the status of the individual into those of the physical environment, social environment (including psychological determinants), the indivdiual's constitution, and the biological environment, particularly the microbiological (table 9/3). The *arrows* imply multiple determinants in each case. The use of *double arrows* pointing in the opposite directions symbolizes the fact that not only do the determinants operate on the individual but also that he can alter the nature or effects of the determinants by his adaptive mechanisms. Man especially has brought adaptation to the point that he adjusts the environment to his advantage, rather than merely adjusting himself to it.

Determinants

Physical Determinants. The physical environment comprises such features as geography, climate, season of the year, and such derived factors as the availability and composition of food and water. Geography, for example, determines the availability of minerals. The relationships of fluoride to dental caries and iodine to thyroid dysfunction are familiar. The seasonal associations of respiratory diseases with winter and poliomyelitis with summer are well known. Streptococcal infections and their rheumatic sequelae seem to be more

Table 9/3

The individual in relation to the determinants of his internal (constitutional) and external environments

Constitutional
Determinants

$\updownarrow$

Determinants
of the Physical $\rightleftharpoons$ The Individual $\rightleftharpoons$ Microbial
Environment   Determinants

$\updownarrow$ $\updownarrow$

Determinants of the   Other Micro-
Social Environment   organisms

serious in the semiarid mountain regions of the western United States than in the low-lying humid areas of the south. Mycotic diseases, on the other hand, become more prevalent in the south.

Cultural Determinants. Under natural conditions, adaptations to the physical environment usually take the form of evolution by selection. We are more concerned here with adaptations of a cultural nature, such as housing, clothing, diet, public sanitation and personal hygiene, occupational conditions, degree of exposure to cases of disease or carriers, and exposure to deleterious chemical and physical agents. The profound possibilities of psychological factors for both benefit and detriment are recognized but are beyond the scope of the present discussion. Cultural habits can be very important. A diet high in marine fish appears to provide beneficial amounts of fluoride and possibly other trace elements. On the other hand, modern preference for diets high in refined sucrose conduces to dental caries. Undoubtedly, the worldwide trend away from agrarian society to urban industrial society has epidemiological consequences that we do not yet suspect.

Constitutional Determinants. Constitutional determinants generally refer to the character of the basic biological equipment with which the individual is born. Specifically, one refers to the factors associated with race, sex, inherent immunity, familial tendencies, mental endowment, and anatomical anomalies. The constitution, however, changes as the individual develops. The physiology changes with age and so does the susceptibility to various infections. The common "childhood" diseases are generally more severe in the adult who escaped them earlier. However, in some instances increasing resistance occurs with age, probably the result of immunization by previous subclinical experience with the given organism or with an organism conferring cross-immunity. Previous experience with disease also may weaken the general resistance by imposing too great a strain. Man can exercise some control over his constitution. Immunity can be built up by artificial immunization (vaccination). Anatomical anomalies and the effects of some diseases can be corrected surgically. Deficiencies such as diabetes and thyroid dysfunction can be met medically. The general well being can be fostered by our knowledge of diet and personal hygiene, and it can be undermined by neglect of this knowledge.

Biological Determinants. The biological environment includes the macroflora and fauna of the external environment as reservoirs and vectors of potentially pathogenic microorganisms. The external and internal microbiota also are important biological determinants. The external microbiota varies quantitatively and qualitatively from region to region. It is sparse in arid regions, at high altitudes, and in frigid climates. It is more abundant and active in humid tropical areas. It probably differs markedly from actively cultivated agricultural regions to the midst of a modern industrial city. The internal (parasitic) micribiota, however, is basically characteristic of the host species, with regional differences superimposed. Both external and internal microbiota are subject to alteration, by the level of public and personal hygiene, by changing agricultural practices (*e.g.*, substitution of chemical fertilizers for animal and human excreta), and by changing customs (the replacement of the horse by the automobile as a means of transportation lowers the incidence of tetanus spores in an urban environment). A thoroughly applied program of active immunization reduces the incidence of the homologous parasite in the community. Another important determinant of the microbial flora is interaction with other microorganisms, which may take the form of indifference (commensalism), antagonism (antibiosis), mutual benefit (symbiosis), or cooperation (synergism), to produce results that are not brought about by any one of them alone.

HUMAN MICROBIOTA

Introduction

In what is considered to be a state of health, the human host normally exists in some reasonable equilibrium with the bacteria, fungi, viruses and protozoa which compose its normal resident microbiota. Under such conditions the resident microorganisms are parasites and they establish either a commensal, symbiotic, or synergistic relationship with each other and with the host. These parasites may establish an antagonistic or antibiotic relationship with other members of the microbiota, which helps to establish an equilibrium within the microbiota and between the host microbiota and microorganisms introduced into it.

However, as long as the resident microbial flora maintains a reasonable equilibrium with the human

host, they are parasites and the host is considered to be healthy (*i.e.*, there is absence of clinical disease).

If host resistance decreases, the equilibrium between host and members of the resident microbiota may be upset and a clinically discernible infection (disease) develops in the host. The parasite causing the disease is then a pathogen. Such an infection is termed endogenous, for it is caused by microorganisms that are components of the normal human microbiota. The principal infectious diseases of the oral cavity, such as dental caries and periodontal disease, are endogenous infections in that the microorganisms causing them are normal residents of this region. Many infectious diseases are exogenous in origin, however, for they are introduced into the normal human microbiota at some point, where they invade the host and interfere with his normal functions. In a human infectious disease it must be emphasized that the infection usually takes place among mixed microbiota present on or in the area of the human body where the pathogen was introduced. This, as well as the actions of the causative agent, influences the course of the disease. An understanding of the normal microbiota of the body areas of the host is required for an understanding of the complex situation that exists in health or disease. In the following sections the indigenous microbiota of the human is discussed, as well as the factors which affect the growth of microorganisms in the different body areas.

Skin

The skin sustains a relatively abundant and somewhat constant microbial flora that is limited to a relatively few species when compared to the microbiota of other body areas. The outer surface or stratum corneum is a rough surface whose scales are constantly being shed into the environment, carrying some of the resident microorganisms with them. The deeper layers contain sebaceous glands and sweat glands, whose ducts pierce the skin, and hair follicles, which also pass through the skin. The sweat glands secrete a saline solution that contains such nutrients as amino acids, carbohydrates and vitamins for bacteria and fungi. An adequate but saline water source is available over most of the skin areas. The average temperature of the skin is maintained at 90 to 93 F (32 to 34 C), near the optimum for most pathogenic microorganisms. Maintenance of the skin microbiota is interfered with by several factors. Sebum, secreted by the sebaceous glands, is composed mostly of lipids that are broken down into fatty acids that are antibacterial to many microorganisms that might otherwise find the skin a suitable habitat. Another factor is the antibiotic activity of the predominantly gram positive flora, especially against gram negative bacteria. The slight acidity (pH 5.2 to 5.8) of the skin also may inhibit prospective microbial residents.

The skin is quite selective in which microorganisms establish temporary or permanent residence. Some fungi and yeast are common residents of the surface of the skin. These include the dermatophytes which are principally species of *Microsporum*, *Trichophyton*, and *Epidermophyton*. The two principal bacterial inhabitants are *Propionibacterium acnes* (*Corynebacterium acnes*) and *Staphylococcus epidermidis*. Although *Mima* species and gram negative bacilli are considered to be skin residents, the skin microbiota is predominantly gram positive and is antagonistic to prospective gram negative residents.

The density of the skin microbiota varies from one region of the integument to another. For example, growth is sparse on the trunk and upper arms and heavy in the axilla, scalp, face, and neck. The average density of microorganisms of the back is about 300 per cm^2, while that of the scalp is about 1.5 million per cm^2, and as much as 2.5 million per cm^2 on the skin of the axilla of the male. On a weight basis, it has been estimated that the microbial population is about 530 million per g of skin scurf.

Mouth

The oral cavity is the residence of a wider variety of microorganisms than any other body area. This complex ecosystem is influenced by the morphology of the mouth, the state of oral hygiene, the nature of saliva and its rate of flow, the abrasiveness and nature of the diet, and the physiological state and health of the individual. While all these factors influence the nature and extent of the oral microbiota, saliva is the major mediating factor. Important salivary factors include rate of flow, viscosity, mineral content, ionic strength, buffering capacity, E_h, pH, essential metabolites, presence or absence of salivary gases, the organic content, and antibacterial properties (lysozyme, secretory antibodies, leukocytes).

The oral microbiota is composed of four primary ecosystems: the tongue; the tooth crown; the gingival crevice, and saliva. Organisms also colonize the buccal and gingival mucosa. Since each of these ecosystems provides a unique environment, the relative numbers and types of certain species can vary from site to site within the same mouth. Thus, some microbes preferentially colonize only certain sites while other species are widely distributed in the mouth. For example, *Streptococcus sanguis* is commonly found within coronal and gingival crevice plaque, on the tongue and buccal mucosa and in saliva while *Streptococcus mutans* is most commonly associated with only the tooth surface.

Approximately 200 billion microbial cells are present in a gram of wet coronal dental plaque. This is an incomprehensible number. In fact, it takes about 6342 years to count to 200 billion at the rate of one numeral every second. Gingival crevice plaque contains a similar concentration of microbes while each epithelial cell on the surface of the tongue and buccal mucosa contains about 110 and 20 microbial cells, respectively. Since whole saliva bathes all of the microbe-laden oral surfaces and is constantly swallowed and replenished with bacteria-free saliva from the various salivary glands, its microbial concentration varies greatly with an average of a few hundred million per milliliter.

Over 80 different microbial species have been recovered at one time or another from the human mouth. On the average about 35 to 40 species are normal oral residents as described later. While the predominant organisms in the mouth are *Steptococcus*, *Actinomyces*, and *Veillonella*, other types include lactobacilli and other gram positive rods or filaments, *Fusobacterium*, *Bacteroides* and other gram negative rods, *Neisseria* and *Branhamella*, micrococci, spirochetes and occasionally yeasts, other fungi, protozoa, viruses and mycoplasmas.

Gastrointestinal Tract

The gastrointestinal tract sustains variable numbers of microorganisms that are consistent with the various regions. Depending on the time of the sampling, the esophagus might contain few bacteria, or an abundant flora that is similar to that of saliva and/or the contaminants of food and drink. At best, however, most, if not all, esophageal bacteria are transients, and the microbial flora fluctuates widely.

The stomach is not a very suitable environment for the growth of most microorganisms due to the high acidity of stomach fluids and the motility of the stomach, which empties itself rather rapidly at periodic intervals following a meal. With the intake of a meal, the microbial flora consists mostly of the salivary bacteria and the contaminants in food and drink. At other times the empty stomach contains a reduced salivary microbiota derived mostly from the swallowing of saliva. It is estimated that about 1 to 2 g of salivary bacteria are swallowed daily.

In the duodenum and the upper jejunum, the intestinal content is also acidic (pH 5 to 6), restricting the microbial population. Below the upper levels of the intestinal tract, the microbiota increases in numbers and complexity, reaching a maximum in the large intestine. Here the intestinal microbiota is predominantly gram negative. Obligate anaerobic bacteria find the lower bowel suitable for growth and counts average more than 10^{10} per g of feces. Facultative and aerobic organisms are also present but in lesser numbers. In the final stages of the digestive process in the lower bowel, the feces is comprised of about 30% bacteria. Over 90% of the fecal flora consists of *Bacteroides* and *Bifidobacterium*. Other principal residents are *Fusobacterium*, *Eubacterium* and *Peptostreptococcus*; with lesser numbers of *Propionibacterium*, *Escherichia coli*, *Clostridium*, *Lactobacillus*, enterococci, streptococci, and others.

Upper Respiratory Tract

Many microbes are filtered from the air as it passes through the upper respiratory tract. Since most of these transient species are trapped on the mucous membranes and swallowed, the sinuses, bronchi and lungs remain bacteria free under normal conditions. Normal residents in the nose include various gram positive rods and filamentous forms and staphylococci. Occasional residents are species of *Haemophilus*, *Neisseria*, and *Branhamella*, as well as pneumococci and moraxellae. The microbiota of the nasopharynx resembles that of the nose, being chiefly staphylococci, streptococci, diphtheroids, and neisseriae, whereas that of the lower pharynx resembles the salivary flora. Here are found most of the microorganisms of the oral cavity, although anaerobic forms are not abundant.

Eye

The eye is remarkably free of a complex resident microbiota probably due to the washing action and high lysozyme content of tears. Residents consist of staphylococci and one or more types of gram positive pleomorphic rods sometimes referred to as diphtheroids. Streptococci, neisseriae and others may be present as transients.

Genitourinary Tract

The microbiota of the male external genitalia includes yeast, gram positive bacilli, gram negative bacilli, cocci, fusiforms, spirochetes, and *Mycobacterium smegmatis*. The microbiota of the vagina varies with age and the physiological conditions. For a month or so after birth, the vaginal epithelium accumulates glycogen as a result of transferred maternal estrogen. This glycogen provides a readily available fermentable substrate for the acidogenic and aciduric flora (principally lactobacilli). Prolif-

eration of these organisms results in a low pH which inhibits growth of many microbial types. As the estrogen is excreted, the utilized glycogen is not replaced and the acidogenic flora decreases. This yields a more alkaline environment and a shift in the types of microbes which can flourish. After puberty, when glycogen is again present, the acidogenic and aciduric flora returns. Microorganisms found in the adult vagina are lactobacilli, diphtheroids, micrococci, staphylococci, streptococci, yeast and an occasional gram negative coccus or rod.

ADDITIONAL READING

BARTELS, H. A. 1961 Host-Parasite Relationships in the Oral Cavity and Their Clinical Significance. N Y State Dent J, **27**, 221.

BURNET, F. M. 1962 *Natural History of Infectious Disease.* Ed. 3. Cambridge University Press, Cambridge, England.

COCKBURN, A. 1963 *The Evolution and Eradication of Infectious Diseases.* The Johns Hopkins Press, Baltimore.

DELOUVOIS, J., STANLEY, V. C., LEASK, B. G. S., AND HURLEY, R. 1975 Ecological Studies of the Microbial Flora of the Female Lower Genital Tract. Proc R Soc Med, **68**, 269.

DUBOS, R. J. 1965 *Biochemical Determinants of Microbial Diseases.* Harvard University Press, Cambridge, Mass.

GUBA, A. M., JR., MULLIKEN, J. B., AND HOOPES, J. E. 1975 The Selection of Antibiotics for Human Bites of the Hand. Plast Reconstr Surg, **56**, 538.

KLOOS, W. E., ZIMMERMAN, R. J., AND SMITH, R. F. 1976 Preliminary Studies on the Characterization and Distribution of *Staphyloccus* and *Micrococcus* Species on Animal Skin. Appl Environ Microbiol, **31**, 53

LAPAGE, G. 1958 *Parasitic Animals*, Ed. 3 W. Heffer and Sons, Cambridge, England.

LIEBERMAN, J., (Ed.). 1958 Animal Disease and Human Health. Ann N Y Acad Sic, **70**, 279.

NOBLE, W. C. 1975 Skin as a Microhabitat. Postgrad Med J, **51**, 151.

ROSEBURY, T. 1962 *Microorganisms Indigenous to Man.* McGraw-Hill, New York.

SMITH, T. 1934 *Parasitism and Disease.* Princeton University Press, Princeton, N. J.

SOCIETY FOR GENERAL MICROBIOLOGY. 1964 Symposium: *Microbial Behaviour, "In Vivo" and "In Vitro."* Cambride University Press, New York.

SKINNER, F. A., AND CARR, J. G. 1974. *The Normal Microbial Flora of Man.* Academic Press, New York.

RUTGERS UNIVERSITY, BUREAU OF BIOLOGICAL RESEARCH. 1960 *Host Influence on Parasite Physiology.* Rutgers University Press, New Brunswick, N. Y.

SIMON, H. J. 1960 *Attenuated Infection. The Germ Theory in Contemporary Perspective.* Lippincott, Philadelphia.

chapter 10

Microbial Pathogenicity and Innate Host Resistance

Chris H. Miller

INTRODUCTION

Pathogenicity is the ability of a microorganism to cause disease. Within the realm of pathogenicity, microbes express degrees of disease-producing ability referred to as virulence. For example, a highly virulent microorganism may cause damage to the host at low dosages while another pathogenic microorganism of low virulence may damage the host only at high dosage levels. In addition, a single pathogenic species actually may contain strains which are highly virulent, of intermediate virulence or avirulent depending upon changes in specific disease producing properties.

As described earlier, the pathogenicity of even a highly virulent microorganism may not be expressed as clinically detectable damage in a host if the host resistance is sufficient. Thus, health and disease are functions of virulence and dosage of the infecting organism versus resistance of the host.

DEVELOPMENT OF AN INFECTIOUS DISEASE

The infectious disease process is very complex and many events must take place before the virulence of an infecting microorganism is actually expressed as clinically detectable damage in the host. This becomes evident upon examination of the stages in the development of an infectious disease (Table 10/1). Of particular importance is that the control of infectious diseases can be approached by interrupting or preventing any one of these stages.

Causative Agent

The requirement for a causative agent in the development of an infectious disease is obvious. The factors listed in table 10/1 in general apply to all types of potentially pathogenic microorganisms; bacteria, viruses, fungi and protozoa. The sources of the causative agents are most often previously infected hosts who are obviously ill or who are natural or asymptomatic transient or chronic carriers of the agent. The inanimate enviroment also may serve as a source of infectious disease agents.

Transmissibility

While microbial properties related to the transmission of pathogens between suitable hosts are not necessarily called pathogenic properties, the transmissibility itself is a vital function of most human disease agents. It is not only important to the parasite which must occasionally find a new host, but also to the human host in relation to the communicability or spread of infectious diseases. Since many human pathogens are obligate parasites, they can survive as a species only if they have a mode of transmission to the new host, a mode of entry into the new host, ability to survive for some period of time within the host and a mode of escape from the host. These stages constitute a typical parasitic life cycle.

While many protozoan and metazoan parasites have intricate life cycles, most fungi, bacteria, and viruses have relatively simple developmental stages. They are transferred, most often from host-to-host of the same species by (a) direct contact, (b) droplet infection (inhalation of droplets from the upper respiratory tract), (c) ingestion (in food and drink contaminated directly or indirectly with infectious materials), and (d) indirect contact with contaminated objects. Some viruses and a few bacteria are transmitted by the bites of arthropods, in whom the agent multiplies and may persist by transovarial transfer.

The importance of a suitable exit for the parasite from a host is well illustrated in cases of aberrant parasitism. Tularemia, brucellosis, rabies, and trichinosis in man are all dead ends for the respective parasites, for there is no effective natural exit and means of transfer from man-to-man. Civilized man is an ineffective host for many insect-borne diseases because his cultural habits minimize con-

Table 10/1
Stages in the development of an infectious disease

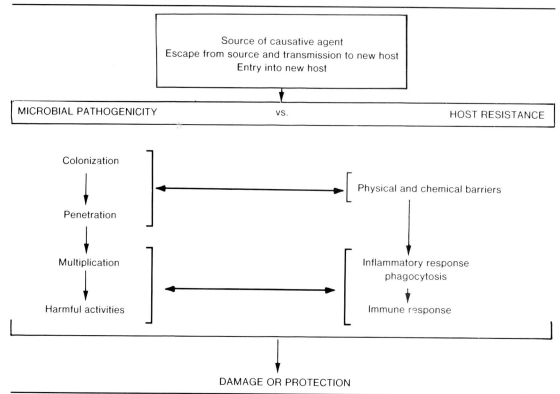

tact with the vectors, and there are no other means for the respective agents to make exit and be transferred to an uninfected individual.

Expression of Virulence Properties

The interaction of pathogens with the host varies from complete destruction of the microorganisms to a complete overwhelming of the host. In between these extremes is the near stalemate that occurs in chronic or residual infections by pathogens. The pathogenic properties of the contaminating microorganisms are categorized by their involvement in (a) colonization of the host, (b) penetration of the host tissues, and (c) damage to host tissue. The host defense system may be directed against any of these groups of pathogenic properties and is divided into two categories (a) innate or nonacquired body defenses and (b) acquired (immunological) body defenses. Specific microbial pathogenic properties and host resistance properties will be described in the following sections.

PATHOGENIC PROPERTIES OF MICROBES

Colonization

The term colonization is synonymous with infection—the establishment and survival of a parasite on or within a host. As described earlier, microbial colonization of man does not always lead to infectious disease as is evident by the existent indigenous body floras. Colonization is, however, a prerequisite for subsequent damage to the body by most pathogens. Food poisoning with microbial toxins would be an exception. This does not require colonization but only ingestion of the harmful products produced in food by growth of some clostridia and staphylococci. Nevertheless, colonization includes initial attachment to a body surface and subsequent multiplication within the body. Thus, attachment mechanisms and ability to multiply within the body are considered as important pathogenic properties of disease-producing microorganisms.

Attachment. Although some pathogens associate with the body by being mechanically trapped on a surface or by being accidently injected or implanted into underlying tissues, most must attach to and multiply on mucous membranes (or teeth in the case of *Streptococcus mutans*) to become established. In doing so they must compete with the indigenous flora already present and with the natural body defense mechanisms active at that site (*e.g.*, cleansing action of saliva, tears, respiratory secretion, urine). Persistent colonization of mucous membranes which continually undergo desquamation presents additional problems. It involves initial attachment, multiplication, dislodgement of the progeny from desquamated epithelial cells and reattachment to newly exposed epithelium.

Microbial attachment to body surfaces or tissues does have some degree of specificity. This helps explain why some organisms colonize or damage only certain tissues of the body. This has long been recognized for many viral diseases and is becoming quite obvious for many bacterial diseases as well. Specific structures or polymers on the bacterial surface are involved in the attachment mechanisms of many potential human pathogens including *Streptococcus mutans*, *Streptococcus pyogenes*, *Neisseria gonorrhoeae*, *Vibrio cholerae*, *Salmonella typhimurium*, enteropathogenic *Escherichia coli*, *Klebsiella pneumoniae*, *Bacteroides asaccharolyticus*, *Fusobacterium nucleatum*, *Corynebacterium parvum*, *Actinomyces viscosus*, *Actinomyces naeslundii*, and mycoplasmas. For example, gonorrhoea is confined to the mucous-secreting epithelial surfaces of man and cannot even be established on such surfaces in animals. Thus, the initial attachment is very specific and involves interaction between specific receptor sites on human epithelial surfaces and pili on the surface of the gonococci.

Multiplication. Multiplication is essential for colonization. It replenishes those attached cells which are removed by the local host defense mechanisms. Multiplication begins soon after attachment and continues as long as suitable conditions exist even after the pathogen may penetrate colonized mucous membranes. The successful colonizer must be able to derive all of its nutritional and physical requirements for growth from a specific host enviroment. Since the mere numbers of a pathogen within a host can determine whether damage to the host will occur (by overwhelming host defenses), the ability to multiply within the host is considered as a virulence determinant. It appears that most pathogens that attach to host surfaces also can multiply there. With human viruses the initial attachment or adsorption to a host cell is an essential step for subsequent multiplication of the virus within that cell. Since a specific virus usually can attach to only certain types of host cells, subsequent multiplication at the initial site of attachment is a common event in viral infections. The relationship is less clear for bacteria but some pathogens may have specific properties which favor their growth *in vivo*. For example, iron is required for growth by bacteria but may not be in a usable form within the host tissue fluids, since it is commonly bound to the protein transferrin. Some pathogenic bacteria such as *Mycobacterium tuberculosis* and some strains of *E. coli* have special iron scavenging systems which may overcome this problem. The tubercle bacillus produces a substance called mycobactin which releases iron from transferrin, and the *E. coli* produces a catechol which can compete with transferrin for iron binding.

Penetration

Viruses and most bacterial pathogens which colonize mucous membranes must penetrate this surface and multiply in the underlying tissues before host damage occurs. Exceptions in the bacterial world are some enteric pathogens like the cholera organisms which colonize the intestinal mucosa, multiply on the surface and produce toxic substances which then penetrate the tissue and cause damage. Little is known about specific mechanisms of microbial penetration. Viruses enter host cells by a process similar to phagocytosis or by direct penetration of the plasma membrane. Bacteria may produce enzymes (*e.g.*, lecithinase, proteases) or other substances (*e.g.*, endotoxin) which cause lysis or degeneration of the host cell, and the bacteria then proceed into the tissue space previously occupied by the host cells. Penetration of intestinal mucosa by *Shigella* is dependent upon the presence and chemical composition of lipopolysaccharide (endotoxin). Some bacteria may produce enzymes like hyaluronidase which may destroy intercellular material and separate the host cells. Other bacteria such as *N. gonorrhoeae* actually may enter epithelial cells through a process similar to phagocytosis and then further invade the epithelium by repeated cycles of exocytosis and phagocytosis.

Resistance to Host Defenses

Successfully virulent pathogens must be able to at least partially withstand preexisting and subsequently mobilized body defense systems. This microbial capacity is especially important in the early stages of an infection when, in most cases, the protective reactions of the host are heavily weighted against the few invading organisms.

Resistance to Phagocytosis. Phagocytosis is one of the most important components of the innate body defense systems. Therefore, pathogens which resist phagocytosis are allowed to accumulate in the body at a less restricted rate. Many of the key factors related to the virulence and pathogenic mechanisms of bacteria involve surface components.

Early investigators observed capsules surrounding a variety of pathogenic bacteria as they occurred in infectious exudates and inferred that these structures were important for virulence. In most instances the capsules consist of polysaccharides in the form of a hydrophilic gel, with a distinct chemical composition for each type of organism. However, peptide and glycoprotein capsules are present on some bacteria. *Streptococcus pneumoniae* is a representative example of a bacterium with a polysaccharide capsule. Virulent strains have capsules and resist phagocytosis (engulfment). The larger the capsule, the more virulent the pneumococcus. Mutants that have lost the power to make capsules also have lost virulence and resistance to phagocytosis. Digestion of the capsule by a specific enzyme leaves the cell viable but avirulent and susceptible to phagocytosis. Ingestion and subsequent intracellular destruction by phagocytes is the main host defense against the pneumococcus. In turn, the presence of a capsule is the main virulence property of the pneumococcus, but once it is engulfed it is readily destroyed by the phagocyte. The antiphagocytic properties of a capsule are destroyed when it reacts with its homologous antibody.

Resistance to phagocytosis may not totally depend upon the presence of a capsule, for similar activity can be expressed by other surface components. For example, some *S. pyogenes* produce hyaluronic acid capsules which are not so readily detectable as are the capsules of the pneumococci. Virulence (resistance to phagocytosis) in these streptococci relates only in minor part to the somewhat labile capsule; it relates even more to a cell wall antigen, the M protein, which is distributed over the surface of a streptococcal cell wall. M protein is involved in virulence since it is antiphagocytic and anti-M antibody is protective. The streptococci also have other surface antigens and components that are not related to virulence.

In most gram negative bacteria, phagocytosis and the lytic action of serum are both neutralized by the cell wall endotoxins.

Although there can be no doubt of the importance of capsular and similarly active surface constituents for the pathogenicity of many bacteria, their presence does not ensure pathogenicity (although it may still confer resistance to phagocytosis), and in some cases is not known to be contributory. Encapsulated but nonvirulent variants of pneumococci, *Haemophilus influenzae*, and *Bacillus anthracis* have been discovered.

Resistance to Phagocytic Digestion. Once pathogenic bacteria invade a host, they may be divided into two types depending upon their resistance to phagocytic digestion. One group, the "intracellular pathogens" offers little resistance to engulfment by phagocytes, but once inside they often establish a complex relationship that allows both phagocyte and intracellular pathogen to exist in balance. Intracellular pathogens such as *M. tuberculosis* and *Brucella* are able to survive and multiply within the phagocytic cells which facilitates their distribution within the body. Such pathogens are relatively inaccessible to chemotherapeutic agents and to antibodies.

Another group of invasive microorganisms are "extracellular pathogens" that are readily destroyed once they are phagocytized. For this group,

which includes *S. pyogenes* and *S. pneumoniae*, the critical act of invasion is to escape or resist phagocytosis, which they do because they produce antiphagocytic capsules or because they have certain types of cell walls. Once phagocytized, however, the majority of such microorganisms are destroyed. As long as such microorganisms can remain outside of phagocytes they can produce diseases. Their position outside of phagocytes allows them to stimulate the production of antibodies, which makes them susceptible to phagocytes and shortens the length of their infection.

Impairment of Neutrophil Functions. During an acute inflammatory reaction induced by an invading pathogen, leukocytes migrate towards the site of microbial proliferation as influenced by chemoattractants released at the infection site. At the site, the neutrophils (polymorphonuclear heterophilic leukocytes, PMNs) attempt to destroy the microorganisms. While some bacteria interfere with phagocyte engulfment or digestion, others may have different effects on PMNs. Strains of several bacteria (*e.g., Staphylococcus, Streptococcus, Pseudomonas aeruginosa, Actinobacillus actinomycetemcomitans*) produce a leukocidin which specifically kills PMNs. The leukocidin from *Staphylococcus* is immunogenic and acts by increasing the permeability of PMNs through changes in the potassium pump. *Capnocytophaga*, a gram negative anaerobic bacterium implicated in the pathogenesis of periodontal disease, produces changes in PMN morphology and impairs complement-induced PMN chemotaxis.

Several bacterial enzymes may damage many types of host cells including PMNs. More specifically, neuraminidase produced by some strains (*e.g., Actinomyces, V. cholerae*) induces cell membrane damage to PMNs.

Exotoxins

Some bacteria produce special soluble proteins called exotoxins which are among the most poisonous group of substances known to man. These include: a potent inhibitor of protein synthesis produced by *Corynebacterium diphtheriae*; the neurotoxins of *Clostridium tetani* and *Clostridium botulinum*; the enterotoxins of *Staphylococcus aureus*, *V. cholerae*, enteropathogenic *E. coli, Clostridium perfringens* and *Shigella dysenteriae*; and the tissue necrosis toxins of *S. aureus, Bordetella pertussis* and *S. pyogenes*.

Properties. Classical exotoxins have several distinctive characteristics, although they sometimes overlap with the characteristics of endotoxins or microbial lytic enzymes. They usually are excreted or readily separated from the bacterial cell that produced them. They are usually labile high molecular weight proteins that resemble enzymes and are strongly antigenic. With the exception of botulinum toxin and the staphylococcus enterotoxin, most exotoxins are sensitive to proteolytic enzymes, particularly those of the gastrointestinal tract. They also are sensitive to heat and acids. Exotoxins are unusually lethal, even in very small amounts, but they do have variable toxicity for different animals. Tetanus and botulinum toxins have more than a million guinea pig LD_{50} per mg. On the other hand, diphtheria toxin contains about 3500 guinea pig LD_{50} per mg. Described in a different fashion, 218 g of botulinim type A toxin, if properly administered, would kill the entire world population. The exposure of exotoxins to various chemicals eliminates their toxicity but preserves their antigenicity, producing toxoids, some of which are used to induce active immunity without the dangers of toxicity.

Pharmacological Actions. At the subcellular level, diphtheria toxin interferes with protein synthesis by the polysomes. At the tissue level, it acts on skeletal muscle, heart muscle, and the muscles of the diaphragm. Cells of *C. diphtheriae* are relatively nontoxic and remain in the localized pharyngeal lesion in typical diphtheria. However, the toxin itself is disseminated throughout the body via the blood. The net effect of the pharmacological action is to cause residual paralysis in individuals who recover, or to cause death from cardiac failure.

The toxins of botulism and tetanus are both neurotoxins. Botulinum toxin affects impulse conduction through both pre- and postsynapses of peripheral autonomic nerves by blocking the release of acetylcholine. This acid ester of choline is released from pre- and postganglionic endings of parasympathetic fibers and from preganglionic regions of sympathetic fibers. If acetylcholine is not released, impulses do not cross the affected synapses. Tetanus toxin produces a peripherial spastic action at the neuromuscular junction of voluntary muscles by suppression of synaptic inhibition. Tetanus toxin also may influence synaptic transmission at myoneural junctions possibly by causing the accumulation of acetylcholine. Typical botulism food poisoning results from ingesting the toxin previously produced in the food, although a recently described condition called infant botulism apparently involves ingestion of the spores with subsequent toxin production. In tetanus, the infecting *C. tetani* remain localized at the site of entry (*e.g.*, puncture wound) but the toxin produced is disseminated to the central nervous system.

The shiga neurotoxin of *S. dysenteriae*, in contrast to tetanus and botulinum toxins, does not act directly on the cells of the central nervous system, but it acts primarily on the small blood vessels of brain and spinal cord. In animals, when introduced parenterally it will cause paralysis, diarrhea, and death. The *S. aureus* enterotoxin of food poisoning apparently acts on neural receptors in the gut causing a stimulation of the central nervous system with increased gut motility and powerful vomiting reactions.

Diarrhea-inducing enterotoxins (*e.g. V. cholerae, E. coli, C. perfringens*) presumably function in a similar manner by increasing movement of water and ions from the intestinal tissues to the lumen of the bowels causing diarrhea. Studies with the cholera toxin have shown that it binds to specific receptors on the mucosal cell membranes and stimulates adenyl cyclase activity which reduces intracellular concentrations of cyclic AMP. This alteration of tissue cAMP apparently causes excretion of water and ions from the tissue.

Besides producing enterotoxins and leukocidins, certain strains of staphlococci also produce exfoliative toxin, an exotoxin which causes exfoliation of skin in the scalded skin syndrome. Another tissue necrotizing exotoxin from *B. pertussis* destroys upper respiratory tract epithelium in whooping cough. The erythrogenic toxin produced by strains of *S. pyogenes* causing scarlet fever produces necrosis of blood vessels.

The significance of exotoxin formation in bacterial physiology is uncertain. In some cases exotoxin production is a dispensable activity which is acquired by or expressed as a result of bacteriophage infection. For example, only those strains of *C. diphtheriae* which are lysogenic for β-phage which contains the tox^+ gene produce the toxin. The erythrogenic toxin of *S. pyogenes* also is under the genetic control of a temperate bacteriophage. The same is probably true for botulinum toxin, since some toxigenic strains yield bacteriophages which infect and convert nontoxigenic strains to toxin producers.

Endotoxins

Properties. Endotoxins are lipopolysaccharides (LPS) complexed to proteins which occur in the outer membrane of the envelope of gram negative bacteria. In contrast to exotoxins, they are heat stable, resistant to proteolytic enzymes, less toxic, have similar biological activities regardless of their source, are released from bacterial cells whose integrity has been disrupted, and cannot be converted to toxoids. The polysaccharide part of LPS is composed of a core, which is similar in all endotoxins, and the O-specific side chain which varies in composition among endotoxins and determines the O-antigen specificity of the bacterial strain. The lipid A portion of LPS is generally accepted to be responsible for the biological activity of endotoxin.

Biological Activities. Endotoxins have a number of biological actions. They elicit fever by causing the release of an endogenous pyrogen from PMNs. A more characteristic pharmacological activity of endotoxins is that they cause an increase in capillary permeability, together with hemorrhages. Another characteristic pharmacological reaction is to elicit inflammation when injected intradermally. Associated with the endotoxins' ability to elicit inflammation is their ability to cause the Shwartzman reaction. If endotoxin is injected into the skin of a rabbit, mild inflammation occurs at the site of the initial injection. If, after a day, the same or another endotoxin is administered intravenously, it provokes at the site of the original infection edema, hemorrhage, and necrosis. This is known as a localized Shwartzman reaction. If both injections are given intravenously, it produces bilateral cortical necrosis of the kidneys and death usually occurs after the second injection. This is known as a generalized Shwartzman reaction. Other reactions elicited by endotoxins are hyperglycemia, leukopenia followed by leukocytosis, and a wide variety of circulatory distrubances.

Other Toxic Substances

Bacterial Enzyme Toxins. Pathogenic bacteria sometimes produce enzymes capable of disorganizing host function by lysing host cells or the constituents of host tissue. Although it is often difficult to assess their exact significance, it usually is accepted that many of them may contribute to the disease process.

Certain invasive strains, such as staphylococci, streptococci and C. perfringens, produce hyaluronidase. This enzyme degrades hyaluronic acid, a mucopolysaccharide that is the cementing substance of connective tissues, thus allowing bacteria to penetrate such tissues and to be disseminated from the site of the initial infection. There are enzymes in the plasma of normal individuals that are antagonistic to hyaluronidase, which often helps establish an equilibrium between pathogen and host.

Pathogenic microorganisms sometimes produce enzymes (e.g., coagulase) that accelerate blood clotting, or they may produce kinases which inhibit clotting or which dissolve fibrin clots once they are formed. Staphylococci are widely known for their ability to produce coagulase. It has been postulated that the ability of staphylococci to produce a fibrin clot assists them in the establishment of a localized circumscribed infection. It is sometimes suggested that staphylococci which produce coagulase are pathogenic and those that do not are not pathogenic, but the distinction is not always clear. A plasma factor, with an action similar to prothrombin, converts a staphylococcal product into active coagulase which then induces fibrin clot formation. Animals that are resistant to staphylococcal infection (e.g., rats or mice) do not have the blood

cofactor necessary for this type of clotting. Another factor involves inhibition of phagocytosis. Staphylococci that produce coagulase become coated with fibrin and are resistant to phagocytosis. The clotting plasma in the outer boundaries of a staphylococcal-induced infection physically restrains the phagocytes and prevents their contacting and engulfing the bacteria.

Bacteria such as the streptococci produce enzymes or enzyme precursors known as kinases that indirectly inhibit fibrin clots by activating plasminogen of the blood plasma to form plasmin, which dissolves the clot. Staphylococci also are able to lyse fibrin clots by producing a staphylokinase, which is distinct from streptokinase. Several other bacteria lyse fibrin clots, probably by producing proteolytic enzymes rather than by producing kinases.

The role of the kinases in the nature of virulence seems rather straightforward with regard to staphylococci and streptococci. The pathogenic staphylococci, all of which produce a potent coagulase, are virulent and produce a localized, circumscribed lesion. They seldom invade the deeper tissue. Those staphylococci that seldom significantly disseminate from the localized infection do not produce significant amounts of staphylokinase, which would allow them to disseminate. On the other hand, streptococci are extremely invasive. They actively produce potent kinases, which may allow them to quickly break out of the local lesion and invade tissues.

Bacterial hemolysins are a group of substances that cause destruction of red blood cells. Hemolysins are antigenic and are often named after the bacteria producing them, e.g., streptolysin or staphylolysin.

In addition to the filterable or soluble bacterial hemolysins described above, bacteria also cause the hemolysis of erythrocytes about colonies on blood agar. Two types of reactions occur, green or α-type hemolysis, and clear or β-type hemolysis. The relationship has not been established between filterable hemolysins and blood-plate hemolysins, but it appears that different enzymes and different actions are involved. In most instances, a direct relationship has not been established between the ability of a microorganism to produce hemolysins and its ability to produce the the symptoms of an infectious disease. A number of nonpathogenic bacteria also produce hemolysins.

Toxic Metabolites. During bacterial growth and metabolism a variety of low molecular weight metabolites are released from the cells. If these substances accumulate in localized environments they may damage host cells or tissues. The best example is the tooth demineralizing acids (e.g., lactic acid) produced by many types of plaque bacteria. Other examples would be hydrogen sulfide and ammonia which are cytotoxic and are products of protein metabolism primarily by anaerobic bacteria.

Virulence of Viruses

The factors involved in the virulence of viruses are not so well defined as those of many bacteria. In general, virulence relates to the cellular changes viruses bring about as a result of their obligate intracellular parasitism. Host cell susceptibility to a given virus is primarily related to the presence or absence of receptors to which the virus particles can attach prior to entering the cell. Susceptibility also may be related to the inability of a virus to replicate within a cell as a result of nonspecific or specific host defense mechanisms such as interferon or antibody.

The cell responses to a viral infection include (a) no apparent damage as in persistent infections, (b) cell transformation (hyperplasia with cell death or hyperplasia without cell death as in transformation to cancer cells), and (c) a cytopathic reaction with death of the infected cell.

The mechanisms of the cytopathic changes caused by viruses relate to a number of possible reactions. Virulent DNA and RNA viruses respectively may inhibit host cell DNA or RNA synthesis. Viruses also act on lysosomes causing either a reversible increase in permeability or an irreversible disruption. The latter results in the discharge of hydrolytic enzymes into the cell cytoplasm, resulting in the disruption and death of the host cell.

During an infection, enveloped viruses may incorporate a portion of their envelope into the cytoplasmic membrane of host cells, or more commonly, alter the host cell. The cell membrane of the altered host cell then has some of the antigenic characteristics of the infecting virus. As immunity to the virus develops during the course of an infection, the antigenically altered host cell reacts with the virus-induced effectors of the immune response, such as antibodies or lymphocytes, causing their inactivation or destruction. With some viruses, adjacent altered cells tend to fuse with each other and form giant cells.

Some viruses must replicate in host cells before they produce a cytopathic reaction. Other viruses in high concentration are toxic and rapidly produce cytopathic effects and death of cells without replicating. Vaccinia virus kills macrophages and mumps virus lyses erythrocytes without replicating in such cells. Syncytial cell formation by mumps virus relates to some action which it has on cytoplasmic membranes. Such actions relate to the viral capsid. Some viruses also may produce cytopathic effects when they replicate, but produce an incomplete, noninfectious virion.

Another cytopathic effect occurring in host cells during virus infections is the development of inclusion bodies. Inclusion bodies consist of an accumulation of incompletely assembled units of viruses, virus-induced products, or of completely assembled virions. They may accumulate only in the nucleus of the host cell (e.g., adenoviruses), only in the cytoplasm of host cells (e.g., rabies virus), or in both nucleus and cytoplasm (e.g., measles virus). In some instances, the inclusion bodies occurring in host cells contain neither unassembled subunits of virions nor completely assembled virions. Instead, these seem to be a type of scar remaining at the site of a previous replication of virions which have departed the area. As example of such an inclusion is the intranuclear eosinophilic inclusion body produced by herpes simplex virus.

Some viruses are oncogenic, causing tumors or leukemia, particularly in animals. In tissue cultures, such viruses are able to transform a normal cell to what resembles a malignant cell. The division of such malignant-type cells is no longer constrained by their contact with adjacent cells. If host cells are transformed by DNA viruses, they no longer continue to synthesize the infectious virus. However, they do retain some functional units of the infecting virus. Cells transformed by RNA viruses continue to produce complete virions. The mechanism of cell transformation by oncogenic viruses is not known, but such viruses stimulate DNA synthesis, they alter the cell surface resulting in the incorporation of new antigens in the transformed cells, they cause chromosomal aberrations, and they remove the control of cell division that is due to a cell contacting adjacent cells (contact inhibition).

Virulence of Fungi

Only a few of the thousands of different fungi are pathogenic for man. The types of infectious diseases caused are classified according to the affected tissues: superficial infections (e.g., piedra); cutaneous infections (e.g., ringworm); subcutaneous infection (e.g., sporotrichosis); systemic infections (e.g., histoplasmosis).

Fungal virulence determinants are not as well defined as those of bacteria (e.g., exotoxin and endotoxins). However, specific molds and yeasts do have known properties which could affect their pathogenicity. The yeast *Cryptococcus neoformans* which causes cryptococcosis has a capsule which does impair phagocytic ingestion. While the fungal world is a source for various pharmacologically active compounds (e.g., vitamins, antibiotics, adrenergic alkaloids, hallucinogens) very little is known about potentially damaging products produced by the pathogenic yeasts and molds. While some may produce potentially damaging enzymes (e.g., *Spo-*

rothrix schenckii produces neuraminidase), in general, they do not produce typical toxins during the infectious disease process. However, some fungi produce mycotoxins which may be fatal if ingested (*e.g.*, the mushroom *Amanita phalloides*). Some strains of the mold *Aspergillus flavus* produce another mycotoxin called aflatoxin which is toxic and carcinogenic for animals. Outbreaks with high fatality in livestock after ingesting infected grain have been reported worldwide. The potential dangers for man also come from ingestion of foodstuffs contaminated with aflatoxins. However, the true risk to the human population is unknown. Sensitive techniques are used to monitor grains, peanuts and other foods potentially contaminated with toxin-producing fungi.

One general property of fungi which may influence the course of mycoses is the relative inertness of the fungal cell wall polysaccharides (*e.g.*, chitin, mannans, β-glucans). The cell walls are highly immunogenic, yet mammalian tissues lack the enzymes necessary to degrade the wall polysaccharides. Therefore, the cell wall is slowly removed from the tissues while continuing to stimulate the immune system. This along with the production of other immunogenic products contribute to the development of hypersensitivity which is a regular occurrence in fungal disease.

INNATE HOST RESISTANCE

Man's defense against infectious diseases is a combination of innate and acquired mechanisms. Innate resistance is the sum of the defense mechanisms that are the genetic endowment of the individual, regardless of his past experience. Acquired resistance is the sum of specific adaptive reactions to previous contact with microorganisms. Innate resistance depends on the integument as a mechanical barrier, on the inhibition or destruction of microorganisms and their products that find their way upon or into tissues, on inflammation and phagocytosis, and on a rather vaguely defined quality of insusceptibility, due to the unresponsiveness of an individual to the microorganism or its products.

First Line of Defense—Physical and Chemical Barriers

Skin. The first line of the body's defense is the skin and mucous membranes which are not, however, impenetrable mechanical barriers. Hair follicles, sweat glands, and sebaceous glands provide potential sites for microbial localization and growth. The ability of some bacteria to produce infection through the apparently intact skin suggests that they can pass through the interstices between the keratinized cells of the epidermis. However, the skin is never entirely free from microscopic breaks owing to normal wear and tear, allowing microorganisms to penetrate and enter the deeper tissues.

The skin also exerts an important bactericidal action. When millions of cells of *Proteus vulgaris*, for example, or *Staphylococcus aureus*, are placed on the skin, nearly all die within 10 minutes to 2 hours. When placed on sterile glass they survive during the same periods. The bactericidal action of the skin relates to the secretion of the sweat glands, which maintain an average dermal pH from 5.2 to 5.8, and to free higher fatty acids, which are bactericidal and fungicidal. A secretion of the apocrine glands that is peculiar to the axillary and inguinal regions of the postpubertal male promotes the growth of fungi. Also contributory to bacterial control in skin is lysozyme, which hydrolyzes the cell walls of many "nonpathogenic" bacteria and kills them. Finally, the indigenous *Propionibacterium acnes* (*Corynebacterium acnes*) and micrococci are antibiotic to the gram negative bacteria. The bactericidal action of the skin is greatly reduced within 15 minutes after death, showing that unidentified mechanisms are also at work.

Alimentary Tract. When particles such as bacteria are caught in the mucus coating of the mouth, they are washed backward and eventually swallowed. Saliva is inhibitory for nonindigenous organisms. Salivary lysozyme definitely lyses many nonpathogenic, nonindigenous bacteria, but it may injure rather than lyse "pathogenic bacteria." It does not affect any of the species indigenous to the mouth. Since the antibacterial activity of saliva is mostly due to antibiotic activities of the indigenous oral flora, it is an adaptive phenomenon rather than an innate defense. In the stomach, microorganisms are exposed to lethal acidity. A small fraction escape by lodging in particles of food or due to the diluting and buffering action of food and drink. Conditions also are not favorable for bacterial survival in the intestines above the lower half of the jejunum. The full normal intestinal flora is not encountered above the ileum, due to inhibition by the washing and bactericidal action of mucus, a low pH, pancreatic secretions, bile, and possibly lysozyme. It is not certain that living bacteria may not be susceptible to the digestive enzymes of the alimentary tract. In the large intestines, as in the mouth, antagonisms of the normal flora assist in the disposal of nonindigenous forms, especially by their production of antibiotics and bacteriocins.

Respiratory Tract. Except under heavy exposure, less than 1% of the bacteria that are inhaled ever reach the terminal bronchioles. They are trapped by the hairs and in the mucus of the nasal passages and on the pharyngeal surfaces. Movement of the ciliated epithelium lining the respiratory tract ("ciliary escalator") keeps the mucus coating in constant motion, from the upper respiratory tract backward and downward and from the trachea and bronchi upward, and the entrapped microorganisms are finally swallowed. Also, as at other sites, the chemical nature of mucus secretion may inhibit many microorganisms, and phagocytosis also contributes to the defenses of the nasal mucosa. Microorganisms that may find their way into the terminal bronchioles and alveoli are removed by phagocytosis and lymphatic drainage. Therefore, the trachea, bronchi, and lungs are normally free of microbes.

Urogenital Tract. The urethra is normally sterile in both sexes, owing in part to the flushing action and slight acidity of the urine. The cellular response to infection of the urogenital tract indicates that phagocytes are readily mobilized in this area. Also, the prostatic secretion is bactericidal. Between puberty and menopause, estrogen causes a marked thickening of the vaginal epithelium and deposition of glycogen, which is fermented by indigenous lactobacilli to lactic acid, so that the pH is too low for most other bacteria. During childhood and after the menopause, the vagina is neutral or slightly alkaline and more susceptible to infection.

Conjunctivae. Except for a few diphtheroid bacilli, the conjunctivae are normally sterile. Much of their resistance must be due to the flushing action of the lachrymal secretion, and the high lysozyme content.

Second Line of Defense—Inflammation and Phagocytosis

General Description. Microorganisms penetrate the skin and mucous membranes of the host by abrasions and wounds. Such microorganisms and their toxic agents injure the cells and tissues, eliciting an inflammatory response. This response involves blood vessels, cells, and organized tissues in a series of complex biochemical and morphological events that result in the homeostatic control and repair of the injury. The inflammatory events are manifested clinically by the typical signs of inflammation: heat, redness, swelling, and pain. The constitutional signs and symptoms induced by the local response relate to its severity, but they usually include fever, weakness, lassitude, headache, and generalized pain. In spite of these reactions, inflammation is essential for the host to combat infection and to contain and dispose of the offending pathogen so repair can take place. If the inflammatory process loses its homeostatic controls, it becomes destructive as in glomerulonephritis, rheumatoid arthritis, systemic hypersensitivity inflammatory reactions, and periodontal disease.

Inflammation is innate in that a similar series of events occurs in all normal human beings. The reactions do not require previous exposure to the eliciting agent, and the same reactions occur regardless of the pathogenic microbial species involved or the nature of the microbial toxic agent. However, the final outcome of the reaction may vary considerably, ranging from relatively rapid control and repair of the injury, to mutilation of tissues and to the loss of homeostasis, profound constitutional signs and symptoms, and even death.

Leukocytic Transmigration and Chemotaxis. One of the key factors in inflammation is the migration of leukocytes across vascular barriers into the infected tissues. Such leukocyte transmigration is a characteristic response of relatively short duration; neutrophils at first marginate along the periphery of the blood vessels in the infected tissues, perhaps in response to some chemotactic substance. They then migrate in increasing numbers from the vessel into adjacent connective tissue until they effectively wall off the infection.

The migration of leukocytes from the blood stream through the endothelial barrier into infected tissue has been related most often to chemotactic mechanisms. *In vitro* studies have shown that neutrophils respond rapidly (within 90 minutes) to chemotactic factors, whereas mononuclear cells require up to several hours. The difference in rate of response may account for the respective early and late appearance of neutrophils and mononuclear cells. Substances that are chemotactic for neutrophils include soluble components of most pathogenic microorganisms and products of the complement system produced during complement activation.

Monocytes respond to chemotactic factors more slowly than neutrophils. Their chemotactic factors include soluble microbial components and lysed neutrophils. The presence of chemotactic factors for mononuclear cells in neutrophils may account for the late arrival of the monocytes. Thus, the monocytes would arrive after the neutrophils were lysed to release the chemotactic factor. Antigen-antibody complexes elicit factors which attract mononuclear cells. Fragmentation products of complement components are chemotactic for mononuclear cells. Also, sensitized lymphocytes react with their specific antigen to produce a chemotactic factor. This latter reaction could account for the presence of lymphocytes in delayed hypersensitivity reactions. One enzyme has been involved in the chemotactic response of mononuclear cells, although there must be others, as evidenced by the diversity of their chemotactic agents.

Reticuloendothelial System. The control of a circumscribed infection in deeper tissues is accomplished chiefly by neutrophils and macrophages. However, if an infection is not self-contained in the deeper tissues, pathogenic microorganisms, their soluble toxic components, and other proteins enter the lymphatics and eventually reach the blood-stream. The cells of the reticuloendothelial system then operate as a clearing mechanism. The mono-nuclear cells of the reticuloendothelial system are derived from bone marrow. They are released into the blood stream as monocytes that are actively phagocytic. They make up from 3 to 7% of the circulating white blood cells. After a few days in the blood stream, the monocytes migrate into extravas-cular tissues as large, actively phagocytic macro-phages that are widely distributed through connec-tive tissue, along the outside of the basement mem-branes of most small blood vessels, liver sinusoids (where they are known as Kupffer cells), in the spleen, lung, bone marrow, and lymph nodes. The reticuloendothelial system and its cells are involved in almost any significantly severe inflammatory response in the body. When pathogenic microor-ganisms elicit a severe localized inflammatory re-sponse, the area is drained by lymphatics which carry off the cellular and fluid exudates. As the infection intensifies, the pathogenic bacteria enter the lymphatics, which dilate and often become inflamed (lymphangitis). Bacteria and inflamma-tory detritus are carried toward the closest regional lymph nodes, which attempt to filter them out of lymphatic circulation. The cells of the lymph nodes undergo hypertrophy and hyperplasia (lymphade-nitis). If containment is not successful, the affected lymph node breaks down and the infection spreads to other lymph nodes. If an infection is sufficiently severe, the reticuloendothelial system may be over-whelmed and the entire body may become involved in a generalized inflammatory reaction.

Exudate. Accumulation of an exudate in the affected tissues is a characteristic feature of inflam-mation. Serous exudates are watery with a low protein content, and fibrinous if they are rich in protein, particularly fibrin. Purulent or suppurative exudates occur if there is much tissue destruction concomitant with pus formation. The exudate is an indicator of the reactions occurring in the inflam-matory response. It also is related to the continued presence of a pathogen in the infection. In acute inflammation, removal of the pathogen results in a reversal of the inflammatory reactions, disappear-ance of the leukocytes, reduced permeability of the blood vessels, the removal of fibrin, protein, and water, and the return of the tissue to a normal state. If the pathogen and acute inflammation per-sist, the lysis of neutrophils releases hydrolytic enzymes which lyse tissue and cause an abscess. Such a reaction in the skin is not so serious but a similar reaction, for example, in the central nervous system is most serious.

An inflammatory reaction that becomes chronic is characterized by proliferation and the presence of monocytes and lymphocytes. Healing is charac-terized by a fibroblastic response that induces the formation of dense, collagenous connective tissue and scars.

The persistence of an exudate may result in a chronic inflammatory focus. This focus is charac-terized by the accumulation of neutrophils, fibrin, and granulation tissue which walls off the affected tissue, producing a persistent lesion.

Healing and Regeneration. When the infec-tion and its inflammatory reaction subside, healing and regeneration occur, with either restoration of the tissue to a normal state or its replacement by scar tissue. The regenerative capacity of tissues varies considerably. Most dental structures, endo-crine glands, retinal tissue, sense organs, neurons of the central nervous system, renal glomeruli, lung parenchyma, and muscle have limited regenerative capacity. Tissues with considerable or unlimited regenerative capacity include cutaneous and mu-cosal epithelium, formed cells of the bone marrow, renal tubular epithelium, ductal epithelium of exo-crine glands, liver parenchyma, lymphoid tissue, endothelium and bone.

Granulomatous Inflammation. Granuloma-tous inflammation occurs in response to infections such as tuberculosis, some fungal infections, syph-ilis, and actinomycosis. Lymphocytes, monocytes, and plasma cells are characteristically present in such a response, as are large epitheloid cells (or histiocytes) which unite to form multinucleated, giant cells. Also characteristic of the reaction is the peculiar clustering of the monocytes (or histiocytes) about the causative microorganisms or, if the infec-tion has persisted for some time, about a central necrotic area. Granulomatous inflammation ordi-narily requires the development of a delayed type hypersensitivity or at least an intact immunocom-petence.

Suppression of Inflammatory Response. A number of factors may suppress the inflammatory response. Any activity which interferes with bone marrow functions and formation of the short-lived neutrophils (e.g., drugs or radiation) will prevent the initiation or interfere with the continuation of the inflammatory response. The inability to form neutrophils renders an individual highly susceptible to uncontrolled infections. Factors which interfere with the formation of lymphocytes or which pro-duce immunologically incompetent lymphocytes (e.g., chronic granulocytic leukemia) also increase susceptibility to infection. In other individuals af-fected by the chronic granulomatous diseases of childhood, the neutrophils may be unable to kill the microorganisms that they have phagocytized. The failure to resolve the infection and the persist-ence of the microorganisms leads to the accumula-tion of lymphocytes and monocytes and to chronic granulomatous inflammation.

Phagocytosis. One of the principal benefits of inflammation induced by an infection is the activities of phagocytes which help to control the infection. The phagocytes involved comprise two principal groups of cells: the polymorphonuclear leukocytes (PMNs) of the blood and the large mononuclear cells (macrophages) that make up the reticuloendothelial system. In addition to particulate matter, phagocytes take in and dispose of soluble and insoluble foreign matter, and detritus of inflammation and tissue degradation.

Phagocytes, by an energy-requiring process, engulf microorganisms at the site of an infection, forming a vacuole in the cytoplasm that contains the microorganism (fig. 10/1). This vacuole usually is enclosed entirely by a portion of the plasma membrane of the phagocyte, isolating the ingested microorganism from the cytoplasm. The ability of phagocytes to engulf microorganisms is increased by a number of factors, such as opsonins, which appear to coat bacteria and make them more easily phagocytized. Some virulent bacteria cannot be phagocytized unless opsonins are present. While most opsonins occur naturally and are innate, some antibodies (IgG and IgM) are opsonins and are acquired defense mechanisms. Other factors considered to be opsonins are some of the components of complement, polypeptides, lysozyme, basic polyamino acids, and noncomplement thermolabile factors in serum.

Once microorganisms are engulfed, several things may happen. Some microorganisms, such as gonococci, tubercle bacilli, vaccinia virus, and the yeast form of *Histoplasma capsulatum*, appear to survive in phagocytes and are well adapted to such an intracellular existence, where they are protected from antibodies and chemotherapeutic agents. In such circumstances, the wandering phagocytes may serve to spread the infectious agents. Occasionally, after being ingested, microorganisms are simply ejected either dead or alive from the phagocyte (egestion). However, the majority of phagocytes that have engulfed microorganisms actively attempt to kill them. This is accomplished by the lysosomes of the phagocytes contacting and fusing with the vacuole containing the microorganism, then ejecting hydrolytic enzymes into the vacuole. These potent enzymes, which are capable of degrading the basic components of microorganisms, then act directly on the microorganism without immediately affecting the cytoplasm of the phagocyte.

Some leukocytes have a specialized activity in innate resistance. The eosinophils, for instance, are attracted to the usually extensive exudate of allergic reactions, and they ingest and dispose of the antigen-antibody complexes which form under such conditions. While doing so they lose their granules, as do the neutrophils. They also seem to produce substances which counteract histamine, serotonin, and bradykinin, and thereby decrease the amount of the exudate which occurs in such allergic reactions.

The structure of the involved tissues may play a role in phagocytosis. Microorganisms such as *Streptococcus pneumoniae* and *Haemophilus influenzae* are not significantly phagocytized unless homologous antibodies are present. In an infection with such microorganisms, at least 5 or 6 days are required before homologous antibodies are detectable in the serum. The question then arises as to how a host can survive the first few days of an infection with microorganisms which require homologous antibodies for phagocytosis. Both PMNs and monocytes phagocytize the resistant bacteria before the appearance of homologous antibodies by trapping them against rough tissue surfaces, between phagocytes if the tissue fluid is viscous, or by trapping them in the interstices of fibrin clots. It becomes evident, then, that tissue architecture greatly influences the efficiency of preantibody phagocytosis. This may partially account for the variances in survival rates of infections in tissues with different architecture. Formation of a walled off necrotic abscess, either acute or chronic, greatly interferes with phagocytosis, and the infecting microorganisms survive quite well in such an environment. Such infections are very resistant to resolution and usually require the establishment of drainage, which removes the barrier and exudate that interferes with phagocytosis.

Other Innate Defenses

Although described in detail in a later chapter, the complement system along with the related properdin system are considered as innate defense mechanisms. Even though they are frequently effectors of the immune system they are preexisting normal body components that may become active during many types of infectious diseases. Activation of complement directly or through the properdin system by certain bacterial cells, microbial products, or antigen-antibody complexes may result in lysis of gram negative bacteria, or enhancement of the inflammatory responses by increasing leukocyte chemotaxis and facilitating phagocytosis.

Many cells in the body after being infected with a virus have an innate capacity to synthesize a substance called interferon which prevents viral replication in other cells. This is an important nonspecific defense mechanism in man, for many different viruses and other substances can induce the formation of interferon which is then protective against replication of many different types of viruses.

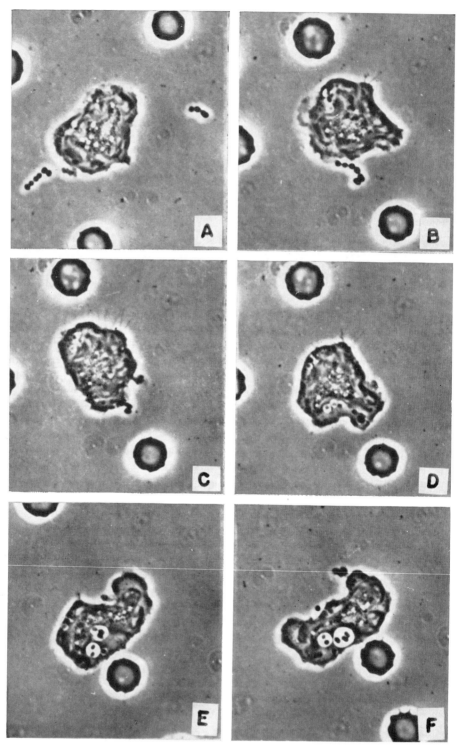

Figure 10/1. Phagocytosis and egestion of streptococci by a mouse polymorphonuclear neutrophil. (*A*) The leukocyte is near two chains of streptococci. (*B*) The shorter chain of streptococci has been phagocytized and is seen in vacuoles in the upper part of the leukocyte. (*C*) The larger chain of streptococci, which has been reproducing by cell division, is being phagocytized. (*D–F*) A streptococcal cell from the small chain is egested from the upper left hand portion of the leukocyte: streptococci from the longer chain are in vacuoles. (From A. T. Wilson 1953 The Egestion of Phagocytized Particles by Leukocytes. *Journal of Experimental Medicine*, **98**, 305.)

MODIFICATION OF RESISTANCE

Nutrition

There is little doubt that, in general, malnutrition adds a stress that contributes to the likelihood of infection. Hypoproteinemia and deficiencies of the B vitamins generally increase susceptibility of experimental animals to bacterial and rickettsial infections. Also deficiency of vitamin C possibly coupled with other nutritional disturbances resulting from, for example, alcoholism and "fad" dieting may enhance the development of gingivitis. The true relation of other vitamins to resistance is undetermined. There is a widespread suspicion that minerals, particularly those ordinarily present in trace amounts, influence innate resistance; except for the protective effect of fluoride against dental caries, unequivocal data for man are scant.

Hormones

The adrenocortical hormones can cause a decrease in host resistance by depressing the inflammatory response. Also, diabetics, unless adequately controlled by insulin, have been recognized for a long time to be unusually susceptible to pyogenic infections of the extremities. The relation of estrogen to vaginal glycogen synthesis and resistance of the vagina to bacteria was discussed earlier.

Miscellaneous

Innate resistance to specific infections also vary with race, age, sex, fatigue, and climate although the specific mechanisms involved are not well understood.

ADDITIONAL READING

AJL, S. J., KADIS, S., AND MONTIE, T. C. 1970 *Microbial Toxins, Vol. 1. Bacterial Protein Toxins.* Academic Press, New York.

BERKELEY, R. C. W., LYNCH, J. M., MELLING, J., RUTTER, P. R., AND VINCENT, B., (Eds.) 1980 *Microbial Adhesions to Surfaces.* Ellis Horwood Ltd., Chichester, England.

BERRY, L. J. 1972 Factors Influencing the Function of the Reticuloendothelial System in Infections. J Reticuloendothel Soc, **11,** 450.

BOYDEN, S. 1962 The Chemotactic Effect of Mixtures of Antibody and Antigen on Polymorphonuclear Leukocytes. J Exp Med, **115,** 453.

DOUGLAS, D. M. 1969 Wound Healing. Proc R Soc Med, **62,** 513.

ELIN, R. J., AND WOLFF, S. M. 1976 Biology of Endotoxins. Annu Rev Med, **27,** 127.

FREEMAN, BOB A. (Ed.) 1979 *Textbook of Microbiology.* Saunders, Philadelphia.

HIRSCH, J. G. 1965 Phagocytosis. Annu Rev Microbiol, **19,** 339.

HO, M., AND ARMSTRONG, J. A. 1975 Interferon. Annu Rev Microbiol, **29,** 131.

LAMANNA, C., AND SAKAGUCHI, G. 1971 Botulinum Toxins and the Problem of Nomenclature of Simple Toxins. Bacteriol Rev, **35,** 342.

LEWIS, G. P. 1964 Plasma Kinins and Other Vasoactive Compounds in Acute Inflammation. Ann N Y Acad Sci, **116,** 846.

MAJNO, G., AND PALADE, G. E. 1961 Studies on Inflammation. I. The Effect of Histamine and Serotonin on Vascular Permeability: An Electron Microscopic Study. J Biophys Biochem Cytol, **11,** 571.

PAGE, A. R., AND GOOD, R. A. 1968 A Clinical and Experimental Study of the Function of Neutrophils in the Inflammatory Response. Am J Pathol, **43,** 645.

PAPPENHEIMER, A. M., JR. 1977 Diphtheria Toxin. Annu Rev Biochem, **46,** 69.

PIERCE, N. F., GREENOUGH, W. B., AND CARPENTER, C. C. J. 1971 Vibrio cholerae Enterotoxin and Its Mode of Action. Bacteriol Rev, **35,** 1.

RABINOVITCH, M. 1968 Phagocytosis: The Engulfment Stage. Semin Hematol, **5,** 134.

SACK, R. B., *et al.* 1971 Enterotoxigenic *Escherichia coli* Isolated from Patients with Severe Cholera-Like Disease. J Infect Dis, **123,** 378.

SHURIN, S. B., SOCRANSKY, S. S., SWEENEY, E., AND STOSSEL, T. P. 1979 A Neutrophil Disorder Induced by Capnocytophaga, a Dental Microorganism. N Engl J Med, **301,** 849.

SMITH, H. 1972 Mechanisms of Viral Pathogenicity. Bacteriol Rev, **36,** 291.

SMITH, H., AND PEARCE, J. H. (Eds.) 1972 Microbial Pathogenicity in Man and Animals. *22nd Symposium, Society of General Microbiology,* Cambridge University Press, London.

SPECTOR, W. G. 1969 The Granulomatous Inflammatory Exudate. Int Rev Exp Pathol, **8,** 1.

SYMPOSIUM. 1975 Pathogenic Mechanisms in Bacterial Disease. In *Microbiology-1975,* edited by D. Schlessinger. p. 105. American Society for Microbiology, Washington, D. C.

WARD, P. A., COCHRANE, C. G., AND MULLER-EBERHARD, H. J. 1965 The Role of Serum Complement in Chemotaxis of Leukocytes in Vitro. J Exp Med, **122,** 327.

chapter 11

Immunoglobulin Structure and Function

Keith R. Volkmann

INTRODUCTION

If one considers infectious diseases as dynamic processes, which indeed they are, then the immune response becomes an extension or second line of defense following nonspecific host defense mechanisms discussed earlier. The intended result of both nonspecific defense and the immune response (specific defense) is to eliminate noxious agents from the body leading to a return of body homeostasis. However, there are significant differences between these two defense mechanisms, particularly in their activation or induction and the specificities of the responses.

Induction

The nonspecific defense is always ready to function whereas the immune system requires time and elaborate intercellular collaboration to become fully functional. In addition, the immune system usually requires prolonged or continuing presence of the stimulus before induction occurs. Thus, infectious agents or toxic substances which are rapidly cleared from the body rarely involve an immune response.

Specificity

As the term implies, the nonspecific defense system will attempt to rid the body of any substance or infectious agent which is not considered a normal body constituent. On the other hand, the immune system is selectively induced to respond to a specific stimulus. Indeed, one of the hallmarks of the immune response is its specificity. In the presence of repeated encounters with the same infectious agent, the nonspecific defense system of an individual responds in exactly the same fashion to each encounter with that agent while the immune system's response is usually faster and more vigorous and longer lasting upon subsequent exposures to the same agent. This last observation is extremely important in the control of infectious diseases since reexposure of the individual to the same infectious agent after an immune response has been elicited can result in a less severe disease process. This same characteristic may be used to prevent clinical disease in individuals prior to their encounter with the infectious agent in nature; it is the basis of deliberate immunization against a specific disease.

GENERAL DESCRIPTION OF THE IMMUNE SYSTEM

Typically, the immune system responds to substances foreign to the body. This includes infectious agents, many chemicals, transplanted tissues or cells, and altered normal or self-components of the body. Collectively, those foreign substances capable of inducing an immune response are referred to as immunogens or antigens. Small- to medium-sized lymphocytes constitute the afferent limb of the immune response and act as a recognition network for immunogens. After an immunogen has been recognized, a complex interplay of several subsets of lymphocytes and macrophages occurs in secondary lymphoid tissues leading to the development of the efferent or effector limb (mediators) of the immune response which interact specifically with the immunogens. These include immunoglobulins (antibodies) and effector lymphocytes. The secondary lymphoid tissue in which these mediators develop include lymph nodes, the spleen, gut-associated lymphoid tissue (GALT) and perhaps lymphoepithelial tissue such as tonsils and the appendix. In the adult, the source of cellular components of the immune response is the bone marrow. Bone marrow-derived lymphocytes require a maturation step before they become immunocompetent (able to respond to immunogens). The maturation function is provided by primary lymphoid organs, namely the thymus and, in man, the bursal equivalent.

Classically, immune reactions have been divided into the humoral immune response, whose function includes the production of immunoglobulins, and the cell-mediated response whose function includes the production of effector lymphocytes. For descriptive purposes this separation will be continued in this text. However, it is becoming increasingly apparent that this pedagogical separation of humoral and cellular responses is probably artificial and misleading when the immune response is viewed in terms of a dynamic biological process *in vivo*. Not only may both occur in response to the same immunologic challenge, but also both responses share common cellular elements and probably common control mechanisms.

MOLECULAR COMPONENTS OF THE HUMORAL IMMUNE SYSTEM

Immunogens

Antigens. Antigens, or the newer term immunogens, refer to substances which possess two important properties: 1) they can elicit an immune response leading to the production of immunoglobulins, and 2) the immunoglobulins formed in response to the immunogen will specifically bind to the immunogen. The array of natural and synthetic substances which can act as immunogens includes: many man-made substances, proteins, polysaccharides, nucleic acids and combinations of these substances such as glycoproteins and glycolipids in addition to synthetic polypeptides. Structurally, antigens must be further defined in order to understand how they interact with elements of the immune system. The portions of a macromolecular antigen which can interact with the recognition elements of the immune system and which also can combine with formed immunoglobulin are called antigenic determinants. In terms of size or mass relative to the entire antigen, antigenic determinants may represent a very small fraction. The remainder and perhaps majority of the antigen is called the carrier. The carrier portion of the antigen may be important for cellular interactions necessary to induce immunoglobulin synthesis.

Haptens. Landsteiner demonstrated that small chemical compounds (MW <1000) when coupled to a larger molecule called a carrier could elicit the formation of immunoglobulins specific for the small compounds. Landsteiner termed these small compounds "haptens." Once bound to the carrier, the hapten-carrier complex formed a complete antigen. The small chemical compounds alone, not coupled to a carrier, were incapable of inducing the formation of immunoglobulins but after the immunoglobulins were formed, these small chemical compounds alone could combine with them. In essence, haptens are single antigenic determinants and their study has been helpful in gaining an understanding of the nature of antigenic determinants and the nature of the antigenic combining site on immunoglobulin molecules.

Characteristics of Antigens. To describe a substance as being an antigen or as possessing antigenicity is to describe the substance in an operational manner. If a substance elicits an immune response in an animal species then it is an antigen. The term antigen does not confer any intrinsic chemical or physical properties on a substance. Antigenicity is as much a characteristic of the responding host species and its genetic make up and the method of antigenic administration as it is a characteristic of the molecule itself. Nonetheless, some general statements can be made with regard to properties of substances which appear to be important in determining their antigenicity or immunogenicity.

Position of Antigenic Determinants. Antigenic determinants must be available to recognition units on small lymphocytes. Usually this means that the determinants are located on the exterior of a macromolecular-complete antigen, but at the very least it means that the determinant must be exposed to the solvent which is suspending the antigen.

Molecular Weight. Experimentally it has been shown that a homologous series of substituted amino acids of 7 to 8 units in length can induce both humoral and cellular immunity in guinea pigs. As a general rule, however, substances with a molecular weight of 10,000 or below are weakly antigenic or not antigenic at all. Some of the most potent antigens are proteins with a molecular weight of 100,000 or greater.

Chemical Complexity. It is generally accepted that the greater the chemical complexity possessed by a substance, the more likely it is to be antigenic. Again, using polypeptides as an example, homopolymers of an amino acid tend to be poorly antigenic. The greater the number of different amino acids present in the polymer, the more likely the polymer is to be antigenic. Aromatic amino acids are more likely to confer antigenicity than are nonaromatic amino acids.

Foreignness. In conjunction with the above properties, perhaps the single most important attribute of an antigen is that is is recognized by the immune system of the responding host as being foreign or not "self," even if the "foreignness" is very subtle.

IMMUNOGLOBULIN STRUCTURE AND FUNCTION

The immunoglobulins represent a heterogenous group of glycoproteins found throughout the body. Nevertheless, they share many common functional and structural features. Based on their structure, immunoglobulins exhibit two characteristic functional areas. One area has the ability to physically combine with the antigenic determinants of antigens. The second area determines its biological

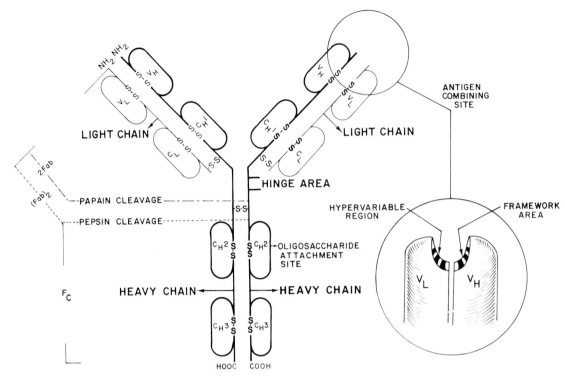

Figure 11/1. Schematic representation of structural features of an IgG molecule. The amino acid sequence of heavy and light chains are arranged in domains, either variable (V_H and V_L) or constant (C_L and C_H1, C_H2 and C_H3). Disulfide bonds (—S—S—) are located within each domain, covalently link light chain to heavy chain, and covalently link heavy chain to heavy chain. Proteolytic enzyme cleavage of the molecule by papain results in three fragments: two identical fragments (2 Fab) and approximately one half of both heavy chains including the interheavy chain disulfide bond (F_c). Proteolytic enzyme cleavage of the molecule by pepsin leaves one large fragment; both light chains and approximately the amino one-half of both heavy chains extending to the interheavy chain disulfide bond (Fab)$_2$. *Inset,* detail of the antigen combining site. The *darkened areas* represent hypervariable regions which actually form the combining site. The *white areas* represent framework areas which maintain the overall structure of the variable domains.

activity before and after it has complexed with antigen. As a basic unit each immunoglobulin (Ig) is composed of a total of four polypeptide chains: two identical chains each of molecular weight 25,000, termed light chains, and two identical chains each of molecular weight 50,000, termed heavy chains. These four polypeptide chains are held together with a variable number of interchain disulfide bonds (fig. 11/1). There are five major classes of immunoglobulins in humans, which can be distinguished by differences in heavy chain structure.

Light Chains

There are two classes of immunoglobulin light chains in man. About 60% of the complete Ig molecules have a type called κ chains and about 40% have a type called λ chains. Although both types are approximately 214 amino acids in length, they differ considerably in their amino acid sequences. Close examination of the amino acid sequences of light chains has revealed the presence of two domains. The first 110 to 112 amino acids beginning from the amino terminal end of the light chain show a high degree of sequence variability, when the sequences of many light chains of the same class (κ or λ) are compared. For this reason, the area composed of the amino terminal half of the light chain has been called the variable domain (V_L). On the other hand, the amino acid sequences of the carboxy terminal half of the light chains (approximately 110 to 112 amino acids) show a high degree of homology, when light chains of the same class (κ or λ) are compared. Therefore, the carboxy terminal half of the molecule is called the constant domain (C_L). Amino acid sequence differences in light chain constant domains specify the light chain class. Each light chain is bound to a heavy chain via a single disulfide bond near the carboxy terminus of the light chain. Functionally, the light chain variable domain, when paired with the variable domain of a heavy chain, constitutes the antigen binding site of the complete immunoglobulin molecule. The amino acid sequences of both light chains on a single Ig molecule are identical.

Our understanding of the amino acid sequence of light chains was greatly increased when it was discovered that some individuals suffering from multiple myeloma (plasma cell tumors) excreted in their urine large quantities of identical light chains, unattached to heavy chains. These free light chains are named *Bence Jones* proteins, after the physician who discovered them. Bence Jones proteins provided a source of homogeneous light chains with quantities large enough to make practical the procedures necessary to determine three-dimensional structure as well as amino acid sequence.

Heavy Chains and Three-Dimensional Structure of Igs

There are five different classes of heavy chains found in human immunoglobulins. These are designated α, γ, μ, δ, ϵ and subclasses of heavy chains have been distinguished within the γ and α classes. Heavy chain classes have been identified on the basis of both differences in amino acid sequences and qualitative and quantitative differences in oligosaccharide side chains which are attached to heavy chain constant domains. Whereas the total polypeptide chain length of light chains can be divided into two domains, variable and constant, both of approximately equal length, the full heavy polypeptide chain is composed of one variable domain and an additional three or four constant domains (C_H1 to C_H4) also of approximately equal length. In the completed Ig molecule, two identical heavy chains are joined together by a minimum of one disulfide bond, located in a linear stretch of amino acids near the midpoint of the polypeptide length.

When the four chains have been joined by disulfide bonds to form an Ig molecule, the variable domains of both light chain (V_L) and heavy chain (V_H) are arranged in a parallel fashion to form the antigen-combining site. The length of heavy chains which extends beyond the attached light chains has been designated the Fc portion. Biological functions which are apparent before and after the Ig has combined with specific antigenic determinants on antigens are due to properties of the Fc portion of the immunoglobulin. Certain cells, macrophages for example, contain receptors for the carboxy terminus of the Fc portion of Igs on their surface membranes. When antigen-Ig complexes are formed, the macrophages can bind the Ig at the receptor to enhance phagocytosis. Also, the Fc portion determines whether or not an immunoglobulin will cross the placenta from maternal to fetal circulation. In addition, after an immunoglobulin has combined with antigen, to form an immune complex, the Fc portion determines whether or not complement will be fixed (Chapter 13).

Based on evidence obtained from a variety of techniques, the shape of the typical monomeric Ig molecule is thought to be T or Y shaped. Midway along the length of the H chains near the inter-H chain disulfide bonds is a "hinge" area which allows the arms of the T or Y to flex (fig. 11/1). Biologically this structure is significant. The monomeric Ig molecule is symmetrical, possessing two antigen-combining sites, and for this reason is termed bivalent. The hinge area allows the antigenic-combining sites some degree of mobility, meaning that the Ig molecule can accommodate to minor variations in the distance between two identical antigenic determinants on the surface of an antigen and still combine in a bivalent fashion.

Proteolytic Enzyme Fragmentation. During early attempts to determine the structure of Ig molecules, proteolytic enzyme cleavage was employed and the resulting fragments were analyzed for biologic activity and shape. Although the details of the analysis are not germane to this presentation, knowledge of the resulting fragment names is indeed helpful because it allows one to identify specific areas of the Ig molecule.

Papain Cleavage. When papain is added to an Ig termed IgG, three fragments are produced, two of which are essentially identical and a third which is unique. The identical fragments each contain a portion of the Ig which can combine with antigenic determinants in a univalent manner. These fragments are designated Fab (antigen-binding fragments) and correspond to the entire light chain and approximately the amino terminal one-half of the heavy chain. The third fragment does not combine with antigen but is so homogeneous that it crystallizes under appropriate conditions and therefore is designated Fc (crystallizable fragment). The Fc portion is composed of the carboxy-terminal half of the heavy chains including the inter-H chain disulfide bonds.

Pepsin Cleavage. Analysis of the IgG fragments which result from pepsin cleavage reveal one rather large fragment with bivalent antigen binding activity (designated $(Fab)_2$) but no Fc fragment. The $(Fab)_2$ fragment is composed of the entire length of both light chains and the amino terminal one-half of both H chains including the inter-H chain disulfide bonds and the hinge region. If the inter-H chain disulfide bonds are cleaved, then univalent fragments result that are about 10% heavier (due to increased H chain length) than the corresponding papain fragment (Fab). Therefore, the cleaved pepsin fragment is designated Fab′ C instead of Fab.

Ig Classes

All immunoglobulin molecules share many structural and some functional features. In the following section, significant differences in structure and biological functions of human immunoglobulins will be emphasized. The nomenclature of complete immunoglobulins is derived from the designation of their component heavy chains. Thus, an immunoglobulin composed of γ heavy chains becomes immunoglobulin G (IgG); immunoglobulins with μ heavy chains become IgM; α heavy chains, IgA; δ heavy chains, IgD and ϵ heavy chains, IgE.

IgG. The IgGs can be divided into four subclasses (IgG-1 through IgG-4) based on distinctive differences found on the Fc segments of their respective heavy chain domains (γ_1 through γ_4). IgG as a class represents about 85% of the total immunoglobulin found in blood. IgG-1 is by far the most prevalent IgG, followed in descending order of blood concentration by IgG-2, IgG-3 and IgG-4. IgG, along with IgM, has the ability to fix complement (Chapter 13). If complement-fixing ability is assessed in terms of IgG subclasses, it is found that IgG-1 and IgG-3 fix complement rather efficiently, IgG-2 fixes complement less efficiently, and IgG-4's ability to fix complement is questionable.

IgG molecules are the only class of antibodies which are bound to, and actively transported across, the placenta. Therefore, maternal IgG provides the humoral source of antibody protection to the developing fetus. After birth, maternal IgG levels gradually diminish and virtually disappear when the infant reaches 6 to 9 months of age.

Considering protective functions within the body, IgG antibodies are perhaps most useful because of their opsonic capacity (ability to enhance phagocytosis). IgG mainly enhances this function in macrophages, one of the cell types which possess receptors for the Fc portion of IgG molecules on their cell surface membranes. Therefore, any antigen to which IgG is bound can be rather efficiently phagocytosed by macrophages due to the presence of the IgG Fc receptor. This phenomenon is particularly important in infectious diseases caused by etiologic agents which by themselves are not easily phagocytosed by macrophages, e.g., encapsulated *Streptococcus pneumoniae*. Specific IgG antibodies play a very important role in viral neutralization and toxin neutralization as well. When a sufficient number of specific IgG antibodies bind to virus particles or virions, the virion is not able to attach to or to penetrate through the cytoplasmic membrane of a susceptible cell. In a similar manner, specific IgG molecules bound to a bacterial exotoxin inhibit the biological activity of the exotoxin. It is of interest that the antigenic determinant on the exotoxin which elicits protective immunoglobulin responses is probably different from the biologically active site of the toxin.

In general, IgGs are thought to be the most important immunoglobulins involved in elimination of extracellular infectious agents under conditions where circulatory patterns allow the IgG access to body compartments which might harbor such agents. Furthermore, most immunization procedures primarily induce an IgG response and therefore, IgG is extremely important in prophylaxis against infectious diseases.

IgM. IgM was originally named macroglobulin because of its high molecular weight (about 900,000). This large size is due to the fact that IgM is present in blood as a pentamer (μ 10 L10) composed of five monomeric subunits each of which is composed of two light chains (either κ or λ) and two heavy chains (μ). The monomeric subunits are held together with two disulfide bonds linking Fc portions of the μ chains. One disulfide bond is located in the C_H3 domain and the second bond is located between penultimate amino acids in the C_H4 domain. In addition to amino acid sequence differences and oligosaccharide differences, μ chains differ structurally from γ heavy chains. μ Chains lack a hinge area and have an additional segment of 130 amino acids between the C_H1 and C_H2 domains. In essence, the additional amino acids amount to another domain. Therefore, μ chains are said to have five domains: one variable domain and four constant domains.

Multimeric forms of immunoglobulins such as IgM possess an additional structure not found on IgG or other monomeric forms of immunoglobulin. This is a 15,000-dalton polypeptide which is structurally different from all classes of Ig and is termed the J chain (joining chain). It is synthesized in the same cell in which IgM is synthesized. There is a single J chain for every multimeric Ig and it is attached to the Fc segment of heavy chains near the carboxy terminus by two disulfide bonds. Because J chains are only seen in association with multimeric Igs, it is believed that the J chain is necessary to stabilize these multimeric forms.

IgM comprises about 10% of the Ig in normal human blood. It fixes complement very efficiently. Biologically, IgM functions in a manner similar to IgG with opsinization being one of its most important functions. IgM and IgG can both be produced in response to the same antigenic stimulus and when this occurs IgM is seen first but is not synthesized as long, nor in as large a quantity, as is IgG. Monomeric subunits of IgM can be found on the surfaces of B lymphocytes and probably function as antigen receptors (chapter 12). Finally, IgM, acts as an isohemagglutinin which can bind to the nonself blood group antigens on the surface of red blood cells and is a normal constituent of blood (Chapter 14).

IgA. IgA can be present in a monomeric as well as various polymeric forms. In human serum, where it represents approximately 15% of the total serum Ig, it is present in a typical monomeric form ($\alpha_2 L_2$). IgA is also present in exocrine secretions primarily saliva, lacrimal secretions, mucous of the gut and respiratory tree, colostrum and urogenital mucosa.

When present in exocrine secretions, IgA is usually present as a dimer ($\alpha_4 L_4$) and like the polymeric form of IgM possess one J chain per dimer. In addition to the J chain, secretory IgA (sIgA) has a glycoprotein (9% carbohydrate, MW 71,000) attached to the Fc component of α chains via noncovalent bonds and disulfide bonds. This additional glycoprotein is called either secretory component (SC) or secretory piece (SP).

Secretory Piece. The secretory piece is not synthesized by the plasma cell which synthesizes IgA but rather is produced by epithelial cells lining the ducts of exocrine glands. Secretory piece appears to play two important functional roles in the maturation of biologically active sIgA. First, secretory piece may act as a transport molecule, binding dimeric IgA on the tissue side of the epithelial lining and then transporting the dimeric IgA across the epithelial cell to be released on the luminal side of the epithelial lining. After release from the epithelial cell, secretory piece remains attached to the IgA. Secondly, secretory piece may increase the resistance of sIgA to proteolytic enzyme activity and low pH found particularly in the gut, and in other body secretions as well. The manner in which the secretory piece is attached to the IgA dimer is not well understood.

Recent evidence suggests that the J chain and epithelial-bound SC represent the receptor-receptor site interaction in the selective transport of dimeric IgA and pentameric IgM. However, it has not been definitely ruled out that the epithelial cells express type-specific Fc receptors for IgA and IgM. Immunoelectron microscopy has revealed that sIgA is transported through the epithelial cell in a secretory vesicle and then extruded on the luminal side of the cell. It is not known how the SC is released from the membrane surface.

There are two subclasses of α heavy chains, designated $\alpha 1$ and $\alpha 2$. Both $\alpha 1$ and $\alpha 2$ polypeptides have four domains (one variable and three constant). However, $\alpha 1$ has a much larger hinge area which is not present in $\alpha 2$ chains. The hinge area of $\alpha 1$ chains is particularly susceptible to cleavage by proteolytic enzymes released from specific strains of streptococci and *Neisseria*. On the other hand, the foreshortened $\alpha 2$ polypeptides seem to be completely resistant to this bacterial proteolytic attack. Therefore, the heavy chain composition of sIgA has definite implications in the ability of sIgA to function extracorporally such as in the oral cavity where these organisms are common. Interestingly, approximately 90% of serum IgA is composed of $\alpha 1$ heavy chains, whereas the composition of sIgA seems to be at least equally distributed between $\alpha 1$ and $\alpha 2$ polypeptides or perhaps a predominance of $\alpha 2$ polypeptides.

Biologically, sIgA acts by interfering with the attachment of bacteria to mucosal surfaces. It also may interfere with the ability of viruses such as influenza, with a trophism for mucosal epithelium, to attach to and then penetrate these cells. Finally, sIgA may prevent the absorption of nonliving antigens first to the mucosa of the lungs and the gut and later prevent the transport of the antigens across the mucosa. sIgA is of great interest to the dental community because it is functionally present in saliva and may be important in resistance to infections by oral microorganisms and in maintaining the balance of the oral microflora.

IgE. IgE is a very minor component of serum. Because of its low serum concentration (approximately 0.3 μg/ml), its discovery was delayed until quite recently. Structurally, IgE is composed of two identical ϵ heavy chains and two identical light chains of either the κ or λ class ($\epsilon_2 L_2$). Like μ heavy chains, ϵ heavy chains have one variable domain and four constant domains. In addition, ϵ heavy chains have a high carbohydrate content (approximately 11.5%). Like IgG, IgE does not tend to form multimeric units.

In terms of biological function, IgE represents a bit of an enigma. The most familiar function of IgE involves its role as a mediator of acute allergic responses as seen in insect venom allergy or hay fever and asthma.

It would be difficult to convince a hay fever sufferer that this condition represented a protective mechanism for some life-threatening antigen. However, there is some speculation that IgE may play a role in protection against percutaneous infections of some parasites. In either event, one very important property of IgE is its ability to bind via its Fc portion ($C_H 4$ and perhaps $C_H 3$) to specific receptors located on the surface of mast cells and basophilic leukocytes. These cells contain vasoactive amines which can be released when surface-bound IgE is cross-linked by specific antigen. IgE does not fix complement in the manner that IgG and IgM do. However, aggregated IgE can activate complement via the "alternate pathway" (Chapter 13).

IgD. Although IgD levels vary somewhat in human sera, on the average they represent about 2% of the total serum Igs present. Their overall structure is similar to IgG except that they do not appear to be as compact as IgG or other immunoglobulins and this may account for their increased sensitivity to proteolysis. IgD is also quite heat labile.

No functional role has been assigned to serum IgD. However, IgD has been found in abundance on the surface of B-lymphocytes linked via its Fc portion. Therefore, IgD may play a role as a specific antigen binding site on B-lymphocytes which are the precursor cells of immunoglobulin-producing cells. Furthermore, IgD appears on the B-lymphocyte surface after the appearance of monomeric IgM and is thought to be a step in the normal maturation of immunocompetent B-lymphocytes.

VARIABLE DOMAINS AND ANTIGEN COMBINING SITES

Variable Domains

Comparison of the amino acid sequences of polypeptide chains from the same class of Ig molecules shows that they differ from each other at many positions in the 110 to 112 residues at the amino-terminal end. For this reason, this amino terminal stretch of 110 to 112 amino acids has been designated the variable region or domain. Closer examination of this sequence has revealed that these differences are more pronounced at certain areas within the variable domain. These highly variable regions consist of 5 to 10 residues located at positions 30 to 35, 50 to 55 and 95 to 100 on both H chains and L chains, and are termed hypervariable regions. These hypervariable regions are what constitutes the antigen-combining site of the Ig molecule. Considering the vast array of antigenic determinants present in nature, it is not surprising that extreme amino acid variability in hypervariable regions would be necessary to form a three-dimensional, complementary site to physically accommodate many different antigenic determinants.

The amino acid sequences on either side of the hypervariable regions of many immunoglobulins are far less variable and these are termed framework regions. Each variable domain on both heavy and light chain consists of four relatively constant framework regions and three hypervariable regions. Because of the relative invariance found in certain framework sequences, variable domains have been divided into three types: one associated with heavy chains, one associated with κ light chains and finally one associated with λ light chains. Whereas the hypervariable regions determine the antigenic specificity of the Ig molecule, the framework regions are extremely important in maintaining a consistent overall shape of the entire variable domain.

Antigen Combining Sites—Light Chain and Heavy Chain Interaction

H chains which have been separated and isolated from a functional immunoglobulin will bind to the antigen, although not as strongly as the original, complete immunoglobulin. Isolated light chains bind antigen even less strongly than do isolated heavy chains. Therefore, it appears certain that the hypervariable regions of both heavy and light chains contribute significantly to the overall binding properties of the intact immunoglobulin. The variable domains of heavy and light chains are arranged in such a way that the hypervariable regions from both chains form a cleft or pocket which will accommodate all or a portion of the corresponding antigenic determinant.

Three Dimensional Structure

Each domain, variable or constant consisting of a stretch of amino acids approximately 110 to 112 residues long, is arranged in a compact globular shape. The polypeptide chain of each domain is folded in such a way that there are three relatively straight stretches in one plane and four relatively straight stretches in a second, antiparallel plane. In addition, each domain has one intrachain disulfide bond which apparently stabilizes the structure. This conformation gives rise to a sandwich-like or barrel-like structure. Domains residing on the same chain are linked to one another by short, linear interdomain polypeptides. The hinge region, located between C_H1 and C_H2 of heavy chains, also is composed of a linear polypeptide. The length of the hinge region varies depending on the class of heavy chain. The hinge region also contains a variable number of cysteine residues which provide the locations for interheavy chain disulfide bonds. The fact that this region consists of single linear stretches of amino acids may explain why the hinge region is so susceptible to proteolytic enzyme cleavage.

The oligosaccharide side chains are linked to either serine or asparagine located on heavy chains. To date, oligosaccharides have only been found on heavy chain constant domains.

GENETICS OF IMMUNOGLOBULINS

Considering the enormous number of different antigenic determinants that the humoral immune system specifically responds to, the question of DNA coding capacity and the question of genetic-controlling mechanisms have intrigued scientists for many years. Unproven hypotheses still abound in many areas but some recent research has increased our understanding of many of the molecular events culminating in the synthesis of a functional immunoglobulin molecule.

Many lines of evidence now suggest that two separate genes code for a single polypeptide chain. Specifically, the genes for the variable domains are distinct and physically separated from genes coding for constant domains. It has been shown that there are three gene clusters which segregate independently. Two clusters involve light chains, κ or λ and the third cluster codes for heavy chains so that variable genes in one cluster exclusively link up with a constant gene to form λ chains, variable genes in the second cluster exclusively link up with a constant gene to form κ light chains and variable genes of the third cluster exclusively link up with the constant genes of any one of five constant genes to form heavy chains.

Another remarkable fact to emerge recently involves the discovery of gene arrangement in cells which are actively producing immunoglobulins for extracellular transport. Hybridization experiments using mRNA as a probe to determine the specific location of the corresponding DNA coding regions have revealed that the distance between DNA coding for the variable domain and the constant domain of λ light was much greater in embryonic cells than it was in a cell actively making λ light chains. This would strongly suggest that an intervening segment of DNA had been excised from the genome. This finding has interesting implications for the long-held notion that all cells in the body contain a complete and identical full gene complement. The extent to which other cells in the body undergo a similar type of gene rearrangement is not known at the present time.

Origin of Variable Gene Sequences

Considering the genetic coding capacity necessary to accommodate all the possible antigens encountered in nature, mention will be made of two of the more popular theories which have been put forward to explain the origins of this great diversity.

Germ Line Theory. The germ line theory states that germ cells carry all the structural genes for all variable and constant domains necessary throughout life. It is further postulated that these genes probably arose through conventional genetic mechanisms such as gene duplication and mutation with concomitant selective pressure preserving the useful mutations. Based on estimates of the amount of DNA necessary to accomplish this task relative to the total amount of DNA available for other necessary functions, the germ line theory is mathematically possible.

Somatic Mutation Theory. The somatic mutation theory suggests that germ cells carry a small number of variable genes which become diversified through mutation in somatic cells. If one considers, the normal mutation rate and the number of cells in vertebrates which can respond to immunogens, somatic mutation is also mathematically possible. In this case, the positive selective pressure for maintaining a mutation would be an encounter with the appropriate immunogen.

ADDITIONAL READING

AMZEL, L. M., AND POLJAK, R. J. 1979 Three-Dimensional Structure of Immunoglobulins. Annu Rev Biochem, **48**, 961.

BIENENSTOCK, J., AND BEFUS, A. D. 1980 Review—Mucosal Immunology. Immunology, **41**, 249.

BELLANTI, J. A. 1978 *Immunology II*, Saunders, Philadelphia.

BRANDTZAEG, P. 1981 Transport Models for Secretory IgA and Secretory IgM. Clin Exp Immunol, **44**, 221.

DAVIS, B. D., DULBECCO, R., EISEN, H. N., AND GINSBERG, H. S. 1980 *Microbiology*, Ed. 3. Harper & Row, Hagerstown, Md.

FUDENBERG, H. H., STITES, D. P., CALDWELL, J. L., AND WELLS, J. V. 1978 *Basic and Clinical Immunology*, Ed. 2. Lange Medical Publications, Los Altos, Calif.

ISHIZAKA, K., AND ISHIZAKA, T. 1978 Mechanisms of Reaginic Hypersensitivity and IgE Antibody Response. Immunol Rev, **41**, 109.

KABAT, E. A. 1976 Structural Concepts in Immunology and Immunochemistry, Ed. 2. Holt, Rinehart & Winston, New York.

KOSHLAND, M. E. 1975 Structure and Function of J Chain. Adv Immunol, **20**, 41.

LIN, L. C., AND PUTNAM, F. W. 1981 Primary Structure of the F_c Region of Human Immunoglobulin D: Implications for Evolutionary Origin and Biological Function. Proc Natl Acad Sci, **78**, 504.

NISONOFF, A., HOPPER, J. E., AND SPRING, S. R. 1975 The Antibody Molecule. Academic Press, New York.

PLAUT, A. G., GILBERT, J. V., AND WISTAR, R. JR. 1977 Loss of Antibody Activity in Human Immunoglobulin A Exposed to Extracellular Immunoglobulin A Proteases of *Neisseria gonorrhoeae* and *Streptococcus sanguis*. Infect Immun, **17**, 130.

ROITT, I. M., AND LEHNER, T. 1980 *Immunology of Oral Diseases*. Blackwell Scientific Publications, Oxford.

ROSENTHAL, A. S. 1980 Regulation of the Immune Response—Role of the Macrophage. N Engl J Med, **303**, 1153.

SAKANO, H., MAKI, R., KUROSAWA, Y., ROEDER, W., AND TONEGAWA, S. 1980 Two Types of Somatic Recombination are Necessary for the Generation of Complete Immunoglobulin Heavy-Chain Genes. Nature, **286**, 676.

SAMTER, M. 1978 *Immunological Diseases*, Ed. 3. Little, Brown, Boston.

SILVERSTEIN, A. M., AND BIALASIEWICZ, A. A. 1980 History of Immunology, A History of Theories of Acquired Immunity. Cellular Immunology, **51**, 151.

TAUBMAN, M. A., SMITH, D. J., AND MURRAY, R. 1978 Immunoglobulin Susceptibility to Proteolytic Effects of Human Dental Plaque Extracts. Arch Oral Biol, **23**, 949.

WEIGERT, M., AND RIBLET, R. 1978 The Genetic Control of Antibody Variable Regions in the Mouse. Springer Semin Immunopathol **1**, 133.

chapter 12

Tissue and Cellular Basis for the Immune Response

Keith R. Volkmann

INTRODUCTION

Lymphocytes, the cells which recognize immunogens, can be found throughout the body in blood circulation, in lymphatic circulation and in either well organized lymphoid tissue such as lymph nodes and spleen or in less well organized tissue such as the mesentery of the gut. Lymphocytes, as a class, represent one of the most numerous cell types in the body. It has been estimated that they comprise about 10% of all cells in the body. Ultrastructurally, all unstimulated lymphocytes are quite similar. They average 6 to 15 μm in diameter and are characterized by possessing a large, centrally located nucleus surrounded by a very thin rim of cytoplasm. Unstimulated lymphocytes reveal a paucity of organelles associated with protein synthesis. Specifically, one finds few mitochondria, very little Golgi apparatus and very little rough endoplasmic reticulum. Functionally, however, lymphocytes can broadly be divided into three very distinct categories. After stimulation by a specific antigen, two of the lymphocyte types can differentiate into effector cells: cells producing immunoglobulins or effectors of the cellular immune response while the third type of lymphocyte can differentiate into regulator cells.

Considering the total complement of an individual's lymphocytes, it has been determined that as a group they can respond to an enormous number of different immunogens. However, mature lymphocytes are not totipotent with regard to the antigens to which they can respond. In fact, an individual lymphocyte usually responds to just one antigenic determinant or, at most, a very limited number of antigenic determinants. Historically, favor has vacillated between two theories which have attempted to explain the seeming limitless ability of lymphocytes to respond to the wide variety of immunogens that may be encountered. At one time it was widely believed that the immunogen itself served as an "instructive template" around which

the antigenic combining site of an immunoglobulin was molded or formed. When it became evident that the shape of a protein molecule was determined by primary amino acid sequence and that the sequence was specified by DNA, "the instructive template" theory became untenable. Present day theories revolve around the concept that individual lymphocytes are preprogrammed to respond to specific antigenic determinants before the lymphocyte ever encounters its specific antigen. When antigen combines with a lymphocyte, the lymphocyte proliferates into a clone of cells that differentiates into two populations: 1) a population of effector cells, and 2) a population of antigen sensitive cells (sometimes called memory cells) which provides an expanded pool of the original, responding small lymphocyte. Even though, at the moment, this clonal selection theory is reasonably satisfactory, the explanation of antigen-sensitive cell diversity remains a problem (Chapter 11).

LYMPHATIC ORGANS AND TISSUES

Primary Lymphoid Tissues

Origin of Lymphocytes. Lymphocytes and other formed blood elements are derived from pluripotent and unipotent, self-renewing hematopoietic stem cells. During human development these cells are found first in the yolk sac and then in the fetal liver. After birth and persisting through adult life, hematopoietic stem cells are located in the bone marrow. Progenitor cells arising from stem cells develop into immature erythroid (which terminally differentiate into erythrocytes), myeloid (which terminally differentiate into granulocytes) and lymphoid cells. In the case of immature lymphocytes, terminal differentiation into B lymphocytes and T lymphocytes (primarily involved in the cellular immune response and regulation) occurs in primary lymphoid organs (the bursa of Fabricius, or its equivalent in humans and the thymus), respectively. (For a more complete discussion of lymphocyte maturation, see below.)

Thymus. The thymus develops from the fourth and fifth brachial pouches in the growing embryo as epithelial tissue migrates from these pouches to the midline of the upper thorax. Eventually the rudimentary thymus is populated with cells, termed thymocytes, derived from hematopoietic stem cells. Thymocytes in the thymus divide rapidly and approximately 10% of this dividing pool matures into immunocompetent (meaning that they can respond to specific immunogens) lymphocytes which have been designated T lymphocytes (thymus derived). Presumably a peptide hormone synthesized by epithelial cells of the thymus induces the differentiation of less mature thymocytes into immunocompetent T lymphocytes. After maturation in the thymus, mature T lymphocytes leave the thymus and go into blood and lymphatic circulation in addition to populating secondary lymphoid tissues such as lymph nodes, spleen and gut-associated lymphoid tissue (GALT).

The thymus is quite large at birth and remains very active up to puberty at which time it begins to involute. The adult thymus is considerably smaller than the prepubescent thymus, but in all likelihood it is still active. Recent experiments in which adult mice were thymectomized suggested that these mice aged more rapidly than did control, intact adult mice. Furthermore, it was postulated that the rapid aging process observed was due to the fact that suppressor T lymphocytes were no longer being formed (see T cell subsets below).

Certainly adult thymectomy does not result in the dire consequences to the host animal that are seen when neonatal thymectomies are performed. Neonatal thymectomy of animals results in a drastically altered immune response. The number of circulating lymphocytes is reduced, the cellular immune response including the ability to reject foreign tissue, the ability to recover from many infectious diseases, and the ability to produce immunoglobulin molecules other than the IgM class are greatly reduced, if not ablated. A situation similar to the animal model can be observed in humans when, for one reason or another, the thymus fails to form embryonically or when the thymus does not function properly.

Bursa of Fabricius (Bursal Equivalent). Birds possess a lymphoepithelial organ which anatomically resembles the thymus. It begins as epithelial tissue from the intestine and is later populated by migratory immature lymphocytes. However, the lymphocytes which mature to become immunocompetent cells in the bursa of Fabricius are quite distinct from mature T lymphocytes which leave the thymus. The cells leaving the bursa have surface immunoglobulins, and when stimulated under the appropriate conditions with specific immunogens will produce immunoglobulins. These immunocompetent cells are designated B lymphocytes (Bursa derived). Mammalian species do not have a bursa of Fabricius as a discrete lymphoepithelial organ. It is presumed, however, that mammals have a bursal equivalent which is necessary to promote the maturation of B lymphocytes. Several candidates for a bursal equivalent have been proposed but to date there is no compelling evidence to favor any one particular area. Some of the proposed bursal equivalents include: gut-associated lymphoepithelial tissue such as the appendix or tonsils, Peyer's patches in the mesentery of the gut, bone marrow, the fetal liver, and lymph nodes.

Extirpation of the bursa of Fabricius from a neonatal chick results in a different set of immunological deficits than results from neonatal thymectomy. Bursectomy of a young chick leaves the cellular immune response intact but does lead to a reduced number of antibody-producing cells, a severe depletion of serum immunoglobulin levels and practically no cells populating germinal centers in lymph nodes and the spleen.

Secondary Lymphoid Tissues

Lymph Nodes. Lymphatic vessels begin in peripheral tissues at the capillary level and are structurally similar to venous circulation in the sense that smaller vessels merge to form large vessels until lymphatic flow finally enters one large vessel, the thoracic duct, which returns all lymph flow back into blood circulation. Interspersed in this network of lymph vessels are lymph nodes. Lymph nodes share many structural features in common with primary lymphoid organs and like the primary lymphoid organs are involved in the maturation of lymphocytes, albeit the terminal stages of differentiation. There is one very striking difference between primary lymphoid tissue and secondary tissue. Whereas primary lymphoid tissue is devoid of any known immunogen, and maturation of precursor lymphocytes appears to be hormonally driven in the thymus at least, secondary lymphoid tissue is very efficient at trapping immunogens and the final stages of lymphocyte differentiation is triggered by the presence of immunogens.

Architecturally, lymph nodes are small ovoid structures which are surrounded by a capsule and are composed of three internal areas: the cortex, the paracortex and the medulla. Many afferent lymph channels join the capsule of the node and empty into a subcapsular sinus located directly under the capsule. The cortex which is located immediately beneath the subcapsular sinus is the major site of B lymphocyte localization. Small B lymphocytes are clustered into areas termed lymphoid follicles. Located within lymphoid follicles are dendritic reticulum cells which have a unique capacity to retain antigens on their plasma membranes. During antigenic stimulation, lymphoid follicles give rise to germinal centers, areas of cellular proliferation and hypertrophy which can result in the physical enlargement of the node.

The paracortex is positioned between the cortex and medulla and is the primary area of T lymphocyte localization. Also located within the paracortex are post capillary venules. Recirculating lymphocytes from the bloodstream are able to pass through the specialized endothelial cells of these postcapillary venules in order to enter lymph nodes. The medulla of the node is comprised of a network of cords and sinuses. The sinuses link the subcapsular sinus with the origin of a single efferent lymph vessel which drains the entire node. The endothelial lining of the medullary sinuses has many macrophages and lymphocytes adherent to it. Following antigenic stimulation, plasma cells, producing large quantities of immunoglobulins, accumulate within medullary cords. With few exceptions, immunogens located within body tissue will eventually localize in lymph nodes.

Spleen. Immunologically, the spleen serves a function for the bloodstream similar to the function served by lymph nodes for lymphatic vessels located in body tissue. Bloodborne immunogens tend to be retained within the spleen. Anatomically, the spleen has two areas referred to as red pulp and white pulp. Lymphoid follicles (B lymphocyte areas) and periarteriolar sheaths (T lymphocyte areas) are found in white pulp. These two areas are analogous to lymphoid follicles/germinal centers and the paracortex of lymph nodes respectively. On the other hand, the red pulp contains cords and sinuses corresponding to similar structures located in the medulla of lymph nodes. Unlike lymph nodes, the spleen has no afferent lymphatic vessels. Instead, all fluid enters the spleen via arteries. In addition to filtering out bloodborne immunogens, the spleen may be important in trapping immunogens carried in blood from areas of the body which lack lymphatic drainage such as the central nervous system, including the spinal cord and the eye.

Gut-Associated Lymphoid Tissue. In addition to rather centrally located lymphoid tissues *e.g.*, lymph nodes and spleen, there are lymphoid tissues arranged in various degrees of organization and associated with mucosal surfaces of the body. The lamina propria of the gastrointestinal tract (gut-associated lymphoid tissue, GALT) possesses lymphocytes and lymphocytic aggregates within the connective tissue subjacent to epithelial cells. The respiratory tree and urogenital mucosa also reveal similar accumulations of lymphoid tissue. The immunoglobulins associated with these are predominantly of the IgA class and it is believed that GALT lymphocytes respond to immunogenic stimulation by substances or infectious agents of the mucous

membranes closest to them. The appendix, tonsils and Peyer's patches represent lymphoepithelial tissue showing a higher degree of organization more analogous to lymph nodes than to the small lymphoid aggregates of the lamina propria. These more organized structures have lymphoid follicles and germinal centers populated with B lymphocytes as well as diffuse areas of T lymphocytes.

In summary, lymphoid tissue and organs have two basic functions: 1) primary lymphoid organs accept precursor lymphocytes and release immunocompetent T and B lymphocytes which are capable of responding to immunogenic stimulation; and 2) secondary lymphoid tissue serves as a site for immunocompetent lymphocytes, antigens and other ancillary cells to localize, then interact in such a way that the effector responses of the immune system can be generated.

CELLS OF THE IMMUNE RESPONSE

When examined by the light microscope, all small lymphocytes look very much alike. However, we do know that lymphocytes can broadly be divided into two large groups, B lymphocytes and T lymphocytes, and recently subsets of both T and B lymphocytes have been identified and associated with highly specific immune functions. The identification of specific cell surface markers has provided the basis for categorizing sets and subsets of lymphocytes and has led to further understanding of the functions associated with these subsets of cells.

B Lymphocytes

The presence of surface immunoglobulins on the cytoplasmic membrane of B lymphocytes and the lack of an antigenic marker termed thy (found on all T lymphocytes) formed the basis for distinguishing B lymphocytes from T lymphocytes. Most B lymphocytes have a modified form of monomeric IgM, bound by the Fc portion, projecting from their cytoplasmic membranes. The modification involves an extension of hydrophobic amino acids on the carboxy termini of the IgM heavy chains that presumably penetrate into and are stably held within the membrane itself. Precursor B cells leaving bone marrow possess surface IgM. In addition to surface IgM, many B cells also have surface IgD. It has been suggested that the presence of IgD on B cells is an indication of a maturation step presumably a bursal function necessary for immunocompetence. Other surface immunoglobulins have been identified on B lymphocyte surfaces but these will be discussed later. The Fab portions of surface immunoglobulins are widely regarded as being the antigen recognition unit of the B lymphocyte. Interestingly, if two different classes of immunoglobulin are on the surface of one cell, the variable domains all possess exactly the same receptor specificity for one antigenic determinant.

Practically all B lymphocytes have receptors on their surface membranes for the Fc portions of aggregated immunoglobulins. Aggregation can occur as a result of immunoglobulins binding to immunogens or it can occur *in vitro* when immunoglobulins are denatured. At the time when surface IgD appears on lymphocyte surfaces, a receptor for the third component of complement also appears (Chapter 13). Again it would seem that the appearance of the complement receptor is linked to a maturation process which results in changing an immature B cell into an immunocompetent B cell.

T Lymphocytes

As surface immunoglobulins were the key surface antigenic markers for B lymphocytes, the thy-1 antigen is the key, distinguishing surface antigen marker for all T lymphocytes. Whereas surface immunoglobulins are considered to be the antigen recognition unit for B lymphocytes, the identity of the antigen recognition unit on T lymphocytes is still very much in question. Some T cells appear to have receptors with exactly the same antigen specificity as Ig molecules. However, Igs which can specifically bind to the heavy chains of immunoglobulins do not react with the surface of T lymphocytes. This would suggest that the antigen recognition site of T lymphocytes may well share variable domains with Ig molecules but it also suggests that the variable domains of T cells are not linked to Ig constant domains. On the other hand, antigen recognition by many other T cells appears to be greatly dependent on cell-surface histocompatibility antigens (Chapter 14).

With regard to other surface markers which further distinguish T lymphocytes from B lymphocytes, research on mouse lymphocytes has revealed surface antigens that characterize subsets of T cells that have different functions. There is presumptive evidence to suggest that a similar system is present in humans. In mice there is a complex of antigens termed the Lyt system which consists of three antagenic determinants, designated Lyt-1, Lyt-2 and Lyt-3. During early postnatal life most peripheral T cells carry all three Lyt antigens and are therefore designated Ly-123. These cells appear to have a regulator function. As T lymphocytes mature and gain effector function, the distribution of Lyt antigens also changes. Cells which express just the Lyt-1 antigen (Ly-1) comprise 35% of peripheral T cells and functionally act as T helper cells (T_h) and the T cells which participate in delayed type hypersensitivity reactions (T_{DTH}). Cells which express the Lyt-2 and Lyt-3 antigens (Ly-23) comprise 5 to 10% of peripheral T cells and function as suppressor cells (T_s) and T killer cells (T_k). T_s cells are involved in regulation of the immune response and T_k cells specifically kill certain target cells.

Null Cells

In addition to typical T and B lymphocytes, a class of lymphocyte has been found in mice which lacks both the Thy-1 marker and surface Igs. It has been suggested that these cells, termed null, represent a heterogeneous mixture of immature hematopoietic cells. Functionally, two subclasses of null cells have been identified in the mouse. One subset has been designated K cells (killer cells). K cells have surface receptors for the Fc portion of Igs which are linked to antigens. If the Igs are linked to antigens on a cell surface, then the binding of a K cell to this surface-bound Ig results in the lysis of the Ig covered cell. The second subset of null cells has been termed NK cells (natural killer cells). NK cells have the ability to lyse various tumor cells without prior immunization.

Macrophages

The macrophage already has been discussed as a very important component of nonspecific host defenses. In addition to their role as nonspecific scavengers, macrophages are intimately involved in specific immune responses. There is good evidence to suggest that macrophages present antigens, perhaps after modifying them, to both T and B lymphocytes. *In vitro* experiments have shown that when macrophages are added to a cell system designed to produce Igs after antigenic stimulation, significantly less antigen is required to drive the system if macrophages are also present. There is also some evidence to suggest that macrophages in close physical proximity to antigen sensitive B and T lymphocytes may secrete a factor which triggers proliferation of these lymphocytes. Finally, macrophages can act as effector cells in an immune response. In certain cell-mediated responses, macrophages become more aggressive phagocytic cells with an enhanced capacity to kill ingested microorganisms. Because macrophages have Fc receptors on their surfaces, antigens with immunoglobulin bound to them are easily phagocytosed (opsinization). Thus, in the body's attempt to rid itself of noxious agents, either nonspecifically or specifically (immune response), the macrophage appears to be ubiquitous.

ANTIBODY FORMATION

When an immunogen is introduced into the body, a very small number (out of a pool of about 10^{12} cells) of mature, immunocompetent B lymphocytes are able to bind the immunogen to their surfaces. A sequence of events is then initiated which culminates in the production of specific immunoglobulin, observed as an increase in its concentration in the blood. The most likely anatomical locations for this series of events to occur are the lymph nodes and spleen.

B Lymphocyte—Immunogen Interaction

Immunogens most likely to interact with and stimulate B lymphocytes are soluble macromolecules with multiple antigenic determinants, blood-borne infectious agents such as bacteria and viruses or subcomponents of infectious agents. When the immunogen comes in contact with a B lymphocyte whose surface antigen receptors, IgD plus either IgM or IgG, can specifically interact the immunogen, it is bound by several surface Ig molecules. It has been shown by the use of labeled immunogens that immunoglobulin receptors which were evenly distributed, aggregate when binding to multivalent immunogens. Univalent antigens (haptens) will not aggregate receptors because a hapten by virtue of its single determinant cannot cross-link surface Igs. Immunogen-aggregated surface Igs then further coalesce to form patches. The patches migrate across the lymphocyte membrane to a polar region of the cell, a process termed polar capping. Polar cap formation appears to be dependent on ATP generation and an intact cytoplasmic microtubule system. After a polar cap has formed, it is internalized within the B lymphocyte by endocytosis. The entire process of immunogen binding, aggregation, migration of aggregated "patches," polar cap formation and internalization of the cap takes just a few minutes to complete.

Little is known about the intracellular molecular events which occur after the polar cap has been internalized. However, at the cellular level, proliferation of the stimulated lymphocyte is the next observable step. The proliferating cells divide at a rapid rate and at some point a signal is received which stops the division cycle and initiates a differentiation sequence. The source and nature of these signal(s) are unknown but there is some evidence to suggest that helper T cells may provide the proliferation signal (see below). At the conclusion of differentiation, two populations of cells emerge. Morphologically, one population looks very much like the original antigen-sensitive B lymphocyte with the exception that the surface immunoglobulins on these "secondary" lymphocytes are predominated by IgG or IgA in addition to IgD. The second population to emerge is morphologically quite distinct from the typical B lymphocyte. The cytoplasm of these cells has an abundance of organelles associated with protein synthesis and no surface immunoglobulin. They are called plasma cells. Plasma cells synthesize immunoglobulins in vast quantities (about 2000 molecules/cell/minute) for secretion. The antigenic specificity of the synthesized immu-

noglobulins is exactly the same as the specificity of the surface immunoglobulin on the B lymphocyte from which it was derived. This means that the heavy and light chain variable domains of plasma cell-produced Igs and lymphocyte-surface Igs are the same. However, the plasma cell can couple the heavy chain variable domain to different heavy chain constant domains. This means that any single plasma cell makes immunoglobulins of a single antigen specificity but it also implies that the single specificity can be linked to more than one heavy chain class. Therefore, the rule is, one plasma cell, one antigen specificity or idiotype of immunoglobulin.

The net result of antigenic stimulation of a single or a few B lymphocytes is: 1) specific antibodies produced by plasma cells are available for systemic circulation, and 2) a greatly expanded pool or clone of antigen-sensitive B lymphocytes (sometimes called memory cells) is created which can respond to that same single antigen. Plasma cells are relatively short-lived since they die within a matter of weeks. On the other hand, antigen sensitive B lymphocytes are long-lived (average life span approximately 5 years) and account for the enhanced ability of the immune system to respond to the same antigen during subsequent encounters.

Synthesis and Secretion of Immunoglobulins

Immunoglobulin synthesis and assembly follow a pattern typical of any protein which ultimately will be transported out of a cell. Heavy and light chains are synthesized on ribosomes associated with the rough endoplasmic reticulum and transferred across the membrane into the lumen of the rough endoplasmic reticulum where the inter- and intra-chain disulfide bonds are completed. From there, the immunoglobulins pass to the Golgi complex where hexosetransferases sequentially add sugars to establish heavy chain oligosaccharides, thus completing the assembly of the immunoglobulin. Finally, membrane-bound vesicles containing completed immunoglobulins and derived from the Golgi complex traverse the cytoplasm, fuse with the cell surface membrane and empty the immunoglobulins to the exterior of the cell.

Cell Interactions and the Humoral Immune Response

With increasingly sophisticated *in vitro* and *in vivo* experiments, it has become quite apparent that the interaction of immunogen with immunocompetent B lymphocytes alone does not necessarily result in antibody production. In addition to specific binding of immunogen to the surface Igs of B lymphocytes, it has been found that most immunogens have a requirement for T lymphocyte cooperation and perhaps macrophage cooperation. These antigens, which constitute the vast majority of antigens in nature are termed T-dependent antigens and are characterized by having many structurally different antigenic determinants available to interact with B lymphocytes.

Helper T Lymphocytes

In order for T-dependent antigens to stimulate B lymphocytes to proliferate, differentiate and release antibody, the cooperation of a particular subclass of regulatory T lymphocytes is required. The co-operating T cells are designated T helpers (T_h) and are distinguished by carrying the Lyt-1 surface alloantigen. Furthermore, there is good evidence to suggest that the stimulation of B lymphocytes requires two signals. The first signal is antigen specific and involves binding of the appropriate antigen to B cell surface Ig. The second signal (a mitogenic signal) induces proliferation of the B cell and this signal appears to be T_h dependent. The exact mechanism of T cell cooperation is not known but there is evidence that this, too, may be a two-step process. A macrophage carrying the appropriate antigen may interact with a precursor T cell resulting in the "activation" of the T lymphocyte. Then the activated T cell interacts with a B lymphocyte with the same antigen bound to its surface Ig and stimulates the proliferation of the antigen-bearing B cell. It appears that the helper T cell is in some fashion also bound to the antigen on the surface of the B lymphocyte. Most investigators indicate that the T cell binds to an area of the antigen which does not involve antigenic determinants (the so-called carrier portion of the antigen molecule). Presumably, there are several different carrier regions on one complete antigen. Therefore, several T cells with different carrier specificities conceivably could all "help" a single B cell.

This partly explains why haptens cannot act as immunogens. First, a hapten, by virtue of the fact that it is composed of just one antigenic determinant, cannot cross-link surface Igs on B lymphocytes and therefore patching and polar migration cannot occur as described earlier. Secondly, because there is no carrier attached to the hapten, helper T cells cannot cooperate with B lymphocytes to the extent necessary to provide the proliferation signal.

Suppressor T Lymphocytes

In addition to T_h cells, there is another subset of regulatory T lymphocytes known as suppressor T cells (T_s). T_s cells carry the Lyt-2,3 alloantigens on their surfaces. As the name implies, suppressor T-cells inhibit the production of antibody. Whereas, antigen bound to macrophages stimulates T helper cells, the suggestion is that antigen not bound to macrophages stimulates T_s cells which in turn in-hibit T_h cells. If the appropriate T_h cells are inhibited, then T-dependent antigens cannot stimulate B cell proliferation and no antibody is produced. This condition may occur in the body when small quantities of antigens are administered with the result that very little antibody is produced (see low zone tolerance below).

IgM-IgG Switch

Some plasma cells secreting Ig, which were derived from a B lymphocyte stimulated by a T cell-dependent antigen have the ability to change the heavy chain class of the immunoglobulins they are synthesizing. *In vitro* experiments designed to follow individual clones of immunoglobulin-secreting plasma cells have revealed that after antigen stimulation there can be a switch in the type of heavy chain class with time. Soon after primary antigenic stimulation, all plasma cells were secreting IgM. Four to five days later plasma cells were found to secrete IgM and IgG, or IgM and IgA. One week after antigenic stimulation, all clones were secreting immunoglobulins of just one heavy chain class: IgM, IgG or IgA. The switch from IgM to IgG production, in particular, is considered as an advantage to the host because IgG binds to antigens with greater tenacity than IgM. It must be stressed that although the constant domains of heavy class chains can change, the entire light chain and the heavy chain variable domain remains constant. Therefore, the specificity of the antigen receptor site of the Ig, regardless of heavy chain class, never changes. Interestingly, if the body is rechallenged (secondary immunization) at a later date with the same antigen, practically no plasma cells secrete IgM. IgG in particular is secreted exclusively (an-amnestic response or memory). If one follows the appearance of free IgG in serum following antigenic challenge, the same IgM-to-IgG switch is observed.

T Lymphocyte—Independent Immunogens

Immunogens which do not require T_h cell cooperation in order to stimulate B lymphocytes to proliferate and differentiate appear to have two important properties. They tend to be high molecular weight polymers, particularly polysaccharides, which have multiple, repeating, identical antigenic determinants. Therefore, they are capable of binding to many surface Ig receptors on B-lymphocytes. This satisfies the antigen-specific signal necessary for B cell activation. These immunogens also have the intrinsic ability to provide the mitogenic signal necessary for B cell proliferation. In fact lipopolysaccharides, released from gram negative bacteria, are such potent B cell mitogens, that they can nonspecifically induce proliferation and antibody secretion of many clones of B lymphocytes.

In contrast to T cell-dependent immunogens,

however, no IgM-to-IgG switch is seen with T-independent antigens. Plasma cells derived from T-independent immunogen stimulated B cells only produce IgM. In addition, immunological memory is lacking. The time course and degree of antibody production after the second and subsequent challenges with T-independent immunogens is exactly the same as is seen after the primary encounter with the immunogen. Finally, in mice at least, there is strong evidence to suggest that B lymphocytes which can respond to T-independent immunogens belong to a separate subset of B lymphocytes which can be distinguished by a distinct cell surface antigen.

HUMORAL IMMUNE RESPONSE IN THE INTACT HOST

When immunogens which will elicit a humoral (antibody) response are introduced into an intact host, under the appropriate conditions a series of molecular and cellular events are initiated (those discussed above) which result in a measurable increase in the amount of specific immunoglobulins which will bind to the immunogens. If the immunogen is located in tissue, with the exception of the CNS, the most likely place for antibody production to occur is the regional lymph node which drains the area of immunogen localization. If on the other hand, the immunogen is primarily located in the blood stream or the CNS, then the most likely place for antibody production to occur is the spleen. As discussed previously, secondary lymphoid tissues (spleen and lymph nodes) are architecturally arranged in such a way as to provide interaction between immunogen bearing macrophages, T_h cells and antigen-sensitive B lymphocytes, to provide a location for plasma cells and to provide a means of distributing secreted antibody (efferent lymph channels leading to the thoracic duct in the case of lymph nodes, and venous circulation in the case of the spleen). Secretory IgA synthesis and secretion varies from this pattern of central processing and distribution. Secretory IgA tends first to be produced locally near the point of immunogen entry through the affected mucosa and later in all exocrine glands. Finally, the systemic increase in concentration of a specific antibody with respect to time (most notably IgM and IgG) can be measured by sampling an individual's serum.

Primary Humoral Immune Response

When an immunologically intact host is challenged for the first time with a T-dependent immunogen, a lag period of several days ensues before any form of specific immunoglobulin is detected in serum. The first class of Ig to appear in serum is IgM. Its production peaks in 2 or 3 days then it disappears and is gradually replaced by IgG of the same antigenic specificity. This change in heavy chain class corresponds to the plasma cell IgM-IgG switch mentioned previously. IgG production peaks 14 to 21 days after the introduction of immunogen, and then gradually declines to a point where residual levels in serum are slightly above the preimmunization level. The biological half-life of IgG in serum is about 23 days whereas the half-life of IgM is about 5 days. As antibody production increases during the primary response, the affinity of the antibodies for the antigenic determinant also increases.

Secondary Humoral Immune Response

When an immunologically intact host is challenged a second time with an immunogen to which the host has mounted a primary response at some previous time, the resulting specific antibody production is different from what was described for the primary response. First, the lag time between immunogen encounter and the appearance of free antibody in serum is shorter than seen in the primary response. Also, antibody production occurs at a higher rate and persists longer than in the primary response, resulting in a much higher serum concentration than is seen in the primary response. Practically no IgM is produced in the secondary response and the affinity of the IgG produced throughout the secondary response is high, similar if not identical to the high affinity IgG produced late in the primary response. The host responds as if it had remembered the first encounter with the immunogen and was able to respond faster and to a greater degree, hence the term memory or anamnestic response.

The increased speed of the secondary response and the larger, more persistent immunoglobulin production can be explained by the increased number of specific antigen-sensitive B lymphocytes (memory cells) resulting from the primary response. The explanation for immediate production of high affinity immunoglobulin is not so obvious but may be due to relative immunogen concentrations (high affinity B cell surface Ig can bind immunogens more efficiently at low immunogen concentration than can low affinity surface Ig). This also may account for the fact that one can elicit a secondary response with lower immunogen concentrations than are required to elicit a primary response.

The biological advantage of such a system is of great significance when one considers the immune response to an infectious agent. During primary exposure to an infectious agent, deliberate or accidental, the immunoglobulins produced may be essential for eliminating the invading organism from the body. On the other hand, reinfection by the same infectious agent at some later date would induce a secondary immune response which, because of its decreased lag time and increased Ig production, in many cases, prevents clinical manifestations of the disease altogether or ameliorates the severity of the disease process.

Immunization

By properly manipulating the immune response, medical science has been able to protect an individual from many dangerous infectious agents. The list of public health immunizations includes many highly communicable viral diseases *e.g.*, measles, diseases produced by potent bacterial exotoxins *e.g.*, tetanus, and many diseases produced by bacteria themselves *e.g.*, bacterial pneumonia. There are two ways in which an individual can be protected by manipulating the humoral immune response: active immunization and passive immunization.

Active Immunization. Active immunization, as the term implies, attempts to stimulate the individual's immune system with a particular antigen in order to produce a primary immune response with its attendant increase in antigen-sensitive B lymphocytes capable of responding to the antigen. The critical factor in primary immunization is to use an antigen which does not cause illness yet is antigenically similar or identical to the agent found in nature which obviously does cause disease. In the case of bacterial exotoxins, the biologically active sites are altered but the antigenicity of the molecule is little altered (Toxoids, Chapter 10). In the case of viruses, either the vaccine virus is "killed" so that it cannot replicate in tissue but the surface antigenicity is not altered or an attenuated vaccine virus is produced in the laboratory which when administered to humans will replicate in tissue but not cause disease, yet which retains the same surface antigenicity as the wild type virus found in nature. In the case of bacterial vaccines, killed or attenuated strains are used, as are cell components. Once a primary response has been mounted against the relatively innocuous vaccine agent, the hope is that when the virulent form of the agent is encountered in nature, little or no clinical disease will result. Based on changing patterns of infectious diseases, we know that this concept is valid and immunization has been extremely effective in controlling many serious diseases. It should be stressed that active immunization is most effective when instituted before the individual is exposed to the natural disease agent or substance. The advantage of active immunization is that the probability that protection will result from properly administered vaccine preparations is high and can last for several years.

Passive Immunization. Passive immunization, unlike active immunization, does not stimulate the individual's own immune system. In fact, in many cases the individual's immune response is inhibited by passive immunization. What then is this technique and what is its rationale? Passive immunization involves the transfer of preformed antibodies, usually from an individual who has recovered from a particular disease, to another individual. The rationale is that transferred antibody will help clear the infectious agent or toxin from the recipient before serious disease results. Passive immunization almost always is done after a nonimmune individual is exposed to a specific disease, *e.g.*, following exposure to hepatitis. The idea is that exogenously administered antibodies are immediately available to the recipient thereby filling the gap between antigen exposure and the appearance of large quantities of naturally produced antibody. However, because the exogenous antibody can quickly clear the offending agent from the recipient, the recipient's own immune system may not have time to respond. The advantage of passive immunization is that it may prevent or lessen the severity of disease in the nonimmune host. The disadvantages are: 1) immunity is of short duration due to the biological half-life of the exogenous immunoglobulins, and 2) the recipient's own immune system may not be stimulated. Interestingly enough, under some circumstances, active and passive immunization are utilized concurrently to prevent disease *e.g.*, following rabies exposure. Historically, hyperimmune serum produced in animal species, most notably the horse, was used for passive immunization. By and large however, this practice has been abandoned because of serious side effects which resulted (see serum sickness).

Passive immunization also occurs in nature. The transfer of maternal IgG across the placenta to fetal circulation is considered passive immunization as is the transfer of secretory IgA found in colostrum and breast milk to nursing infants.

Antigen Administration. Although little detailed information concerning the exact mechanisms of natural immunization is available, deliberate immunization of people and animals has yielded some broad generalizations about effective antigen administration. Immunogens have been administered into the skin (intradermally), subcutaneously or in the muscle. Determination of the best site of antigen administration has occurred empirically considering such factors as the irritancy and the volume of the substance being injected. In animal experiments, immunogens have been injected intravenously and intraperitoneally with success. With a few notable exceptions, ingestion of immunogens is not particularly successful because they are easily degraded in the digestive tract. Inhalation also has been used as a route of administration, particularly when preferential synthesis of secretory IgA is desired. Inhalation of immunogens carries with it the increased risk of IgE synthesis and a resultant allergic reaction, however.

Adjuvants. One very important factor necessary

for immunization to take place is persistence of the immunogen once it has entered the body. A portion of immunogen is catabolized, phagocytized or otherwise degraded soon after it enters the body and is obviously unavailable to stimulate the immune system. Therefore, some crucial minimum amount must persist for some ill-defined but nevertheless essential period of time in order to stimulate the immune system.

One way to enhance the persistence of immunogens, particularly the soluble ones, is to inject a mixture of the immunogen and adjuvant. Adjuvants, many of which are inorganic gels, absorb the antigen, act as a depot and slowly release the antigen over a relatively long period of time. Therefore antigen persistence is enhanced. Many years ago, Freund developed some very effective adjuvants consisting of water-oil emulsions. Freund's complete adjuvant consists of a water-oil emulsion in which is suspended living or dead mycobacteria. This complete adjuvant can cause an intense chronic inflammatory response at the site of deposit, which precludes its use in man. Freund's incomplete adjuvant (without mycobacteria), although not as effective as complete adjuvant has been successfully used clinically.

Tolerance

Going back in history, practically to the point when the immune system was discovered, it was recognized that an individual did not respond to his own or self-antigens. The recognition of self-antigens and the lack of immune response against them is termed self-tolerance. Experimentally it is possible to take a substance which is usually immunogenic and present it to the immunocompetent host in such a way that the host fails to respond to the antigen. Once induced, this type of tolerance is antigen specific, meaning that the host is only immunologically unresponsive to the antigen which was used to induce the tolerant state. Immunity or tolerance then are alternative responses to the same substance. Investigation of the laboratory phenomenon of tolerance has aided our understanding of the more important phenomenon of self-tolerance and the circumstances which may be important in loss of self-tolerance.

Factors Which Favor Induction of Tolerance. It is easier to induce tolerance in fetal and newborn members of a species than in mature adults. This is probably due to the fact that immature B cells in the neonate are more easily made tolerant than mature B cells from the adult. The dose of antigen given appears to be another important factor. Every immunogen has an optimum dose range which is needed to elicit an immune response. Doses which greatly exceed the optimal . dose tend to result in high zone tolerance. B cells

are susceptible to high zone tolerance and therefore, T-independent and T-dependent antigens can be used to induce high zone tolerance. On the other hand, tolerance also can be produced with quantities of antigen on an order of magnitude below the optimal immunizing dose. This so-called low zone tolerance only effects T cells. Therefore, low zone tolerance can only be induced with T-dependent antigens. A third factor involves the physical state of the immunogen. The more soluble or the less aggregated an immunogen is the more likely it is to induce tolerance. On the other hand, particulate immunogens such as bacteria and viruses are usually always immunogenic and therefore it is very difficult to make them tolerigenic. Finally, the route of antigen administration can be a factor, especially in the case of soluble antigens. These antigens tend to be immunogenic when they are injected into tissue but tolerigenic when they are injected intravenously.

Possible Mechanisms of Tolerance. Although tolerance, particularly self-tolerance, is well recognized and can routinely be produced in the laboratory, the cellular mechanisms controlling this phenomenon are not well understood. Empirically it is known that T cell tolerance can be induced with quantities of antigen well below those required for immunity. It has been proposed that either T_h cells are inhibited directly in this situation or that T_s cells are selectively activated, thereby indirectly inhibiting T_h cells. Because T_h cells require an interaction with antigen-bearing macrophages, it may be that T_s cells interact with antigens present in small quantities before macrophages can interact with the same antigen and therefore T_h cells respond to T_s cell suppression rather than to antigen-bearing macrophage activation. In this model, potential helper T cells are not destroyed or lost which implies that if the antigen is presented under appropriate conditions, an immune response could occur. In experimental protocols, it has been found that it is easier to induce T cell tolerance than it is to induce B cell tolerance. In addition to requiring less antigen, tolerance in T cells occurs in a shorter period of time and lasts longer than tolerance in B cells.

B lymphocyte tolerance also is difficult to explain. At one time it was believed that exposure to large quantities of multivalent antigen somehow physically eliminated or destroyed responding B lymphocytes. Because it is difficult to explain how interaction with a noncytotoxic antigen could cause the death of B cells, current theories predict a functional destruction of B cells. During typical activation of a B cell, it has been pointed out that multivalent antigen is bound to surface Ig molecules and these antigen-bearing Igs migrate to a polar cap which is ingested by the B cell, followed by cellular proliferation and differentiation. However, alternatively the polar cap, instead of being ingested, can be sloughed off the surface of the B cell leaving the surface devoid of antigen-binding surface immunoglobulins and therefore the cell would be unable to respond to additional antigen. Mature B cells from adults are relatively difficult to strip of their surface Igs. Furthermore, mature B cells have the ability to regenerate surface Igs in a relatively short period of time. On the other hand, immature B lymphocytes from fetal or neonatal animals can be stripped of their surface Igs more quickly and more completely than mature B cells and regeneration tends not to occur. This may explain why it is easier to induce high zone tolerance in the newborn than in the adult.

Two important factors must be kept in mind concerning tolerance. First, tolerance is antigen specific, meaning that it can be produced to a specific antigen; it is not a state of central unresponsiveness to all immunogens. Secondly, in most circumstances, tolerance can only be maintained by the continuous presence of the immunogen. New antigen reactive B and T cells are constantly being generated and their function can only be inhibited by the constant presence of antigen. This brings the discussion of tolerance to its final point. The easiest way to break tolerance is simply to withhold the antigen, in which case it will in all likelihood be degraded and metabolized within the body, or to eliminate it from the body by adding preformed specific immunoglobulin.

Maturation of the Humoral Immune Response. As might be expected, the immune system begins to develop and mature during fetal development. However, all elements of the humoral immune response do not function at adult levels until 9 to 10 years after birth. B lymphocytes bearing surface IgM or IgG immunoglobulins can be detected in the fetus by the 10th week of gestation. If a fetal spleen is examined at the 15th week of gestation, the proportion of lymphocytes bearing surface immunoglobulins of all classes is essentially similar to the distribution seen in adults. However, secretion of immunoglobulins is not observed until the 20th week of development and then IgM is the predominant immunoglobulin secreted in addition to perhaps sparse secretions of IgG. Secretion of IgA is seen at some point after birth.

Even though secreted immunoglobulins can be detected in a relatively young fetus, it should not be inferred that the fetus can respond to a wide variety of immunogenic challenges. Protective quantities of immunoglobulins are not seen until after birth and although fetal B cells can respond to antigens *in vitro*, the limited responsiveness *in vivo* may be due to the maturational state of macrophages. On the other hand, plasma cell development with concomitant Ig secretion (IgM) can be quite vigorous in the fetus in response to congenital infections such as syphilis.

At birth, the highest concentration of serum immunoglobulin is of the IgG class. However, the majority of this IgG is of maternal origin because that Ig is the only one which is selectively transported across the placenta. Therefore, at birth the infant possesses an IgG repertoire equivalent to that of its mother. During the first 8 to 10 weeks of neonatal life there is a continuous net loss of IgG due to normal turnover and loss of maternal IgG and then total IgG levels begin to rise again as the infant begins to secrete his own IgG. Adult concentrations of serum IgM are found in the infant at about 10 months of age and this is followed by IgG at 3 to 4 years, by IgA at 9 to 10 years and finally by IgE at about 10 to 15 years. The significance of this sequential accretion of immunoglobulin levels coupled with the rapid loss of maternal IgG is that the infant is particularly vulnerable to infectious diseases from the 2nd to the 6th month of life.

IMMUNODEFICIENCY STATES

Immune deficiency states have been discovered which are due to defects in the functional capacities of both B and T lymphocytes. If the condition is due to a B cell defect, then one can expect impaired function of all or a part of the humoral response but T cell-mediated responses should be intact. On the other hand, if the defect impairs the ability of T lymphocytes to function properly, then one would expect not only T cell responses to function poorly but in addition, T-dependent humoral responses would also be affected adversely.

Infantile X-linked Agammaglobulinemia

This X-linked genetic condition occurs overtly in males and is carried symptom-free in heterozygous females. Male infants with congenital agammaglobulinemia usually remain in general good health for the first 9 months of life and then, depending on their environment and exposure to various infectious agents, become ill, particularly with the pyogenic organisms: staphylococci, pneumococci, streptococci and *Haemophilus influenzae*. The disease states can be controlled with appropriate antibiotic therapy, but persistent recurrences are common. Interestingly enough, these children do not seem to have any unusual difficulty with common childhood viral diseases and are not unduly susceptible to protozoal or mycotic infections.

The sera of children with X-linked agammaglobulinemia show a profound reduction of immunoglobulin levels of all classes compared to the normal child. Even more striking is the finding that these children have practically no lymphocytes which have surface immunoglobulins. Therefore, their B cells cannot respond to immunogens. There appears to be either a stem cell defect or a defect in the process leading to mature, functional B lymphocytes. The sure diagnosis of this condition involves lymph node biopsy after deliberate immunization procedures. The histological picture reveals a highly disorganized cellular arrangement and a striking lack of plasma cells. The purely cellular immune responses are intact although in some individuals at a reduced level. Other serum constituents involved in resistance to infection are normal, *i.e.*, complement, lysozyme and properdin levels are within normal limits. The most effective treatment for these individuals is monthly injection of commercially available γ-globulin preparations (passive immunization).

Selective IgA Deficiency

Selective IgA deficiency is the most common immunoglobulin deficiency occurring in 0.1% of the population, and is more correctly termed a dysgammaglobulinemia. The condition is heritable and can be transmitted as either an autosomal recessive trait or an autosomal dominant trait. In addition, there is evidence the selective IgA deficiency can be acquired because it has been associated with congenital infections including rubella. Patients with this condition have a normal complement of IgA bearing B lymphocytes, and *in vitro* these cells can be induced to proliferate when exposed to immunologically nonspecific mitogens such as the lectin derived from the pokeweed plant. The defect in these cells appears to involve an inability to respond to the antigenic signal for terminal differentiation normally elicited by immunogen binding to surface Ig.

Most individuals with selective IgA deficiency suffer no apparent increased susceptibility to disease. One explanation for this paradox is based on recent evidence which suggested that there is a compensatory, secretory IgM produced.

ADDITIONAL READING

ABBAS, A. K. 1979 Hypothesis: Two Distinct Mechanisms of B-Lymphocyte Tolerance. Cell Immunol, **46**, 178.

BIENENSTOCK, J., AND BEFUS, A. D. 1980 Review. Mucosal Immunology. Immunology, **41**, 249.

BELLANTI, J. A. 1978 *Immunology II*, Saunders, Philadelphia.

CHANOCK, R. M. 1981 Strategy for Development of Respiratory and Gastrointestinal Tract Viral Vaccines in the 1980s. J Infect Dis, **143**, 364.

CLAMAN, H. N. 1979 Hypothesis: T-Cell Tolerance—One Signal? Cell Immunol, **48**, 201.

CONGER, J. D., LEWIS, G. K., AND GOODMAN, J. W. 1981 Idiotype Profile of an Immune Response I. Contrasts in Idiotype Dominance between Primary and Secondary Responses and between IgM and IgG Plaque-Forming Cells. J Exp Med, **153**, 1173.

COTNER, T., MASHIMO, H., KUNG, P. C., GOLDSTEIN, G., AND STROMINGER, J. L. 1981 Human T Cell Surface Antigens Bearing a Structural Relationship to HLA Antigens. Proc Natl Acad Sci, **78**, 3858.

DAVIS, B. D., DULBECCO, R., EISEN, H. N., AND GINSBERG, H. S. 1980 *Microbiology*, Ed. 3. Harper & Row, Hagerstown, Md.

EDELMAN, R. 1980 Vaccine Adjuvants. Rev Infect Dis, **2**, 370.

FITCHEN, J. H., FOON, K. A., AND CLINE, M. J. 1981 The Antigenic Characteristics of Hematopoietic Stem Cells. N Engl J Med, **305**, 17.

FUDENBERG, H. H., STITES, D. P., CALDWELL, J. L., AND WELLS, J. V. 1978 *Basic & Clinical Immunology*, Ed. 2. Lange Medical Publishers, Los Altos, Calif.

HASEK, M., AND CHUTNA, J. 1979 Complexity of the State of Immunological Tolerance. Immunol Rev, **46**, 3.

HEDDLE, R. J., KWITKO, A. O., AND SHEARMAN, D. J. C. 1980 Specific IgM and IgG Antibodies in IgA Deficiency. Clinical Exp Immunol, **41**, 453.

LU, C. Y., CALAMAI, E. G., AND UNANUE, E. R. 1979 A Defect in the Antigen-Presenting Function of Macrophages from Neonatal Mice. Nature, **282**, 327.

MANDEL, T. E., PHIPPS, R. P., ABBOT, A., AND TEW, J. G. 1980 The Follicular Dendritic Cell: Long Term Antigen Retention During Immunity. Immunol Rev, **53**, 29.

MARTINEZ, A. C., AND COUTINHO, A. 1981 B-Cell Activation by Helper Cells in a Two-Step Process. Nature, **290**, 60.

MIYAWAKI, T., MORIYA, N., NAGAOKI, T., AND TANIGUCHI, N. 1981 Maturation of B-Cell Differentiation Ability and T-Cell Regulatory Function in Infancy and Childhood. Immunol Rev, **57**, 61.

QUESENBERRY, P., AND LEVITT, L. 1979 Hematopoietic Stem Cells. N Engl J Med, **301**, 755, 819, 868.

ROITT, I. M., AND LEHNER, T. 1980 *Immunology of Oral Diseases*, Blackwell Scientific Publications, Oxford.

ROSENTHAL, A. S. 1980 Regulation of the Immune Response—Role of the Macrophage. N Engl J Med, **303**, 1153.

SABIN, A. B. 1981 Immunization. Evaluation of Some Currently Available and Prospective Vaccines. J Am Med Assoc, **246**, 236.

SAMTER, M. 1978 *Immunological Diseases*, Ed. 3. Little, Brown, Boston.

SUBBARAO, B., MOSIER, D. E., AHMED, A., MOND, J. J., SCHER, I., AND PAUL, W. E. 1979 Role of a Nonimmunoglobulin Cell Surface Determinant in the Activation of B Lymphocytes by Thymus-Independent Antigens. J Exp Med, **149**, 495.

TEW, J. G., PHIPPS, R. P., AND MANDEL, T. E. 1980 The Maintenance and Regulation of the Humoral Immune Response: Persisting Antigen and the Role of Follicular Antigen-Binding Dendritic Cells as Accessory Cells. Immunol Rev, **53**, 175.

chapter 13

Antibody-Mediated Disease, Complement and Serology

Keith R. Volkmann

INTRODUCTION

Up to this point, the immune response, particularly the humoral immune response, has been presented as a beneficial component of the body's defense against invading microorganisms and other noxious substances. However, the immunological sword can cut in two directions. The injection of a small amount of bee venom into the skin of man hardly seems to constitute a serious problem, yet the immune response to that venom can kill a man within minutes. Similarly it is difficult to understand why a protective system should produce acute glomerulonephritis in the process of ridding the body of an infectious agent. In the following sections, these unfavorable phenomena will be discussed and an attempt made to explain these phenomena in terms of an inappropriate, over-vigorous response or insufficient immune response.

IMMEDIATE-TYPE HYPERSENSITIVITY— ANAPHYLAXIS

Most immune responses categorized as immediate-type hypersensitivity or allergic responses are mediated by IgE. The details of why IgE should be produced in response to certain immunogens instead of IgG are not clear, but some general observations may be made. There appear to be at least two groups of antigens which tend to elicit an IgE response. One group consists of haptens: for example, penicillin or its metabolic products which are very efficient in binding to circulating carriers necessary to make the hapten immunogenic. The other broad group of immunogens can be found in the environment and includes various plant pollens, spores and animal danders which are unusually resistant to enzymatic degradation after entering the body. Those immunogens which usually elicit an IgE rather than an IgG response are called sensitizers, reagins or allergens and usually, very low antigen doses stimulate the IgE response.

IgE-producing plasma cells have routinely been found in the intestinal mucosa, respiratory mucosa and mesenteric lymph nodes. Even in these locations however, IgE-bearing B lymphocytes are outnumbered by IgA-bearing lymphocytes. IgE-producing plasma cells or IgE-bearing B lymphocytes are rarely found in other regional lymph nodes or in the spleen, accounting for the extremely low levels of IgE found in serum. The paucity of IgE production and the relatively few incidents of IgE-mediated disease both suggest that IgE production is under stringent regulation. Considering all immunoglobulin production, IgE production is the most dependent on T cell helper activity. Furthermore, IgE production is considerably more susceptible to T cell suppressor activity than is IgG production. Nevertheless, when IgE is produced, all these inhibitory factors not withstanding, a series of events is set into motion which is quite different from any of the humoral responses discussed previously.

Cytotropic Nature of IgE

Several lines of investigation have demonstrated that IgE has the ability to bind to mast cells and basophilic polymorphonuclear leukocytes (basophils). Mast cells are nonmotile connective tissue cells found peripheral to capillaries. They are especially prevalent in skin, lungs, gastrointestinal and genitourinary tracts. Basophils are derived from hematopoietic stem cells of the white cell series and are motile. IgE is bound via specific IgE (Fc) receptors on the surface of mast cells and basophils via the Fc portion of its heavy chains. The high affinity of IgE for these receptors accounts for the long term sensitivity to IgE eliciting antigens.

Mast Cell/Basophil Activation

In order for mast cells or basophils to be activated, two conditions have to be met: 1) IgE must be bound to mast cell or basophil surface receptors. This implies that the individual has had at least one previous exposure to the antigen to induce initial synthesis of IgE, and 2) antigen during a second or subsequent exposure, must specifically cross-link a minimum of two surface-bound IgE molecules which, in turn, causes the aggregation of surface Fc receptors. When receptor aggregation has occurred, mast cells are said to degranulate meaning that preformed granules residing within the cytoplasm of these cells and containing histamine, heparin and other substances fuse with the cytoplasmic membrane, emptying their contents to the exterior of the cell. Degranulation does not involve destruction of the cell. The substances released from granules are pharmacologically active and because they are preformed they are classified as primary mediators of immediate hypersensitivity. In addition, after degranulation begins, other pharmacologically active mediators are rapidly synthesized by the cell and secreted into the surrounding environment. Because these substances are not preformed, they are classified as secondary mediators. The released mediators, be they primary or secondary, actually cause the physical manifestations which are observed in immediate-type hypersensitivity.

Primary Mediators

Histamine. Histamine is formed from L-histidine and is found throughout the body but is present in high concentrations in granules of mast cells and basophils in addition to platelets. Physiologically, the action of histamine is exerted by its interaction with two distinct cell surface receptors. The H-1 receptor controls the inflammatory responses including increased capillary permeability, presumably due to decreasing the adherence of adjacent endothelial cells, smooth muscle contraction of bronchi that results in a profound increase in airway resistance, and smooth muscle contraction of the intestines. Histamine effects, mediated through H-1 receptors, can be reversed by antihistamines. The noninflammatory effects of histamine are mediated through H-2 receptors. These include increased gastric secretion of HCl and cardiac stimulation. These actions cannot be blocked by antihistamines but rather require thiourea derivatives. Species vary in their sensitivity to histamine but unfortunately man is exquisitely sensitive to its actions. Therefore, histamine release is a major contributor to the manifestations of immediate-type hypersensitivity.

Serotonin (5-hydroxytryptamine, 5-HT). Serotonin is formed from L-tryptophan and its body distribution varies in different species. In some rodent species it is found preformed in the granules of mast cells and basophils and is released during typical IgE-antigen complex formation. In humans, serotonin is not found in mast cells or basophils, but rather is located in platelets, the brain and the enterochromaffin cells of the gastrointestinal tract. In humans, serotonin can be released from platelets during an IgE-mediated response by a secondary mediator (see below) produced in mast cells and basophils after degranulation. The pharmacological effects of serotonin are very similar to those of histamine, i.e., smooth muscle contraction and venule leakiness. Many rodents are quite sensitive to this substance but humans are rather resistant to serotonin. Therefore, its role as an active mediator in human immediate-type hypersensitivity responses has come into question.

Eosinophil Chemotactic Factor of Anaphylaxis (ECF-A). ECF-A, a highly selective chemoattractant for eosinophils, is found preformed in human mast cells and basophils. The best characterized ECF-As consist of two acidic tetrapeptides but a much larger polypeptide with the same function also is known to exist in granules. ECF-A is important because eosinophils release a substance which inhibits the actions of slow reaction substance of anaphylaxis (SRS-A), which is a secondary mediator of immediate-type hypersensitivity reactions and will be more fully discussed in that section.

Heparin. Heparin is a proteoglycan which is located in granules of human mast cells. Heparin has the ability to block complement activity and inhibits both coagulation and fibrinolysis.

Secondary Mediators

Slow Reacting Substance of Anaphylaxis. (SRS-A). SRS-A, a sulfur-containing acidic lipid, appears in an immediate type hypersensitivity response after mast cell and basophil degranulation is complete (approximately 5 minutes). Because SRS-A is not preformed prior to IgE-antigen complex formation on the surface of mast cells and basophils, it is classified as a secondary mediator. Nonetheless, degranulation must in some way trigger its synthesis. The most notable pharmacological effect of SRS-A in humans is a profound ability to cause bronchiolar constriction and vascular permeability. The smooth muscle contraction is greater and of longer duration than that produced by histamine. For this reason, SRS-A is considered to be the most important cause of asthma. Furthermore, the action of SRS-A is not blocked by antihistamines, and exogenously administered epinephrine may be required to reduce bronchiole constriction. However, the body does have substances which will block the action of SRS-A, namely the arylsulfatases released by eosinophils. It now becomes clear why ECF-A release is important since this substance and the subsequent release of arylsulfatases provide a mechanism for bringing the system back to homeostasis.

Platelet Activating Factors. (PAF). Platelet activating factors also are synthesized and released from mast cells and basophils after these cells have been degranulated. The major PAFs are phospholipids which, when released, both aggregate platelets and stimulate the release of serotonin from platelets.

Physical Manifestations of Immediate-type Hypersensitivity

The degree and severity of physical manifestations resulting from an IgE-mediated response is dependent on several factors: the total number of mast cells and/or basophils which are coated with surface IgE specific for a particular antigen (usually a function of the number of exposures a responding individual has had to the sensitizing antigen); the site of antigen administration (skin, inhaled into the lung, ingested, or systemically administered); and to some extent the amount of antigen administered. In individuals who are mildly sensitized, local skin administration of the sensitizing antigen would typically produce localized symptoms beginning as soon as 2 to 3 minutes after antigen administration. The first symptom usually experienced is itching at the site of penetration, very quickly followed by a pale edematous raised zone surrounded by a halo of erythema termed a wheal and flare. The response reaches maximal intensity by about 10 minutes, persists for another 10 to 20 minutes and then gradually subsides. This phenomenon is referred to as cutaneous anaphylaxis. At the other end of the spectrum, injection, deliberate or otherwise, of the same amount of antigen in a hypersensitive individual can result in a dramatic increase in the speed of onset, the distribution and the intensity of the anaphylactic response. In generalized or systemic anaphylaxis, massive edema can develop around the site of antigen injection. Difficulty in breathing and swallowing is encountered due to bronchial and laryngeal constriction and edema and there may be profound hypovolemic shock due to peripheral capillary permeability and vasodilation. Anaphylactic death in humans can occur very rapidly and is due primarily to asphyxia. After a response of this intensity, if the individual does not die, recovery is usually complete within an hour. The important points for clinicians to keep in mind are: demonstration on the part of patients of any of these symptoms is cause for concern and demonstration of difficulty in breathing demands rapid and decisive intervention.

Atopy. There appears to be a heritable predisposition for some individuals to easily become hypersensitive to a few or many environmental allergens. Hypersensitivity develops spontaneously when these allergens are either inhaled or ingested. Airborne plant pollens, particularly ragweed pollen, represent the most common and well studied allergens in this country. In addition, tree and grass pollens, microbial spores, house dust (which is composed of epidermal products of man and animals, bacteria, molds and insect parts), bovine milk constituents and egg albumin all can be potent allergens. The two most common physical manifestations of inhalation allergy are hay fever, more properly termed allergic rhinitis, and asthma. Allergic rhinitis is characterized by sneezing, nasal congestion and watery discharge, as well as increased lacrimation, periorbital edema and conjunctival itching. On the other hand, symptoms of bronchial asthma are paroxysmal seizures of dyspnea associated with coughing and wheezing. Chest tightness is an early symptom and in some cases is preceded by allergic rhinitis. Unlike emphysema, asthma is episodic, leaves no permanent tissue damage and usually is not brought on by exertion.

Desensitization. One way of preventing allergic responses is avoidance of the allergen. Since avoidance may not be a practical solution, a common strategy involves active treatment of an individual with the hope of preventing IgE-mediated responses. This involves induction of noncytotropic-blocking antibodies by repeated injections of small and increasing amounts of the allergen to induce the production of IgG. The rationale for this procedure is predicated on the notion that in the presence of high concentrations of IgG, the allergen would be bound by the IgG before it had the opportunity to bind either to mast cell and basophil-bound IgE, or the opportunity to elicit more IgE production. The clinical results of this procedure are somewhat unpredictable and by no means universally successful. As a very rough estimate, approximately 50% of the atopic individuals who have been through a desensitization series demonstrate clinical improvement. Interestingly, many individuals who do not show improvement do have high levels of allergen-specific serum IgG.

Passive Transfer of IgE

Because immediate-type hypersensitivity is mediated by an immunoglobulin, it would seem reasonable to expect that sensitivity to a particular allergen could be transferred by serum from a sensitized to a nonsensitized individual. Indeed this is the case. The guinea pig has been a consistently reliable model for human anaphylactic responses and passive transfer of hypersensitivity has been studied in great detail in this animal species.

Passive Cutaneous Anaphylaxis (PCA). If a small quantity of dilute serum from a previously sensitized guinea pig is injected into the skin of a normal guinea pig and if this transfer is followed the next day by an injection of the sensitizing allergen at the same site, then a typical wheal and flare will be observed within minutes of injection of the allergen. A minimal latent period of 3 to 6 hours between serum injection and allergen injection is required, however, presumably to allow time for the transferred IgE to become bound to the surfaces of mast cells and basophils in the immediate vicinity of the injection site. The PCA phenomenon can be made more visible if a dye such as Evans blue is injected intravenously just prior to the injection of antigen. Because of the mediator-induced increase in capillary permeability, the bloodborne dye leaks into the tissue surrounding the antigen injection site. In fact, measurement of the diameter of the blue-stained area has been used as a semiqualitative measure of IgE concentration.

Prausnitz-Küstner Reaction. Passive cutaneous anaphylaxis can be demonstrated in humans by following essentially the same procedure used to demonstrate PCA in guinea pigs. PCA in humans is termed the Prausnitz-Küstner (P-K) reaction after those who first described it in 1921. Again a small amount of diluted serum from an atopic individual is injected into the skin of a nonsensitized person. In humans, the latent period required between serum injection and allergen injection is 10 to 20 hours. As in PCA in the guinea pig, if the donor's serum contains IgE specific for the allergen, a typical wheal and flare will develop very quickly at the injection site. The P-K reaction was used in humans as a safe alternative to direct skin testing of atopic individuals.

Schultz-Dale Reaction. Returning to the guinea pig model, there is one additional method used for demonstrating immediate-type hypersensitivity induced either actively or passively. The Schultz-Dale reaction occurs when isolated uterine or intestinal strips from a sensitized animal contract *in vitro* with the addition of antigen to the bathing solution.

COMPLEMENT

It has long been recognized that a normal constituent of serum contributes to host defenses in the presence of antigen-antibody complexes. Historically, it was noted that cholera vibrios were lysed within a short period of time when added to the serum from an immunized animal. It was also noted that this constituent was heat labile because the lytic activity of immune serum was destroyed after heating it to 56 C for a few minutes. After heat treatment, lytic activity was restored to the immune serum by adding fresh serum from a normal animal. Therefore, lysis appeared to be dependent on two factors: 1) specific antigen-antibody complex formation; and 2) the presence of a normal constituent

of serum, which is now termed complement. It is now known that complement is not a single entity in serum but rather constitutes a collection of 14 separate proteins which act in an ordered sequence. If the complement sequence is initiated by antigen-antibody complexes, then the term used to describe the initiation is the "classic complement pathway." On the other hand, we now know that the complement sequence can be initiated by substances other than antigen-antibody complexes and when this occurs the term used to describe the initiation is the "alternate complement pathway." Regardless of the initiation circumstance, classic or alternate, completion of the complement sequence results in alterations to cell cytoplasmic membranes, which in turn frequently leads to lysis of the cell. In the aforementioned example, the lysed cells were bacteria and therefore complement was considered as a host defense. However, complement-mediated lysis, under the appropriate conditions, also can destroy normal tissue in which case it would be viewed as a liability to the host rather than as an asset.

The components of complement, designated by a C followed by the number of the component, are a heterogeneous group of proteins which circulate in blood in an inactive form and as a group comprise about 10% of the globulins found in normal serum of humans. When activated, complement proteins acting early in the ordered sequence are cleaved so that one cleavage product becomes a proteolytic enzyme to cleave specifically and only the next complement protein in the sequence. The second cleavage product may have nonenzymatic biological activity such as causing inflammatory tissue changes. Complement proteins acting late in the ordered sequence do not behave as enzymes, but rather aggregate to form a complex which actually alters the permeability characteristics of cytoplasmic membranes.

Early Steps of Complement Sequence

Initiation of Classic Complement Pathway. The classic complement pathway can be initiated by antigen-antibody complexes formed by IgM, IgG-1 or IgG-3. For the sake of this discussion we will assume the antigen is a gram negative bacterial cell wall component located very near the bacterial cell membrane. In the case of IgG complexes, individual IgGs must be aggregated in sufficient numbers and compactness to ensure that two adjacent IgGs are close enough together in order for the first complement protein to physically bridge the distance between adjacent Fc regions. Because IgM is a pentamer with five closely apposed Fc regions, the interaction of just one IgM with an antigen is sufficient to bind the first complement protein (C1). When the appropriate Ig complexes with antigen, a conformational change occurs within the Ig molecule which opens up a C1 receptor located on the C_H2 domain of heavy chains.

C1, the first component to be activated in the classic pathway is actually a complex of three separate proteins designated C1q, C1r and C1s (fig. 13/1). C1q is the recognition unit of the complex and is an unusual protein. It is composed of six stalk-like proteins, all joined at one end of the stalk. The free ends of the stalks are capped with a globular protein such that one could visualize C1q as resembling a hand-held bouquet of six tulips. The globular ends of C1q spontaneously bind to exposed receptors on the C_H2 domains of Igs (no prior activation step is necessary other than the requisite antigen-antibody complex formation). Binding of C1q causes a conformational change in the molecule which results in the activation of C1r and then C1s. First, C1r is cleaved and becomes a proteolytic enzyme ($\overline{C1r}$) which in turn cleaves C1s whose active form is also a proteolytic enzyme ($\overline{C1s}$). A bar over a complement component or complex designates the enzymatically active form, *e.g.*, $\overline{C1s}$, $\overline{C4b2a}$. One additional requirement for the proper functioning of C1 is Ca^{2+} which is necessary to stabilize the complex.

The next component to react in the sequence is C4 (complement proteins were numbered in the order of their discovery, not in the sequence in which they react). $\overline{C1s}$ cleaves C4 into two fragments: a small fragment, C4a, and a larger fragment, C4b. A single C1s activates hundreds of C4 molecules with the result that some C4b remains attached to the Ag-Ab$\overline{C1}$ complex and some C4b becomes bound to the nearby bacterial cell membrane. Membrane-bound C4b enhances the cleavage of, and acts as a receptor for, the split product of the next protein in the sequence, C2 (C2 like C4 is a natural substrate for C1s). When C2 is cleaved, two fragments result: C2a, the major fragment, binds to membrane-bound C4b in the presence of Mg^{2+} and C2b, the minor fragment, is biologically inactive and diffuses away.

The membrane-bound, bimolecular $\overline{C4b,2a}$ complex (also called C3 convertase) which is physically separated from the Ag-Ab$\overline{C1}$ complex, acts as a proteolytic enzyme which is specific for C3, the next protein to be activated in the sequence. The enzymatically active site of C3 convertase is the C2a moiety which cleaves C3 into a small C3a fragment and a larger C3b fragment which joins the membrane-bound $\overline{C4b,2a}$ complex to form the larger $\overline{C4b,2a,3b}$ complex which in turn will activate the next component, C5.

There is another sequence of events which culminates in the cleavage of C3 and which does not require specific antigen-antibody complex formation to initiate the complement cascade. The alternate complement pathway does not utilize C1, C2, or C4, but it does depend on other normal constituents of serum which also react in sequence before C3 is cleaved. This alternative initiation pathway will be discussed before returning to the common remaining late steps in the complete complement sequence.

Initiation of the Alternate Complement Pathway. Complex polysaccharides of bacterial and fungal origin, lipopolysaccharides from gram negative bacteria and aggregated IgA and IgG4 all can initiate the alternate complement pathway. Unlike the classic pathway, in which C1, C2, and C4 are normally present in an inactive form and require specific activation, the early proteins of the alternate pathway are normal constituents of serum which are always active and depend on the activity of normal inhibitors to keep the system in check. It is only when these inhibitors can be by-passed that significant quantities of C3 are cleaved and the complement sequence can go to completion. The continuously active serum proteins in the alternate pathway are: factor B, factor D, properdin (P) and trace amounts of C3b which are also normally found in serum. Factor B binds to C3b to form the complex C3b,B. Factor D, an active protease cleaves factor B in the complex into Ba which is inactive and Bb. The $\overline{C3b,Bb}$ complex in turn cleaves C3 into C3a and C3b, perhaps accounting for everpresent small quantities of C3b in serum. In addition the $\overline{C3b,Bb}$ complex is rather unstable and readily dissociates into its inactive components. However, if the complex binds to properdin, the resulting new complex, P,$\overline{C3b,Bb}$ becomes a relatively stable C3 splitting enzyme, which if left unchecked could trigger the remaining components of the complement sequence. Under normal circumstances, however, there are two regulatory proteins which, working in concert, first inactivates C3b and then dissociates the P,$\overline{C3b,Bb}$ complex.

Returning to the bacterial cell used as an example of the triggering antigen in the classic pathway, the P,$\overline{C3b,Bb}$ complex can bind to complex polysaccharides or lipopolysaccharides. Binding of the complex under these conditions apparently protects C3b from the regulatory proteins and now C3 can be cleaved in sufficient quantities to trigger the rest of the complement sequence, due to the formation of a new enzymatically active complex, P,$\overline{C3b_2,Bb}$.

Late Steps of Complement Sequence

Up to this point, we recognize that there exist two enzyme complexes both of which can activate C5, the next complement protein in the sequence, *i.e.*, the C$\overline{4b,2a,3b}$ complex from the antigen-antibody complex-driven classic pathway and the P,$\overline{C3b_2,Bb}$ complex from the alternate pathway. Recall also, that in the examples given, both of

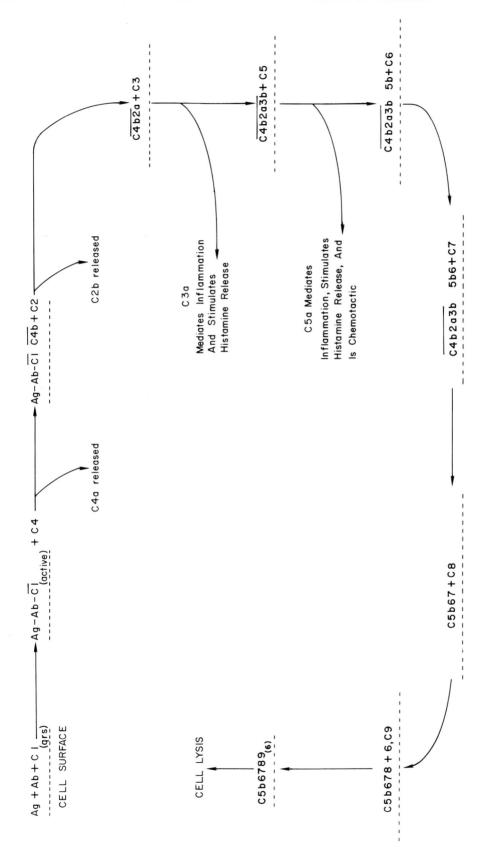

Figure 13/1. Sequential component reactions in the classic complement pathway. A cell surface component is indicated by the dashed line (– – –). Antibody specific for a cell surface component is designated *Ab*. Binding of Ab to Ag and binding of subsequent complement components is indicated by a single dash (—), and consecutive numbered components, respectively. Enzymatically active complement components and complexes are indicated by a *bar* drawn over the component.

these complexes are located near a bacterial cytoplasmic membrane.

Regardless of which enzymatic complex is involved, C5 is cleaved into two fragments: C5a and C5b. If C5 is split by the membrane-bound $C\overline{4b,2a,3b}$ enzyme, then C5b binds to the bacterial cell membrane at a topographical site independent of the enzyme site (fig. 13/1). If, on the other hand, C5 is split by the $P,\overline{C3b_2,Bb}$ complex, C5b also adheres to the bacterial cell membrane even though the enzyme complex may not be in direct contact with the membrane.

The sequence which follows C5 cleavage is quite different from what preceded. Instead of enzymatic cleavage to activate succeeding components, there is an aggregation of succeeding components, one to another. After C5b has become membrane-bound, one molecule of C6 joins each C5b followed by one molecule of C7 joining to C6. The C5b,6,7 aggregate provides a binding site for one molecule of C8 to which up to six molecules of C9 attach by adsorption.

Membrane Injury. Permeability changes are first seen in the affected cell membrane when component C8 is bound to the C5b,6,7 complex and intracellular constituents slowly begin to leak out of the cell. When C9s are added, the flow rate increases 10-fold. Considering the target bacterial cell example, lysis occurs with the passage of water into the cell. Complement-mediated lysis of red blood cells occurs in the same fashion. However, complement attachment to nucleated cells results first in the slow release of small intracellular substances followed by larger substances such as nucleotides and finally proteins. An unambigious mechanism which would explain these observations is currently not available. The suggestion has been made that, as the complex assembles, hydrophobic regions of the proteins are exposed which interact with lipids of the cell membrane creating a transmembrane channel which enlarges with addition of C9s.

C3a and C5a. It was mentioned previously that the two small split fragments C3a and C5a, although not a part of the continuing complement sequence, do possess biological activity. Originally called anaphylatoxins, because they caused inflammatory tissue changes, C3a and C5a stimulate mast cells to secrete histamine resulting in a marked increase in capillary permeability. In addition, C5a along with the C5b,6,7 complex are chemotactic for polymorphonuclear leukocytes and eosinophils. Furthermore, C3a has been shown to cause smooth muscle contraction *in vitro* independent of histamine.

Summary

Although a gram negative bacterial cell was used as an example to introduce the complement system,

it must be pointed out that complement-mediated cell lysis is a far more generalized phenomenon than is indicated by this restricted example. Any cell within the body to which an appropriate antigen-antibody complex may attach or to which a complex polysaccharide may attach is a potential target cell for complement-mediated lysis. The medical importance of this will become more apparent in the following section. Secondly, it should be kept in mind that just one $C\overline{4a,2b,3b}$ complex or just one $P,\overline{C3B_2,Bb}$ complex on a cell surface can result in the formation of many C5b,6,7,8,9 lytic complexes on a single cell. This amplification of the system is based on the fact that many C5s can be split by just one of the aforementioned complexes. Finally, recall that macrophages and neutrophils have specific receptors on their cell surfaces for C3b, perhaps accounting for the opsonic properties of complement.

IMMUNE COMPLEX DISEASES

Soon after the discovery of anaphylaxis, another type of antibody-dependent tissue reaction was described which when compared with immediate-type hypersensitivity differed in the time of onset, was not mediated by IgE, and which differed in histopathology at the tissue reaction site. Although tissue injury caused by immune complexes can manifest itself in many parts of the body, the principals of the reaction can be well illustrated by the cutaneous Arthus reaction, named after the French physiologist who first described the response.

Arthus Reaction (Passive Cutaneous Form)

In order to demonstrate an Arthus reaction, immune serum from one individual is injected intravenously into a nonimmune recipient, then the specific antigen used to induce the immune serum is injected into the recipient's skin. One to two hours later the skin injection site appears edematous and erythematous. This is followed by punctuate hemorrhages which reach a maximum 6 to 12 hours after injection and then the reaction slowly subsides. During severe cutaneous Arthus reactions, one finds evidence of tissue necrosis at the injection site.

It is now known that there are three essential elements which must be present simultaneously in order to produce this lesion: soluble antigen-antibody complexes, complement and polymorphonuclear leukocytes (PMNs). The appropriate soluble antigen-antibody complexes are produced when the concentration of antigen is greater than the concentration of corresponding antibody (slight antigen excess) and they are small so that they can remain suspended in circulating blood. These small complexes are of the configuration Ag_3Ab_2 or Ag_5Ab_3 and easily settle out of circulation along the walls of small blood vessels between endothelial cells and in contact with the elastic lamina. The final condition which these complexes must satisfy is that the complexed antibodies must be able to fix complement, *e.g.*, IgG-1, IgG-3 or IgM.

After the antigen-antibody complexes have settled along vessel walls, complement is fixed via the classic pathway and the attendant release of C5a and perhaps C3a attract and localize PMNs. In their attempt to phagocytize the immune complexes, lysosomal contents of the PMNs which include acid phosphatases, neutral and acid proteases, collagenase, elastase and acid lipases, are released and cause focal necrosis of the vessel wall. This accounts for the hemorrhage seen at the injection site. Necrotic PMNs are gradually replaced by macrophages and eosinophils and because they are able to phagocytize and degrade the immune complexes the inflammation disappears. Even though histamine is probably released from mast cells because of the action of C5a and C3a, the administration of antihistamines does not block the Arthus reaction.

Serum Sickness and Serum Sickness-like Syndromes

During the early days of clinical passive immunity procedures, it was common to induce the production of immunoglobulins specific for many infectious disease agents in rabbits and horses. Subsequently, these animal sera were passively administered to humans. After repeated injections, or in some cases after a single injection, some of the human recipients developed a syndrome which was characterized by: enlarged lymph nodes and spleen, fever, erythematous and urticarial rashes, arthritis, and fever. In most cases the disease subsided in a few days, but in some cases these individuals died. Autopsy revealed disseminated vascular inflammatory lesions very similar to those observed in an Arthus reaction.

Because of subtle differences in the structure of animal serum proteins, they are recognized as foreign antigens by the immune systems of the human hosts. However, again because they are serum proteins, they enjoy a normal biological half-life and remain in circulation for a relatively long period of time. As complement-fixing antibodies begin to appear in the host, the foreign serum proteins are present in antigen excess and therefore the necessary conditions prevail for the formation of soluble antigen-antibody complexes. Under these conditions however, unlike the localized, cutaneous Arthus reaction, any small vessel in the body is a potential target for antigen-antibody complex deposition, complement fixation and localized vascular necrosis. The systemic scope of immune complex deposition provides some explanation for the symptoms which were earlier listed. Vessel damage near skin surfaces explains the rash. Systemic release of endogenous pyrogen from PMNs explains the fever, while systemic production of immunoglobulins is the basis for lymph node and spleen enlargement. Finally, for some unknown reason, synovial joints are a preferred location for complex deposition, accounting for arthritic symptoms. In addition to synovial joints, other tissues which are primarily involved include the heart, which may reveal endocardial proliferation, valvular vegetations along with myocarditis, and pericarditis; the arteries which reveal necrosis involving all layers of the arterial wall; and the kidneys. The latter will be discussed separately.

Because of the obvious potential danger of administering foreign serum proteins, use of animal serum preparations largely have been abandoned with the exception of duck serum which to some extent is still used for rabies prophylaxis. Even though serum sickness was first recognized as a sequel to injection of foreign serum proteins, it is important to realize that any antigen which can, for one reason or another, remain in circulation for relatively long periods of time can also cause a serum sickness-like syndrome. As examples, chronic viral and bacterial diseases provide a continuous source of antigenic material capable of forming soluble complexes.

Glomerulonephritis

For reasons that are poorly understood the basement membrane of glomerular capillaries of the kidney are particularly susceptible to localization of soluble immune complexes regardless of the antigen. Furthermore, because glomerulonephritis is a common sequel of untreated streptococcal disease caused especially by a nephritogenic strain, it deserves separate attention. During immune complex disease in the kidney, the glomerular basement membrane is the primary site of injury. Microscopic examination reveals necrotic lesions in the basement membrane, while urinalyses reveal proteinuria followed by hematuria. If the damage is severe enough, the afflicted individual may experience renal failure. As the degenerative inflammatory process continues, endothelial proliferation occurs along with slight basement membrane thickening. In the case of poststreptococcal glomerulonephritis, streptococcal antigens have been demonstrated in basement membrane immune complexes. In addition antigens from the malarial strain *Plasmodium malariae* and hepatitis B viral antigens both commonly form soluble complexes with antibodies which localize in the kidney. In the case of chronic hepatitis B infection, the suggestion has been made that long-standing immune complex disease including glomerulonephritis occurs in individuals who are unable to mount a massive immunoglobulin response which would clear circulating antigens. Instead, these individuals appear to mount an intermediate response which, coupled with constant antigen production, leaves them in chronic antigen excess without antigen clearance.

SEROLOGY

The specificity with which immunoglobulins can discriminate between antigens of similar structure and selectively bind to the single antigen which induced Ig formation should be abundantly clear at this point. In addition to the high degree of specificity, immunoglobulins possess an extraordinary degree of sensitivity *in vitro*. If a test is properly designed, immunoglobulins can complex with nanogram quantities of antigens. Many important medical diagnostic tests take advantage of these two properties in order to detect minute quantities of either antigens or antibodies in biological specimens. The sensitivity of these diagnostic tests has been increased over the years as sophisticated indicator systems have been developed which detect the presence of extremely small quantities of antigen-antibody complexes.

Quantitative Precipitin Curve

The first visual demonstration of specific antigen-antibody interaction occurred when it was found that antigen and antibody mixed in correct proportions in a test tube yielded a white flocculent precipitate which was relatively stable. This observation led to the development of the quantitative precipitin curve. The curve is experimentally developed by starting with a series of tubes each of which contains a known, constant amount of antibody. To each tube in this series is added a sequentially increasing amount of a single antigen so that the first tube in the series has the least amount of antigen and the last tube contains the greatest amount of antigen. These reaction mixtures are incubated to allow precipitates to form. If one then quantitatively measures the amount of precipitate formed in each tube a curve is generated as shown in figure 13/2. This curve shows that the maximum amount of precipitate is formed in tubes where the concentration of antigen is roughly equivalent to the concentration of antibody, termed the equivalence zone. Moving in either direction away from the equivalence zone (antibody excess or antigen excess) progressively less precipitate is detected. To account for the observed precipitation, it is assumed that as equivalence is approached, each antigen molecule is linked to more than one antibody molecule and each antibody molecule is linked to more than one antigen molecule. When the growing aggregate reaches some critical size it falls out of solution. In both antibody and antigen excess zones, aggregates of this critical size cannot develop.

Precipitin Reactions in Gels

A modification of the precipitin reaction which allows one to analyze multiple antigen systems involves diffusion of antigens through a semisolid agar gel rather than a liquid medium. Depending on the procedure employed, diffusion of antigen or antibody can occur in a single dimension or in two dimensions. Regardless of the procedure the principal is the same. Multiple antigens diffuse at different rates depending on their diffusion coefficients which in turn are partially determined by their molecular weights and three-dimensional shape. The same is true for the diffusion of immunoglobulins. At some point during diffusion, antigen and specific antibody will meet at concentrations corresponding to the equivalence zone of the quantitative precipitin curve and a precipitate will be formed which is manifest as an opaque, opalescent line. Each antigen in the original mixture, for which there is a specific immunoglobulin, will appear as a separate line.

Oudin developed a technique whereby antiserum is mixed with agar in the liquid state and poured into a small tube. When the agar has solidified, a solution of antigen is poured over the antiserum containing agar and precipitin lines develop as the antigen diffuses into the gel. A modification of this technique was introduced in which antiserum is first added to a tube, followed by a column of agar and, finally, antigen is layered over the top of the agar gel. Antiserum diffuses upward into the gel and antigens diffuse downward into the gel and, again, precipitin bands develop in the gel where antigen and antibody meet in a zone of relative equivalence.

Ouchterlony developed one of the most useful agar diffusion techniques which allows one to determine the degree of identity existing between antigens from different sources (fig. 13/3). Agar is poured to a uniform thickness on a glass plate and when the gel has solidified, small cylinders of agar are removed which create wells in the remaining agar. Antigens and antibodies are then added to wells and both constituents diffuse out from the wells in all directions and precipitin lines also are produced at a point where the advancing fronts meet.

Immunoelectrophoresis is another variation of agar diffusion which is particularly useful for analyzing complicated mixtures of antigens such as serum. Serum is first placed in a well cut in an agar slab and then a difference of potential is applied across the agar. Serum proteins are separated according to their respective net electrical charges, molecular weights and diffusion constants. After separation has been accomplished a long trough is created in the agar, parallel to the applied difference of potential and the trough is filled with anti-

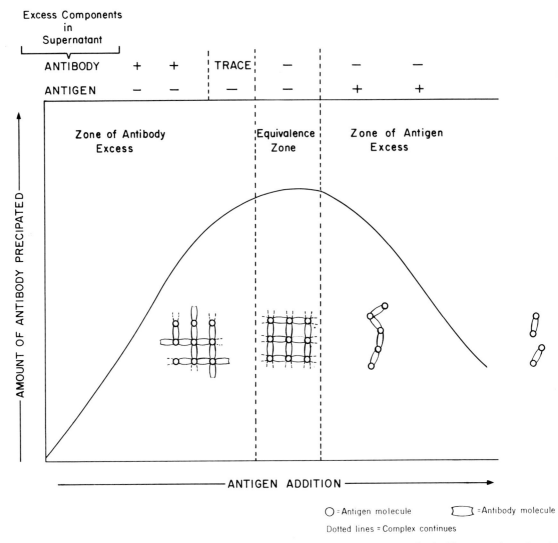

Figure 13/2. Quantitative precipitin curve for a single antigen and its homologous antibody. The curve rises sharply as more antigen is added in the zone of antibody excess, reaching a maximum level with a plateau in the equivalence zone and then declining in the zone of antigen excess. The presumed antigen-antibody lattice configuration is depicted under the precipitin curve, for each zone.

serum (serum-containing antibodies raised against the test serum proteins). The electrically separated proteins and the antiserum diffuse toward each other and precipitin lines are formed (fig. 13/4). This technique is particularly useful for detecting deficiencies in, or absences of, normal serum constituents. In fact, all the gel methods described so far can be viewed as qualitative tests. They measure presence or absence of an antigen rather than indicating how much antigen is present.

On the other hand, radial immunodiffusion can be used to quantitate antigen concentration. In this technique, monospecific antibody is incorporated into an agar gel. Again, wells are created in the agar and the antigen is added. If the antiserum is specific for the antigen a precipitin ring will develop around and at some distance from the antigen well. The diameter of the precipitin ring can be correlated with antigen concentration by comparing the diameters of rings developed from known antigen concentrations.

Agglutination Reactions

Under the appropriate conditions, bacteria, fungi and red blood cells can be agglutinated (clumped) in the presence of immunoglobulins specific for some surface antigen on these cells. Furthermore, the presence or absence of agglutination is easily visualized either microscopically or macroscopically. Therefore agglutination provides an easily observed indicator of the presence or absence of

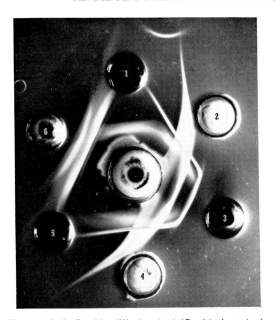

Figure 13/3. Double diffusion test (Ouchterlony technique) between antisaliva serum from a rabbit (*center well*) and six antigen solutions, showing the presence of amylase and several serum proteins in saliva. (*1*) Cohn Fraction V, human serum. (*2*) Whole human serum. (*3*) Human parotid saliva. (*4*) Whole human serum. (*5*) Cohn Fraction II-1, 2, human serum. (*6*) Whole human saliva. The heavy arc from well (*3*) is due to amylase + anti-amylase. (From S. A. Ellison.)

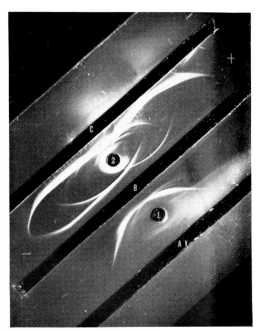

Figure 13/4. Immunoelectrophoretic test with human saliva, human serum, and respective rabbit antisera. A layer of buffered agar about 1 mm thick was formed on a glass plate. Wells (*1, 2*) and troughs (*A, B, C*) were cut from the agar. Saliva in (*1*) and whole serum in (*2*) were subjected to electrophoresis along the strips of agar by electrodes applied across the plate at + and −. The current was interrupted and rabbit antiserum against human saliva was placed in trough (*B*); rabbit antiserum against human serum, in troughs (*A*) and (*C*). Between (*B*) and (*1*) is the amylase band and two minor bands. Serum proteins in the saliva were too dilute to give bands between (*A*) and (*1*). However, antibodies against several serum proteins were present in the antisaliva serum, as shown by the three bands between (*B*) and (*2*). (From S. A. Ellison.)

immune complex formation. In principal, agglutination is very similar to observable precipitation, *i.e.*, at the appropriate concentrations one immunoglobulin is attached to more than one cell and each cell is bound by more than one immunoglobulin so that a large aggregate is formed.

Agglutination forms the basis for some of the most clinically useful diagnostic tests available because not only do they reveal the presence or absence of a specific immune complex but they also can reveal relative concentrations of either antigen or antibody. Usually these tests are employed to determine whether or not an individual has been exposed to a specific infectious agent. This can be determined by measuring an increase in specific antibody to a particular agent over background levels. In many cases this provides a retrospective diagnosis because significant increases in unbound immunoglobulins may only be present in serum after the acute phase of clinical illness. In order to determine the relative concentration of specific immunoglobulins present in an individual's serum, the serum is serially diluted in a 2-fold fashion and the last dilution of the serum which yields a "positive reaction" with a constant amount of antigen is taken as the end point. The relative concentration of immunoglobulins is expressed as a titer which is the reciprocal of the highest dilution that caused

agglutination of the antigen. For example, if a dilution of 1:256 causes agglutination but a dilution of 1:512 does not, then the titer is expressed as 256.

Passive Agglutination

Although the direct agglutination of some bacteria and fungi by serum can be used in the diagnosis of some diseases, by and large the majority of agglutination tests take advantage of the fact that a wide variety of antigens can be passively coupled to the surfaces of red blood cells or latex spheres, to produce an easily observable agglutination or lack thereof. Many antigens including some viruses, bacterial antigens, endotoxins and proteins will spontaneously adsorb to the surface of red blood cells. In addition, the repertoire of antigens can be expanded by using coupling agents such as tannic acid, glutaraldehyde and carbodiimides to passively bind antigens to red blood cell surfaces.

Regardless of the antigen, the mechanics of the

test are the same. A constant amount of antigen-covered red blood cells is placed in a series of small test tubes or the wells of microtiter plates. Increasing dilutions of a patient's serum are added to the tubes or wells and the mixture is incubated to allow agglutination to occur. In some cases, sera with high specific titers fail to agglutinate red blood cells at low serum dilutions. This seemingly false negative reaction is termed the prozone phenomenon and is analogous to the lack of precipitation found in the antibody excess zone of the precipitin curve. In essence, there is such an abundance of antibody that significant cross-linking of red blood cells does not occur. At higher serum dilutions, however agglutination does occur.

Hemagglutination Inhibition

Many viruses, for instance the influenza and parainfluenza viruses, have the ability to spontaneously agglutinate red blood cells. One method of determining the specific antiviral serum titers to these viruses is the hemagglutination inhibition test, which involves two steps. In the first step, a constant amount of virus is mixed with increasing dilutions of the test serum. In the second step, a constant number of red blood cells is added to each reaction mixture. If specific antibody is present, it will bind with the viral surface, thereby interfering with the ability of the virus to agglutinate the red cells. Therefore, the titer of the serum is determined by the highest dilution at which no agglutination is observed. Small quantities of antigen also can be detected by this method. In this case the first step involves mixing the test antigen with a known amount of specific antibody. In the second step, a known number of red blood cells coated with the same antigen is added to the test mixtures. If antigen was indeed present in the test solution, it will bind the available antibody and hemagglutination of the antigen-coated red blood cells will not occur. The degree to which antigen in the test solution successfully competes for the available antibody gives a measure of the amount of antigen present.

Antiglobulin Test (Coombs' Test).

During the development and testing of many hemagglutinating systems, it was found that many specific antibody preparations failed to agglutinate antigen-coated red blood cells. Either the antibody concentration was too low to cause large aggregate formation or, for some reason, the immunoglobulin molecules did not form a bridge between antigen-coated red blood cells. A typical example of such a nonagglutinating antibody is the antibody specific for the Rh determinants on human red blood cells. Coombs discovered that RBCs coated with antibodies specific for a surface antigen could be agglu-

tinated if antibody specific for the cell-bound immunoglobulin was added to the mixture. Furthermore, one can determine the immunoglobulin class of bound antibody by adding antiglobulin specific for each heavy chain class.

Complement Fixation

As has been mentioned previously, many antigen-antibody complexes fix complement. Thus the consumption of complement *in vitro* can be used to detect and measure antigens, antibodies or both. This test also depends on a two-stage procedure. In the first stage, antigen, antibody and a known amount of complement (usually of guinea pig origin) is mixed. If antigen-antibody complexes form, then complement will be consumed. In the second stage, antibody-coated sheep red blood cells are added to the test mixtures. If complement has been consumed in the test mixture, it will be unavailable to lyse the antibody-coated sheep red blood cells. Therefore, absence of red blood cell lysis is a positive test result. On the other hand, if antigen and antibody did not complex in the test mixture, then complement will be available to lyse the red blood cells in the indicator system. Therefore, lysis of red blood cells is a negative result.

Fluorescent Antibody Techniques

Fluorescent antibody tests are particularly useful for detecting the presence of cell-bound antigens or antibodies. The cells can be of bacterial, fungal or human origin. Regardless of the cell origin, the first step in all of these tests involves fixing the cells to a microscope slide. In the direct fluorescent antibody technique, a fluorescent dye, either fluorescein isothyocyanate which appears green under ultraviolet light or tetramethylrodamine isothiocyanate which appears red when excited by ultraviolet light, is covalently coupled to specific antibody. The resulting conjugated antibody is allowed to react with the cell preparation and then the slide is thoroughly washed to remove any unbound antibody. The specimen is then examined microscopically with ultraviolet illumination. Bound antibody is detected by the presence of the characteristic dye color which is seen against a dark background (fig. 13/5).

A modification of this technique which enhances the sensitivity of the test as well as reduces the number of different conjugated antibodies necessary is the indirect immunofluorescent test. In the first stage of this test, specific antibody is added which does not have a fluorescent dye conjugated to it. After thorough washing, an antibody preparation which reacts specifically with human immunoglobulins is added. This second antibody is conjugated with a fluorescent dye and then the

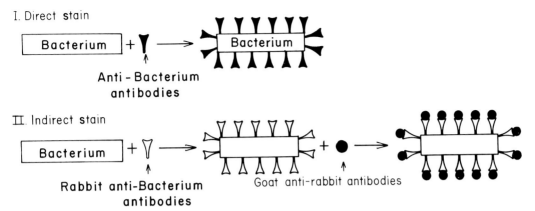

I. Direct stain

Bacterium + Y → Bacterium

Anti-Bacterium
antibodies

II. Indirect stain

Bacterium + Y → + ● →

Rabbit anti-Bacterium   Goat anti-rabbit antibodies
antibodies

Figure 13/5. Immunofluorescence, direct and indirect techniques. In the direct procedure, the antigens on the bacterial cell react with specific antibodies that are labeled with a fluorescent dye (*black*). In the indirect staining procedure, the antigens on the bacterial cell react with unlabeled antibodies (*white*) produced in a rabbit. Antibodies against rabbit immunoglobulins, produced in a goat, are labeled with a fluorescent dye (*black*) and react with the rabbit antibacterial cell antibodies, resulting in a visible complex. Thus, one labeled antibody preparation can be used as a stain for a variety of serologically specific reactions.

slide is observed for specific dye color. The advantage of the indirect method lies in the fact that one conjugated antihuman serum preparation can be used for all test systems which use specific human immunoglobulins (fig. 13/5). Both of these methods are very useful. However, careful attention must be paid to technical details and appropriate positive and negative controls.

Radioimmunoassays

Radioimmunoassays (RIA) are a fairly recent development and are the most sensitive immunological tests now available. If properly used, RIAs can detect less than 1.0 pg of material. They have been employed to detect the hepatitis B virus surface antigen and serum IgE for specific allergens. There are many variations of this technique, but one of the most popular methods is based on the observation that almost all antibodies and some antigens can be adsorbed to the surface of plastic, *e.g.*, polystyrene spheres or tubes. After antibody is bound to the plastic, then a solution of unknown antigen is added. If that antigen is bound to the solid phase antibody, then two methods can be used to detect the presence of the antigen-antibody complexes. In one scheme, a second antibody is added which is radioactively labeled and also is specific for the test antigen. If antigen is bound to the solid phase antibody then the radioactively labeled antibody will bind to the antigen as well. Thus, the antigen is sandwiched between two layers of antibody, and antigen-antibody complex is detected in a radiodetector. In the second scheme, a mixture of antigens is added to the solid phase antibody which consists of a known quantity of radio-labeled antigen and an unknown quantity of the test antigen.

In this case, labeled and unlabeled antigen compete for a limited number of antibodies. The amount of labeled antigen bound is dependent on the concentration of antigen in the unknown solution, *e.g.*, the higher the concentration of unlabeled antigen present, the less labeled antigen will be bound by antibody.

ADDITIONAL READING

BARNETT, E. V., KNUTSON, D. W., ABRASS, C. K., CHIA, D. S., YOUNG, L. S., 1979 AND LIEBLING, M. R. Circulating Immune Complexes: Their Immunochemistry, Detection, and Importance. Annals Int Med, **91**, 430.

BELLANTI, J. A. 1978 *Immunology II*, Saunders, Philadelphia.

DAVIS, B. D., DULBECCO, R., EISEN, H. N., AND GINSBERG, H. S. 1980 *Microbiology*, Ed. 3. Harper & Row, Hagerstown, Md.

FEY, G., AND COLTEN, H. R. 1981 Biosynthesis of Complement Components. Fed Proc, **40**, 2099.

FUDENBERG, H. H., STITES, D. P., CALDWELL, J. L., AND WELLS, J. V. 1978 *Basic & Clinical Immunology*, Ed. 2. Lange Medical Publishers, Los Altos, Calif.

FRANK, M. M. 1979 The Complement System in Host Defense and Inflammation. Rev Infect Dis, **1**, 483.

JOHNSTONE, D. E. 1981 Immunotherapy in Children: Past, Present and Future (Part I–Part II) Ann Allergy, **46**, 1, 59.

KULCZYCKI, A. 1981 Role of Immunoglobulin E and Immunoglobulin E Receptors in Bronchial Asthma. J Allergy Clin Immunol, **68**, 5.

MARSH, D. G., HSU, S. H., HUSSAIN, R., MEYERS, D. A., FREIDHOFF, L. R., AND BIAS, W. B. 1980 Genetics of Human Immune Response to Allergens. J Allergy Clin Immunol, **65**, 322.

ROCKLIN, R. E., SHEFFER, A. L., GREINEDER, D. K., AND MELMON, K. L. 1980 Generation of Antigen-Specific Suppressor Cells During Allergy Desensitization. N Engl J Med, **302**, 1213.

ROITT, I. M., AND LEHNER, T. 1980 Immunology of Oral Diseases, Blackwell Scientific Publications, Oxford.

SAMTER, M. 1978 *Immunological Diseases*, Ed. 3. Little, Brown, Boston.

SCHREIBER, R. D., MORRISON, D. C., PODACK, E. R., AND MULLER-EKERHARD, H. J. 1979 Bactericidal Activity of the Alternative Complement Pathway Generated from 11 Isolated Plasma Proteins. J Exp Med, **149,** 870.

TRANUM-JENSEN, J., BHAKDI, S., BHAKDI-LEHNEN, B., BJERRUM, O. J., AND SPETH, V. 1978 Complement Lysis: The Ultrastructure and Orientation of the C5b-9 Complex on Target Sheep Erythrocyte Membranes. Scand J Immunol, **7,** 45.

WEISSMAN, G., SMOLEN, J. E., AND KORCHAK, H. M. 1980 Release of Inflammatory Mediators from Stimulated Neutrophils. N Engl J Med, **303,** 27.

WILLIAMS, R. C. 1981 Immune Complexes in Human Diseases. Ann Rev Med, **32,** 13.

chapter 14

Cell-Mediated, Tumor and Transplantation Immunity

Keith R. Volkmann

INTRODUCTION

Up to this point the discussion of the immune system has dealt primarily with B lymphocyte responses mediated by immunoglobulin molecules. T lymphocytes have only been mentioned to the extent that they can be distinguished from B lymphocytes and to the extent that they cooperate with or inhibit B cell function. In this section, the functional role played by T cells in the immune system will be more fully developed. There are several immune responses such as delayed-type hypersensitivity, rejection of transplanted tissue and tumor immunology which appear to be mediated primarily by T lymphocytes and their secreted products, all of which are quite necessary for optimum function of specific host defenses.

MAJOR HISTOCOMPATIBILITY ANTIGENS

All nucleated cells of the body have a group of surface antigens coded for by genes associated with immune response functions and, as a class of antigens, they are referred to as the major histocompatibility complex (MHC). In humans, this complex is termed HLA (human leukocyte antigens) and is composed of four antigens which are coded for by four genetic loci, with many different alleles (a series of two or more different genes which may occupy the same position on a specific chromosome) possible at each locus. Although all nucleated cells have these antigens, their density varies greatly from one cell type to another. For instance, leukocytes have a high surface density of HLA antigens whereas heart muscle cells have a low surface density. In a given individual all HLA antigens are identical and they, in all likelihood, form the basis of self-recognition by the immune system. T lymphocytes are particularly sensitive in recognizing subtle differences in, or alterations to, self-HLA antigens. Immunologically, T cells are activated to become effector cells either when they encounter foreign HLA antigens or when they encounter small cell-bound antigens which alter the character of self-HLA antigens.

Genetics for Human MHC

HLA-A–HLA-C loci. Human population studies have revealed that HLA antigens can be arranged into three groups HLA-A, B and C. Recently there were 20 known alleles at the A locus, 33 alleles at the B locus and 6 alleles at the C locus; however, the list may continue to grow. The gene products of these alleles can be identified by specific antisera developed against human leukocytes. Each individual in the population is heterozygous for two alleles specified by each of the three loci and, at fertilization, each parent contributes one allele from each locus to the offspring. The point to be stressed is that in an outbred human population there exists tremendous diversity in HLA antigens due to the combinations of alleles possible at each locus. Conversely, the chances of finding phenotypic identity at each of these three loci in two nonrelated individuals are indeed remote.

HLA-D and HLA-DR. In addition to HLA-A, B and C antigens, a fourth set of antigens, HLA-D and DR (D-related) are found exclusively on the surface of B lymphocytes and perhaps macrophages. Again recently, 11 D and 7 DR antigens have been recognized. These antigens also can be recognized by specific antisera and are considered important in determining whether or not B and T cell interactions will occur. Individuals are usually heterozygous for the two alleles at this locus but individuals homozygous for D alleles are common in reproductively isolated communities.

Structure of MHC Products

HLA-A–HLA-C. The A, B and C loci each code for a polypeptide chain of approximately 45,000 daltons. In addition, there is an oligosaccharide component which is attached to the polypeptide comprising about 10% of the total molecular weight. The oligosaccharide can be enzymatically removed resulting in no change to the antigenicity of the molecule. This finding implies that the varied antigenicity of these polypeptides resides exclusively in the amino acid sequence. The carboxy end of the heavy chain has a hydrophobic segment which apparently interacts stably with lipids of the cell membrane. Interestingly, portions of the heavy chain structurally resemble Ig heavy chain domains.

On the cell membrane each heavy chain is associated noncovalently with a lighter chain, β_2-microglobulin (12,000 daltons). The light chain also shares properties with Ig molecules, in that portions of its amino acid sequence are homologous with those of C_H domains. Unlike the amino acid-sequence heterogeneity seen in HLA heavy chains, the light chains associated with all heavy chains are identical within one specie and, furthermore, do not extend into the cell membrane.

HLA-D. The HLA-D gene product is also a glycoprotein composed of two chains (α and β) per molecule and are of about equal molecular weight. Both chains extend into the cell membrane and some chain pairs have interchain disulfide bonds while others do not.

As mentioned previously, a distinct antigen recognition unit, such as immunoglobulin, has not been discovered on T cells. Nonetheless, the manner in which T lymphocytes recognize MHC gene products, self, nonself or altered self, has great significance in terms of how or if they will respond. The most familiar example involves T cell-mediated destruction of transplanted tissue bearing foreign (nonself) histocompatibility antigens. However, other T cell interactions are affected as well. T cell cooperation in response to T cell-dependent antigen stimulation of B cells only occurs if the MHC antigens on macrophage, T cell, and B cell are identical. An antigen-bearing macrophage will only stimulate T cell proliferation in a delayed type hypersensitivity response if the macrophage and T cell share the same MHC antigens. Therefore, it appears that, in addition to recognizing specific antigenic determinants, T cells recognize MHC antigens. This dependence on MHC recognition is termed MHC restriction.

CELL-MEDIATED IMMUNITY AND INFECTIOUS DISEASE

Antigens which primarily elicit a cell-mediated response have one important common feature. Unlike the rather large particulate (bacterial) and macromolecular antigens of extracellular parasites which tend to stimulate B cells, antigens which stimulate antigen-reactive T cells are usually small and are cell bound. In particular, small antigens derived from parasites capable of intracellular life such as the tubercle bacillus easily become bound to infected cell surfaces and virally infected cells have virus-coded antigens inserted in their surface membranes. When a circulating, antigen-sensitive T cell comes in contact with an antigen-bearing cell, it recognizes the altered surface of the infected cell. It may recognize the new surface antigen in addition to the "self" HLA antigens or, if the new antigen is on or near the "self" HLA antigens, it may recognize an alteration to the HLA antigens themselves.

Generation of Effector T Lymphocytes

Once stimulated by an altered cell surface antigen, the antigen-reactive T cell migrates to either a regional lymph node or the spleen where cellular proliferation occurs in predominantly T cell areas. The result of proliferation is an expanded pool of two subsets of effector cells. One effector subset is termed T_{DTH} (for delayed-type hypersensitivity) which secretes biologically active substances termed lymphokines when it comes in contact with its specific antigen-bearing cell. Both the T_{DHT} and T helper cell carry the Lyt-1 alloantigen (see Chapter 12) but from a functional standpoint, they appear to be quite different cells. The second effector subset is termed cytotoxic T lymphocyte (CTL) or T killer cell (T_k) which specifically lyses target cells carrying the appropriate surface antigen. During the generation of these cells in lymphoid tissue it is not known whether pluripotent precursor cells proliferate and then differentiate (as seen in the B cell response) or whether proliferation of each unipotent subset occurs obviating the need for differentiation. Nonetheless, after proliferation, effector cells return to the site or sites of infected cells.

Tissue Response Mediated by T_{DTH} Cells

When T_{DTH} cells specifically recognize antigen-bearing cells, they release lymphokines which are soluble factors active over short distances. Many different lymphokine functions have been described, but it is not known how many unique molecular species are in fact responsible for all the observed functions. An interesting property of lymphokines is the fact that a specific T_{DTH} cell-antigen interaction is necessary for their release but, once released, the actions of lymphokines are totally nonspecific in an immunologic sense. Representative examples of a few well characterized lymphokine functions will be described.

Migration Inhibitory Factor (MIF). MIF was the first lymphokine to be described. Biochemically it is probably a glycoprotein. When MIF is released at the site of T_{DTH} cell-target cell interaction, it inhibits the migration of macrophages *in vitro* and presumably *in vivo* as well. Therefore, migrating macrophages remain localized at the antigen site.

Macrophage Activating Factor (MAF). Macrophages which have been incubated with MAF *in vitro* develop a number of morphological, metabolic and functional changes and are then termed activated macrophages. Activated macrophages are more aggressive and efficient phagocytes and possess an enhanced ability to kill phagocytosed microorganisms compared to nonactivated macrophages. In addition, activated macrophages exhibit the interesting property of an enhanced ability to kill certain tumor cells, but not their normal counterparts. There is strong, suggestive evidence to indicate that a single glycoprotein performs both MIF and MAF functions.

Leukocyte Inhibitory Factor (LIF). LIF inhibits the migration of polymorphonuclear leukocytes in much the same manner that MIF inhibits macrophage motility. However, LIF is specific only for polymorphonuclear leucocytes (PMNs). It also may enhance the phagocytic ability of PMNs.

Lymphocyte Mitogenic Factor (LMF). T_{DTH} cells release a factor or factors that nonspecifically stimulate other noncommitted T lymphocytes to undergo blast transformation and proliferation at the local peripheral site of antigen-bearing target cell. The result is a local expansion of the number of specific T_{DTH} cells. The proliferation may be quite similar to the proliferation which also takes place in regional lymph nodes.

The three aforementioned lymphokines: MIF/MAF, LIF and LMF, all illustrate the remarkable efficiency and economy of cell-mediated responses. A very small number of T_{DTH} cells migrating from a lymph node or spleen and localizing at some distant antigen site can locally recruit and activate a large number of uncommitted phagocytic cells and lymphocytes which attempt to clear the infectious agent from the area. Histologically, an intense inflammatory response is seen which causes a considerable amount of nonspecific tissue destruction, due to the release of cytolytic enzymes from the accumulated phagocytic cells. In the case of intracellular bacterial and fungal pathogens and considering the entire local cellular infiltrate, perhaps the most important defensive cells are the activated macrophages because these cells now have an enhanced ability to kill phagocytosed organisms. Recall that these same pathogens grow with impunity in nonactivated phagocytic cells.

Osteoclast Activating Factor (OAF). Osteoclast activating factor is an interesting lymphokine whose presence and functional capacities have been described *in vitro* but whose *in vivo* significance remains to be determined. OAF is of particular interest to the dental community because its *in vitro* production stimulates the differentiation of osteoclasts which in turn resorb bone. OAF can be elicited by specific antigen stimulation of T cells or by nonspecific polyclonal T cell mitogens such as phytohemagglutinin. OAF release by stimulated T_{DTH} cells requires intimate interaction of the T_{DTH} cell with a macrophage. This cellular interaction is not seen in the release of other lymphokines. It would be interesting to know whether or not T_{DTH} cell stimulation by subgingival bacterial antigens with subsequent release of OAF plays a role in the pathogenic bone resorbtion seen in aggressive periodontal disease.

Tissue Response Mediated by CTLs

Cytotoxic lymphocytes or killer T cells carry the Lyt-2,3 antigens as do suppressor T cells but again, functionally, these cells appear to be quite different. These effector T cells have the ability to specifically lyse target cells with new, nonself antigens such as virally specified glycoproteins on their surfaces. Recognition of virally infected cells depends on recognition of both viral antigens and HLA antigens. Contact between CTL and target cell is required for lysis but interaction with accessory cells such as macrophages is not required. Because cell lysis is so specific in a pure CTL response, generalized tissue destruction as was caused by T_{DTH} cells is not observed. Several steps in the lytic process can be distinguished. In a Mg^{2+}-dependent step, the CTL binds to the target cell forming a conjugate which persists for several minutes. During the conjugate stage, the target cell seems to become programmed to undergo lysis. The CTL then leaves the first target cell and moves on to another one, repeating the cyle. It has been estimated that one CTL can kill 10 to 12 target cells in the course of a few hours. The "programmed" target cells rupture anywhere from a few minutes to a few hours after contact with the CTL. Again considering the defensive properties of cell-mediated responses against intracellular parasites, CTLs appear to be particularly advantageous in viral diseases. Cells in which viruses are replicating can be specifically killed and any infectious virus which is released during lysis can be cleared by specific antibodies. On the other hand, CTLs would seem to offer no defensive advantage by lysing cells harboring intracellular bacteria or fungi. Lysis of these cells would simply release more organisms which could invade surrounding cells.

Cell-mediated immunity directed against infectious agents, in terms of time course and memory, is very similar to the humoral response. Effector cells in a primary response are first seen experimentally 5 to 7 days after exposure to the antigen. If reexposure to the same antigen occurs, a secondary (anamnestic) response occurs faster, with greater intensity and with longer duration than the primary response. Like the secondary humoral response, this is presumably due to an expanded pool of specific antigen-reactive T lymphocytes. In any given cell-mediated response both T_{DTH} cells and CTLs are probably produced. Finally, like the humoral immune response, tissue damage can be directly linked to the cellular immune response itself. For example, the large inflammatory lesions in response to infection by *Mycobacterium tuberculosis* causing the destruction of large areas of lung parenchyma are probably due to T_{DTH} cells and the sequence of events following their release of lymphokines.

Cutaneous Delayed-Type Hypersensitivity

If partially purified proteins extracted from an organism such as *M. tuberculosis* are injected into the skin of an individual who at some previous time had been exposed to live *M. tuberculosis*, a skin lesion develops (fig. 14/1). Usually no reaction can be seen for at least 10 hours after the protein preparation has been injected. Then erythema, swelling and induration gradually appear with maximal size and intensity being reached at 24 to 72 hours. The lesion then slowly resolves over the next several days. In a highly sensitive human, injection of this substance can cause local necrosis, ulceration and scarring. Historically, the time course of this response distinguished it from immediate-type hypersensitivity, and the cutaneous Arthus response, hence the term delayed-type hypersensitivity (DTH).

Histologically, DTH is readily distinguished from both immediate-type hypersensitivity and the Arthus response. In a mild-to-moderate DTH reaction, the earliest cellular infiltrate consists of small-to-medium sized lymphocytes, neutrophils, monocytes and macrophages which accumulate around postcapillary venules. At the time of maximal tissue

response, the entire dermis is involved and mononuclear cells may be found in the epidermis. Necrosis of blood vessels, muscle, connective tissue and epidermis may occur to varying degrees, depending on the sensitivity of the individual.

Presumably the injected proteins became bound to cells in the dermis and were recognized by antigen-reactive T cells, which had become sensitized during the first exposure to *M. tuberculosis*. The resulting inflammatory lesion is a secondary cellular immune response and represents a localized cutaneous counterpart of the T_{DTH} cell-mediated response mentioned previously. Similar responses may be induced by other antigens to which an individual has been sensitized.

Contact Skin Sensitivity

A variety of small molecular weight chemicals (<1000 daltons) can cause an allergic skin reaction in man simply by coming in contact with skin. The catechols of the poison ivy plant, soaps and detergents, drugs, many dental materials, and cosmetics can all commonly cause an allergic contact dermatitis. The initial exposure to a potential sensitizing substance usually does not elicit any visible skin response. In some individuals however, if reexposure to the same substance occurs anywhere on the skin surface just 4 to 5 days after initial exposure, a localized delayed-type hypersensitivity response is elicited. In other individuals, several exposures to the substance may be required before any visible manifestation is observed.

The time course of contact dermatitis is the same as that for cutaneous delayed-type hypersensitivity of the tuberculin type. Erythema and swelling appear at about 10 to 12 hours and increase to a maximum level between 24 and 72 hours. Unusually intense reactions can produce necrosis, but even in the absence of necrosis complete recovery can take several weeks. The dermis at the site of contact is invaded by macrophages, lymphocytes and basophils resembling the delayed-type response to tuberculin. The superficial epidermis, however looks different. It becomes hyperplastic, invaded by macrophages and lymphocytes and, in man, intraepidermal vesicles or blisters form which are filled with serous fluid and a variety of cell types. Histologically, these lesions develop slowly reaching a peak 3 to 6 days after contact (figs. 14/2 and 14/3).

According to the general properties of antigens (Chapter 11), it would seen that these substances are too small to act as antigens. In fact these substances are not true antigens, but rather act as quasihaptens which covalently bind to skin cell proteins. The covalent skin protein derivatives then behave as the complete antigen. Like other cell-mediated responses, antigen-reactive T cells recognize both the antigen and MHC gene products

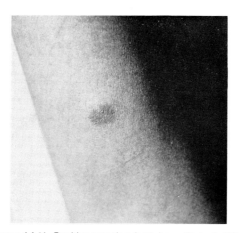

Figure 14/1. Positive reaction for tuberculin test. (AFIP 53-1280.)

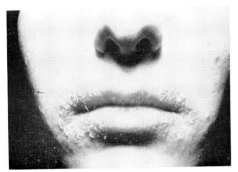

Figure 14/2. Contact dermatitis, an acute allergic reaction about the lips, cause unknown. (AFIP 57-7757-1.)

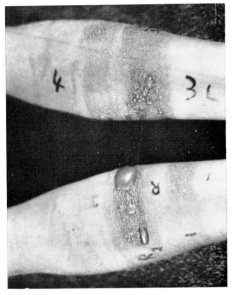

Figure 14/3. Dermatitis due to reaction to drugs. (AFIP 54-1548; 1st MFL-104.)

and, like all immune responses, reactions become more intense and last longer with each succeeding exposure. Once established, contact sensitivity can last for several years and then slowly diminish.

TRANSPLANTATION

The study of tissue transplantation began as an unwelcomed consequence of early cancer studies. It was found that when some tumors were transplanted to recipients in an outbred animal population, the tumor cells were killed. This observation led many people to believe that the immune control of cancer was a rather easily attainable goal. However, more rigorous experiments demonstrated that transplanted normal tissue was rejected as fast or faster than was tumor tissue. Although a cellular-immune phenomenon caused tissue destruction in both cases, it was quickly appreciated that the critical antigens were not specific tumor antigens

but rather normal cell surface antigens. Experimental work in transplantation immunology has led to our understanding of histocompatibility antigens and the role they play in all cell-mediated responses in general and the role they play in tissue rejection in particular. It hardly seems probable that the immune system has evolved for centuries in anticipation of thwarting medical transplantation procedures developed recently. Rather, if the cellular-immune response is viewed in broad perspective, tissue rejection is a minor consequence of the much broader protective functions of cellular-immune surveillance against deleterious nonself antigens, including infectious agents.

Types of Tissue Grafts

Autografts are transplants of tissue from one region to another on the same individual. If the surgical procedure employed is sound, autographs usually survive.

Isografts are transplants of tissue from one individual to a genetically identical individual. In humans, isografts are only possible between monozygotic twins. In animal populations, inbred strains can be produced by a series of brother/sister matings which results in an entire population of genetically identical individuals. Again, isografts, if performed correctly, usually survive in the recipient.

Allografts or homografts are transplants of tissue from one individual to a genetically nonidentical individual of the same species. These transplants represent the bulk of human transplant procedures. Their success or failure is based on degree of similarity between the major histocompatibility antigens as well as minor antigens of donor and recipient.

Heterografts or xenografts are transplants of tissue from one species to another and usually do not survive unless extraordinary measures are taken to eliminate cell surface antigens.

Thus, tissue grafts are permanently accepted only when essentially all of its histocompatibility antigens are identical with the antigens of the recipient.

Responses to Transplantation

Typical rejection phenomena are well illustrated in mice of genetically different strains when skin is transplanted from a mouse of one strain to another. Technically, skin is relatively easy to transplant, its macroscopic fate is easy to observe and tissue specimens are easily obtained for microscopic examination. The median survival time of the grafted tissue gives an indication of the intensity of the recipient's immune response. However, the same principals are involved in grafts of other tissues in other species, including man.

When a skin allograft is placed on a surgically prepared bed on the recipient animal, the graft is vascularized and cells within the graft proliferate. Host and graft tissue also attempt to heal the surgical site. However, several days later (ranging from 10 to 180 days), an intense inflammatory reaction can be observed in the allograft which results in death of the transplanted tissue and finally the entire allograft is sloughed. If a second allograft is performed between the same donor and recipient, the rejection process is accelerated, perhaps beginning as early as 5 to 6 days after transplantation, and is more intense, meaning that once the rejection is started it is completed faster than the first rejection. This second-set rejection is histocompatibility antigen specific, because an allograft from a second donor does not result in an accelerated rejection reaction. Second-set rejection also can be elicited by prior injection of virtually any donor cells other than red blood cells. The cellular nature of this response can be demonstrated by two techniques. Transplantation immunity can be passively transferred by giving the prospective recipient presensitized genetically identical lymphocytes, but not by transferring serum or immunoglobulins. Secondly, if a semipermeable membrane which inhibits cell migration but not fluid flow is placed between the grafted tissue and the recipient, the graft survives.

During rejection the histological picture resembles a typical delayed-type hypersensitivity response with its massive accumulation of inflammatory cells and is, in all likelihood, directly mediated by both T_{DTH} cells and CTLs.

Graft-*Versus*-Host Reactions

In newborn animals which are immunologically unresponsive or in animals which lack T cell function, transplanted lymphocytes from immunocompetent adult donors are not rejected. However, the *donor* lymphocytes can and do respond to the recipient's histocompatibility antigens. In the ensuing graft-*versus*-host reaction the recipient animal fails to gain weight normally, develops skin lesions and diarrhea, and usually dies within a few weeks. In this situation the transplanted tissue literally has destroyed the recipient. This same phenomenon can occur in humans who are given bone marrow transplants in an attempt to repopulate their immune system as a result of congenital immunological defects or as a result of sublethal whole body irradiation or cytotoxic drugs given during leukemia therapy.

A similar response can be demonstrated *in vitro* when peripheral lymphocytes from two genetically different individuals are present in the same culture. The mixed lymphocyte reaction (MLR) occurs when each set of lymphocytes recognizes different MHC antigens on the other, and both sets of lymphocytes undergo blast formation, incorporate radioactively labeled thymidine, and begin proliferating. In humans, this response appears to be particularly dependent on differences in HLA-D and HLA-DR antigens. The reaction can be made unidirectional (just one set of lymphocytes proliferate) by pretreating the lymphocytes of one donor with inhibitors of DNA synthesis or mitosis. This technique has been used as a method for checking the D/DR compatibility of potential tissue donors and recipients in humans.

Human Transplantation

As in any transplantation situation, the long-term survival of transplanted tissue in humans depends upon the degree to which HLA-A, B, C, D and DR gene products are matched between donor and recipient. An extensive bank of specific antisera against most of the known HLA alleles is available which, in addition to MLR tests, can accurately identify histocompatibility markers. These procedures have greatly enhanced our ability to find reasonably compatible tissue and organ donors, but it must be kept in mind that, except for homozygotic twins, exact matches are difficult to achieve. The best matches are usually to be found within the immediate family, either between parents and children or between siblings.

Paradoxically, prior immunization with cells from a prospective donor can sometimes lead to longer graft survival. Although this enhancement is poorly understood, two mechanisms have been postulated to explain the phenomenon. As in the case of B cell tolerance, it could be that specific suppressor T cells are activated which inhibit the activity and proliferation of T_{DTH} cells and CTLs. The second possibility involves the production of specific antibodies which, when combined with cell surface HLA antigens, mask or block the ability of antigen-reactive T cells to recognize the foreign antigens. This enhanced transplant survival is particularly apparent in cadaveric kidney transplants. Kidney recipients who have received multiple blood transfusions prior to transplantation seem to tolerate allografts much longer than recipients who have not received transfusions. Clearly transfusions result in antigenic stimulation by transfused lymphocytes from a variety of genetically disparate donors.

Finally, increased allograft survival in humans can be achieved by modifying the immune system of the recipient. It is not unusual to administer antilymphocyte serum (antibodies which destroy T lymphocytes) either directly after transplantation or at the earliest signs of graft rejection. In addition, immunosuppressive drugs usually are administered such as 11-oxycorticosteroids and cytolytic drugs such as azathioprine (Imuran) or 6-mercaptopurine. The timing of drug therapy appears to be crucial in order to achieve maximum effectiveness and at the moment a great deal of controversy surrounds the clinical circumstances which indicate the best time to intervene with drugs.

TUMOR IMMUNOLOGY

Neoantigens Expressed by Tumor Cells

In spite of the observation made long ago that rejection of a transplanted tumor was more dependent on histoincompatibility of normal cell antigens than on the immune recognition of tumor-specific antigens, experimental tumors in animal systems have revealed the presence of neoantigens on the surfaces of tumor cells. For instance chemical carcinogens induce the appearance of tumor-specific antigens. Curiously enough, the same chemical carcinogen does not result in the appearance of the same antigen when given to different members of the same animal species. Furthermore, the degree to which these varied neoantigens appear seems to be somewhat dose dependent. On the other hand, oncogenic animal viruses are also capable of inducing neoantigens on the surface of tumor cells and in this case the tumor antigens are the same from individual to individual and unique to each virus. Even though there are no definitively established tumor viruses for man, and even though it is difficult to demonstrate tumor specific antigens on tumors induced by chemical carcinogens in man, a few neoantigens have been found on human tumor cells.

Two of the neoantigens found on certain human tumor cells are expressed in fetal development but are rarely if ever produced after birth. α-Fetoprotein (AFP) is synthesized at maximum levels between the 3rd and 6th month of gestation and then gradually disappears. However, high serum levels of AFP are seen in humans with primary liver cancer, teratomas and in some individuals with cancer of the stomach and pancreas. AFP is not immunogenic in the species of origin but, experimentally, rabbits immunized with human AFP develop antibodies which cross-react with their own AFP. For some reason, the cross-reacting antibodies do not seem to influence the growth of the tumor, however. Carcinoembryonic antigen (CEA) is found at elevated serum levels in individuals who have primary cancers of the colon and pancreas and can be isolated from metatases to the liver. Specific isolated antibodies produced by injecting human CEA into rabbits will bind to human tumor cells. Perhaps due to the heterogeneity of CEA antibodies, they seem to have little effect on tumor

growth. The continued decrease in serum CEA is used as a measure of the success of surgically excised primary tumors, however. Even though the search for specific tumor-associated antigens which can elicit an immune response has been disappointing to date, the search continues for antigens similar to those which frequently appear in animal systems.

Again returning to animal models, a variety of immune mechanisms have been described which lead to the destruction of tumor cells. T_{DTH} cells, CTLs and activated macrophages, under the appropriate conditions, all can kill tumor cells. In addition, complement-fixing antibodies specific for animal cell tumor-specific antigens can lyse tumor cells via the classic complement pathway. Another antibody dependent cytolytic process involves null or k cells. Recall that these cells do not express the Lyt 1, 2 or 3 alloantigens of typical T cells and they do not have surface immunoglobulins of typical B cells (Chapter 12). However, null cells do have surface receptors for the Fc portions of immunoglobulins. If antibody is bound to tumor-specific antigens on tumor cells, null cells then can bind to the immunoglobulin and the result of this interaction is tumor cell lysis. This process, termed antibody-dependent cell-mediated cytotoxicity, is not dependent on complement. Finally, a population of lymphocytes have been found in mice which do not resemble B cells, T cells, k cells, or macrophages in surface antigens. These cells, termed natural killer cells, are tumoricidal for a variety of mouse leukemias, particularly those produced by tumor viruses.

Even though tumor-specific antigens can be found on animal tumor cells and even though isolated tumoricidal immune mechanisms can be demonstrated, we know that in the majority of cases tumors appear to grow in an uninterrupted manner, eventually killing the host. How is it that tumors so successfully escape immune surveillance? There is good evidence to suggest that tumor-specific antigens (TSA) readily elicit T-suppressor cells which would block any further response. It also is possible that the more aggressive tumors have TSAs which are only weakly immunogenic or not immunogenic at all. Blocking antibodies may appear in the absence of null cells which effectively interfere with recognition by T cells. This situation would be similar to the enhancing antibodies discussed under transplantation. Finally, successful tumors may escape immune recognition until they reach some critical mass, at which point the immune system is ovehelmed in its attempt to destroy the tumor.

T CELL DEFICIENCY STATES

In addition to immunodeficiency states that primarily effect B cells leading to immunoglobulin deficiencies, there are also deficiency states which primarily effect T cell functions.

Thymic Aplasia

Thymic aplasia, also called Di George syndrome, is caused by a defect in the development of the third and fourth pharyngeal pouches which give rise to the thymus, parathyroid and thyroid glands. In addition to hormonal disorders, these children suffer from a severely compromised immune system. Their blood lymphocytes are virtually all Ig-bearing B cells. They lack practically all T cell-mediated functions and suffer from severe recurring infections; they show no DTH responses to common bacterial antigens and do not develop contact sensitivity to potent sensitizers. If these infants live beyond their first 2 years, they show a surprisingly sound IgG response even to antigens considered to be T cell dependent. The probable explanation for this is that these individuals do in fact have some thymus function.

Severe Combined Immunodeficiency Disease

Individuals with severe combined immunodeficiency disease have a crippling absence of both T and B cell functions. This probably is due to a profound hematopoetic stem cell defect. Without heroic efforts to protect these infants from infection, death at an early age is a common fate. Attempts have been made to reconstitute the immune system of these individuals with bone marrow transplants. Success depends on an excellent histocompatibility match between donor and recipient. Because of the vulnerability of the recipient, graft-versus-host disease is a constant problem in bone marrow transplants of this type.

BLOOD GROUPS AND TRANSFUSION

Human red blood cells (RBCs) do not express either HLA or minor histocompatibility antigens on their surfaces but they do express blood-group antigens which are capable of inducing an immune

Table 14/1
The major human blood groups

Group	Antigen in Erythrocyte	Isoagglutinin in Serum	Erythrocytes Agglutinated by Serum of Group	Serum Agglutinates Erythrocytes of Group
A	A	Anti-B (β)	B and O	B and AB
B	B	Anti-A (α)	A and O	A and AB
AB	AB	None	A, B, and O	None
O	O*	Anti-A, anti-B (α and β)	None	A, B, and AB

* Group O erythrocytes possess a specific antigen (H) but the homologous isoagglutinin rarely appears in human sera.

response in an incompatible host. The major blood-group antigens belong to the ABO system and there are an additional eight minor surface antigens. Family studies revealed that the ABO gene has three alleles, A, B and O, with A and B being codominant over O. An individual receives one allele from each parent. Furthermore, individuals naturally possess agglutinating antibodies of the IgM class in their serum for ABO antigens they do not possess, e.g., type A individuals have isoagglutinins for B, type B individuals have isoagglutinins for A, type AB have no isoagglutinins and type O individuals have isoagglutinins for A and B (table 14/1). There are no isoagglutinins for the O marker, it apparently is not immunogenic in man.

Chemically, the blood group substances are derived from a single large glycopeptide on which various sugars that correspond to the A and B specificities are sequentially added (the glycoprotein corresponding to the blood group O substance is termed H). As each sugar is added it introduces a new antigenic specificity masking the previous one. Why IgM isoagglutinins appear for specific AB substances not present in the body is poorly understood. One speculation is that the antigenic determinants of the A and B substance may be shared by antigenic determinants on polysaccharides of common gut bacteria which, in turn, provide the necessary antigenic stimulation. In addition, A,B substances are found on other cells of the body and are secreted in saliva.

Transfusion of mismatched A,B blood types can lead to hemolytic destruction of the transfused RBCs. Type A blood will be lysed in a type B or a type O recipient. Type B blood will be lysed in a type A or a type O recipient. An individual with type AB blood will not respond to any ABO group and a type O individual will respond to both A and B. Furthermore, after transfusion of ABO-incompatible blood, IgG immunoglobulins are elicited in addition to the preexisting IgM. Because normal isoglutinins are IgM which cannot cross the placenta, a developing fetus with a blood type differing from the maternal type will be relatively safe from hemolytic disease.

Rh Antigen

In addition to the ABO substance, approximately 85% of the population express an Rh antigen (Rh$^+$) and 15% do not (Rh$^-$). This was discovered serendipitously when rabbit antiserum prepared against Rhesus monkey RBCs agglutinated 85% of the samples of human RBCs (thus Rhesus monkeys and humans share a common RBC surface antigen). The Rh factor also must be matched for transfusion because it is more immunogenic than are the A,B substances. Parental couples in which the mother is Rh$^-$ and the father if Rh$^+$ run the risk of serious hemolytic disease in their newborn. During normal development, some fetal RBCs cross the placenta and since the fetal blood is Rh$^+$ and maternal blood is Rh$^-$ the mother will respond with IgG directed against the Rh factor. Before birth, during a first pregnancy, the degree of anti-Rh stimulation is usually not great enough to cause the fetus serious harm. However, at the time of birth, when the placenta separates from the uterine wall, a significant "shower" of fetal RBCs occurs which are absorbed into maternal circulation. This may result in a significant antigenic challenge. The risk of serious hemolytic disease (erythroblastosis fetalis) in the fetus during succeeding pregnancies is therefore greatly increased. In its most severe manifestation, erythroblastosis fetalis can kill the infant.

Prevention of Rh Disease

The incidence of Rh disease is less when the Rh$^-$ mother and the Rh$^+$ baby also differ in ABO type. Rapid removal of fetal cells from maternal circulation by anti-A or anti-B apparently reduces the likelihood of anti-Rh stimulation. This observation has led to an effective method of reducing the incidence of erythroblastosis fetalis. At each delivery, the mother is injected with anti-Rh antibodies causing rapid elimination of Rh$^+$ cells from maternal circulation.

ADDITIONAL READING

BELLANTI, J. A. 1978 *Immunology II*, Saunders, Philadelphia.

BLUME, K. G., BEUTLER, E., BROSS, K. J., CHILLAR, R. K., ELLINGTON, O. B., FAHEY, J. L., FARBSTEIN, M. J., FORMAN, S. J., SCHMIDT, G. M., SCOTT, E. P., SPRUCE, W. E., TURNER, M. A., AND WOLFE, J. L. 1980 Bone-Marrow Ablation and Allogeneic Marrow Transplantation in Acute Leukemia. N Engl J Med, **302**, 1041.

CARPENTER, C. B. 1981 The Cellular Basis of Allograft Rejection. Immunol Today, **2**, 50.

COSIMI, A. B. 1981 The Clinical Value of Antilymphocyte Antibodies. Transplant Proc, **13**, 462.

DAVIS, B. D., DULBECCO, R., EISEN, H. N., AND GINSBERG, H. S. 1980 *Microbiology*, Ed. 3. Harper & Row, Hagerstown, Md.

DOHERTY, P. C., AND BENNINK, J. R. 1981 Monitoring the Integrity of Self: Biology of MHC-Restriction of Virus-Immune T Cells. Fed Proc, **40**, 218.

FIDLER, I. J., AND KRIPKE, M. L. 1980 Tumor Cell Antigenicity, Host Immunity and Cancer Metastasis. Cancer Immunol Immunother, **7**, 201.

FUDENBERG, H. H., STITES, D. P., CALDWELL, J. L., AND WELLS, J. V. 1978 *Basic & Clinical Immunology*, Ed. 2. Lange Medical Publications, Los Altos, Calif.

HERBERMAN, R. B., DJEU, J. Y., KAY, H. D., ORTALDO, J. R., RICCARDI, C., BONNARD, G. D., HOLDEN, H. T., FAGNANI, R., AND PUCCETTI, S. AND P. 1979 Natural Killer Cells: Characteristics and Regulation of Activity. Immunol Rev, **44**, 43.

HORTON, J. E., KOOPMAN, W. J., FARRAR, J. J., FULLER-BONAR, J. AND MERGENHAGEN, S. E. 1979 Partial Purification of a Bone-Resorbing Factor Elaborated from Human Allogeneic Cultures. Cellular Immunol, **43**, 1.

HORTON, J. E., OPPENHEIM, J. J., MERGENHAGEN, S. E., AND RAISZ, L. G. 1974. Macrophage-Lymphocyte Synergy in the Production of Osteoclast Activating Factor. J Immunol, **113**, 1278.

JOHNSEN, H. E., AND MADSEN, M. 1979 Lymphocyte Subpopulations in Man: Characterization of Human Killer Cells Against Allogeneic Targets Sensitized with HLA Antibodies. Scand J Immunol, **9**, 429.

KRANGEL, M. S., ORR, H. T., AND STROMINGER, J. L. 1979 Assembly and Maturation of HLA-A and HLA-B Antigens *In Vivo*. Cell, **18**, 979.

McDONALD, J. C. 1981 The Biologic Implications of HLA. Arch Intern Med, **141**, 100.

MOEN, T., ALBRECHTSEN, D., FLATMARK, A., JAKOBSEN, A., JERVELL, J., HALVORSEN, S., SOLHEIM, B. G., AND THORSBY, E. 1980 Importance of HLA-DR Matching in Cadaveric Renal Transplantation—A Prospective One-Center Study of 170 Transplants. N Engl J Med, **303**, 850.

MOORE, S. B. 1979 HLA. Mayo Clin Proc, **54**, 385.

NAJARIAN, J. S., SUTHERLAND, D. E. R., FERGUSON, R. M., SIMMONS, R. L., KERSEY, J., MAUER, S. M., SLAVIN, S., AND KIM, T. H. 1981 Total Lymphoid Irradiation and Kidney Transplantation: A Clinical Experience. Transplant Proc, **13**, 417.

O'REILLY, R. J., KAPOOR, N., POLLACK, M., SORELL, M., CHAGANTI, R. S. K., BLAESE, R. M., WANK, R., GOOD, R. A., AND DUPONT, B. 1979 Reconstitution of Immunologic Function in a Patient with Severe Combined Immunodeficiency Following Transplantation of Bone Marrow From an HLA-A, B, C Nonidentical But MLC-Compatible Paternal Donor. Transplant Proc, **11**, 1934.

ROITT, I. M., AND LEHNER, T. 1980 *Immunology of Oral Diseases*, Blackwell Scientific Publications, Oxford.

RUSSELL, J. H., MASAKOWSKI, V. R., AND DOBOS, C. B. 1980. Mechanisms of Immune Lysis I. Physiological Distinction between Target Cell Death Mediated by Cytotoxic T Lymphocytes and Antibody Plus Complement. J Immunol, **124**, 1100.

SALAMAN, J. R. 1981 Pharmacologic Immunosuppresion. Transplant Proc, **13**, 311.

SAMTER, M. 1978 *Immunological Diseases*, Ed. 3. Little, Brown, Boston.

SHILLITOE, E. J. AND RAPP, F. 1979 Virus-Induced Cell Surface Antigens and Cell-Mediated Immune Responses. Springer Semin Immunopathol, **2**, 237.

STUART, F. P., McKEARN, T. J., WEISS, A., AND FITCH, F. W. 1980 Suppression of Rat Renal Allograft Rejection by Antigen and Antibody. Immunol Rev, **49**, 127.

TING, C. C., AND RODRIGUES, D. 1980 Switching on the Macrophage-Mediated Suppressor Mechanism by Tumor Cells to Evade Host Immune Surveillance. Proc Natl Acad Sci, **77**, 4265.

VAN ES, A., PERSIGN, G. G., VAN HOOF-EIJKENBOOM, Y. E. A., KALFF, M. W., AND VAN HOOF, J. P. 1981 Blood Transfusions, HLA-A, and B, DR Matching, Graft Survival, and Clinical Course After Cadaveric Kidney Transplantation. Transplant Proc, **13**, 172.

5 ORAL MICROBIOTA AND ITS DISEASES

---

chapter 15

Microbial Flora of the Oral Cavity

Jeremy Hardie

ACQUISITION OF AN ORAL MICROBIOTA

The human is edentulous at birth and has a flora which is characteristic for this condition. When the primary teeth begin to erupt, there is a significant change in the environment which is reflected by changes in the oral flora. When the primary dentition is complete, the conditions are relatively stable until the permanent teeth begin to erupt. During the period of mixed dentition, conditions vary as teeth are lost and new ones erupt, producing varied environmental conditions which can affect the oral flora. Once the permanent dentition is present, conditions become somewhat more stable.

The oral cavity normally supports one of the most concentrated and varied of microbial populations of any area of the body. Particularly high numbers of microorganisms are associated with the dorsum of the tongue, around the gingival sulcus and on the tooth surface. In the latter situation, the soft noncalcified accumulations of bacteria and their products are referred to as dental plaque.

The total microscopic count of saliva, which is derived mainly from the tongue, has been given as anything from 43 million to 5.5 billion per ml, with an average of 750 million. The microbial concentration about the gingival sulcus and in plaque is approximately 200 billion cells per g of sample. This is equivalent to the density of centrifugally packed sediment of a broth culture or of a bacterial colony on solid medium.[1]

In utero the fetus is normally germ free. During birth, the child is exposed to the normal flora of the mother's genital tract, including lactobacilli, corynebacteria, micrococci, coliforms, facultative streptococci, anaerobic cocci, yeasts, protozoa, and possibly viruses. Nevertheless, the oral cavity usually appears to be sterile at birth. From about 8 hours following birth there is a rapid increase in the number of detectable organisms. However, the composition of the bacterial flora varies considerably for the first few days of life. Several species of lactobacilli, streptococci, staphylococci, pneumococci, enterococci, coliforms, sarcinae and neisseriae can be detected, but with the exception of *Streptococcus salivarius*, most of these organisms are found sporadically and not in high numbers. Even though it is exposed to a wide range of organisms during the first few days, the mouth of a newborn infant is a selective habitat. Consequently, few of the bacteria common to adult mouths become established and practically none of the species present in the general environment, except occasionally as transients. Organisms different from those harbored by immediate contacts may be acquired; for example, identical twins may harbor different strains of the same species. Some selectivity continues into adulthood.

At least by the end of the 3rd month, all mouths support a recognizable resident microflora. Even at the end of a year, however, only streptococci, staph-

---

[1] By convention, dental plaque is considered to be those tenacious deposits which cannot be dislodged from the teeth by a spray of water. The term materia alba is sometimes used to include both dental plaque and more loosely attached soft material, which may or may not be bacterial in origin. Calcified dental plaque deposits are termed calculus (tartar).

ylococci, veillonellae, and neisseriae are generally found in all mouths; actinomyces, rothiae, lactobacilli and fusobacteria can be isolated from about half of the mouths, while bacteroides, leptotrichiae, corynebacteria and coliforms are present in less than half of the mouths. By this time streptococci, although still numerically dominant, account for only about 70% of the viable count. The early period is dominated by facultative and aerobic species, to which are added gradually the various obligate anaerobes, but numerically the facultative types generally dominate at all ages.

One of the major changes in the oral environment which occurs at around the age of 6 months is the eruption of the first deciduous teeth. The appearance of hard enamel surfaces in the mouth apparently favors the establishment of *Streptococcus*

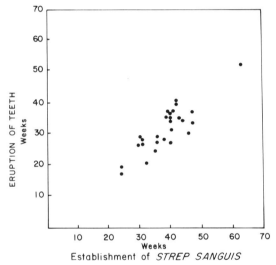

Figure 15/1. The relation between the eruption time of the teeth and the time when *Streptococcus sanguis* was established in the mouth of 27 infants. (Reproduced with permission from J. Carlsson, H. Grahnen, G. Jonsson, and S. Wilkner. Establishment of *Streptococcus sanguis* in the mouth of infants. Arch. Oral Biol., **15**, 1143, 1970.)

sanguis, an organism not usually isolated prior to the eruption of the deciduous incisors (fig. 15/1). Other organisms, including *Streptococcus mutans*, also preferentially colonize the tooth surface and become regular oral inhabitants from about the age of 1 year. In one Swedish study, lactobacilli were only recovered in low numbers from infants and below the age of 2 years appeared to be mostly transients (fig. 15/2). Throughout childhood the bacterial populations increase. Black pigmented organisms (such as *Bacteroides melaninogenicus*) and spirochetes, both of which are strict anaerobes, are not present in the gingival crevice of all children. By adolescence, *B. melaninogenicus* is present in virtually all individuals, and spirochetes also increase in incidence with age. The increase in isolation of these and other anaerobic organisms may be related to the concurrent increase in the prevalence of gingivitis which is seen during the same period. Development of dental caries creates a new set of environmental conditions for microorganisms. The resulting cavities provide a protected and retentive niche, thus favoring those organsisms with little adhesive capability and which are poorly adapted for colonization of exposed tooth surfaces. The lesion also provides new substrates, a more acid pH and, probably, decreased exposure to salivary antimicrobial factors. As indicated in table 15/1, showing the predominant genera and species found in various sites, the cultivable microbiota of different regions of the oral cavity of the adult is quite complex. Certain species have a predilection for particular sites, probably because some nutritional or physical requirement is met at that site. As the individual ages, some changes occur in the microflora, primarily associated with the loss of teeth. Spirochetes, lactobacilli and some strains of streptococci are reduced. Presence of various forms of oral disease further alters the flora, the specific changes depending on which disease processes occur.

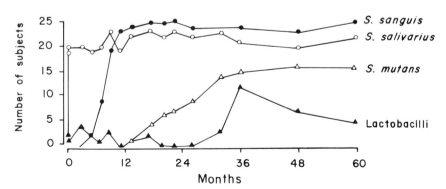

Figure 15/2. Presence of S. salivarius, S. sanguis, S. mutans and lactobacilli in samples taken from the mouth of infants during a 5-year period. (Reproduced with permission from J. Carlsson, H. Grahnen, and G. Jonsson. Lactobacilli and streptococci in the mouth of children. Caries Res., **9**, 333, 1975.)

Table 15/1
Mean percentages of cultivable organisms in the adult oral cavity

	Gingival Crevice Area	Dental Plaque	Tongue	Saliva
Gram Positive Facultative Cocci	28.8	28.2	44.8	46.2
Streptococci	27.1	27.9	38.3	41.0
S. salivarius	N.D.	N.D.	8.2	4.6
Enterococci	7.2		N.D.	1.3
Staphylococci	1.7	0.3	6.5	4.0
Gram Positive Anaerobic Cocci	7.4	12.6	4.2	13.0
Gram Negative Facultative Cocci	0.4	0.4	3.4	1.2
Gram Negative Anaerobic Cocci	10.7	6.4	16.0	15.9
Gram Positive Facultative Rods	15.3	23.8	13.0	11.8
Gram Positive Anaerobic Rods	20.2	18.4	8.2	4.8
Gram Negative Facultative Rods	1.2	N.D.	3.2	2.3
Gram Negative Anaerobic Rods	16.1	10.4	8.2	4.8
Fusobacterium	1.9	4.1	0.7	0.3
B. melaninogenicus	4.7	N.D.	0.2	N.D.
V. sputorum	3.8	1.3	2.2	2.1
other Bacteroides	5.6	4.8	5.1	2.4
Spirochetes	1.0	N.D.	N.D.	N.D.

N.D. = not detected.
(From SOCRANSKY, S. S. AND MANGANIELLO, S.D. 1971 The Oral Microbiota of Man from Birth to Senility. J Periodontol, **42**, 485.)

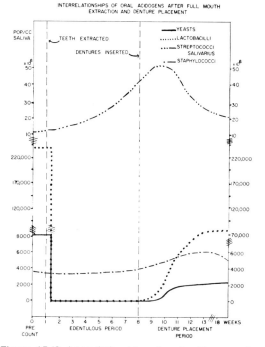

Figure 15/3. Interrelationships of oral acidogens after full mouth extraction and denture placement. (Reproduced with permission from I. L. Shklair, and M. A. Mazzarella. 1960 Salivary Microbial Changes as a Result of Full Mouth Extraction. Dental Research Facility. U. S. Naval Training Center, Great Lakes, Ill. Project MR-005. 12-5004 NM 750127.)

Not only does the extraction of all remaining teeth and placement of complete dentures influence the total numbers of the oral microorganisms, but it also influences the prevalence of particular species (fig. 15/3). Various studies have demonstrated that Streptococcus mutans, Streptococcus sanguis, yeasts, lactobacilli and spirochetes are reduced or virtually eliminated during the edentulous period. The studies of Shklair and Mazzerella (fig. 15/3) indicate that lactobacilli and yeasts virtually disappear during the edentulous period and that Streptococcus salivarius increases. During the first 2 weeks after placement of the denture, streptococci remain at a high level while lactobacilli and yeasts gradually return but remain at a low level. After 3 to 5 weeks the lactobacilli and yeasts increase and the streptococci decrease to preextraction levels. Throughout the entire period of this study, little fluctuation was observed in the number of staphylococci.

A study on full denture wearers by Carlsson et al. (1969) showed that S. sanguis, S. mutans and S. salivarius were present in samples of plaque from the dentures and in saliva from most subjects. When the dentures were left out of the mouth for 2 days, S. sanguis and S. mutans could no longer be detected in saliva, whereas the prevalence of S. salivarius was unaffected. After the dentures had been worn again for 2 to 4 days, S. sanguis was once again found in all subjects and S. mutans was found in five out of seven.

PROBLEMS ATTENDING THE STUDY OF THE ORAL MICROBIAL FLORA

It is difficult to obtain precise and definitive information concerning the distribution, numbers and types of microorganisms which inhabit the oral cavity. This is due partly to the variability of the oral flora itself, and because of technical problems associated with sampling, isolation, enumeration and identification of this complex microflora. As a consequence of these inherent difficulties, and as indicated by the data already presented, it is only realistic to attempt a rather general definition of the oral microflora. Even in a single mouth the microbial population varies in different anatomical situations and undergoes progressive changes throughout the life of the individual.

Variability

Variability of the oral microbiota is demonstrated by comparing the microbial composition of samples taken from similar sites in different mouths. Samples from the various areas, such as dental plaque, may show both qualitative and quantitative differences between individuals. Similarly, different sites in the oral cavity of one individual are colonized by a different microflora. Although each anatomical site may harbor most or all of the different types of organisms at some time, particular organisms tend to predominate in their preferred ecological situations. For example, *Streptococcus mutans* resides primarily on the tooth surface, while *Streptococcus salivarius* resides primarily on the tongue and is washed off into the saliva where it is found in high concentration. However, repeated sampling from the same site in a single individual will often, on different occasions, demonstrate a marked variation, both qualitative and quantitiative, in the composition of the microflora.

In order to be a part of the indigenous microbiota, organisms must be retained in the oral cavity. Bacteria may be retained by adhesion to oral structures, by attachment to other organisms, or by mechanical retention. Several different mechanisms are probably involved in microbial adhesion and it has been demonstrated that different bacteria have different affinities for particular types of surfaces. Production of extracellular polymers by the organisms and interaction of bacterial surface components with salivary macromolecules (including glycoproteins) are both involved in microbial adherence; in addition, some species produce surface appendages (pili) which may aid surface retention. Another possible method of adhesion between bacteria is specific interaction between the surface layers of organisms of different species. For example, the anaerobic species *Bacteroides asaccharolyticus* has been shown to adhere very weakly to clean tooth surfaces but does attach readily to preexisting deposits of dental plaque bacteria.

Nonadherent organisms, or those with low affinity for various oral structures, may be retained mechanically, as in the pits and fissures of teeth, in the gingival crevice, in the periodontal pocket, or in carious lesions. For example, lactobacilli appear to have a low affinity for the tooth surface compared to other bacteria, such as *S. sanguis*. The observed association between lactobacilli and carious lesions may, therefore, be due primarily to mechanical retention within the altered tooth structure.

Physiological Conditions

As is the case with any habitat, the composition of the oral microflora is a reflection of its environment. The organisms which inhabit the mouth have a series of physicochemical and nutrition requirements and must be able to survive various physiological, mechanical and defense activities of the host. The growth requirements of the microorganisms can be provided by the diet and tissues of the host, or by other microorganisms. The nature and amount of carbohydrates or proteins will determine which organisms will flourish and which will simply "exist." For example, the amount of sucrose in the diet can influence the amount of plaque formed on the teeth, its population density, and the proportions of *S. mutans* and *S. sanguis* in the plaque.

Some bacteria can obtain essential metabolites from other species. For example, formic and lactic acids produced by bacteria in the oral cavity in part supply the energy sources for *Veillonella alcalescens*. It is likely that there are a number of similar "food chains" within oral microbial communities.

Bacteria from the human oral cavity have a wide variety of oxygen tension requirements. Obligate aerobes and anaerobes, facultative anaerobes, microaerophilic and capnophilic (*i.e.*, carbon-dioxide requiring) organisms have all been found. Similarly, different organisms require different oxidation-reduction potentials (E_h) for growth. It has been demonstrated that there are variations in oxygen tension and E_h in different parts of the mouth, although it is not entirely clear how such widely divergent potentials are established.

Source of Oral Microorganisms

Which microorganisms become established in the oral cavity depends upon the number of organisms introduced, the frequency of introduction, the nutritional and physicochemical conditions at the time of introduction, and the nature of the existing microbiota. Any incoming bacteria must be present in sufficient numbers and in favorable conditions in order to survive and compete successfully with established organisms. Adequate nutritional requirements must be available to give such incoming organisms enough of an advantage to become established in such a highly competitive situation.

The importance of these factors in establishing a microbiota has been illustrated by *in vitro* studies of antagonistic activities amongst plaque bacteria. *Streptococcus sanguis* has been shown to have a broad inhibitory effect on other streptococci, filamentous organisms and rods. *Lactobacillus casei* and certain *Corynebacterium* species are active against filamentous organisms; and *Bacterionema matruchotii* inhibits some strains of *Rothia dentocariosa*. Some strains of *S. mutans* produce bacterioncins (see Chapter 4), and this property may confer some competitive advantage in the oral cavity. The exact mechanisms for these inhibitory actions are not known in most cases and their clinical implications are difficult to evaluate. However, the ability of the flora to change may be associated with the development of oral disease.

Sampling

No single specimen can be taken as fully representative of the oral flora as a whole, since the microbial composition is known to vary from site to site. A good overall picture of the flora can be obtained by examining the flora associated with three principle foci: the dorsum of the tongue, the gingival crevice region, and the coronal (supragingival) dental plaque. Available evidence indicates that the salivary microflora represents mainly the organisms which colonize the dorsum of the tongue. Saliva samples vary considerably in their bacterial content because of variations in the rate of salivary secretion by individuals and will be affected by the method used for stimulation of salivary flow. Saliva probably never gives an accurate representation of the microflora present on the tooth surface or in the gingival crevice. A good example of the variations which occur is provided by *S. salivarius*. The species averages about half the facultative streptococci isolated from the saliva and scrapings from the dorsum of the tongue, whereas it usually comprises less than 1% of those found in plaque or gingival crevice samples. The latter sites are best sampled by taking scrapings of material with appropriate instruments. Since the concentration of bacteria in these specimens is about 100 times that of saliva, salivary bacterial contamination is unlikely to affect the results to any great extent. Swabbing the oral cavity, either locally or generally, has proved useful in particular situations, as with infants (table 15/2). However, soft cotton swabs are only appropriate for soft tissue surfaces. Other techniques, such as impression cultures, have also been used by some investigators.

Enumeration and Cultivation

Total microscopic counts of the numbers of bacteria in oral specimens can be made relatively easily by conventional techniques, either with stained or unstained material. However, difficulty does arise when attempts are made to quantify the oral flora by means of viable (cultivable) counts. Here it is generally found that the total viable count accounts only for a fraction of the total microscopic count. Part of the discrepancy arises from the fact that oral organisms grow and accumulate in aggregates which, in the case of dental plaque, are embedded in a gelatinous organic matrix. The viable count can be increased significantly by mechanical disruption of specimens, but such gain is offset by the concominant killing effect of many dispersion methods. For example, prolonged ultrasonic treatment of plaque specimens may increase the yield of some gram positive organisms, such as streptococci and actinomyces, while destroying the more sensitive gram negatives originally present.

Serious loss of cultivable bacteria also occurs, unless specimens are cultured promptly using appropriate aerobic and anaerobic techniques and media, or are preserved in a suitable holding (transport) medium which will neither be toxic to the organisms nor support their growth. Technical developments in the methods used for isolation of obligate anaerobes, such as the anaerobic chamber and the roll-tube method with prereduced anaerobically sterilized (PRAS) culture media, have allowed significant improvements to be made in the proportion of total organisms recovered.

The multitide and variety of microorganisms in the oral cavity makes isolation of every species technically most difficult. Even though they flourish in the mouth, some of them present such exacting cultural requirements that they have not been cultivated satisfactorily on artificial media. Some of the species are in such numerical minority that they may be overgrown on culture plates by the more numerous organisms. Dilution techniques that are normally employed in order to achieve optimum numbers of colonies per plate for counting (commonly in the range 30 to 300) may result in the less numerous bacteria being diluted out. Thus, species present as less than about 1% of the total cultivable flora may well be missed, unless appropriate selective media are used in conjunction with lower dilutions of the original specimen. Many of the reported studies, therefore, give useful estimates of the predominant cultivable flora, but may have missed the minor components.

Various selective media have been used for studies on the oral flora. However, it should be remembered that all selective media inhibit, to some degree, even the organisms they are supposed to support. Thus, quantitative studies using such media may produce an underestimate of the numbers of particular species.

By the use of various selective and nonselective media, over 25 bacterial genera have been detected in oral samples (table 15/3). Some of these are regular members of the oral flora which are almost invariably present, others have been recovered only occasionally and are either present in very low

Table 15/2

Incidence and range of viable counts of 13 bacterial genera per milligram of oral sample isolated from infants at four age levels during the first year of life

Genera	Mean Age in Days (No. of Subjects)							
	1.8 (51)		101 (44)		248 (29)		365 (29)	
	No. positive	Range	No. positive	Range	No. positive	Range	No. positive	Range
Aerobic incubation								
Total	42	0.8–1,600,000	44	11,000–1,900,000	29	12,000–2,400,000	29	15,000–690,000
Streptococcus sali-varius	26	1.1–110,000	33	10–39,000	28	1.1–68,000	29	310–84,000
Staphylococcus	23	0.2–270	42	0.2–520	29	0.7–1,900	29	0.5–6,300
Neisseria	4	1.4–1,200	30	2–3,600	29	1.3–54,000	29	4–81,000
Nocardia	0	None	1	540	13	100–14,000	18	0.5–40,000
Lactobacillus	0	None	6	0.8–54	10	0.5–480	14	0.4–310
Corynebacterium	0	None	6	0.7–5	14	0.2–910	10	0.2–600
Candida	3	1.3–6	18	0.2–590	7	0.2–160	14	0.2–51
Coliforms	4	1–630,000	13	0.2–680	13	0.3–81,000	6	0.7–11
Anaerobic incubation								
Total	42	3–3,600,000	44	14,000–2,400,000	29	24,000–1,600,000	29	15,000–1,000,000
Streptococcus	38	2–1,100,000	44	2,200–860,000	29	17,000–1,300,000	29	7,000–690,000
Lactobacillus	9	1–14,000	16	1.4–150	16	0.2–30,000	15	0.2–7,700
Actinomyces	0	None	1	340	6	12–3,600	17	4.6–27,000
Veillonella	1	390	33	1.4–3,100	24	0.2–41,000	29	34–40,000
Fusobacterium	0	None	2	0.4–3	8	0.4–15,000	16	0.2–70,000
Bacteroides	0	None	2	5–100	3	49–580	13	22–2,700
Leptotrichia	0	None	3	0.2–9	15	0.2–5.9	12	0.1–80

(From McCarthy, C., Snyder, M. L., and Parker, R. B. 1965 The Indigenous Oral Flora of Man. I. The Newborn to the 1-Year-Old Infant. Arch Oral Biol, **10**, 61.)

Table 15/3
Genera found in the oral cavity [a]

Gram Positive Genera	Gram Negative Genera
Streptococcus	Neisseria
Micrococcus	Veillonella
Peptostreptococcus	Haemophilus
Peptococcus	Bacteroides
Actinomyces	Fusobacterium
Lactobacillus	Capnocytophaga
Bacterionema	Actinobacillus
Rothia	Eikenella
Arachnia	Campylobacter
Propionibacterium	Vibrio (Wollinella)
Bifidobacterium	Selenomonas
Eubacterium	Leptotrichia
	Treponema

[a] Other genera have been reported occasionally, but do not appear to be regular oral inhabitants. These include *Clostridium, Corynebacterium, Bacillus* and various members of the Enterobacteriaceae.

numbers or, possibly, should be regarded as transient inhabitants of the mouth.

Identification

The current imperfect state of microbial taxonomy does not allow all isolates from the oral cavity to be identified precisely. Many strains can be allocated to the appropriate genus, species or subspecies by comparison of their properties to the descriptions which appear in *Bergey's Manual* and other publications, but there remains a substantial minority of oral organisms which have not been adequately described and classified. However, significant progress is being made in this complex area and new species descriptions appear fairly regularly in the scientific journals.

Under these circumstances of taxonomic uncertainty, some investigators have compromised by simply allocating organisms to broad groups on the basis of microscopic morphology, gram staining reaction and general cultural characteristics. This approach has the advantage of analyzing the total flora, but causes some difficulty in practice because many oral organisms tend to be pleomorphic and many vary in their gram reaction. Consequently, some errors and confusion may arise in allocating organisms to groups according to morphological criteria alone.

NATURE OF THE ORAL MICROBIOTA

Over 40 named species have been recorded in the literature as forming part of the indigenous oral microflora. Notwithstanding the inherent difficulties in sampling, enumerating and identifying oral microorganisms, a general picture of the composition of the normal flora of the dentulous mouth can be discerned. Regardless of variations from person to person and from site to site, facultative and anaerobic streptococci, veillonellae, and pleomorphic gram positive rods (often referred to as "diphtheroids") usually comprise up to about 80% of the total viable count. Facultative streptococci plus veillonellae constitute the major components of the salivary flora, and this appears to represent mostly those organisms which colonize the dorsum of the tongue. In plaque and gingival sulcus, the proportions of gram positive rods (mainly *Actinomyces* species) and gram negative anaerobic rods (bacteroides, fusobacteria, vibrios) are higher. Neisseriae are regularly present, averaging 3 to 5% of the viable count. Lactobacilli, staphylococci and filamentous forms usually each add up to 1% or less of the total. Black-pigmented *Bacteroides* species, spirochetes and some other anaerobic species appear to be indigenous to the gingival sulcus. These organisms may increase in numbers significantly when periodontal disease develops (see Chapter 17).

Yeasts (*Candida* species) and coliforms are indigenous to about half of adult mouths, but usually occur in small numbers. Mycoplasmas can be demonstrated in all adult mouths, but their numbers are uncertain. Few workers have attempted to isolate these organisms routinely, special isolation media and conditions being required for this purpose. However, mycoplasmas have been isolated from saliva, plaque, and calculus samples from both healthy and diseased gingival crevices, and from carious lesions. Protozoa can be demonstrated in small numbers in nearly half of clean and healthy adult mouths; their presence in abundance may signify bad oral hygiene and periodontitis.

For comparative purposes, the distribution of different groups of microorganisms in various parts of the body is summarized in table 15/4. However, it is possible that the picture may change with the application of more sophisticated sampling and isolation techniques to normal flora studies. Some of the characteristics of microorganisms known to be regular members of the oral flora are described briefly in the sections which follow.

GRAM POSITIVE COCCI

Streptococci

Facultative streptococci form the most numerous single group in the oral cavity. Most surveys have shown these organisms to average nearly half of the total viable counts of saliva and the dorsum of the tongue and about a quarter of the viable counts of plaque and gingival sulcus samples (fig. 15/4).

The pyogenic species, such as *Streptococcus pyogenes* (Lancefield Group A) are not commonly found in the oral cavity and they rarely cause local

Table 15/4
Distribution of indigenous microorganisms in man

Organism	Mouth	Oropharynx	Nasophar-ynx	Intestine	Skin	Eye	External Genitalia	Vagina
α-Streptococcus	1	1	2	2	0	0	2	2'
β-Streptococcus	tr	3	tr	2*	0	0	0	tr
γ-Streptococcus	2	2	tr	2	0	0	2	2
Anaerobic streptococcus	2	2	0	2	0	0	2	2
Pneumococcus	tr	3	tr	0	0	0	0	0
Staphylococcus epidermidis	2	tr	3	2	1	2	2	2
Staphylococcus aureus	2	2	3	2	0	0	0	tr
Other staphylococci	2	2	tr	2	tr	tr	tr	2
Corynebacterium†	1	2	2	2	1	1	2	2‡
Lactobacillus	2	0	0	2	0	0	0	1
Leptotrichia	2	0	0	0	0	0	0	0
Actinomyces	2	2	0	0	0	0	0	0
Bacteroides	2	tr	tr	1	0	0	tr	tr
Fusobacterium	2	tr	0	2	0	0	2	0
Spirochetes	2	tr	0	2	0	0	2	0
Anaerobic vibrios	2	tr	tr	0	0	0	0	tr
Neisseria meningitidis	0	3	3	0	0	0	0	0
Other neisseriae	2	1	1	0	0	0	tr	tr
Veillonella	1	2	2	0	0	0	0	2
Haemophilus	tr	3	3	0	0	0	0	0
Mycoplasmas	2	2	0	2	0	0	2	2
Coliform bacteria	tr	tr	tr	1	0	0	2	2
Proteus	0	0	0	2	0	0	tr	0
Pseudomonas	tr	0	0	tr	0	0	tr	0
Clostridium	0	0	0	2	0	0	0	0
Bacillus	0	0	0	0	0	0	0	0
Mycobacterium	0	0	0	tr	tr	0	3	0
Yeasts	2	2	0	2	2	0	2	2‡
Protozoa	2	tr	0	3	0	0	3	3

1 = Generally present and constituting a principal fraction of the regional microbial flora.
2 = Generally present but constituting a minor fraction of the regional microbial flora.
3 = Carriers found frequently, in whom the organisms may constitute a prominent fraction of the regional microbial flora.
tr = Often found, usually in small numbers, as a trace component or a transient.
0 = If found, may be assumed to be a transient.
* = Group D hemolytic enterococci.
† = A very small proportion of the populace acts as the reservoir of diphtheria, owing to the persistence of *C. diphtheriae* in the nasopharynx.
‡ = During the period of ovarian activity.

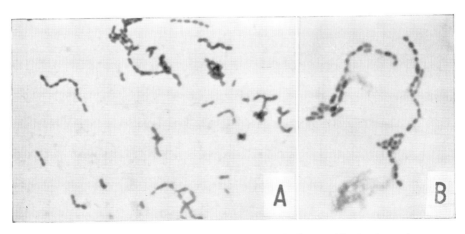

Figure 15/4. (*A*) Oral aerobic streptococci. (*B*) Oral anaerobic streptococci.

oral infections. On the occasions when such strep-tococci are isolated from the mouth they probably derive from the oronasopharynx and should not be regarded as part of the resident flora. Enterococci (Lancefield Group D) may be present in the human oral cavity of up to 75% of people, although usually in low number. These organisms are scarce on the tongue and average less than 10% of the strepto-cocci from the gingival crevice. Enterococci are distinguished by their ability to grow under condi-tions that are inhibitory to most other streptococci (table 15/5) and by the presence of the Lancefield Group D antigen. *Streptococcus faecalis* has been encountered more frequently than other enterococ-cus species. *Streptococcus bovis*, an extracellular dextran producer which also belongs to Lancefield Group D, has not been reported as part of the normal oral flora. This streptococcus inhabits the human gut, is an occasional source of infective endocarditis and is also one of the species associated with bovine mastitis.

The most abundant of the oral streptococci are those referred to collectively as the viridans group. Historically, these have been classified by a variety of criteria over the years and considerable confusion has surrounded their taxonomy and nomenclature. In addition to α-hemolytic varieties, from which the name "viridans" is derived, some of the strep-tococci in this group may display either complete (β) hemolysis or be totally nonhemolytic. The char-acter of hemolysis is, in any case, not completely reliable and depends upon the type of blood used and the cultural conditions employed. Recent stud-ies have clarified the taxonomy of the viridans

streptococci considerably; on the basis of physiolog-ical and biochemical tests they can be divided into several distinct species. Some of these species can be further subdivided into serotypes, biotypes or bacteriocin types.

The tests which have been employed for char-acterizing the streptococci include some commonly used biochemical tests, cell-wall analysis and sero-logical methods. Some of the oral streptococci, in-cluding strains of *S. sanguis*, *S. salivarius* and *S. mutans*, form distinctive colonies on media contain-ing 5% (or more) sucrose. One such medium, mitis-salivarius agar, has been widely used for selective isolation of oral streptococci. In addition to sucrose, this medium contains trypan blue, crystal violet and tellurite which inhibit the growth of most of the organisms other than streptococci. Several other selective media have also been developed for isolation of oral streptococci.

S. sanguis may comprise up to half of the total count of facultative streptococci in plaque, which seems to be the primary habitat of this species. Although previously recognized as the causative agent in a substantial number of cases of subacute bacterial endocarditis, the source of the organism was not defined until more recently. As shown in table 15/5, *S. sanguis* can be distinguished from other streptococci by the following combination of characteristics; production of ammonia from argi-nine, hydrolysis of aesculin and production of hy-drogen peroxide. Most isolates produce extracellu-lar glucans from sucrose, although some negative variants are also recognized. A certain amount of confusion surrounds the serology and antigenic

Table 15/5
Some characteristics for identifying oral streptococci

	S. faecalis	S. sanguis	S. mitis/ mitior	"S. mutans group"	S. milleri	S. salivarius
Acid production from						
Mannitol	+	−	−	+	−	−
Sorbitol	+	−	−	+	−	−
Glycerol	+	−	−	−	−	−
Production of						
Acetoin from glucose	V	−	− *	+	+	V
Hydrogen peroxide	−	+	+	− *	−	−
Ammonia from argi-nine	+	+	−	− * *	+	−
Extracellular polysac-charide from su-crose	−	Glucan	V	Glucan	−	Fructan
Hydrolysis of aescu-lin	+	+	−	+	+	V
Growth in 6.5% NaCl	+	−	−	− *	−	−

+ = usually positive
− = usually negative
V = variable reactions
* some strains positive
** Serotype *b* strains (*S. rattus*) positive

structure of *S. sanguis*, although attempts have been made to define specific antigens. Some strains react with Lancefield Group H antiserum, but this reaction is known to vary according to the commercial source of the antiserum used in the test. Typical isolates from human dental plaque are distinguished on mitis-salivarius agar incubated aerobically as small (0.5- to 0.9-mm diameter), sometimes mucoid, colonies that deform the surrounding agar and have such a firm consistency and attachment to the medium that they are difficult to remove with a wire loop. Similar hard, "rubbery" and adherent colonies of *S. sanguis* are observed on other sucrose-containing solid media. On blood agar, colonies are usually α-hemolytic, but occasional β-hemolytic strains are also found.

There is considerable controversy over the nomenclature and classification of streptococci variously described as *Streptococcus mitis, S. sanguis* type II and *Streptococcus mitior*. In the United States, the first two of these names are generally preferred, the species being separated on the basis of a single sugar fermentation reaction (raffinose). British workers tend to group these variants together and refer to them both as *S. mitior*. At present, the term *S. mitior* is officially recognized in the *Approved List of Bacterial Names* (Skerman et al., 1980). It would appear that *S. mitis* (and/or *S. mitior*) consists of a rather heterogeneous collection of strains which are generally arginine and aesculin negative, produce hydrogen peroxide and may or may not produce extracellular glucans from sucrose. Such strains usually lack rhamnose in their cell walls. The glucan positive strains give rise to hard, adherent colonies on sucrose agar, similar to those of *S. sanguis*. Whatever the correct name should be, strains resembling *S. mitis* are found in relatively high numbers on the tongue and cheek, in plaque and in saliva, with somewhat lower levels in the gingival crevice. Like *S. sanguis*, this species is also recovered quite commonly from blood cultures of patients with infective endocarditis.

Streptococcus salivarius averages about half the viable count of facultative streptococci from saliva or tongue scrapings, yet this organism usually numbers less than 1% of the viable count in plaque and gingival sulcus material. The major distinguishing feature of this species is the production of extracellular levan (a fructose polymer) from sucrose. This property leads to the development of large, often mucoid, colonies on mitis-salivarius agar and other sucrose-containing media. Some strains of *S. salivarius* react with Lancefield group K antisera. Other characteristic properties are given in table 15/5.

The strains described as *Streptococcus milleri* were originally isolated from dental infections and are commonly present in dental plaque. This organism is not listed as such in the eighth edition of *Bergey's Manual* nor in the *Approved List of Bacterial Names*, although the name is quite widely used in practice for strains with the properties listed in table 15/5. This species is probably synonymous with strains described as *Streptococcus anginosus, Streptococcus intermedius, Streptococcus constellatus* and *Streptococcus MG*. In one study, *S. milleri* was present in highest numbers in the gingival crevice (as a percentage of total streptococci), second highest in plaque, and less than 1% from tongue, cheeks, and saliva. In addition to being isolated from dental abscesses, *S. milleri* has been implicated, with increasing frequency, as a significant agent in infections at other sites in the body, including liver and brain abscesses. This species has also been shown recently to be cariogenic in gnotobiotic rats.

Streptococcus mutans was originally described in 1924 by Clarke, who isolated the organism from carious teeth. Although this species was not mentioned in the eighth edition of *Bergey's Manual* (published in 1974), it is now generally recognized as a distinct entity and has been included in the *Approved List of Bacterial Names* (1980). In fact, streptococci grouped together as *S. mutans* are genetically heterogeneous and may be subdivided into several types on the basis of DNA base composition and antigenic structure. It has been suggested that the various subgroups within *S. mutans* actually represent different taxa and separate species names have been proposed (table 15/6). Although these organisms share a number of common characteristics, some, but not all, of these subgroups can be differentiated by simple biochemical and physiological tests. For example, strains of the apparently rare *Streptococcus rattus* (*S. mutans* serotype *b*) hydrolyse arginine, unlike other organisms in the "*S. mutans* group."

In cultures on mitis-salivarius agar, typical *S. mutans* strains can readily be differentiated by

Table 15/6
Sub-divisions of *Streptococcus mutans*[a]

Serotype	Biotype	Proposed Species name	Animal Source
c, e, f	I	*S. mutans*	Humans
b	II	*S. rattus*	Rats
a	III	*S. cricetus*	Hamsters, humans
d, g	IV	*S. sobrinus*	Humans
c		*S. ferus*	Wild rats
e	V	(*S. mutans*)	Humans
h	VI	(*S. mutans*)	Monkeys

[a] Data from: Bratthall (1970), Perch et al. (1974), Shklair and Keene (1974) Coykendall (1977), Beighton et al. (1981) and Hamada and Slade (1980).

their high convex to pulvinate, light blue colonies, 0.5 to 1 mm in diameter, which are opaque and have an appearance reminiscent of frosted glass. Smooth and mucoid colonial variants of *S. mutans* have also been described. On other sucrose-containing selective media, fragile, rough, crumbly colonies are often observed. As a concomitant of extracellular glucan synthesis from sucrose, a watery exudate may collect on top of these colonies, often abundant enough to run off and form a puddle beside the colony. Polysaccharide production can also be detected in sucrose broth by addition of one volume of ethanol which yields an insoluble precipitate. Some of the properties which distinguish *S. mutans* from other oral streptococci are shown in table 15/5. Fermentation of mannitol and sorbitol are often used in identification schemes, but it should be remembered that *S. faecalis* and other Lancefield Group D streptococci (including *S. bovis*) frequently give positive reactions in either or both of these tests.

In dental plaque, *S. mutans* may number only a few percent of the total colony count on mitis-salivarius medium particularly in subjects with a relatively low sucrose intake. In the presence of high levels of dietary sucrose, the proportion of *S. mutans* can rise to 50% or more of the streptococcal count. The proportions of *S. mutans* in human plaque have been reported to correlate with caries activity and the organism may be isolated from carious lesions. The oral streptococci differ in their ability to elicit caries in experimental animals. Although most species have the potential to produce caries in pits and fissures of teeth, *S. mutans* strains have been shown consistently to induce severe to moderate caries activity if implanted in a suitable animal system. The cariogenic potential of this organism is associated with its ability to attach to and accumulate on the tooth surfaces, forming large plaque deposits. The synthesis of high molecular weight glucans from sucrose, which contribute towards the plaque matrix, is thought to aid the adherence and retention of *S. mutans* to the tooth surface. Mutant strains which have lost the ability to synthesize extracellular glucans have been shown to be less cariogenic in animals than the glucan-positive parent strains from which they were derived.

Not all strains of streptococci isolated from the mouth are easy to identify by existing criteria, and it is likely that some additional species will be described in the future. Strains which give test reactions intermediate between those of *S. sanguis* and *S. mitior* are sometimes found, and there are some isolates which appear to resemble "atypical" *S. mutans.* Such difficulties can only be resolved by further detailed taxonomic studies into the characteristics of these and other "problem strains."

Anaerobic Cocci

Obligately anaerobic gram positive cocci of the genus *Peptostreptococcus* (family Peptococcaceae) have been estimated to average from 4 to 13% of the viable count in different sites in the oral cavity. There is considerable confusion surrounding the classification of this apparently heterogeneous genus. Several species previously regarded as peptostreptococci have subsequently been found to be facultatively anaerobic or carbon dioxide dependent and have been transferred to other genera and species, while others are only poorly characterized and described. Five named species were included in the eighth edition of *Bergey's Manual* and four of these (*Peptostreptococcus anaerobius, Peptostreptococcus micros, Peptostreptococcus parvulus* and *Peptostreptococcus productus*) appear in the *Approved List of Bacterial Names*. Examples of these, including *P. anaerobius* and *P. micros*, have been reported from infected root canals and dental abscesses. One useful method for differentiating obligately anaerobic cocci from facultative cocci is to demonstrate their sensitivity to the antibiotic metronidazole, using a simple disc-sensitivity test. Streptococci are invariably resistant to this agent.

Peptostreptococci are spherical to ovoid, 0.7 to 1.0 μm in diameter, and may occur in pairs or short or long chains. They are nonmotile, do not form spores, and are rarely hemolytic. The organisms are anaerobic, require complex media, and have pH and temperature optima of 7.0 to 7.5 and 35 to 37 C, respectively. They are generally quite sensitive to penicillins.

In addition to peptostreptococci, isolates belonging to the genus *Peptococcus* have also been reported from the oral cavity. In view of the confusion surrounding the taxonomy of these two genera, and the lack of information about their role in oral ecology and disease, there is clearly a need for more detailed studies on anaerobic cocci from the mouth.

Staphylococci and Micrococci

Nearly every mouth harbors facultative, catalase positive, gram positive cocci that ferment glucose and nitrate, and are accordingly identified as staphylococci or micrococci. Available data indicate that they average about 2% of the viable count from the gingival sulcus and up to 6.5% from the dorsum of the tongue. Staphylococci are not common in dental plaque and, when found, usually only comprise a small proportion of the viable count. Such isolates, when found, are usually coagulase-negative.

The tongue appears to provide the main ecological niche for one oral organism, *Micrococcus mucilagenosus* (formerly called *Staphylococcus salivarius*). This large coccus produces considerable amounts of an extracellular polysaccharide slime.

A number of reports agree that staphylococci range from 0 to around 50,000 per ml of saliva, with a mean of 5000. About half of subjects examined using single salivary samples yield some *Staphylococcus aureus*. If swabbings of nose, throat and mouth were cultured simultaneously, the total *S. aureus* carrier rate increased to about 80%. Although the number of salivary carriers equaled the number of nasal carriers, the anterior nares were judged to harbor much larger quantities of *S. aureus*. Exchange of *S. aureus* between dentists and patients does not seem to be a special public health problem. In 19 trials, transfer of *S. aureus* from a carrier dentist to a noncarrier patient could not be demonstrated during oral prophylaxis lasting half an hour. Likewise, the carrier rate of *S. aureus* by dental students did not increase during the clinical years of training.

GRAM NEGATIVE COCCI
Veillonellae

Gram negative, obligately anaerobic cocci of the genus *Veillonella* are among the most numerous oral bacteria. These organisms comprise between 5 and 10% of the cultivable flora of saliva and on tongue surfaces; estimates for their proportion in dental plaque vary from 0.1 to 28%, these differences possibly reflecting variations in sampling and laboratory methods. Two species are generally recognized, *Veillonella parvula* and *Veillonella alcalescens*, although as discussed below, new proposals have recently been made concerning the taxonomy of this genus.

Veillonellae are nonmotile, nonsporulating cocci averaging 0.3 to 0.5 μm in diameter. In culture they occur as spherical masses of diplococci, or as short chains. Growth is good from 30 to 37 C at pH 6.5 to 8.0; cells do not survive at 60 C for 30 minutes. Veillonellae cannot ferment carbohydrates because they lack glucokinase and fructokinase, but evidently they have the other enzymes of a glycolytic system. Accordingly, they require for growth certain intermediate metabolites such as lactate, pyruvate, malate, fumarate, or oxalacetate. Carbon dioxide is indispensable for growth. Lactate is utilized with production of propionate, acetate, carbon dioxide, and hydrogen. Hydrogen sulfide is produced if the medium is supplemented with such substrates as cystine, glutathione, or thiosulfate. Gelatin is not liquefied.

The veillonellae are parasitic in the mouth and in the respiratory and intestinal tracts of humans and various animals. Serological tests have established seven groups, divisible into two species. *V. parvula*, the type species, comprises serogroups II, V, and VI, the latter being exclusively of human origin. *V. alcalescens* comprises serogroups I, III, IV, and VII, the latter two being primarily of human origin. The veillonellae contain serologically specific lipopolysaccharide endotoxins which induce pyrogenicity and the Shwartzman reaction in rabbits.

Recent taxonomic studies, using the technique of DNA-DNA homology in addition to other criteria, indicate that *V. alcalescens* and *V. parvula* are probably identical and should be combined under the latter name which has priority. Other species which have been redefined as a result of these investigations are *Veillonella dispar*, *Veillonella atypica*, *Veillonella rodentium*, *Veillonella rattii*, *Veillonella criceti* and *Veillonella carviae*. Several of these have only been isolated from animals (guinea pigs, rats, rabbits and hamsters), but *V. parvula*, *V. dispar* and *V. atypica* have all been recovered from human sources.

Neisseriae

Microorganisms designated as *Neisseria* have been found at several sites in the oral cavity, including the lips, tongue, cheek, plaque and saliva. However, the mean proportions reported have generally been less than 1 to 2% of the cultivable flora, and the organisms do not appear to have any particular affinity for specific surfaces or sites within the mouth. As with many other groups of oral bacteria, the taxonomy of the genus *Neisseria* is far from being fully understood. Two species were previously considered to be the predominant ones in the oral cavity, *Neisseria sicca* and *Neisseria catarrhalis*. The latter has more recently been transferred to the genus *Branhamella* and is now designated *Branhamella catarrhalis*, since it has been shown on the basis of biochemical, physiological and genetic data to differ significantly from members of the genus *Neisseria*. The two genera may be distinguished by demonstrating the presence or absence of the enzyme glucose-6-phosphate dehydrogenase (absent in *B. catarrhalis*). Although oral *Neisseria* strains may be divided into broad groups according to their ability to produce polysaccharide and to ferment carbohydrates, it is not possible to assign unknown isolates to named species with any confidence at present.

GRAM POSITIVE ROD-SHAPED BACTERIA

Large numbers of gram positive rod-shaped or filamentous bacteria are found in the oral cavity, particularly in supragingival plaque. These include aerobic, facultative and obligately anaerobic species.

Lactobacilli

Lactobacilli are a characteristic group of oral bacteria, although numerically a minor fraction. Their numbers vary according to circumstances to be discussed later in relation to dental caries, but it is probable that some are present in all human oral cavities soon after birth, although probably not in significant proportions. The salivary *Lactobacillus* count in adults ranges from nearly 0 to about 100,000 per ml or more, with a mean of about 70,000 per ml, which is only a small fraction of a percent of the mean total viable count. Lactobacilli are widely distributed, also being found in the intestinal tracts of both infants and adults, and in the vagina after puberty; in addition they are found in milk and milk products (including pasteurized milk), compressed yeast, sour beer, soil, manure, feces of invertebrates, fishes, mammals, sewage, and many fermenting plant and animal products.

Lactobacilli are gram positive, nonmotile except for rare strains, nonsporing, sometimes pleomorphic rods which divide in one plane only without branching. They tend to become gram negative in older cultures. A few species produce orange, rust, or brick-red pigment. In general they have very complex nutritional requirements for carbohydrates, fatty acids, inorganic ions, vitamins, nucleic acid precursors, peptides, and amino acids; in fact, many species are so specific in their amino acid requirements that they can be used for amino acid determination. Most oral lactobacilli grow best in or require a reducing medium containing a surface tension-reducing agent, adequately supplied with carbohydrate, and at a wide temperature range (15 to 45 C). They are aciduric with an optimal pH of usually 5.5 to 5.8. Isolation and enumeration of oral lactobacilli are greatly facilitated by selective agar media, which suppress the growth of practically all other oral microorganisms, owing to a high content of acetate and other salts, a surface tension depressant, and an acid pH (5.4), while providing adequate nourishment for lactobacilli. Most lactobacilli are not proteolytic. Carbohydrate fermentation by lactobacilli is variable with the species, although they are generally quite active. Differences in the action of oral lactobacilli on glucose divide them into homofermentative species which produce principally lactic acid (above 65%) and heterofermentative species which produce less lactic acid (less than 65%) and a considerable number of other end products (principally acetic acid and ethanol) including gas (usually carbon dioxide).

The eighth edition of *Bergey's Manual* recognizes 27 homofermentative and heterofermentative species, grouped principally on the basis of optimum temperature and metabolic patterns such as type of lactic acid produced and differential fermentation of sugars (table 15/7). Previous classifications have been quite different from the present one. Indeed, almost from the time that lactobacilli were first found in the oral cavity until relatively recently, there has been a tendency to assign all oral lactobacilli to the species *Lactobacillus acid-*ophilus* usually without supporting data. This is a most inaccurate practice, although it must be admitted that differentiation is often difficult. Although it is unusual for lactobacilli to be pathogenic, many attempts have been made to establish lactobacilli as *the* causative agent of dental caries. It does seem that a fair correlation has been established between the state of caries activity and the numbers of salivary lactobacilli, but these bacteria are only one of the microbial factors involved in the disease.

PLEOMORPHIC GRAM POSITIVE RODS AND FILAMENTS

The oral cavity supports the growth of large numbers of a surprisingly wide variety of gram positive rods. Many of these are pleomorphic, assuming a range of microscopic forms from coccobacillary to filamentous. Some of these rods are club shaped and many show evidence of branching. Because of the morphological appearance of such organisms, they have often been grouped together for descriptive purposes and referred to simply as "diphtheroids" or "coryneforms." This broad morphological group of bacteria includes both facultative and anaerobic representatives. Facultative diphtheroids have been estimated to comprise 13% of the viable count from the dorsum of the tongue, 15% in the gingival sulcus, and 24% in plaque; obligately anaerobic strains were found to average, respectively, 8, 20 and 18%.

Identification of this group of oral bacteria to the generic and species level can be difficult on occasions, but their classification has been greatly facilitated in recent years by the application of chemotaxonomic techniques. Most of the strains initially isolated as diphtheroids appear not to be true *Corynebacterium* species; many turn out to be *Actinomyces*, including the catalase positive species *Actinomyces viscosus* which may account for many of the unidentified strains reported in earlier studies. Other genera which are found are *Arachnia*, *Propionibacterium*, *Bifidobacterium*, *Eubacterium*, *Rothia* and *Bacterionema*. Some of the distinguishing features of the various genera of pleomorphic gram positive rods are summarized in table 15/8.

Spore-forming genera, such as *Clostridium* and *Bacillus*, do not seem to be part of the normal oral flora according to most investigators. However, there have been a few published reports of the isolation of such organisms from particular population groups.

Actinomyces

Filamentous forms are seen in oral smears, especially those from the gingival crevice and the dental plaque, in numbers far in excess of the

Table 15/7
Some characteristics used to classify oral lactobacilli

Lactobacillus species	Optimum temperature	Guanine and Cytosine content of DNA	Type of lactic acid	Fermentation				
		(moles %)		Lactose	Sucrose	Raffinose	Arabinose	Maltose
Homofermentative:								
L. acidophilus	35–38	36.7	DL	+	+	Some strains +	–	+
L. salivarius	35–40	34.7	Mainly L (+)	+	+	+	–	+
L. casei		46.4	Mainly L (+)	Some subspecies +	Some strains +	–	–	Some strains +
L. plantarum	30–35	45	DL	+	+	+	Some strains +	+
Heterofermentative:								
L. fermentum	41–42	53.4	DL	+	+	+	Some strains +	+
L. cellobiosus	30–35	53.1	DL		+	+	+	+
L. brevis	30	42.7–46.4	DL	Weak	Some strains +	Weak	+	+
L. buchneri	30	44.8	DL	Weak	Some strains +	Weak	+	+

Table 15/8
Some distinguishing chemical characteristics of oral pleomorphic gram positive rods[a]

Genus	Cell Wall Components						Mycolic Acid	Acid End Products from Glucose						DNA %GC
	Dibasic amino acids				Sugars									
	ORN	LYS	DL-DAP	LL-DAP	GAL	ARAB		A	P	B	C	L	S	
Actinomyces	+	+	–	–	V	–	–	+	–	–	–	+	+	60–63
Arachnia	–	–	V	V	+	–	–	+	+	–	–	–	±	63–65
Propionibacterium	–	–	–	+	+	–	–	+	+	–	–	–	–	57–60
Bifidobacterium	+	+	–	–	+	–	–	+	–	+	–	+	–	57–64
Eubacterium	–	–	+	–	V	–	NA	+	–	+	V	V	V	NA
Rothia	+	+	–	–	+	–	–	+	–	–	–	+	±	65–69
Bacterionema	–	–	+	–	+	+	+	+	+	–	–	±	–	55–57
Corynebacterium	–	–	+	–	+	+	+	+	+	–	–	±	–	57–60

[a] Data from Bowden and Hardie (1978).

ORN = ornithine
LYS = lysine
DAP = diaminopimelic acid
GAL = galactose
ARAB = arabinose

A = acetic
P = propionic
B = butyric
C = caproic
L = lactic
S = succinic

+ = usually positive
– = usually negative
V = variable results reported
NA = data not available

number of colonies of filamentous microorganisms obtainable by any known cultural methods. Branched, filamentous *Actinomyces* strains are regular inhabitants of the oral cavity—in fact, they have not been found in nature apart from a parasitic habitat—but ordinarily they are not present in large numbers. They are facultative anaerobes, although most are preferentially anaerobic. The first *Actinomyces* species from a normal human mouth was isolated by Bergey in 1907. Since then investigators have isolated oral strains apparently identical with the pathogenic strains causing clinical actinomycosis such as *Actinomyces israelii*. Most of the isolates from normal individuals, however, were studied insufficiently to identify them or differentiate them from those isolated from frank disease. More recently, some success has been achieved in the delineation of the oral strains of *Actinomyces*. Filamentous oral organisms have been isolated which differed sufficiently from those causing frank disease to be designated as *Actinomyces naeslundii*. The species designation *Actinomyces odontolyticus* has been given to filamentous, aerobic or facultatively anaerobic organisms isolated from human dentinal caries. Pathogenic species, *A. israelii* and *Actinomyces bovis*, will be discussed in Chapter 32. Therefore, this section will concentrate more on *Actinomyces naeslundii*, *Actinomyces odontolyticus*, and *Actinomyces viscosus*.

A. naeslundii (fig. 15/5) produces microcolonies which have a dense mass of diphtheroid cells and tangled filaments at their centers surrounded by a periphery of radiating, curved, and branched filaments. In liquid media, growth usually appears as a floculent mass toward the top with some soft granules below. Although *A. naeslundii* is a facultative anaerobe, most strains will grow in air on solid media. The optimum temperature is 35 to 37 C. The normal habitat is the oral cavity, including tonsillar crypts and dental calculus. Although human infections with this organism have been reported, its role is unproved, but seems to be minor. Mice have been infected experimentally and periodontal destruction has been produced in rats.

Colonies of *A. odontolyticus* on blood agar may produce an area of greening around the colonies, resembling α-hemolytic streptococci. Some strains of *A. odontolyticus* may grow aerobically on blood agar. Colonies characteristically have a reddish brown center. Growth in liquid media is usually turbid and even, but sometimes may be flocculent. The normal habitat of this organism is the oral cavity of man; it may be isolated from deep dentinal caries.

A. viscosus has been isolated from the oral cavity of hamsters, rats, and man. In liquid media, growth of this organism occurs with a viscosus (although strain-variable) sediment. This produces a muci-

nous "string" when the media are swirled. *A. viscosus* is a facultative anaerobe which grows better with CO_2. The organism produces periodontal disease with subgingival plaque in hamsters, and iso-

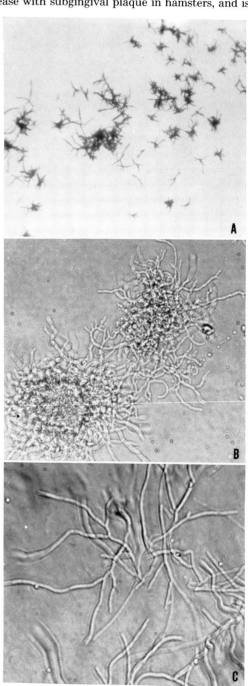

Figure 15/5. (*A*) Gram stain of *Actinomyces naeslundii* grown in thioglycolate medium. (*B*) Microcolony of *Actinomyces naeslundii* on 24-hour anaerobic brain-heart infusion agar culture. (*C*) Microcolony of *Actinomyces israelii* on 48-hour anaerobic brain-heart infusion agar culture. (Reproduced with permission from A. Howell, Jr., W. C. Murphy, E. Paul, and R. M. Stephan. 1959 Oral Strains of Actinomyces. Journal of Bacteriology, **78,** 82.)

lates from these animals will induce the disease in other hamsters. Strains of *A. viscosus* have been isolated in human dental calculus and root surface caries. Human and rodent strains of *A. viscosus* are serologically distinct.

Recent taxonomic studies have shown that human *A. naeslundii* and *A. viscosus* strains are very similar to one another biochemically, the most obvious distinguishing feature being the positive catalase reaction given by the latter named species. It has been argued that these species should be combined, since they differ less than the animal and human isolates of *A. viscosus* or even the different serotypes of *A. israelii*.

Two species of *Actinomyces* have been isolated from frank human and bovine infections. The organism from human infections, commonly termed *A. israelii*, produces sparse or no growth aerobically. The source of infection generally is endogenous, as the normal habitat of the organism is the oral cavity of man, including the tonsillar crypts and dental calculus.

The actinomycete usually isolated from bovine infections, *Actinomyces bovis*, causes actinomycosis in cattle. Similar infections have been described in other animals, but in the latter cases the species involved were inadequately described.

Rothiae

The genus *Rothia* is currently listed as a member of the family Actinomycetaceae. The organisms have a branching, filamentous morphology but may appear in culture as coccoid, diphtheroid, or bacillary forms, or a mixture of these. Largely because of these morphological features, Rothiae were at one time considered to belong to *Nocardia*, but they are now recognized as a clearly distinct genus. *Rothia* is aerobic, although some strains may grow under anaerobic conditions. CO_2 is not stimulatory. Characteristic, usually white or cream pigmented colonies are produced which often give a raised, rough appearance and may grow to several millimeters in diameter on aerobic blood agar plates.

At present only one species is recognized, *Rothia dentocariosa*. However, several biotypes and serotypes have been described and it is likely that one or more new species designations will be proposed. Rothiae are commonly isolated from the normal human mouth, particularly from saliva, dental plaque and calculus, and they have also been found in animals. No natural infections have been reported in man or animals but abscess formation has been demonstrated experimentally in mice.

Bacterionemae

The genus *Bacterionema* was proposed to separate these branching filamentous organisms from the different *Leptotrichia*. There is a single species within the genus, *Bacterionema matruchotii*, which appears to be biochemically and serologically homogeneous. It is a gram positive, nonacid-fast, nonmotile, usually facultative organism (some anaerobic strains have been described) with a characteristic cellular morphology. The cells are pleomorphic filaments 1 to 2 μm wide by 20 to 200 μm long, typically attached to a rectangular rod-shaped body 1.5 to 2.5 μm wide by 3 to 10 μm long. This combination of rod and filament gives rise to the so-called, "whip handle" cells. Filamentous and rod forms also occur singly in microscopic preparations, and branching may be observed. *B. matruchotii* ferments carbohydrates to yield acid (predominantly acetic and propionic, with smaller amounts of lactic acid) and some CO_2. Their optimal pH range is 6.5 to 7.5 and optimal temperature is 37 C.

Bacterionema has been shown to be distinct from *Actinomyces*, *Nocardia* and *Rothia*. Recent chemotaxonomic data, including cell-wall composition, DNA-base ratios and the presence of low molecular weight mycolic acid, indicate that *B. matruchotii* is closely related to *Corynebacterium* and should be reclassified with that genus.

Injection of live organisms into mice produces nodules or abscesses. Similar lesions are produced following intraperitoneal or intravenous inoculation. *B. matruchotii* is found in the oral cavity of man and other primates, particularly in dental plaque and calculus.

Corynebacteria

True animal corynebacteria have a typical cell wall composition, containing DL-DAP, galactose, and arabinose, possess a low molecular weight mycolic acid, and have a GC ratio of 55 to 60%. With the exception of *B. matruchotii*, which may be a true *Corynebacterium*, presence of corynebacteria in the mouth is uncertain. It is likely that many of the organisms described in the earlier literature as "diphtheroids" were not true corynebacteria, but a few isolates reported in more recent studies do appear to fit the description. It is clear that further research is required to clarify the uncertainty which exists in this area.

Propionibacteria

This genus includes many of the organisms which were previously described as "anaerobic coryneforms." They are anaerobic, gram positive rods which produce a major peak of propionic acid when grown in glucose broth, and are catalase positive. Although primarily inhabitants of the skin, propionibacteria have been isolated from the mouth by a number of different workers and can, therefore, be regarded as part of the regular oral flora. Strains identified as *Propionibacterium acnes* have been isolated from dental plaque, carious dentin and necrotic pulps and have also been detected microscopically in oral samples by immunofluorescence.

Arachniae

The organisms now designated *Archnia propionica* are anaerobic gram positive, pleomorphic bacteria which can resemble *Actinomyces israelii* both in colonial and microscopic appearance. They are catalase negative. This species was originally isolated from a case of lachrymal canaliculitis and has also been found in patients presenting with actinomycosis-like symptoms. Chemotaxonomic data indicate that this genus is distinct from *Actinomyces*, and also from *Propionibacterium* which it superficially resembles by virtue of producing propionic acid from glucose. Differences between strains of *Arachnia* indicate that there may be more than the one named species currently accepted. *Arachnia* has been isolated from dental plaque, carious dentin and necrotic pulps, but the organism does not appear to be a numerically dominant member of the oral flora in most situations.

Bifidobacteria

These pleomorphic anaerobic gram positive rods typically have bifid ends and have been classified at various times either with the Actinomycetaceae or the Lactobacillaceae. The characteristic ratio of fermentation products of the genus is three parts acetic to two parts lactic acid. Isolation of bifidobacteria from the mouth has been reported by several authors, the species found being *Bifidobacterium eriksonii* and *Bifidobacterium dentium*. Strains have been recovered from dental plaque and carious dentin, but their numbers appear to be relatively low.

Eubacteria

Anaerobic, nonspore-forming, pleomorphic, gram positive, rod-shaped or filamentous bacteria which cannot be allocated to any of the foregoing named genera may be classified in the genus *Eubacterium*. This is one of the least well explored areas of bacterial taxonomy at present, and further studies are required before the situation can be clarified. Of the 29 species names listed in the *Approved List of Bacterial Names*, *Eubacterium saburreum* and *Eubacterium alactolyticum* are the two most certainly associated with the oral cavity, although other species are almost certainly present. *E. saburreum* is commonly isolated from dental plaque where it contributes to the mass of filamentous organisms present in mature supragingival deposits. Eubacteria have also been reported from calculus, carious dentin and necrotic pulps.

A recent report from the Virginia Polytechnic Institute (VPI) Anaerobe Laboratory describes three new species of *Eubacterium* isolated from patients with periodontitis. The names *Eubacterium timidum*, *Eubacterium brachy* and *Eubacterium nodatum* have been proposed for these oral isolates. *E. timidum* cells are described as "small diphtheroids" which may produce trace amounts of acetate, formate, succinate or lactate when grown in peptone-yeast extract broth. Unlike *Actinomyces* species, they do not ferment sugars. The cells of *E. brachy* are very short gram positive rods arranged in chains and those of *E. nodatum* are said to resemble *Actinomyces* morphologically. *E. nodatum* can be distinguished from *Actinomyces* species by its inability to ferment sugars and by the detection of butyric acid as a metabolic end product.

GRAM NEGATIVE ANAEROBIC BACTERIA

Our knowledge of this important group of organisms has increased considerably in recent years, largely as a result of the application of more sophisticated anaerobic isolation techniques to studies on the oral flora. In particular, several groups of investigators have been using anaerobic roll tube and anaerobic chamber methods for the microbiological examination of material from periodontal pockets. As a consequence of such improved isolation methods, many organisms have been found which cannot readily be identified by existing criteria and which may represent new taxa. Isolation of such previously undescribed organisms has stimulated a considerable amount of basic taxonomic work as research investigators attempt to characterize and classify the new isolates.

Anaerobic gram negative rods generally belong to the family Bacteroidaceae which at present consists of three genera, *Bacteroides*, *Fusobacterium* and *Leptotrichia*. Most of the recent changes and additions to the taxonomy of this family have been related to the genus *Bacteroides*.

Bacteroides

This genus comprises obligately anaerobic, gram negative, sometimes pleomorphic rods with rounded ends and diameters greater than 0.3 μm. Most species produce acetic and succinic acid as end products of glucose metabolism, together with varying amounts of other acids. The eighth edition of *Bergey's Manual* recognized 22 species, which are primarily inhabitants of the intestinal tracts and mucous membranes of warm-blooded animals. This number was increased to 29 species, two of which were subdivided into several named subspecies by 1980 when the *Approved List of Bacterial Names* was published. Since then descriptions of several additional species of *Bacteroides* have been published, including some from the oral cavity. To add to the confusion which surrounds this rapidly changing area of bacterial taxonomy, it seems, in some cases, as if different authors have given different names to the same "new species."

The *Bacteroides* species currently considered to comprise part of the oral microflora are listed in table 15/9. These can be broadly divided into black (or brown)—pigmented and nonpigmented varieties. Members of the important group of *Bacteroides* associated with the intestinal tract, the "*B. fragilis* group," which are frequently implicated in anaerobic infections, do not seem to be found as regular inhabitants of the oral cavity.

Pigmented *Bacteroides* species. At one time, not very long ago, all gram negative anaerobic rods which yielded black or brown colonies on blood agar were referred to simply as *Bacteroides melaninogenicus*. Such strains were generally found to require hemin and menadione for growth; pigmentation varied both in shade and speed of development. There was considerable interest in the potential pathogenic role of this "species" since it was often isolated from human infections and played an indispensable role in experimental mixed anaerobic infections in guinea pigs. Pigmented *Bacteroides* are frequently isolated from the mouth, particularly from the region of the gingival sulcus or periodontal pocket. In the early studies many strains were found to produce collagenase and it was suggested that this enzyme might contribute significantly to the destruction of collagen in the periodontal tissues.

A few years ago it became clear that there were important biochemical differences between strains which produced black colonies. Consequently, it was proposed that the species *B. melaninogenicus* be subdivided into several subspecies, namely *B. melaninogenicus* ss. *intermedius*, *B. melaninogenicus* ss. *asaccharolyticus*, *B. melaninogenicus* ss. *melaninogenicus* and *B. melaninogenicus* ss. *levii*. The asaccharolyticus subspecies was subsequently found to be heterogeneous and has now been further split into two entities which have each been

elevated to separate species status, namely *Bacteroides gingivalis* and *Bacteroides asaccharolyticus*. These differ from one another in the electrophoretic mobility of their malate dehydrogenase (MDH) enzymes, lipid composition, and DNA base ratio (46.5 to 48.5% G + C and 51 to 52% G + C, respectively). *B. gingivalis* appears to be the more common of the two in the mouth and may be an important pathogen in human periodontal disease. Another variety of black-pigmented, asaccharolytic *Bacteroides* has also been isolated from the mouths of monkeys and named *Bacteroides macacae*.

Very recently, further proposals have been made concerning the reclassification of *B. melaninogenicus* ss. *intermedius* and ss. *melaninogenicus*. It is likely that the subspecies designations will be replaced by the species names *Bacteroides intermedius*, *Bacteroides melaninogenicus*, together with the new epithets *Bacteroides corporis*, *Bacteriodes socranskii* and *Bacteroides loescheii*.

Nonpigmented *Bacteriodes* species. The taxonomic status of oral nonpigmented gram negative rods is no less confusing and changeable than that of the pigmented species. *Bacteroides oralis* was described several years ago but there has been some difficulty over recent years in deciding upon internationally-agreed type and reference strains. However, the species is recognized and included in the *Approved List of Bacterial Names*. Several new species have been described by different authors since 1980, including *Bacteroides oris*, *Bacteriodes buccae*, *Bacteroides pentosaceus*, *Bacteroides denticola*, *Bacteriodes buccalis*, *Bacteroides capillus* and *Bacteroides gracilis*. The last mentioned in this list is one of several oral organisms which cause pitting or corrosion of the agar surface. Another corroding anaerobe is now called *Bacteroides ureolyticus*; this species was formerly designated *Bacteroides corrodens* and is quite distinct from the facultative anaerobic gram negative rod, *Eikenella corrodens*.

Unfortunately, the taxonomic situation has not been helped by independent authors proposing different names for what are, apparently, the same organisms. Thus, *B. oris*, *B. buccae*, *B. pentosaceus* and *B. capillus* are all new species names for bacteria previously referred to as *B. ruminicola* ss. *brevis*.

In view of the rapidly changing classification and nomenclature of the oral *Bacteroides* species, it is not possible at the moment to make much useful comment about their distribution in the mouth or their role in dental disease. Clearly the earlier view that only two or three species of *Bacteroides* were present was a gross over-simplification and new studies are required on the ecology and pathogenicity of the recently described taxa, using up-to-date criteria for identifying the organisms isolated.

Table 15/9

List of proposed names of *Bacteroides* species in the mouth

Nonpigmented Species	Pigmented Species
B. oris[a]	B. gingivalis
B. buccae[a]	B. asaccharolyticus
B. pentosaceus[a]	B. levii
B. denticola	B. intermedius
B. buccalis	B. corporis
B. capillus[a]	B. melaninogenicus
B. gracilis	B. socranskii
B. zoogleoformans	B. loescheii
B. ureolyticus	B. macacae
B. oralis	

[a] *B. oris*, *B. buccae*, *B. pentosaceus* and *B. capillus* may represent different names for the same species.

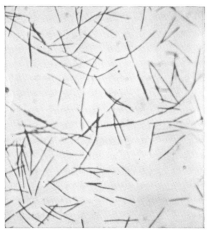

Figure 15/6. Oral fusiform organisms from the gingiva ✕ 900 (from Stig Schultz-Haudt).

Fusobacteria

Members of the genus *Fusobacterium* are obligately anaerobic, gram negative, nonspore-forming rods (fig. 15/6).

The classification and nomenclature of the fusiform bacteria have changed considerably in recent years, and various species have had a variety of names and designations at various times. Therefore, those bearing a particular name may not be the same organism as originally described and given that designation. The eighth edition of *Bergey's Manual* recognized 16 species, with *Fusobacterium nucleatum* designated as the type species. Of these, 11 named species are retained in the *Approved List of Bacterial Names*. *F. nucleatum* and *Fusobacterium plauti* are the recognized species isolated from the oral cavity. *F. nucleatum* produces small translucent colonies on horse blood agar. They are usually nonhemolytic and nonmotile. *F. plauti* is a motile organism which produces 0.5-mm colonies which are gray-white and smooth. It also is nonhemolytic. In the laboratory, fusobacteria are distinguished from other morphologically similar organisms by the production of major amounts of butyric acid from glucose. *F. nucleatum* has been isolated from infections of the upper respiratory tract and pleural cavity, as well as the oral cavity.

Fusobacteria were first observed in ulcerative gingivitis in the 1880s and later they were associated with spirochetes in angina. Considerable impetus was given to the role of fusiform bacteria in the etiology of oral gangrenous lesions when they were associated with spirochetes in 40 of 47 cases of hospital gangrene (commonly, Vincent's infection or angina or more properly, acute ulcerative gingivitis). Consequently, the fusobacteria have long been associated etiologically with fusospirochetal disease (acute necrotizing gingivitis) but within recent years their significance has been questioned, principally because of their inability to produce a serially transmissible infection when introduced concurrently with spirochetes into experimental animals, particularly guinea pigs. Nevertheless, the fusobacteria and spirochetes greatly increase in inflammatory periodontal disease and decrease with the abatement of the disease. Reports of the fusobacterial oral population have varied considerably, depending in part on the media used for cultivation. These figures range from 26,000 to 854,000 per ml of saliva; approximately 5% of salivary cultures were negative.

Leptotrichiae

The position of the genus *Leptotrichia* (a thin hair) has been ambiguous. Very early in the development of bacteriology, oral thread-like filamentous bacteria, differentiated almost entirely on the basis of their structure and oral habitat, were described by many and, after 1843, were generally classified in the genus *Leptothrix*, which originally referred to filamentous iron bacteria. In 1879, because of the obvious misnomer, Trevisan proposed the name *Leptotrichia buccalis* for these organisms and in following years the status of the species was further confused by investigators placing any unbranched filamentous organisms, even sporulating bacilli, in it. Subsequently, *L. buccalis* was confused with *Bacillus fusiformis*, a synonym of *Fusobacterium nucleatum*, and *Fusobacterium plauti-vincenti* and even *Bacterionema matruchotii*. Some authors have described *L. buccalis* as gram positive and related to the lactobacilli. However, early descriptions considered *Leptotrichia* to be gram negative and related to *Fusobacterium*. Also, the fine structure and lipopolysaccharides are characteristic of gram negative organisms. In the eighth edition of *Bergey's Manual*, *Leptotrichia* is recognized as a valid genus, with a single species, *Leptotrichia buccalis*, as the type species. This is retained in the *Approved List of Bacterial Names*.

L. buccalis (fig. 15/7) is an unbranching, nonmotile, nonsporulating straight or slightly curved rod with a tendency for one or both ends to point. In young cultures it grows into short chains but in older cultures filaments of considerable length can be seen twisting around each other. Although cells in cultures less than 6 hours old are gram positive, by 24 hours they are gram negative but contain gram positive granules. *L. buccalis* is anaerobic, but 5% carbon dioxide is essential for isolation and optimal growth. Carbohydrate fermentation follows a metabolic pattern similar to that of homofermentative lactobacilli.

FACULTATIVE GRAM NEGATIVE RODS

There are a number of facultatively anaerobic gram negative rods in the oral cavity; many of these are described as capnophilic because growth of colonies on solid media is enhanced by the addition

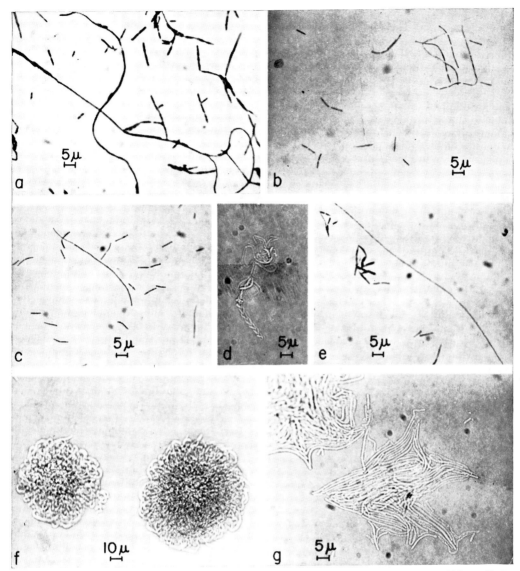

Figure 15/7. Cellular and colonial morphologies of *Leptotrichia buccalis*, originally described by Thiøtta, Hartmann, and Boe, 1939. (*A*) Gram stain of 12-hour thioglycolate broth culture with morphology ranging from short rods to long filaments, with branching evident. The cells are mostly gram positive but some are gram negative with gram positive granules. (*B*) Gram stain of 48-hour anaerobic brain-heart infusion agar culture, showing trichome formation and gram negative cells. (*C*) Gram stain of 20-hour anaerobic brain-heart infusion agar culture, showing gram positive rods and short filaments. (*D*) Unstained microcolony on 12-hour anaerobic brain-heart infusion agar culture showing a braided filament. (*E*) Gram stain of a 20-hour anaerobic brain-heart infusion broth culture showing short gram positive and gram negative rods and one-third of a filament. (*F*) Colony on a 48-hour, anaerobic brain-heart infusion agar culture. (*G*) Microcolony on a 16-hour anaerobic brain-heart infusion agar plate showing characteristic parallel arrangement of the cells. (Reproduced with permission from M. N. Gilmour, A. Howell, Jr., and B. G. Bibby. 1961 The Classification of Organisms Termed *Leptotrichia (Leptothrix) buccalis*. Bacteriological Review, **25**, 131.)

of 5 to 10% CO_2 to the atmosphere. This group of bacteria has tended to be overlooked by most oral microbiologists until a few years ago, but recent studies on oral ecology and the flora associated with various types of periodontal disease have drawn attention to their presence and potential pathogenicity. The organisms included in this category include members of the genera *Haemophilus, Eikenella, Actinobacillus* and *Capnocytophaga.*

Some of the distinguishing features of these bacteria are shown in Table 15/10.

Haemophili

Haemophili are regularly present in dental plaque, saliva and on soft tissue surfaces. The mean salivary level has been found to be of the order of 4×10 haemophili per ml. The majority of strains isolated from the mouth are V-factor (nicotinamide adenine dinucleotide, NAD)-dependent, but do not require X-factor (hemin). Good growth is usually obtained on heated-blood (chocolate) agar plates at 35 to 37 C, and most strains are enhanced by a moist atmosphere with the addition of 5 to 10% CO_2. The species most commonly isolated from the mouth are *Haemophilus parainfluenzae*, *Haemophilus paraphrophilus* and *Haemophilus segnis*. *Haemophilus aphrophilus* is also found occasionally in dental plaque. *Haemophilus segnis* is a recently described species from dental plaque. It forms smooth or granular, high convex, greyish-white colonies, up to 0.5 mm in diameter on chocolate agar and is nonhemolytic on blood-containing media. The cells are pleomorphic, nonmotile and noncapsulated, forming mainly irregular filaments with a few bacillary forms. Colonies of some strains of *H. parainfluenzae* ("*H. parahaemolyticus*") are surrounded by zones of hemolysis on blood agar and many resemble those of β-hemolytic streptococci.

Eikenella corrodens

This species is a facultatively anaerobic organism which characteristically "corrodes" or causes "pitting" of the surface of agar media. Several other bacterial species also produce similar corroding colonies, and this property has caused some confusion in the past. In particular, *E. corrodens* has been confused with the obligately anaerobic organism *Bacteroides corrodens* (now designated *Bacteroides ureolyticus*), although it is known that they differ in several important respects, including DNA base ratio.

The cells of *E. corrodens* are small, nonspore-forming, nonencapsulated, nonmotile, microaerophilic, gram negative coccobacilli. The organism grows on blood or chocolate agar and is enhanced by the presence of 3 to 10% CO_2. It is found in the mouth and upper respiratory tract as part of the normal commensal flora, and has also been isolated from abscesses in various parts of the body, usually in mixed infections. Strains are usually sensitive to penicillin, ampicillin, chloramphenicol and tetracycline, but resistant to clindamycin and aminoglycosides. DNA homology studies indicate that strains designated *E. corrodens* comprise a genetically homogeneous species, although some antigenic and biotype differences have been demonstrated. This organism can be recovered from "active" periodontal pockets in humans and has also been shown to induce a particular type of periodontal disease in gnotobiotic rats.

Actinobacilli

Only one of five known species of the genus *Actinobacillus*, *Actinobacillus actinomycetemcomitans*, is found as a regular inhabitant of the oral cavity. Since its original description in 1912, it has frequently been reported from cases of actinomycosis, usually in association with *Actinomyces israelii*. This organism has also been isolated from various abscesses and from patients with infective endocarditis. *A. actinomycetemcomitans* is a small, gram negative, coccoid or coccobacillary organism which morphologically resembles *Haemophilus aphrophilus*. Like other facultative gram negative rods, growth on solid media, such as blood agar, is enhanced by an atmosphere with 5 to 10% CO_2. Distinguishing biochemical and physiological features are shown in table 15/10. Although not definitely established, it is possible that *A. actinomycetemcomitans* may be one of the organisms implicated in destructive periodontal disease. It is commonly isolated from patients with juvenile periodontitis, less frequently from adult periodontitis and is found only occasionally in children and adults with a healthy periodontium.

Capnocytophagae

Capnocytophaga is the genus name which has been proposed for a group of fastidious, CO_2-requiring, gram negative, fusiform rods isolated from the oral cavity. These canophilic organisms are characteristically described as gliding or surface translocating bacteria. Colonies tend to have a spreading, fringelike edge and may be gray-white, pink or yellow in color. Some strains produce pitting of the agar surface. Three species have been described within the new genus, *Capnocytophaga ochracea*, *Capnocytophaga sputigena* and *Capnocytophaga gingivalis*; these can be distinguished on the basis of lactose and galactose fermentation and nitrate reduction. Although the names are new, *C. ochracea* in fact corresponds to an organism previously known by various other titles (including *Fusiformis nucleatus* var. *ochraceus*; *Bacteroides ochraceus*). Isolates of *Capnocytophaga* are clearly differentiated from both *Fusobacterium* and *Bacteroides* on the basis of their ability to grown in air + CO_2, fermentation of carbohydrates, end products of glucose metabolism, and DNA base composition. Interest has been aroused in these organisms because of their association with juvenile periodontitis and, possibly, other forms of destructive periodontal disease.

CURVED GRAM NEGATIVE RODS

Motile curved rods and spiral microorganisms have long been recognized as part of the oral microbiota. Leeuwenhoek described an oral, curved, comma-shaped, motile rod to which Miller in 1890 gave the name *Spirillum sputigenum* (fig. 15/8). Several other early investigators also observed oral comma-like rods, but these have often been found to be difficult, if not impossible, to culture in the

Table 15.10
Some characteristics of oral facultative gram negative rods[a]

Characteristic	Eikenella corrodens	Actinobacillus actinomycetem-comitans	Capnocytophaga species	Haemophilus species
Oxidase	+	V	−	V
Catalase	−	+	−	− or V
Urease	−	−	−	− or V
Indole	−	−	−	−
Motility	−	−	V[b]	−
Acid from				
Glucose	−	+	+	+
Mannitol	−	V	−	−
Lactose	−	−	V	V
Sucrose	−	−	+	+
Nitrate reduction	+	+	V	+
Pitting of agar	+	−	V	−
Major acid end products	A	A, S	A, S	A,S, L
Require V-factor	−	−	−	+[c]
% G + C	56	43	33–41	40–44

[a] Growth of all species is enhanced by 5 to 10% CO_2 in atmosphere
[b] 1 = Capnocytophaga species display "gliding" motility
[c] 2 = Haemophilus aphrophilus does not require V-factor unlike H. segnis, H. paraphrophilus and H. parainfluenzae
+ = most strains positive A = acetic acid
− = most strains negative S = succinic acid
V = variable reactions   L = lactic acid

laboratory. As a result of these difficulties, a variety of names have been employed to describe organisms characterized solely according to their microscopic appearance.

The current taxonomic situation regarding this group of oral bacteria is not completely clear, although recent studies have shed some light on the matter. Under the heading of curved rods can be included both facultative (or microaerophilic) and obligately anaerobic species. Many of these are motile organisms and some cause "pitting" or "corrosion" of the agar surface. Among the known oral representatives of this group are bacteria classified in the genera *Selenomonas, Wolinella* and *Campylobacter*.

Selenomonas

The genus *Selenomonas* is of uncertain affiliation. The *Approved List of Bacterial Names* includes three subspecies of *Selenomonas ruminantium*, together with the one recognized oral species, *Selenonomonas sputigena*. This is composed of gram negative curved cells about 1 μm wide and 3 to 5.5 μm long; some cells may exceed 500 μm in length. The cells sometimes form an "S" curve but more often they have from two to five curves, hence the spiroid appearance. They are motile by a cluster of flagella attached on the concave side of the cells. The organisms are strictly anaerobic. Acid is produced from a variety of sugars. This organism is

found in the oral cavity, and it has been suggested that some strains cause periodontal destruction in animals.

Wolinellae

This new genus name has recently been proposed to accommodate organisms previously called *Vibrio succinogenes* (renamed *Wolinella succinogenes*) and a new group of similar bacteria isolated from periodontal pockets, *Wolinella recta*.

Cells of this genus are helical, curved or straight, 0.5 to 1 × 2 to 6 μm, with round or tapered ends. They have a single, polar flagellum and display a rapid, darting motility when examined in wet films. They are anaerobic; some strains will grow in the presence of up to 5% oxygen, but not in air + CO_2. They neither require nor ferment carbohydates, but growth is stimulated in fluid cultures by the presence of formate and fumarate. Hydrogen and formate can be used as energy sources, formate being oxidized to hydrogen and carbon dioxide. The G + C ratio of the genus is 42 to 49 mol percent.

The two species, *W. succinogenes* and *W. recta*, differ from one another in cellular and ultrastructural morphology, antigenic structure and their susceptibility to dyes and antibiotics. They have also been shown to be distinct by DNA-DNA homology studies. *W. recta* is found in the human gingival crevice, but its pathogenicity is unknown. *W. succinogenes* has been isolated from a variety of sources, including the bovine rumen, human abdominal infections, blood cultures, dental abscesses and root canals.

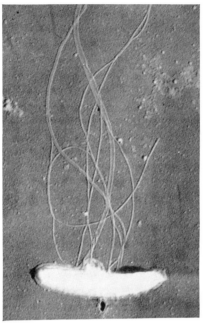

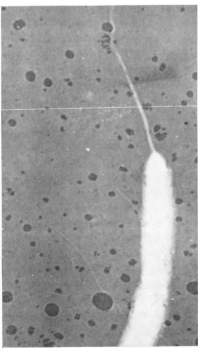

Figure 15/8. Electron micrograph of *Sprillum sputigenum* (*Selenomonas sputigena*), showing flagella originating, respectively, on the concave side and terminally. (Reproduced with permission from J. B. MacDonald, E. M. Madlener, and S. S. Socransky, 1959 Observations on *Spirillum sputigenum* and its Relationship to *Selenomonas* Species with Special Reference to Flagellation. Journal of Bacteriology, **77**, 559.)

Campylobacter

This genus contains some species which are not found in the oral cavity (*Campylobacter fetus* and *Campylobacter faecalis*) and at least two species which are common oral inhabitants, *Campylobacter sputorum* and the recently described *Campylobacter concisus*. These organisms are thin, gram negative, curved rods, 0.2 to 0.8 × 0.5 to 5 µm. The cells occasionally assume long spiral, S-shapes or "gull-winged" forms. They are motile, having a single polar flagellum at one or both ends. The organisms neither ferment nor oxidize carbohydrates. All strains are oxidase positive, but catalase varies between species. Some strains are microaerophilic (requiring 3 to 15% oxygen in the atmosphere), some are anaerobic and others are facultative. Species can be differentiated on the basis of biochemical tests, resistance to various antibiotics and growth inhibitors, and temperature tolerance.

C. concisus will grow in up to 5% oxygen and forms small curved cells 0.5 to 1 × 4 µm with rounded ends. Convex, translucent, entire colonies, approximately 1 mm in diameter are produced, without pitting of the agar surface. This species was found to have a G + C content of 34 to 38 mol per cent; there was no significant DNA homology between *C. concisus* and reference strains of *C. sputorum* ss. *sputorum*. Both species have been isolated from the human gingival crevice.

SPIROCHETES

Oral Spirochetes

Spirochetes are common inhabitants of the oral cavity, particularly of the gingival crevices and interproximal areas. Together with the fusiform bacilli, they have been implicated as causal organisms in several forms of periodontal disease. In 1875 one of the first references was made to an oral spirochete, *Treponema buccale*, and in 1877 another oral spirochete was given the name *Treponema dentium* by Koch. W. D. Miller made numerous microscopic observations of the oral spirochetes, referring to them collectively under the name *Spirochaeta dentium*, but was unable to culture any of them. Among the first references to a possible association between the oral spirochetes and diseases of the oral cavity or upper respiratory tract was that of Plaut in 1894, who observed such organisms in angina caused by a throat infection. Vincent, in 1896 and 1898, also observed spirochetes and fusiform bacilli in "hospital gangrene" and in angina. Later Noguchi isolated and described six species, based on morphological characteristics and the motions of the organisms in fluid culture media. Noguchi's classification of the oral spirochetes gradually fell into disrepute because other workers could not substantiate his findings. Subsequently, so many new strains were described that more than 40 names for oral spirochetes were recorded in an appendix to the family Treponemataceae in the sixth edition of *Bergey's Manual*. Only four species were given recognition in the seventh edition: *Treponema microdentium, Treponema mucosum, Borrelia buccalis,* and *Borrelia vincentii*. Even this limited number of species, however, has not received the concurrence of present-day investigators, who are reluctant to classify the oral spirochetes on the basis of size, shape, and motility, all of which are apt to be variable characteristics.

The eighth edition of *Bergey's Manual* lists seven oral species of the genus *Treponema*. Five species, *Treponema macrodentium, Treponema denticola, Treponema orale, Treponema scoliodontum,* and *Treponema vincentii,* have been more thoroughly characterized than *T. mucosum* and *T. buccale,* which, while being legitimate, have been poorly described. Thus, their taxonomic relationships are not clear. *T. vincentii* and *T. buccale* were classified as *B. vincentii* and *B. buccalis* respectively in the seventh edition of *Bergey's Manual*.

The oral *Treponema* species are helical cells 5 to 16 μm long and 0.10 to 0.30 μm wide. The ends of the cells taper to a point and one to several axial fibrils are inserted into the ends of the cells. They are actively motile, with a rapid, jerky motion. The organisms are gram negative but stain well with silver impregnation methods. They are best observed under phase-contract or dark-field microscopy. Cultivation of most oral spirochetes has not been particularly difficult but since they are slow-growing and motile, isolation by the usual techniques has not been feasible. Anaerobic conditions must be observed and a medium enriched with serum, blood, or ascitic fluid is needed for growth.

Spirochetes are almost always present in the oral cavity of adults with normal dentition but they are seldom present in infants before the teeth erupt or in edentulous adults. They have been found in approximately half of school children and young adults and in almost 100% of older adults. The morphology of the mouth, particularly with regard to the teeth, seems to determine the prevalence of the spirochetes. In infants before the teeth erupt and in the edentulous adult, there are no areas where conditions are particularly suitable for growth of the spirochetes. With the eruption of the teeth, the gingival crevices provide suitable areas for the spirochetes and hence their prevalence increases. As gingival recession and pocket formation occur in adults, the environment becomes even more suitable and the prevalence of the spirochetes approaches 100%. Spirochetes similar, if not identical, to those of the oral cavity and upper respiratory tract spirochetes are found in the intestinal tract and on the external genitalia of humans and in the oral cavities of monkeys, cats, dogs, and guinea pigs.

The pathogenicity of the oral spirochetes has been the subject of much speculation and some investigation. It is difficult to discuss the pathogenicity of the oral spirochetes apart from that of other oral bacteria, particularly the fusiform bacilli, for these two groups occur together consistently in lesions. Furthermore, pure cultures of oral spirochetes do not cause a characteristic or serially transferable infection when inoculated into experimental animals, in contrast to the suppurative necrotic lesions produced by the mixed flora containing spirochetes, fusiforms, and other common oral bacteria. One of the most common infections with which the fusospirochetal complex is associated is Vincent's infection, in which the gingivae and other oral mucous membranes are swollen and ulcerous and covered by a necrotic membrane, which, when removed, leaves a raw, bleeding surface. In the lesions of Vincent's infection, the fusospirochetal complex predominates, although accompanied by other species of common oral bacteria. The inoculation of the mixed flora of such lesions into the groins of guinea pigs results in a serially transferable infection with a lesion containing a mixed microbial flora, predominantly of the fusospirochetal type. Admittedly this experimental disease cannot necessarily be compared to the original human disease and it gives no information about the possible specific pathogenic function of the spirochetes. Nevertheless, it does provide an indication of the general pathogenicity of the mixed flora from the lesion of Vincent's infection. In addition, upper respiratory tract infections occur with lesions containing a predominance of spirochetes and fusiform bacilli. Infections of a very serious nature may result from the transfer of fusospirochetes from the oral cavity to subcutaneous tissue by biting, or wounding the fist on the teeth during fights. Lung abscesses are also caused by fusospirochetes. Noma is another type of infection either caused by, or greatly influenced by, the fusospirochetal complex. It is a slowly spreading gangrenous stomatitis that develops mostly in children whose physical condition is weakened by improper nutrition or by a debilitating disease. Finally, a widespread form of cutaneous "tropical ulcer" is caused by the fusospirochetal complex.

MYCOPLASMA

The highly pleomorphic organisms of the genus *Mycoplasma* are regular oral residents. Mycoplasma species have been isolated from throat swabs, dental plaque and calculus, root canals, inflamed pulp, carious lesions, and from healthy and diseased gingival crevices. These organisms are found more frequently in the gingival area than at other sites. Those species isolated seem to be mainly either *Mycoplasma orale* or *Mycoplasma salivarium*. In one study, *M. salivarium* was the only species isolated from the gingival area, and serological identification of the isolates indicated that there were no appropriate differences between the incidence and species of mycoplasmas isolated from normal and diseased gingival crevices. Most studies indicate that mycoplasmas are ubiquitous in the oral cavity.

YEASTS

While considerable variation has been reported in the occurrence of oral yeasts (fig. 1519), there is general agreement that *Candida albicans* is the most common one. Until recently the habitat of *C. albicans* was considered to be restricted to the animal body, but since 1954 it has been isolated from soil and vegetables where it is considered to be a chance invader. The reported incidence of *C. albicans* in the oral cavity and throat of healthy individuals varies considerably, ranging from 10 to 80%. The range of counts in positive mouths is from 10 to 10,000; in 90.3% the count is 1000 or less. Of the yeasts isolated, the great majority were *C. albicans*, with smaller percentages of *Candida tropicalis*, *Candida stellatoidea*, *Cryptococcus* species, *Candida pseudotropicalis*, and various unidentified *Candida* species. A direct relationship has been found between the occurrence of yeasts and the acidity of saliva, but some yeasts were present in the salivas at all pH levels:

pH	Percentage Occurrence
5	100
5.5	83
6.0	67
6.5	52
7.0	29
7.5	14

C. albicans has been reported to be more common in persons with untreated caries than in those with caries-free dentition. Following antibiotic therapy the frequency was reported to range from 5 to 80%. One study examined the occurrence in winter and summer of fungi in plaque on noncarious teeth in a group whose ages ranged from 7 to 20 years but who were mostly in the 13- to 19-year age group. The frequency in women in the winter was 33.3 ± 8.0% and in summer 58.3 ± 7%. The frequency in men in the winter was 20.8 ± 8.2% and in summer 34.6 ± 6.8%. The summer sex differences are significant but the winter sex differences are not. Of the fungi isolated, 58% were *C. albicans* and 11.6% were *Penicillium* species. Other fungi occasionally isolated were *Scopulariopsis brevicularis*,

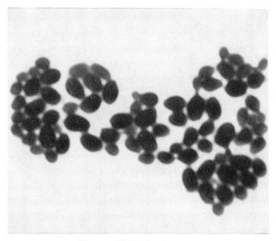

Figure 15/9. Oral yeast.

Geotrichum asteroides, *Hormodendrum compactum*, *Aspergillus* species, and *Hemispora stellata*, but these could not be considered as normal oral inhabitants.

Studies of the role of *Candida* species in the ecology of the oral microbiota indicate a number of symbiotic and antagonistic relationships. Symbiosis exists between *C. albicans* and *C. tropicalis* and *Staphylococcus aureus* and *Staphylococcus epidermidis*, the former prolonging the viability of the latter. *C. albicans* also prolongs the viability of *Corynebacterium diphtheriae* and β-hemolytic streptococci; if these pathogens are placed alone on a cotton swab they survive only for a few days, but together with *C. albicans* they survive for up to 10 weeks. *Lactobacillus acidophilus* will grow in vitamin-deficient media in which single omissions of thiamine, folic acid, riboflavin, and niacin are supplemented by a mixed culture with *C. albicans*. The growth of lactobacilli in deficient media is proportional to the amount of thiamine, riboflavin calcium pantothenate, and pyridoxamine liberated in *C. albicans*.

While *Candida* species generally have a stimulatory effect on lactobacilli *in vitro* by furnishing essential growth factors, the latter have an inhibitory effect on the yeast due to the accumulation of lactic or other acids. However, such a mechanism has not been demonstrated *in vivo*.

C. albicans also stimulates growth of *Mycobacterium tuberculosis* by an unidentified factor in the polysaccharide fraction of cell-free extracts of the yeast. Some fraction of the cell-free extract also protects the tubercle bacillus against isoniazide and streptomycin. *In vitro*, *M. tuberculosis* either metabolizes or neutralizes dyes toxic for *C. albicans*, allowing the latter to grow.

PROTOZOA

Protozoa are not uncommon in the oral cavity, the most common being *Entamoeba gingivalis* and

Trichomonas tenax. It was found that the oral cavities of 39% of 700 patients contained *E. gingivalis*, while 23% had *T. tenax* and 17.7% had both. Distribution was also related to the condition of the oral cavity. In "clean and healthy" mouths, 26.4% contained *E. gingivalis*, 11.2% contained *T. tenax*, and 6.4% contained both. In early periodontal disease, 62.5% contained *E. gingivalis*, 48.2% contained *T. tenax*, and 39% contained both. In advanced periodontal disease 100% contained *E. gingivalis*, 80% contained *T. tenax*, and 80% contained both. *E. gingivalis* and *T. tenax* were absent from the oral cavities of children 6 to 12 years of age, but were present in increasing proportions with age. There was no relationship between the number of carious lesions and the prevalence of the protozoa. Protozoal infestation was approximately equally prevalent in men and women.

VIRUSES

With some exceptions, notably herpes simplex virus, viruses, based on available data, appear to be oral transients. Herpes simplex virus infection occurs in a large proportion of the population, for approximately 70 to 90% of adults continuously maintain significant levels of homologous circulating antibody. This fact and the recurrent nature of vesicular lesions in or near the oral cavity indicate persistence of the virus throughout life. The manner or exact site in which the herpes simplex virus is maintained between the recurrent episodes has not been definitely determined, but it seems likely that it persists in the trigeminal ganglia during latency. Herpes simplex virus is excreted in saliva for as long as 2 months after complete recovery from the infection. It has been demonstrated in the saliva of slightly less than 3% of asymptomatic adults.

Rabies virus has been demonstrated in the salivas of rabid animals and human beings. Many investigators have also demonstrated this virus in parotid, sublingual, and submaxillary glands of infected human beings. Rabies virus is more likely to be present in saliva during convulsive rabid seizures when copious amounts of saliva are excreted. There is no evidence that rabies virus persists in the saliva of asymptomatic human beings. However, an asymptomatic infection of indefinite duration occurs in the salivary glands of vampire and probably other species of bats, during which their saliva is infectious.

Mumps virus also occurs in saliva during the course of the disease, as evidenced by the infectivity of mumps saliva for both experimental animals and susceptible human beings.

A "salivary gland virus" infection of man and animals has been recognized for nearly 60 years. The viruses are the cytomegaloviruses and the infection is termed cytomegalic inclusion disease because the infected cells, usually in epithelial tissue, become greatly enlarged, while their nuclei contain prominent inclusions and their cytoplasms may contain inclusions of a different nature. The virus has been recovered from adenoids, liver, and urine, as well as from salivary glands. Also, in fatal cases lesions have been found in various other organs. Recovery of cytomegalovirus from adenoids and urine of apparently healthy persons, and the occurrence of homologous antibody in a large proportion of sera from normal adults, indicate that subclinical infection is quite widespread.

FUNCTIONAL GROUPS OF MICROORGANISMS IN THE ORAL CAVITY

In addition to the studies that have been made of the numbers, kinds, and localization of microorganisms in the oral cavity, much useful information has been obtained concerning the functions of various groups of oral bacteria. Early studies revealed the presence of chromogenic, acidogenic, and proteolytic types, to which was soon added the aciduric group. The chromogens have never been investigated in much detail, although discoloration is a prominent feature in dental caries. Interest has centered on the acidogenic and aciduric types and the proteolytic organisms.

Aciduric oral microorganisms usually are defined as those that will grow on a suitable medium at pH 5.0. When this condition is maintained in a medium, lactobacilli, yeasts, some streptococci, and some staphylococci are the only oral microorganisms that grow. No clear distinction has been established between the aciduric and acidogenic qualities. In the study of the etiology of oral disease, particularly of dental caries, undue emphasis may have been placed upon the aciduric property in contrast to the acidogenic and even the proteolytic activities. For example, the yeasts not only resist acid conditions but grow well under them, yet they are not significantly acidogenic. The streptococci usually are not considered to be very aciduric, yet they seem to be a very important acidogenic group of the oral cavity, owing to their predominance and to their rapid rates of growth and acid production. Streptococci and various filamentous microorganisms, which also are not considered to be aciduric, have been found in locations in the oral cavity where the lactobacilli occur, including the advancing carious lesions from deep in dentin. Furthermore, the aciduric bacteria constitute only a very small fraction of the total oral microbial flora. In mouths without carious lesions, the lactobacilli and other aciduric bacteria have been found to account for less than 0.05% of the total cultivable organisms. When carious lesions were present, the lactobacilli might increase as much as 20 times and other aciduric bacteria as much as 8 times but they would still constitute not more than 0.5% of the total. The acidogenic quality usually has not been precisely analyzed. The lactobacilli must derive most of their energy from the conversion of a carbohydrate to organic acids; hence, they are correctly considered to be typically acidogenic. The streptococci, although very closely related metabolically to the lactobacilli, are not obligatorily acidogenic. Many of them produce proteolytic enzymes and they can utilize a predominantly nitrogenous rather than a glycolytic metabolism, in which case basic rather than acidic products are produced. Even further removed from the purely acidogenic lactobacilli are those bacteria such as the genera *Veillonella, Neisseria,* and *Branhamella,* some of which are apparently nonsaccharolytic. Another limiting condition is the ability to utilize acid intermediates. Lactic acid is the end of the metabolic road for homofermentative lactobacilli, whereas heterofermentative lactobacilli and many streptococci are able to some extent to carry the glycolytic process to the two-carbon or one-carbon stage, with the formation of such end products as ethanol, acetaldehyde, acetoin, acetic acid, formic acid, and carbon dioxide. Such facultatively anaerobic bacteria as micrococci and diphtheroids accumulate acid approximately in proportion to the restriction of the oxygen supply. We may conclude that under natural conditions in the mouth the actual production of acids is not necessarily what we would predict from test tube observations.

The proteolytic microorganisms of the oral cavity also have been investigated. Proteolysis, like acidogenesis, is not an all-or-none reaction. Various microorganisms produce enzymes that can act on some proteins but not on others, or only under restricted circumstances. Some of the bacterial enzymes can degrade proteins only one step, whereas others can carry the process to the peptide stage or even completely to amino acids. Other microorganisms act only on amino acids. Therefore, proteolytic microorganisms should, if possible, be described in terms of the types of proteins or peptide linkage upon which they act. Thus, gelatin liquefaction, the commonest bacteriological criterion of proteolysis, gives a most inadequate picture of oral conditions. In the oral cavity at large there are many microorganisms that liquefy gelatin, fewer than can digest casein, still fewer that can lyse the protein of coagulated egg, and very few that can lyse decalcified dentin or enamel. The latter group, however, abounds in the outer layers of decalcified dentin in the carious lesion. There is doubt that any known oral microorganisms, or combination of them, have been shown to attack *in situ* the protein constituents of the calcified portions of intact dentin or enamel.

An important additional consideration is the utilization of lactic acid by organisms such as *Veillonella.* In situations where acidogenic organisms exist side-by-side with acid utilizers, such as in dental plaque, the amount of free lactic acid may be less than that present in an environment entirely dominated by saccharolytic bacteria. Furthermore the types and amounts of acids produced vary in response to changes in availability of substrate and other factors such as growth rate.

Bacterial Adherence

In recent years it has been appreciated that microorganisms must be retained in the oral cavity to become a functioning part of the oral microbiota and potentially play a role in oral disease. Bacteria may be retained in the mouth by adhering to various oral structures or to one another. The phenomenon of bacterial adherence to surfaces is a central issue in microbial ecology which has attracted the interest of scientists from a variety of backgrounds. Much of this current interest has been stimulated by fundamental work in the field of oral microbiology, notably the excellent studies by Dr. R. J. Gibbons and his colleagues at the Forsyth Dental Center. The extent of scientific activity in the field is illustrated by the considerable number of symposia held in recent years, several of which have resulted in the publication of books on bacterial adherence and microbial-surface interactions (see list of Additional Reading).

Oral bacteria exhibit different abilities to attach to structures such as the teeth and the epithelial cells of the oral cavity. Thus *Streptococcus salivarius* has a high affinity for the dorsum of the tongue, where it is found in abundance naturally, but relatively low ability to adhere to the tooth surface. In contrast, strains of *Streptococcus sanguis* have been shown to attach strongly to the coronal surfaces of the teeth and in moderate degree to oral epithelial surfaces. Other species, such as *Bacteroides gingivalis* (formerly called *Bacteroides asaccharolyticus*), have only very limited ability to adhere to clean oral surfaces, but can attach readily to the bacteria present in preformed aggregations of dental plaque.

The exact mechanisms whereby different bacteria attach themselves to and colonize surfaces are not fully understood, but appear to be complex. A variety of physicochemical attractive and repulsive forces may be operative and the surface characteristics in terms of shape, charge, chemical composition, etc., vary from organism to organism and according to environmental conditions. Once an organism has attached itself initially, retention may be enhanced by the formation of polymer bridges. The production of extracellular glucans by several of the oral streptococci, including *Streptococcus mutans,* is thought to be particularly important for their establishment and survival on the tooth surface and has been studied in considerable detail. Other factors of importance are the production, by some oral bacteria, of surface fibrils which participate in their attachment to surfaces, and the interactions which occur between bacterial surface components, salivary macromolecules (such as glycoproteins) and the various anatomical structures in the mouth.

Bacterial polymers such as glucans enhance the initial attachment of strains of S. mutans to the tooth surface, although these organisms can attach, albeit weakly, in the absence of these polymers. However, it appears that in order to effect this enhanced attachment the glucans must be synthesized by the bacteria at the tooth surface: preformed polymers do not appear to be effective.

Colonization in retention areas such as the fissures of teeth probably occurs in part by mechanical entrapment of organisms which find such sites favorable for growth. However it is likely that cell-to-cell and cell-to-tooth interactions play a major role in colonization of such areas, particularly the more open or superficial portions such as the entrances to fissures. Since these areas, particularly the deeper portions, are inaccessible to cleaning mechanisms such as the bristles of a toothbrush or a free flow of saliva, organisms which have a relatively low affinity for the tooth surface or other organisms are likely able to persist and colonize.

In the gingival crevice many organisms can persist even if their adherence abilities are relatively low because the site is retentive, fluid flow is minimal, and there is a good supply of nutrients. These factors may account for the diversity of bacterial types found in the crevicular area.

REGULATION OF THE ORAL MICROBIOTA

From the foregoing discussion, it is seen that many microorganisms are introduced into the oral cavity from time to time, and that some survive and become permanent residents. The simple introduction of microorganisms that are not normal residents seldom results in their establishment, unless conditions are altered to favor the intruder. For example, even if large numbers of the saprophytic chromogen, Serratia marcescens, are introduced into the oral cavity as indicator organisms, they soon disappear. For establishment, a usable substrate in the form of accessible carbohydrate is necessary, together with a proper environment, all of the factors of which have not been defined. Similarly, it appears that the development of many of the diseases of the tissues of the oral cavity depends upon the development of conditions that favor the manifestation of the pathogenic potentialities of the usually harmless resident microorganisms. It is important, therefore, to discuss what we know of the factors that regulate the oral microbiota.

The oral environment at birth seems to favor microorganisms tolerant of oxygen because of the absence, in the edentulous mouth, of areas where anaerobiosis can be readily achieved. When the teeth erupt, numerous areas become available, most importantly the interproximal surfaces, the gingival sulci, and to some extent the enamel pits and fissures, where a degree of anaerobiosis can be maintained suitable for the growth of the most exacting microorganisms. Most of the early investigations found evidence of a predominantly aerobic and anaerobic microbiota after eruption of the teeth. However, although it is evident that the eruption of the teeth favors an anaerobic microbiota, the absence of the teeth does not preclude the establishment and growth of some strictly anaerobic species. The establishment of an E_h favorable to strict anaerobes could be accomplished in the edentulous infant or adult by symbiotic growth with aerobes. One study indicated that the mucous membrane of the tonsillar region is the chief resident site in infants of anaerobic bacteria before eruption of teeth. Other investigations seem to confirm this, for strictly anaerobic gram negative bacteria were isolated from 58% of 18 infants without teeth. The proportion of mouths positive increased with age, even in the edentulous infant. Other investigations also confirm the appearance of anaerobic microorganisms in the oral cavity before the eruption of the teeth but show that they are present in small numbers and fail to establish permanent residency until the eruption of the teeth.

Several factors tend to effect an increase or decrease of the total oral microbial flora or of individual species. The state of oral hygiene appears to have a distinct influence. With good oral hygiene, the total number of microorganisms in the oral cavity decreases and is predominantly composed of microorganisms tolerant of oxygen. Neglect of oral hygiene results in an increase of the total microbial flora and an anaerobic and putrefactive character, probably owing to the accumulation of food and tissue debris in the gingival sulci and to increased plaque formation. In this connection, it has been shown that cultivable proteolytic microorganisms may increase as much as 37-fold in the saliva from oral cavities where there are open carious lesions. This is most likely attributable to an accompanying poor state of general oral hygiene (fig. 15/10).

The density of the oral microbial population changes temporarily with the time of day. One responsible factor is the flow of salia, which is greater under the stimuli of the waking hours than during the sleeping hours. The character of the saliva is probably different at night than in the day.

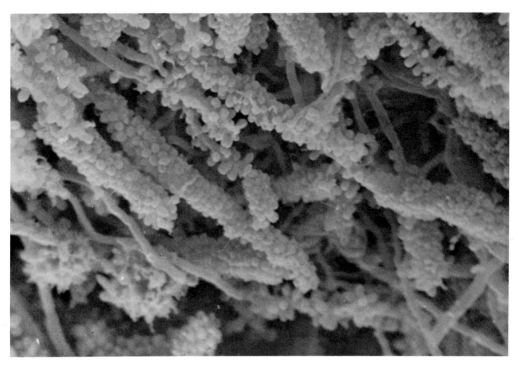

Figure 15/10. "Corn-on-the-cob" formations in plaque, with coccoid forms coating filamentous organisms. (Photograph courtesy of Dr. Sheila Jones, University College, London). (Adapted from: Jones, S. A. Special Relationship Between Spherical and Filamentous Microorganisms in Mature Human Dental Plaque. Arch Oral Biol, **17**, 613.)

Also, the abrasive activity associated with eating certain types of foods tends to deplete temporarily the microorganisms that are accessible to removal during this process. The net effect of the diurnal flow of saliva and the abrasive action of chewing during waking hours is that the total number of microorganisms is usually greatest at night and before each meal, and least after each meal.

Another factor affecting the total as well as the nature of the microbial population, albeit an extreme one, is aptyalism. The suppression of salivary secretion results in a significant increase in the total microbial population probably because of the undue accumulation of food debris and the loss of the mediating factors inherent in saliva.

The complete loss of teeth also causes a decrease in the total numbers of oral bacteria in comparison to those with a normal dentition or complete dentures.

In addition to factors which significantly increase or decrease the total microbiota are factors that cause temporary or permanent shifts among the individual members of the microbiota. Among these factors are antibiotics, change of diet, physiological changes, restoration of all carious teeth, and the extraction of all teeth. Each antibiotic suppresses a more or less specific group of organisms. Furthermore, the overall balance of the oral microbiota is upset owing to an increase in those sensitive species normally controlled or greatly influenced by the presence of the suppressed organisms. Thus, sufficient administration of penicillin decreases many sensitive gram positive oral bacteria and allows overgrowth of the insensitive gram negative organisms ordinarily held in balance by the suppressed gram positive bacteria. Sufficient administration of a broad-spectrum antibiotic suppresses both gram positive and gram negative microorganisms so that the insensitive yeasts and fungi overgrow and become the predominant microbial flora.

That large amounts of refined sugar in the diet favor those organisms with a metabolism dependent on the degradation of sugars has been confirmed by both animal and human experimentation. Similarly, it is likely that alterations of other dietary components will affect the oral microbiota. For example, rats fed a high protein diet had more than twice as high a percentage of facultative, gram positive rods as did litter mates fed a standard lab diet. Likewise, many oral organisms have strict vitamin requirements, so that their growth and activity could be influenced by deficient diets.

So far we know little of the effects of subtle or even drastic physiological changes in the host on the oral microbiota, but undoubtedly they would be mediated largely by salivary flow and constitution or by changes in the oral tissues. *Candida albicans* occurs more frequently in diabetics (80%) than in nondiabetics (50%). Many investigations have found that the average concentration of oral lactobacilli increases in the presence of carious lesions, decreases with the restoration of carious lesions, and remains low or nil until the appearance of new lesions.

The examples discussed above illustrate the fact that numerous interrelated factors combine to regulate the composition and metabolic activities of the oral microflora. Some of the factors either known or believed to influence this complex ecosystem are listed in table 15/11. These include both host-related and microorganism-related variables. In some cases, such as racial factors and hormonal factors, the evidence is largely speculative at present.

RELATIONSHIP OF SALIVA TO THE MICROBIOLOGY OF THE ORAL CAVITY

To a great extent, the oral microbiota is regulated by the saliva since it is the culture medium in which the oral microorganisms must live, grow, reproduce, and carry out their various functions. "Whole saliva" is a complex mixture of the secretions of the parotid, the submaxillary, and the sublingual glands, and of numerous lesser glands of the mucous membranes of the oral cavity; other substances which may be taken into the mouth from time to time, and their degradation products; leukocytes, shed epithelial cells, and their products; and the oral microbiota and its metabolic products. Since the secretions of the various salivary glands are distinctive and subject to change by various reflex stimulations, the composition and amount of saliva secreted varies. Furthermore, the enzymatic activity of the oral microbiota must produce profound but extremely variable changes in the excreted saliva, and its dissolved foods. On the average, saliva is composed of about 99.5% water and 0.5% solid, of which about half is inorganic (mostly chloride, bicarbonate, phosphate, sodium, calcium, potassium, trace elements, and dissolved carbon dioxide, oxygen, and nitrogen), and about half is organic (proteins, cholesterol, hormone-like substances,

Table 15/11
Some environmental factors which may affect the oral microflora

Anatomical factors	Antimicrobial agents and other drugs
Salivary secretions	Oral and dental diseases
Crevicular fluid	Systemic diseases
Diet	Dental treatment and appliances
Oxidation-reduction potential	Oral hygiene procedures
Microbial nutrition and metabolism	Genetic and Racial factors
Microbial interactions	Smoking and other habits
Microbial adherence	Hormonal secretions

free amino acids, urea, ammonia, vitamins, and antibacterial and antienzymatic factors). In addition, various foods and their breakdown products are transitorily present in saliva during and after their ingestion.

Mineral Content and Ionic Strength

The mineral content of saliva has been extensively investigated, although not in relation to its influence on the oral microbiota. Salivary minerals influence the microbiota through osmotic pressure, buffering capacity, E_h and pH, as essential metabolites, and as activators or inhibitors of enzymes. Based on the mean inorganic content of saliva, derived from the literature, the calculated ionic strength of saliva is 0.046. The salivary proteins presumably contribute slightly but not enough to bring the ionic strength up to isotonicity. Although this is only about one-fourth to one-third that of tissue fluids or common bacterial culture media, the osmotic tolerance of bacteria is quite great, for many can grow in either an extremely hypo- or hypertonic environment.

Individual Ions. The values for concentrations of inorganic constituents of saliva vary considerably. Only potassium and phosphate ions are more concentrated in saliva than in blood; the significance of this is obscure. Most attention has been given to salivary calcium and phosphate, because of their relationship to the teeth and to calculus formation. Their mean concentrations are respectively 5.8 mg per 100 ml (range, 2.2 to 11.3) and 52.0 mg per 100 ml (range 19 to 220). The calcium is about 60% ionized, the remainder being probably mostly bound to protein. Saliva is probably saturated with calcium phosphate. This assists in preventing the dissolution of the calcified tissues of the tooth. On the other hand, saturation leads to precipitation of calcium phosphate as dental calculus but, strangely, not to significant reformation of any dissolved portions of the tooth. Although it is true that an increase in alkalinity of saliva causes the precipitation of calcium phosphate, this seems to occur locally (i.e., calculus formation) rather than generally. The specific mechanisms causing the local precipitation of calcium phosphate have not been determined precisely. A number of investigators have suggested that it is due to the action of the oral microbiota, particularly the filamentous microorganisms.

The specific influence of inorganic ions upon the oral microbiota is difficult to evaluate because we lack adequate information about the inorganic ion requirements of bacteria. Most culture media contain at least available sodium, potassium, magnesium, manganese, calcium, iron, chloride, sulfate, phosphate, and carbonate. It is difficult to determine the essentiality of each of these ions, for some, such as sodium chloride and sodium and potassium phosphates, are present in part to give the medium sufficient ionic strength and osmotic pressure and to provide a balanced ionic environment. Others have been shown definitely to be either essential or stimulatory to certain microbial species. Iron for instance, is required particularly for microorganisms having a high cytochrome content, e.g., strongly aerobic bacteria such as *Pseudomonas aeruginosa*.

Most of the inorganic ions required for or stimulatory to bacteria operate as activators or essential components of enzymes. If such ions were deficient in saliva, bacteria requiring them would be severely limited. Such ions, particularly trace ions, could be supplied via foodstuffs. Also, inorganic ions could indirectly influence the oral microbiota by activating salivary enzymes which would help supply the necessary substrates for growth.

Fluoride. Other inorganic ions could influence the oral microbiota by inhibiting enzymes. Fluoride is considered a trace ion in saliva, for it seldom exceeds 2 ppm regardless of the amount normally supplied in drinking water or food. Primarily by inhibiting enolase, fluoride in low concentrations inhibits acid production and in higher concentrations inhibits growth and reproduction of bacteria that are obliged to obtain energy by glycolysis. The inhibitory action of fluoride is enhanced by increased concentrations of hydrogen, potassium, magnesium, and phosphate ions. Hence, it is often postulated that conditions obtain locally or even generally in saliva which are conducive to inhibition by fluoride of bacterial activity including that related to anaerobic degradation of carbohydrates.

Buffer System

Salivary buffering capacity is directly related to the secretion rate, for more buffer is available per unit of time in rapid than in slow secretors. Most agree that the buffering capacity of saliva is mainly related to its bicarbonate system, which contributes about 64 to 85% of the total capacity. Microorganisms, mucoids, and proteins contribute little buffering capacity between pH 4.0 and 7.0. Most of the buffering capacity of salivary sediment is due to adsorbed bicarbonate. The buffering capacity of dental plaque is not due to bicarbonate, but probably to bacterial products. It is generally agreed that the excretion of carbon dioxide and hence the buffering capacity of the saliva is increased 4- to 5-fold by stimulation of the glands and that it returns to its previous level within about half an hour after cessation of stimulation. Hence, at meals the buffering capacity of saliva is maximal and between meals it is minimal. As a corollary, the abrasive action of food ingested during a meal reduces the total microbial flora to a minimum during the period of greatest buffering, after which the flora increases to a maximum in the interval between meals, when buffering capacity is minimal. On the other hand,

local acid production as in dental plaque or in carious lesions would be greatest when buffering capacity is maximal.

The pH of the saliva is thought to have an important influence in the regulation of the oral microbial flora. The pH of freshly collected saliva varies between 5.7 and 7.0 with the mean near 6.7, which is satisfactory for the growth of a wide variety of microorganisms. It may vary by as much as 1 unit in normal circumstances of chewing, fatigue, change in breathing rate, and general metabolic influences. Such changes, if prolonged, would affect the oral microbial flora, since most bacteria grow only within a restricted pH range. If the saliva became too alkaline, acidophilic organisms would be unable to grow; if too acid, such proteolytic bacteria as staphylococci, streptococci, and *Bacillus* species could not maintain themselves. However, no relationship has been established between the pH of saliva and the incidence of caries, which would reflect changes in the microbial flora. The actual pH is determined by the ratio between the concentrations of bicarbonate ion and dissolved carbon dioxide, whereas the buffer capacity at a given pH depends upon their total amounts. Ultimately, both depend upon the carbon dioxide-secreting capacity of the salivary glands. Thus, an increase in carbon dioxide would lower the pH and at the same time increase the buffer capacity. Since carbon dioxide is essential for the growth of all bacteria and stimulates some species more than others, an increase in the buffer capacity of the saliva may favor certain oral microorganisms indirectly by increasing the content of carbon dioxide, as well as directly stabilizing the pH at a favorable value. Of course, the effective buffer capacity of saliva is enhanced by its rate of flow, whereby the buffer is continually renewed. Consequently, in areas of stagnation the production of acids or alkalis by bacterial action soon exceeds the effective buffer capacity of the saliva and favors the establishment of those bacteria that grow best in an acid or alkaline environment, as the case may be. Thus, despite its own considerable additional buffer capacity, the dental plaque rapidly becomes quite acid in response to the ingestion of sugars and tends to favor aciduric microorganisms. Conversely, the gingival crevice is definitely alkaline and is characterized by proteolysis and putrefaction.

Oxidation-Reduction Potential

Another indirect effect of pH is through the oxidation-reduction potential (E_h), which becomes more positive (oxidative) as the pH decreases and vice versa, although the relationship appears not to hold as rigidly in saliva as in simple systems.

Although the E_h of saliva has been shown to vary over a considerable range, there was no significant variation in the E_h of the saliva of individuals tested under identical conditions. The E_h did not vary greatly during the day although the pH did. Determination of the E_h for stimulated saliva in open vessels showed that the mean E_h for 50 caries-resistant persons was $+309 \pm 4.7$ mv, and for 50 caries-active persons it was $+237 \pm 9.9$ mv, the difference between the two groups being statistically significant. The salivas of the caries-resistant persons were oxygen saturated, whence the strongly oxidative E_h, which could not be raised by passing pure oxygen through the saliva. Nevertheless, the high oxidative potential of all salivas favors aerobic microorganisms. A typical aerobic culture broth has an E_h of $+300$ mv, and cultures of bacteria that produce hydrogen peroxide may go as high as $+429$ mv. Facultative and obligate anaerobes require a negative E_h. For instance, cultures of oral lactobacilli have an E_h from -130 to -240 mg, and of clostridia, from -300 to -400 mv. The question must be asked, therefore, how do so many anaerobes grow in saliva? Saliva does, of course, possess reducing substances and tends to drift fairly rapidly toward a negative E_h. More important, it is unlikely that the freely flowing saliva is the primary habitat of the oral anaerobes, for, as we have noted previously, they are scarce in the edentulous mouth. Dental plaque has E_h levels as low as -200 mv and the gingival crevice area has E_h levels over the range of $+100$ to -300 mv.

Gases

The principal gases in saliva are carbon dioxide, oxygen, and nitrogen. The carbon dioxide content of saliva ranges from about 13 to 85 ml per 100 ml, depending largely on the degree of stimulation of the salivary glands. About half of the carbon dioxide in stimulated saliva is in the form of bicarbonate at pH 6.9. The remaining portion is extremely labile. Being present in saliva in greater concentration than in air, it tends to escape, with concomitant changes in salivary pH, E_h, and buffering capacity. Not only does carbon dioxide influence the oral microbiota by regulating the physical environment (cell permeability, pH, E_h, and buffering capacity), but it is also an essential metabolite for all microorganisms that have been tested.

The oxygen content of saliva from caries-inactive or -resistant and caries-active persons differs, averaging respectively about 1.35 and 0.51 ml per 100 ml. The high oxygen content of the saliva of caries-inactive persons may be associated with a predominantly aerobic oral microbiota, for oxygen uptake by the microbiota of unstimulated saliva of caries-resistant persons is greater than that of the saliva of caries-susceptible persons. The predominantly aerobic flora of caries-resistant persons may also influence the oral microbiota by rapid oxidation of the acids formed by the anaerobic degradation of carbohydrates by the anaerobic components of the flora.

The nitrogen content of saliva, ranging from 0.48 to 2.78 ml per 100 ml, has not been shown to relate to caries activity or to any component of the oral microbial flora.

Organic Content

As it is secreted, saliva contains many organic constituents. Some are derived from or similar to those of plasma, whereas others are distinctive secretions of the glands. In addition, a multitude of organic substances are introduced into saliva via the diet and the metabolism of the oral microbiota. Some of these substances are transitory but others remain in the oral environment for sufficient time to influence the oral microbiota. Some, such as amino acids and proteins, carbohydrates, vitamins, purines, and pyrimidines, serve as nutrients for the oral microbiota, limiting or promoting various bacterial species, depending on their availability and on the degree of nutritional dependence of the bacteria. Enzymes such as lysozyme may limit bacterial growth. Other salivary enzymes (table 15/12) promote bacterial growth by breaking down complex salivary or dietary substances into components that are suitable nutrients. Salivary organic constituents may also affect the oral microbiota by their influence on the physical environment (viscosity, ionic strength, osmotic pressure).

Proteins. Proteins comprise the major portion of the organic constituents of saliva. The exact nature of each of the salivary proteins has not been determined due to difficulties in isolating them in unchanged form. The principal salivary protein-containing material is mucin, composed of about two-thirds protein and one-third polysaccharide. It is derived principally but not exclusively from sublingual and submaxillary glands. Mucin imparts viscosity to saliva, primarily due to its bound polysaccharide. Whether under the conditions that exist in the oral cavity mucin serves as a nutrient for the oral microbiota is not known, for mucin preparations have generally been found to be poor culture media for bacteria. However, mucin breaks down considerably if saliva stands for any length of time, in which case its components are available for bacterial nutrition. It had been theorized that precipitation of mucinous material was a major factor in formation of plaque. Subsequent studies have cast doubt on the validity of this theory, at least as the major mechanism of plaque formation. However, it does appear that some salivary constituents can bind to certain types of plaque bacteria. For example, mucinous polymers appear to be involved in the aggregation of *Streptococcus mitis* and *Streptococcus sanguis*. The salivary polymers may become incorporated into plaque by binding to bacteria, and as the bacteria proliferate, more salivary constituents attach, building up the mass of material. The binding of bacterial cells and salivary

Table 15/12
Salivary enzymes

Enzyme	Source		
	Glands	Micro-organisms	Leuko-cytes
Carbohydrases			
Amylase	+		
Maltase		+	+
Invertase		+	
β-Glucuronidase	+	+	+
β-D-Galactosidase		+	+
β-D-Glucosidase		+	
Lysozyme	+		+
Hyaluronidase		+	
Mucinase		+	
Esterases			
Acid phosphatase	+	+	+
Alkaline phosphatase	+	+	+
Hexosediphosphatase		+	
Aliesterase	+	+	+
Lipase	+	+	+
Acetylcholinesterase	+		+
Pseudo-cholinesterase	+	+	+
Chondrosulfatase		+	
Arylsulfatase		+	
Transferring enzymes			
Catalase		+	
Peroxidase	+		+
Phenyloxidase		+	
Succinic dehydrogen-ase	+	+	+
Hexokinase		+	+
Proteolytic enzymes			
Proteinase		+	+
Peptidase		+	+
Urease		+	
Other enzymes			
Carbonic anhydrase	+		
Pyrophosphatase		+	
Aldolase	+	+	+

(From Chauncey, H. H. 1961 Salivary Enzymes. J Am Dental Assoc, **63**, 360.)

components probably contribute to the cohesive nature of the plaque.

Mucin is also a resistance-lowering substance, for when it is injected into animals together with bacteria of low virulence, it protects them, thereby lowering the number required to produce a fatal infection. It is likely that salivary mucins influence the oral microbiota in a similar fashion, protecting some of the oral microbiota from salivary inhibitors and phagocytosis probably by a coating effect.

Immunological and electrophoretic analyses reveal many other proteins in the salivary secretions. Serum albumin and α-, β-, and γ-globulins account for about 25% of the protein, but except for some enzymes the other proteins in these secretions have not been identified. We know little of the regulatory effects of these salivary proteins on the oral microbiota.

Carbohydrates. Hydrolysis of parotid secretion yields the following sugars: hexosamine, methyl pentose, galactose, mannose, deoxyribose, and glu-cose. Sialic acid also is present, indicating some mucin even in parotid secretions. The free carbohydrate in saliva as it is secreted (about 0.5 mg per 100 ml) does not appear sufficient to sustain the optimal growth of oral bacteria requiring it. Saliva, therefore, tends to favor those microorganisms that utilize nitrogenous compounds and produce an alkaline reaction, unless accessible carbohydrates come in with the food.

The carbohydrates most probably available for oral bacteria are dietary refined sugars (sucrose and glucose) and maltose, released by the hydrolysis of starchy foods by salivary amylase. Although starch is a principal carbohydrate in food, it cannot be used by most bacteria. Salivary amylase is a powerful, rapidly acting enzyme, but the rapid passage of most foods through the mouth and the solvent action of saliva may preclude the digestion of starch as a very significant source of nutrient for the oral microbiota, except (importantly) when food is retained about the teeth. Dietary refined sugars are probably more significant because of their proved relationship to caries activity.

Urea and Ammonia. Ammonia is the simplest salivary nitrogen source available to the oral microbiota, although apparently few use it significantly. Urea appears to be derived by the salivary glands by filtration from blood, but ammonia is not secreted by them in significant amounts. Rather, it is considered to be derived from urea or by deamination of amino acids by bacterial enzymes. Staphylococci produce considerable urease while many of the common oral gram negative bacteria produce deaminases. These enzymes are not present in the glandular secretion, for ammonia is not produced in saliva that has been filtered to remove the bacteria.

Amino Acids. For those oral bacteria whose nutritional requirements have been even partially defined, amino acids are essential. Aspartic and glutamic acids, threonine, serine, glycine, alanine, phenylalanine, leucine, and isoleucine are regularly present in whole saliva but there is considerable variation in proline, cystine, valine, methionine, tyrosine, tryptophan, histidine, lysine, and arginine. The free amino acids in whole saliva ranged from 3.44 to 4.78 mg per 100 ml. Amino acids may provide a source of substrate for salivary microorganisms in the absence of dietary substrates. In addition to free amino acids in saliva, peptides and proteins also may act as a potential source of amino acids.

Vitamins. Vitamins of the B group are essential for the growth of many members of the oral microbiota, particularly streptococci and lactobacilli. Hence, the vitamin B content of saliva could either enhance or limit microbial growth as well as determine the nature of the oral microbiota. Little or no vitamin A is normally present in saliva. The ascorbic acid (vitamin C) content of saliva averages less than that of whole blood, urine, or gastric juice. There is no correlation between the vitamin C contents of saliva and other body fluids. The concentrations of B vitamins present in whole saliva, as reported by various investigators, shows considerable variation. One study found pantothenate in whole saliva only after it was incubated, suggesting that microbial activity is a source of vitamins in saliva. Oral yeast, particularly *Candida albicans*, are a potent source of vitamins essential to oral lactic acid bacteria, particularly lactobacilli. Many other common oral bacteria are sources of B vitamins. Nevertheless, the actual amounts of these vitamins in saliva are barely adequate, particularly for lactic acid bacteria.

As demonstrated in a study of 18 strains of oral streptococci, vitamin requirements do not appear to be related to cariogenicity, nor do they account for the preferential colonization of various sites in the oral cavity. However, they may affect the overall ecological picture of the oral flora.

ANTIBACTERIAL PROPERTIES

Bacterial Antagonism

Saliva has a number of antibacterial properties whose origin and specificity are difficult to define; undoubtedly some are attributable to antagonisms between particular microorganisms. Thus, oral streptococci are antagonistic to some other streptococci and to common airborne bacteria such as staphylococci, gram positive spore-forming bacilli, and gram negative bacilli; streptococci, staphylococci, and pneumococci are antagonistic to lactobacilli; staphylococci are antagonistic to encapsulated bacteria such as *Klebsiella pneumoniae*; and so on *ad infinitum*. Despite this, many organisms can exist in environments where their antagonists are present.

Although bacterial antagonisms are generally believed to be of great importance in the regulation of the oral microbiota, there has only been a limited amount of direct experimental proof of their effect. In gnotobiotic experimental animals, for example, bacteriocin-producing strains of streptococci have been shown to have a competitive advantage over nonproducers when inoculated together.

Notwithstanding the paucity of detailed information about the role of bacterial antagonistic activities in the mouth, it is probable that many bacteria not normally present may be unable to become inhabitants because of them.

Lysozyme and Peroxidase

Although whole saliva inhibits such organisms as streptococci or lactobacilli, there is little evidence to indicate the origin of the inhibitory factors. A notable exception is salivary lysozyme, derived from salivary glands and leukocytes, which tends to limit the oral flora because it lyses some species of common bacteria by hydrolysis of the cell wall mureins. The lysozyme content of saliva is about the same as that of blood but much less than that of other areas of the body where bacteria are not abundant; it is about 1/300 that of tears and about 1/45 that of nasal mucus.

Another system in saliva which inhibits the growth of a number of microorganisms is salivary peroxidase. This system consists of peroxidase, thiocyanate, and hydrogen peroxide. The levels of thiocyanate in the saliva have been shown to be more than adequate for this system to function and the requirement for hydrogen peroxide may be met by microbial metabolism. Under these conditions, growth inhibition is limited to those bacteria which accumulate hydrogen peroxide, or to adjacent organisms. Introduction of an exogenous source of peroxide can make other organisms susceptible.

Antibodies

A possible role for antibodies in defense mechanisms has been discussed for many years. Presently, salivary immunoglobulins are recognized as potentially important factors for local host resistance to oral disease. IgA is the predominant immunoglobulin class in saliva and other secretions, although other classes have also been demonstrated.

Secretory IgA has been demonstrated to provide protection in viral infection, and it also plays a role in bacterial infections. One role may be its effect on bacterial adherence. Secretory IgA has been reported to bind to and agglutinate bacteria. It is not generally considered to be bactericidal or opsonic, but may exert its protective function by aggregating bacteria, altering their ability to adhere to and colonize surfaces. This function could serve, in part, to control the balance of the indigenous flora, as well as exerting a protective function by limiting exogenous pathogens. While pathogens may enter the oral cavity, adhere to various structures and multiply, their advantage would be only temporary. Once IgA increases to a sufficient level, the bacteria would be aggregated and their colonization impaired, permitting them to be washed away and eliminated.

An interesting recent finding has been the production of proteases which are able to break down immunoglobulin A1 by certain pathogenic bacteria. This property has been observed in meningitis-producing species, such as *Neisseria meningitidis*, *Haemophilus influenzae* and *Streptococcus pneumoniae* and in the etiological agent of gonorrhoea. It has also been found in the oral streptococcal species, *Streptococcus sanguis* and *Streptococcus mitior*. Further studies have revealed proteases capable of degrading IgA, IgA2 and IgG in several gram negative species suspected as periodontal pathogens, and it has been suggested that these enzymes may be significant virulence factors.

SALIVA AS A CULTURE MEDIUM

Throughout the preceding discussion of saliva we have indicated wherever possible the role of individual components in the ecology of the oral microbiota. Generally speaking, whole saliva seems to be a poor culture medium for many oral microorganisms, particularly *in vitro*. For example, it does not sustain growth of resident lactobacilli unless appropriate carbohydrates are added; even with added carbohydrates, the resident lactobacilli grow suboptimally. Also, there is doubt whether whole saliva *in vitro* is able to supply the nitrogenous components necessary for growth of lactobacilli. A strain of *Lactobacillus acidophilus* which grew on a medium composed of casein hydrolysate, tryptophane, mono- and dipotassium phosphates, thiamine hydrochloride, nicotinic acid, calcium pantothenate, and dextrose did not grow at all in whole saliva and grew less than optimally in saliva concentrated as much as 7-fold. It was suggested that whole saliva failed to sustain *in vitro* growth because of deficiencies in amino acids and other nitrogenous components that were supplied by the casein hydrolysate. However, acid or alkaline hydrolysis liberates sufficient amino acids to sustain growth of lactobacilli. Thus, slow bacterial hydrolysis of protein occurring in incubated whole saliva may supply sufficient amino acids, accounting for the slow growth of lactobacilli in incubated saliva.

Many, but not all, samples of bacteria-free parotid secretions are able to serve as a source of nutrients for several species of bacteria to sustain a limited growth of staphylococci, enterococci, *Aerobacter* strains, yeasts, and the spores and vegetative cells of the *Bacillus* species, but none supports the growth of lactobacilli, β- or viridans streptococci, and *Corynebacterium diphtheriae*. A portion of the deficiency of the parotid secretion is attributable to the unfavorably alkaline pH, correction of which with buffer makes a more favorable culture medium. Considering the amino acid deficiency of parotid secretion, it is not surprising that it does not support the growth of bacteria requiring amino acids; it is perhaps surprising that it supports germination of spores, which require a nitrogen source, carbon source, and precursors of nucleic acid. The organic acids in saliva are used only to a slight extent by the oral flora. Carbohydrates derived from salivary glycoproteins can be used by the oral flora. However, the proportion of metabolic activity that could be attributed to this source was not more than 20%.

Clearly, in spite of our considerable knowledge of the physiology of saliva, we can explain only in small part how the oral environment supports such an extraordinarily heterogeneous, yet generally balanced, group of microorganisms, many of which have some of the most exacting nutritional and environmental requirements known.

ADDITIONAL READINGS

Ashamaony, L., Goodfellow, M., Minnikin, D. E., Bowden, G. H. W., and Hardie, J. M. 1977 Fatty and Mycolic Acid Composition of *Bacterionema matruchotii* and Related Organisms. J Gen Microbiol, **98**, 205.

Beighton, D., Russell, R. R. B., and Hayday, H. 1981 The Isolation and Characterization of *Streptococcus mutans* Serotype *h* from Dental Plaque of Monkeys (*Macaca fascicularis*) J Gen Microbiol, **124**, 271.

Berg, J-O., and Nord, C-E. 1972 Isolation of Peptococci and Peptostreptococci in Developing Human Dental Plaque by Maintaining Continuous Anaerobiosis. Acta Odont Scand, **30**, 503.

Berkeley, R. C. W., Lynch, J. M., Melling, J., Rutter, P. R., and Vincent, B., (Eds.) 1980 Microbial Adhesion to Surfaces. Ellis Horwood.

Berkowitz, R. J., Jordan, H. V., and White, G. 1975 The Early Establishment of *Streptococcus mutans* in the Mouths of Infants. Arch Oral Biol, **20**, 171.

Bowden, G. H., and Hardie, J. M. 1973 Commensal and Pathogenic *Actinomyces* Species in Man. In *Actinomycetales: Characteristics and Practical Importance*, p. 277. G. Sykes and F. A. Skinner, eds. Academic Press.

Bowden, G. H., Hardie, J. M., and Slack, G. L. 1975 Microbial Variations in Approximal Dental Plaque. Caries Res, **9**, 253.

Bowden, G. H., and Hardie, J. M. 1978 Oral Pleomorphic (coryneform) Gram-Positive Rods. In *Coryneform Bacteria.*, p. 235. I. J. Bousefield and A. G. Cally, eds. Academic Press.

Bowden, G. H. W., Ellwood, D. C., and Hamilton, I. R. 1979 Microbial Ecology of the Oral Cavity. In *Advances in Microbial Ecology*, vol., 3, M. Alexander, ed. Plenum Press.

Bowden, W. H. 1970 Effects of Foods on Oral Bacterial Populations in Man and Animals. J Dent Res, **49**, 1276.

Bratthall, D. 1970 Demonstration of Five Serological Groups of Streptococcal Strains Resembling *Streptococcus mutans*. Odontol Rev, **21**, 143.

Brooks, G. F., O'Donoghue, J. M., Rissing, J. P., Soapes, K., and Smith, J. W. 1974 *Eikenella corrodens*, a Recently Recognized Pathogen. Medicine, **53**, 325.

Carlsson, J. 1967 Presence of Various Types of Nonhaemolytic Streptococci in Dental Plaque and in Other Sites of the Oral Cavity in Man. Odontol Rev, **18**, 55.

Carlsson, J., Soderholm, G., and Almfelt, I. 1969 Prevalence of *Streptococcus sanguis* and *Streptococcus mutans* in the Mouth of Persons Wearing Full Dentures. Arch Oral Biol, **14**, 243.

Carlsson, J., Grahnen, H. Jonsson, G., and Wikner, S. 1970 Establishment of *Streptococcus sanguis* in the Mouth of Infants. Arch Oral Biol, **15**, 1143.

Carlsson, J., and Gothefors, L. 1975 Transmission of *Lactobacillus jensenii* and *Lactobacillus acidophilus* from Mother to Child at Time of Delivery. J Clin Microbiol, **1**, 124.

Carlsson, J., Grahnen, H., and Jonsson, G. 1975 Lactobacilli and Streptococci in the Mouth of Children. Caries Res, **9**, 333.

Collins, P. A., Gerencser, M. A., and Slack, J. M. 1973 Enumeration and Identification of Actinomycetaceae in Human Dental Calculus Using the Fluorescent Antibody Technique. Arch Oral Biol, **18**, 145.

Cowman, R. A., Perrella, M. M., and Fitzgerald, R. J. 1974 Influence of Incubation Atmosphere on Growth and Amino Acid Requirements of *Streptococcus mutans*. Appl Microbiol, **27**, 86.

Coykendall, A. L. 1977 Proposal to Elevate the Subspecies of *Streptococcus mutans* to Species Status, Based on Their Molecular Composition. Int J Syst Bacteriol, **27**, 26.

COYKENDALL, A. L., AND MUNZENMAIER, A. J. 1979 Deoxyribonucleic Acid Hybridization Among Strains of *Actimomyces viscosus* and *Actinomyces naeslundii.* Int J Syst Bacteriol, **29,** 234.

COYKENDALL, A. L., KACZMAREK, F. S., AND SLOTS, J. 1980 Genetic Heterogeneity in *Bacteroides asaccharolyticus* (Holdeman and Moore, 1970) Finegold and Barnes, 1977 (Approved Lists, 1980) and Proposal of *Bacteroides gingivalis* sp. nov. and *Bacteroides macacae* (Slots and Genco) comb. nov. Int J Syst Bacteriol. **30,** 559.

DENT, V. E. 1982 Identification of Oral *Neisseria* Species of Animals. J Appl Bacteriol, **52,** 21.

DREIZEN, S., SPIRAKIS, C. N., AND STONE, R. E. 1966 Human Tooth Structure as a Bacterial Culture Medium. J Dent Res, **45,** 976.

ELLWOOD, D. C., MELLING, J., AND RUTTER, P. (Eds.) 1979 Adhesion of Microorganisms to Surfaces. Academic Press.

ESKOW, R. N., AND LOESCH, W. J. 1971 Oxygen Tensions in the Human Oral Cavity. Arch Oral Biol, **16,** 1127.

FILLERY, E. D., BOWDEN, G. H., AND HARDIE, J. M. 1978 A Comparison of Strains of Bacteria Designated *Actinomyces viscosus* and *Actinomyces naeslundii.* Caries Res, **12,** 299.

GIBBONS, R. J., AND BANGHART, S. B. 1967 Synthesis of Extracellular Dextran by Cariogenic Bacteria and Its Presence in Human Dental Plaque. Arch Oral Biol, **12,** 11.

GIBBONS, R. J., AND VAN HOUTE, J. 1975 Bacterial Adherence in Oral Microbial Ecology. Annu Rev Microbiol, **29,** 19.

GIBBONS, R. J., SPINELL, D. M., AND SKOBE, Z. 1976 Selective Adherence as a Determinant of the Host Tropisms of Certain Indigenous and Pathogenic Bacteria. Infect Immun, **13,** 238.

GOLD, O. G., JORDAN, H. V., AND VAN HOUTE, J. 1975 The Prevalence of Enterococci in the Human Mouth and their Pathogenicity in Animal Models. Arch Oral Biol, **20,** 473.

GREEN, G. E. 1966 Inherent Defense Mechanism in Saliva. J Dent Res, **45,** 624.

GUGGENHEIM, B. 1968 Streptococci of Dental Plaques. Caries Res, **2,** 147.

HAMADA, S., AND SLADE, J. D. 1980 Biology, Immunology, and Cariogenicity of *Streptococcus mutans.* Microbiol Rev, **44,** 331.

HAMMOND, B. F. 1967 Studies on Encapsulated Lactobacilli. III. Human Oral Strains. J Dent Res, **46,** 340.

HARDIE, J. M., AND BOWDEN, G. H. 1971 Carbohydrate Components of the Cell Walls of *Streptococcus mutans* and the Possible Value in Serological Grouping. Caries Res, **6,** 80.

HARDIE, J. M., AND BOWDEN, G. H. 1974 The Normal Microbial Flora of the Mouth. In *The Normal Microbial Flora of Man*, p. 47, F. A. Skinner and J. G. Carr, eds. Academic Press, London.

HARDIE, J. M., AND BOWDEN, G. H. 1976 Physiological Classification of Oral Viridans Streptococci. J Dent Res, **55,** A166.

HARDIE, J. M., AND MARSH, P. D. 1978 Streptococci and the Human Oral Flora. In *Streptococci*, p. 157. F. A. Skinner and L. Quesnell, eds. Academic Press, New York.

HARDIE, J. M., AND SHAH, H. N. 1982 Factors Controlling the Microbial Flora of the Mouth. Eur J Chemother Antibiot, **2,** 3.

HAY, D. I., AND HARTLES, R. L. 1965 Effect of Saliva on Metabolism of the Oral Flora. Arch Oral Biol, **10,** 485.

HEIMDAHL, A., AND NORD, C-E. 1979 Effect of Phenoxymethylpenicillin and Clindamycin on the Oral, Throat and Faecal Microflora of Man. Scand J Infect Dis, **11,** 233.

HOLDEMAN, L. V., CATO, E. P., AND MOORE, W. E. C. (Eds.) 1977 *Anaerobe Laboratory Manual.* 4th edition. Virginia Polytechnic Institute and State University Anaerobe Laboratory, Blacksburg.

HOLDEMAN, L. V., CATO., E. P. BURMEISTER, J. A., AND MOORE, W. E. C. 1980 Descriptions of *Eubacterium timidum* sp. Nov., *Eubacterium brachy* sp. nov. and *Eubacterium nodatum* sp. nov., isolated from human periodontitis. Int J Sys Bacteriol, **30,** 163.

HOLDEMAN, L. V., JOHNSON, J. L., AND MOORE, W. E. C. 1981 Pigmenting *Bacteroides* in Periodontal Samples. J Dent Res, **60,** Special Issue A, 414.

HOLDEMAN, L. V., MOORE, W. E. C., CHURN, P. J., AND JOHNSON, J. L. 1982 *Bacteroides oris* and *Bacteroides buccae*, New Species from Human Periodontitis and Other Human Infections. Int J Syst Bacteriol, **32,** 125.

HOLMBERG, K., AND HALLANDER, H. O. 1972 Interference Between Gram-Positive Microorganisms in Dental Plaque. J Dent Res, **51,** 588.

HUXLEY, H. G. 1973 The Effect of Inoculating Strains of *Streptococcus mutans* and *Streptococcus sanguis* Upon Caries Incidence and Bacterial Content of Plaque in Rats. Arch Oral Biol, **18,** 1215.

JACKSON, F. L., AND GOODMAN, Y. E. 1978 *Bacteroides ureolyticus*, a new species to accomodate strains previously identified as "*Bacteroides corrodens* anaerobic." Int J Syst Bacteriol, **28,** 197.

JORDAN, H. V., AND HAMMOND, B. F. 1972 Filamentous Bacteria Isolated from Human Root Surface Caries. Arch Oral Biol, **17,** 1333.

KASHKET, S., AND DONALDSON, C. G. 1972 Saliva-Induced Aggregation of Oral Streptococci. J Bacteriol, **112,** 1127.

KELLSTRUP, J. 1966 The Incidence of *Bacteroides melaninogenicus* in Human Gingival Sulci and Its Prevalence in the Oral Cavity at Different Ages. Periodontics, **4,** 14.

KILIAN, M. 1976 A Taxonomic Study of the Genus *Haemophilus.* with the Proposal of a New Species. J Gen Microbiol, **93,** 9.

KILIAN, M. 1981 Degradation of Immunoglobulins A1, A2 and G by Suspected Principal Periodontal Pathogens. Infect Immun, **34,** 757.

KLEINBERG, I., CHATTERJEE, R., REDDY, J., AND CRAW, D. 1977 Effects of Fluoride on the Metabolism of the Mixed Oral Flora. Caries Res, **11,** (Suppl 1) 292.

KLEINBERG, I., ELLISON, S. A., AND MANDEL, I. D. (eds.) 1979 *Saliva and Dental Caries.* Information Retrieval Inc., New York.

KORNMAN, K. S., AND HOLT, S. C. 1981 Physiological and Ultrastructural Characterization of a New *Bacteroides* Species (*B. capillus*) Isolated from Severe Periodontitis. J Peridont Res, **16,** 542.

KUMAGAI, K., IWABUCHI, T., HINUMA, Y., YURI, K., AND ISHIDA, N. 1971 Incidence, Species, and Significance of *Mycoplasma* Species in the Mouth. J Infect Dis, **123,** 16.

LAMBE, D. W., GENCO, R. J., AND MAYBERRY-CARSON, K. J. (Eds.) 1980 *Anaerobic Bacteria: Selected Topics.* Plenum Press, New York.

LEACH, S. A. ed. 1980 Dental Plaque and Surface Interactions in the Oral Cavity. Information Retrieval Inc., London.

LEADBETTER, E. R., HOLT, S. C., AND SOCRANSKY, S. S. 1979 *Capnocytophaga*: New Genus of Gram Negative Gliding Bacteria. I. General Characteristics, Taxonomic Considerations and Significance. Arch Microbiol, **122,** 9.

LENNETTE, E. H., BALOWS, A., HAUSLER, W. J., AND TRUANT, J. P. (Eds.) 1980 *Manual of Clinical Microbiology*, 3rd edition, American Society for Microbiology, Washington, D.C.

LESHER, R. J., GERENCSER, M. A., AND GERENCSER, V.

F. 1974 Morphological, Biochemical, and Serological Characterization of *Rothia dentocariosa*. Int J Syst Bacteriol, **24**, 154.

LILJEMARK, W. F., AND GIBBONS, R. J. 1971 Ability of *Veillonella* and *Neisseria* Species to Attach to Oral Surfaces and Their Proportions Present Indigenously. Infect Immun, **4**, 264.

LOESCHE, W. J., AND SYED, S. A. 1973 The Predominant Cultivable Flora of Carious Plaque and Carious Dentine. Caries Res, **7**, 201.

LONG, S. S., AND SWENSON, R. M. 1976 Determinants of the Developing Oral Flora in Normal Newborns. Appl Environ Microbiol, **32**, 494.

MANDEL, I. D., THOMPSON, R. H., JR., AND ELLISON, S. A. 1965 Studies of the Mucoproteins of Human Parotid Saliva. Arch Oral Biol, **10**, 499.

MARSH, P. D. 1980 *Oral Microbiology*. Thomas Nelson and Sons Ltd., London.

MAYS, T. D., HOLDEMAN, L. V., MOORE, W. E. C., ROGOSA, M., AND JOHNSON, J. L. 1982 Taxonomy of the Genus *Veillonella* Prévot. Int J Syst Bacteriol, **32**, 28.

MCCARTHY, C., SNYDER, M. L., AND PARKER, R. B. 1965 The Indigenous Oral Flora of Man. I. The Newborn to the 1-year-old Infant. Arch Oral Biol, **10**, 61.

MEJARE, B., AND EDWARDSSON, S. 1975 *Streptococcus milleri* (Guthof); An Indigenous Organism of the Human Oral Cavity. Arch Oral Biol, **20**, 757.

MOLAN, P. C., AND HARTLES, R. L. 1971 The Nature of the Intrinsic Salivary Substrates Used by the Human Oral Flora. Arch Oral Biol, **16**, 1449.

MORHART, R. E., AND FITZGERALD, R. J. 1976 Nutritional Determinants of the Ecology of the Oral Flora. Dent Clin North Am, **20**, 473.

NEWMAN, H. N., AND McKAY, G. S. 1973 An Unusual Microbial Configuration in Human Dental Plaque. Microbios, **8**, 117.

OFEK, I., BEACHEY, E. H., EYAL, F., AND MORRISON, J. C. 1977 Postnatal Development of Binding of Streptococci and Lipoteichoic Acid by Oral Mucosal Cells of Humans. J Infect Dis, **135**, 267.

PARKER, R. B. 1970 Paired Culture Interaction of the Oral Microbiota. J Dent Res, **49**, 804.

PERCH, B. E., KJEMS, E., AND RAVN, T. 1974 Biochemical and serological properties of *Streptococcus mutans* from various human and animal sources. Acta Pathol Microbiol Scand, **82**, 357.

RASMUSSEN, E. G., GIBBONS, R. J., AND SOCRANSKY, S. S. 1966 Taxonomic Study of 50 Gram-positive Anaerobic Diphtheroids Isolated from the Oral Cavity. Arch Oral Biol, **11**, 573.

ROGERS, A. H. 1973 The Vitamin Requirements of Some Oral Streptococci. Arch Oral Biol, **18**, 227.

RØLLA, G., SØNJU, T., AND EMBERY, G. (Eds.) 1980 Tooth Surface Interactions and Preventive Dentistry. IRL Press Ltd.

ROTH, G. D., AND FLANAGAN, V. 1969 The Pathogenicity of *Rothia dentocariosa* Inoculated into Mice. J Dent Res, **48**, 957.

SCHOFIELD, G. M., AND SCHAAL, K. P. 1981 A Numerical Taxonomic Study of Members of the Actinomycetaceae and Related Taxa. J Gen Microbiol, **127**, 237.

SHAH, H. N., WILLIAMS, R. A. D., BOWDEN, G. H., AND HARDIE, J. M. 1976 Comparison of Biochemical Properties of *Bacteroides melaninogenicus* from Human Dental Plaque and Other Sites. J Appl Bacteriol, **41**, 473.

SHAH, H. N., BONNETT, R., MATEEN, B., AND WILLIAMS, R. A. D. 1979 The Porphyrin Pigmentation of Subspecies of *B. melaninogenicus*. Biochem J, **180**, 45.

SHAH, H. N., AND COLLINS, M. D. 1980 Fatty Acid and Isoprenoid Quinon Composition in the Classification of *Bacteroides melaninogenicus* and Related Taxa. J Appl Bacteriol, **48**, 78.

SHAH, H. N., AND COLLINS, M. D. 1981 *Bacteroides buccalis*, sp. nov., *Bacteroides denticola*, sp. nov., and *Bacteroides pentosaceus*, sp. nov., New Species of the Genus *Bacteroides* from the Oral Cavity. Zentralbl Bakteriol Mikrobiol Hyg, I. Abt. Orig. C2, 235.

SHAH, H. N., VAN STEENBERGEN, T. J. M., HARDIE, J. M., AND DE GRAAFF, J. 1982 DNA Base Composition, DNA-DNA Reassociation and Isoelectric-Focusing of Proteins of Strains Designated *Bacteroides oralis*. FEMS. Lett **13**, 125.

SHARPE, M. E. 1979 Identification of the Lactic Acid Bacteria. In *Identification Methods for Microbiologists*, 2nd edition, F. A. Skinner and D. W. Lovelock, eds. Academic Press.

SHKLAIR, I. L., AND KEENE, H. J. 1974 A Biochemical Scheme for the separation of the Five Varieties of *Streptococcus mutans* Arch Oral Biol, **19**, 1079.

SIRISINHA, S., AND CHARUPATANA, C. 1971 Antibodies to Indigenous Bacteria in Human Serum, Secretions, and Urine. Can J Microbiol, **17**, 1471.

SKERMAN, V. D. B., McGOWAN, V., AND SNEATH, P. H. A. (Eds.) 1980 *Approved List of Bacterial Names*. Int J Syst Bacteriol, **30**, 225.

SLACK, J. M., AND GERENCSER, M. A. 1975 *Actinomyces, Filamentous Bacteria. Biology and Pathogenicity*. Burgess Publishing Company, Minneapolis.

SLOTS, J., REYNOLDS, H. S., AND GENCO, R. J. 1980 *Actinobacillus actinomycetemcomitans* in Human Periodontal Disease: a Cross Sectional Microbiological Investigation. Infect Immun, **29**, 1013.

SMIBERT, R. M. 1978 The genus *Campylobacter*. Annu Rev Microbiol, **32**, 673.

SOCRANSKY, S. S., AND MANGANIELLO, S. D. 1971 The Oral Microbiota of Man from Birth to Senility. J Periodontol, **42**, 485.

SOCRANSKY, S. S., HOLT, S. C., LEADBETTER, E. R., TANNER, A. C. R., SAVITT, E., AND HAMMOND, B. F. 1979 *Capnocytophaga*: A New Genus of Gram-Negative Gliding Bacteria. III. Physiological Characterization. Arch Microbiol, **122**, 29.

SYED, S. A., AND LOESCHE, W. J. 1973 Efficiency of Various Growth Media in Recovering Oral Bacterial Flora from Human Dental Plaque. Appl Microbiol, **26**, 459.

TANNER, A. C. R., BADGER, S., LAI, C-H., LISTGARTEN, M. A., VISCONTI, R. A., AND SOCRANSKY, S. S. 1981 *Wolinella* gen. nov., *Wolinella succinogenes* (*Vibrio succinogenes* Wolin *et al.*) comb. nov., and Description of *Bacteroides gracilis* sp. nov., *Wolinella recta* sp. nov., *Campylobacter concisus* sp. nov. and *Eikenella corrodens* from Humans with Periodontal Disease. Int J Syst Bacteriol, **31**, 432.

TAUBMAN, M. A. 1974 Immunoglobulins of Human Dental Plaque. Arch Oral Biol, **19**, 439.

VAN HOUTE, J., GIBBONS, R. J., AND PULKKINEN, A. J. 1972 Ecology of Human Oral Lactobacilli. Infect Immun, **6**, 723.

VAN STEENBERGEN, T. J. M., VLAANDEREN, C. A., AND DE GRAAFF, J. 1981 Confirmation of *Bacteroides gingivalis* as a Species Distinct from *Bacteroides asaccharolyticus*. Int J Syst Bacteriol, **31**, 236.

WATT, B., AND JACK, E. P. 1977 What are Anaerobic Cocci? J Med Microbiol, **10**, 461.

WILLIAMS, R. C., AND GIBBONS, R. J. 1972 Inhibition of Bacterial Adherence by Secretory Immunoglobulin A: A Mechanism of Antigen Disposal. Science, **177**, 697.

WILLIAMS, R. C., AND GIBBONS, R. J. 1975 Inhibition of Streptococcal Attachment to Receptors on Human Buccal Epithelial Cells by Antigenically Similar Salivary Glycoproteins. Infect Immun, **11**, 711.

chapter 16

Dental Caries

Charles F. Schachtele

DEFINITION AND MAGNITUDE OF THE PROBLEM

In dentistry, the term caries (Latin, decay; rottenness; dry rot) refers to a disease where the calcified tissues of the teeth are modified and eventually dissolved. Due to the frequency of occurrence of this destructive process dental caries must be ranked as one of the more significant diseases affecting humans. In the United States greater than 95% of the population has experienced caries. In spite of the minimal life-threatening potential of this disease the consequences of caries development are great. The disease is costly, can cause considerable discomfort and can have a significant effect on personality and overall health.

Dental scientists have made great progress toward understanding the etiology of caries formation in humans. Starting with the basic premise that carious lesions result from "localized, progressive decay of the teeth, initiated by demineralization of the outer surface of the tooth due to organic acids produced locally by bacteria that ferment deposits of dietary carbohydrates" knowledge has evolved to where it is known that this disease involves a unique complexity of interactions. These are between the dentition, as a part of the entire oral cavity, the oral bacterial flora, as a part of the total human indigenous microbiota, and the diet, as an essential intermittent source of cariogenic substrates and anticariogenic components. By elucidating the intimate details of these interactions dental researchers are continuously supplying new leads for disease control and/or prevention. In order to evaluate the status of current attempts to eliminate caries as a public health problem we must have an understanding of the status of research on each facet of the disease process as well as an appreciation for the unique status of caries as an infectious disease.

In the context of oral microbiology and infectious disease it must be emphasized that dental caries is considered to be an endogenous bacterial disease. This is in contrast to an exogenous microbial disease where the pathogen is relatively foreign to the host and creates an infection upon colonization of a susceptible site or sites. Caries involves bacteria that have latent pathogenic potential and which are indigenous to and ubiquitously found in the human oral cavity. The disease results from the development of conditions where the resistance of the host is lowered and specific bacterial strains can proliferate to elevated levels and express detrimental traits. The challenge to oral microbiologists and other dental scientists is to understand how and why this transition from a friendly symbiotic state to a harmful relationship takes place at specific times and at unique locations in the human dentition.

THE CARIOUS PROCESS

Tooth Structure and Chemistry

The mature erupted human tooth is made up of four distinct tissues: pulp, dentin, cementum and enamel (fig. 16/1). Each of these tissues has been biochemically analyzed and their detailed ultrastructure studied using sophisticated instrumentation. Although much of our understanding of the details of carious lesion development have resulted from studies on the outermost tissue, the enamel, the other three tissues have been shown to have important roles in lesions as they progress from the incipient to the cavitation stage. Indeed, as the disease progresses through the enamel toward the pulp the microenvironment of the lesion changes. This may be reflected in the complex microbial etiology of caries where various types of bacteria appear to be involved in the different phases of tooth destruction.

Pulp. This tissue makes up the core of the tooth and it has been described as a special type of connective tissue. It is like most other soft tissues which, on the average, contain 25% organic material and 75% water. The basic structural entities of the dental pulp are connective tissue cells, fibers and ground substance. The cells of this tissue are predominantly fibroblasts but undifferentiated mesenchymal cells, macrophages, lymphocytes, plasma cells and eosinophilic granulocytes can occasionally

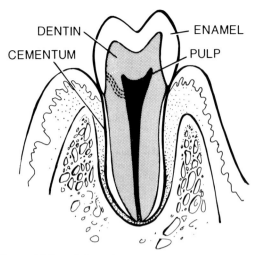

DENTIN — ENAMEL
CEMENTUM — PULP

Figure 16/1. Schematic drawing illustrating the four tissues of a human tooth. The *dashed lines* indicate the relative location of representative dentinal tubules.

be observed. In inflammed pulps mast cells can be found. The fibers in the pulp are mainly collagenous in nature, are not predominant in young pulp, but increase in number with age. The ground substance of the pulp includes a complexity of molecules including complex carbohydrates, glycoproteins and acid mucopolysaccharides. The carbohydrate complexes are more predominant during tooth development and decrease in quantity during tooth aging. It is important to emphasize that the presence of this wide range of materials which can provide many bacterial growth substrates and water under conditions where the pulp is exposed to the oral environment, due to caries or an accident, sets up a situation where serious bacterial infections can occur. Since the pulp contains arteries, veins, lymphatic vessels and nerves, entering through an apical foramen, infections of this tissue provide a portal to the rest of the body and an immediate problem which must be treated.

Dentin. Encasing and physically protecting the pulp is a calcified collagenous tissue called dentin. On a wet weight basis this tissue contains approximately 70% inorganic material, 18% organic material and 12% water. The water phase is labile and its *in situ* concentration is not known. The basic structural entities of dentin are the odontoblast, the odontoblast process, the dentinal tubule, the periodontoblastic space, the peritubular dentin and the intertubular dentin. The odontoblasts are specialized cells whose long cytoplasmic processes, the odontoblast processes, are located within the dentinal tubules and extend through the entire width of the dentin (fig. 16/1). The diameter and volume of the dentinal tubules vary depending on location in the dentin and the age of the tooth. In young teeth the diameter of the tubules may be 4 to 5 μm.

Close to the pulp the lumens of the tubules may make up 80% of the total volume of the dentin. In the peripheral dentin they may make up only about 4% of the dentin volume. On the average there are about 35,000 tubules per square millimeter of dentin. With regard to caries the tubules are clearly large enough and nutritive enough to be invaded by bacteria and serve as a pathway for lesion progression. Although bacteria do not normally penetrate dentin due to the presence of a fine layer of "microcrystalline debris," under conditions where acid has modified the surface bacterial invasion can occur. Acid etching of dentin could occur either from the carious process or during restorative procedures.

The periodontoblastic space intervenes between the wall of the dentinal tubule and the odontoblast process. This region contains tissue fluid and some organic components such as collagen fibers. This is an important area because tissue changes in dentin occur in this location. The peritubular and intertubular dentin are mineralized with the latter containing abundant quantities of collagen. Dentin collagen normally exists tightly complexed to the mineral phase and is not accessible to stains or proteases. It is important that dentin is a vital tissue in that its odontoblasts exchange solutes through their extensions into the tubules. In addition, the odontoblasts can lay down a layer of secondary dentin, relatively lacking in tubules, in response to irritation resulting from caries, operative procedures, erosion and attrition.

The inorganic portion of dentin consists mainly of hydroxyapatite crystals. The crystals are similar in size to those found in cementum and bone but are significantly smaller than those found in enamel. Of the dry weight, dentin contains 26% calcium and 13% phosphorus. Compared to enamel, the Ca-P weight ratio averages 2.05 vs. 2.11. Since dentin forms the structural bulk of the tooth and has a unique chemical and structural composition caries of the dentin is a very critical phase in destruction of the tooth.

Cementum. Radicular dentin is covered by a 20- to 200-μm thick layer of calcified tissue, called cementum, which is laid down in incremental zones of high and low mineral content by cementoblasts derived from the periodontal ligament. Cementum is the least mineralized of the three dental hard tissues being slightly less calcified than dentin. On a wet weight basis the mineral content of cementum is approximately 65%, the organic content constitutes 23%, and the remaining 12% is water.

Like dentin and bone, the organic material of cementum is largely insoluble collagen which is highly cross linked. Cementum anchors the periodontal ligament fibers to the tooth. From midroot to the cementoenamel junction, cementum is acellular; increasingly toward the apex, the cemento-blasts become embedded in the developing mineral phase and are then referred to as cementocytes. Cementum is continuously deposited throughout life and can triple in thickness from 10 to 70 years of age.

Enamel. Coronal dentin is covered by the hardest and most highly calcified tissue normally found in the body, the enamel. Greater than 95% of the mass of enamel is inorganic material which is essentially all in the crystalline state. Mature enamel is acellular and contains minimal amounts, less than 1%, of organic matter. Only about 3% of this tissue is water. It is important that enamel is not the inert system that one would predict from its chemical composition. In fact, within the oral cavity the tooth enamel is an active chemical system participating in ion and solute transport from saliva to dentin, ion-exchange reactions with saliva, and demineralization-remineralization processes. All of these reactions can have an influence on the rate of caries development. To appreciate the formation of carious lesions we must have an understanding of the structural and chemical nature of this unique tissue.

The largest structural components of enamel are the rods or prisms. These entities are approximately 4 to 6 μm in diameter and can be up to 3 mm long. In most cases the rods extend perpendicularly from the enamel-dentin junction to the tooth surface. In cross section the rods have a characteristic "keyhole" shape. The dense packing of the rods give enamel most of its physical properties, such as hardness, which we normally associate with the teeth. Closer inspection reveals that the rods are composed of millions of small elongated crystallites arranged in a characteristic pattern. The crystallites are approximately 1,000 angstroms in length and are thus 5 to 10 times larger than crystallites in bone. The large size of the enamel crystallites is an important factor in maintaining the structural integrity of enamel and markedly influences the ability of teeth to resist the disruptive effects of the continuously changing conditions in the oral cavity.

The enamel crystallites are made up of thousands of stacked subunits called unit cells. These cells are about 10 angstroms across and are made up of a highly ordered arrangement of atoms including oxygen, hydrogen, calcium and phosphorus. X-ray diffraction analysis of enamel reveals patterns that are characteristic of apatite structures. Apatite represents a general class of minerals characterized by similar stoichiometry and crystal structure. Chemically, apatites have compositions that are variants of the formula D_5T_3M where D is a divalent cation; T is a trivalent, tetrahedral, compound anion, and M is a monovalent anion. The unit cell of apatite crystals contain two of the formula units and thus

has the formula $D_{10}T_6M_2$. The mineral components of enamel are often described as impure forms of hydroxyapatite $Ca_{10}(PO_4)_6(OH)_2$. The basic formula of hydroxyapatite allows many partial substitutions without changing the crystal lattice. To some extent calcium may be replaced by strontium, barium, lead and radium; phosphate may be partially replaced by carbonate, arsenate, and vanadate; hydroxyl may be replaced by fluoride and chloride. A broad range of ions can be incorporated secondarily 1) in the hydration shell that surrounds each crystal, 2) absorbed to the crystal surface, and 3) within the body of the crystal. Since hydroxyapatite behaves as a highly active ion-exchange medium, after eruption the outer layer of enamel acquires a number of ions, depending mainly on dietary intake.

With regard to caries it is important that variations in enamel composition extend over broader ranges than from unit cell to unit cell. The chemical composition of enamel varies considerably from person to person, from tooth to tooth, and from site to site within a given section of enamel. In addition to the influence of ions present in the oral cavity at any given time the enamel composition is also determined by the presence and concentration of various ions at different stages of tooth development. Concentrations of several of the components can be shown to vary depending upon the distance from the tooth surface. For example, the concentration of fluoride is normally higher in samples of enamel close to the tooth surface and the concentration decreases toward the enamel-dentin junction. On the other hand, carbonate concentrations follow a reverse pattern, where the level is lower at the tooth surface and the concentration increases toward the enamel-dentin junction. Some ions such as strontium appear to be uniformly distributed through enamel. It is clear that dental enamel is not a simple substance, but contains a large variety of minor components that can be distributed in various patterns within the mineral. The solubility of the enamel has been shown to be influenced by the presence of the minor components in that carbonate, magnesium, sodium and citrate can increase dissolution while fluoride decreases it.

Hydroxyapatite can exist in equilibrium with an aqueous phase at neutrality where its solubility is such that the product of calcium and phosphate ion activities in the solution is equivalent to about 100 mg per liter of the ions. The daily oral passage of more than a liter of saliva might be expected to leach out tooth mineral. Significant leaching does not occur because saliva is normally supersaturated with respect to calcium and phosphate. Only when the pH of the environment reaches about 5.2 will the supersaturation of saliva be overcome and loss of mineral from the enamel commence. This level of acidity has been termed the critical pH for initiation of caries but it is an operational concept and not subject to exact calculation. The exact pH at which tooth mineral begins to be lost *in situ* is an important issue which will be discussed with regard to attempts to evaluate the cariogenic potential of various foods.

Caries Mechanism

Chemical analyses have clearly demonstrated that the main process occurring in caries development is one of demineralization followed by replacement of the dissolved mineral with loosely bound water. For simplicity one can discuss the mechanism of caries formation as involving acid dissolution of enamel. The alternate but unproven mechanism, primary dissolution of the protein phase followed by demineralization, cannot be absolutely excluded, but to date no one has succeeded in biologically degrading tooth protein without demineralizing it. In enamel, demineralization suffices also to destroy the protein phase. Enamel protein evidently goes into solution concomitantly with sufficient loss of mineral. In dentin, demineralization leaves the collagenous matrix intact. This residue is either digested by proteolytic bacteria or converted to a leathery material.

To the unaided eye, caries first becomes discernible as a "white spot" (incipient caries), an apparent opacity of partially demineralized subsurface enamel. Early white spot lesions are not easily distinguishable from areas of developmental hypocalcification. Long before this stage, however, the initiation of coronal caries is delineated by microscopic changes.

Demineralization does not proceed uniformly within enamel but selectively along regular pathways. The earliest structural changes include roughening of exposed ends of enamel rods, resulting in grain-like defects and spreading to the inter-rod area. Individual crystallites become smaller, widening the spaces between them. These spaces tend to fill with organic matter (acquired pellicle), which might actually slow the carious process. Surface indentations appear in the acquired pellicle and underlying enamel surface, conforming to the shape and location of plaque bacteria. Even as demineralization proceeds, a relatively intact surface zone averaging 30 μm deep remains over an increasingly radiolucent area. Demineralizing agents apparently diffuse through an outer, less readily soluble layer of involved enamel at one or more undefined microscopic points of entry. Whatever the points of entry, demineralization radiates primarily laterally along striae of Retzius beneath the intact surface zone, gradually creating a roughly cone-shaped lesion with its base parallel to the surface. Examination by transmitted polarized light

reveals a translucent zone at the advancing edge of the lesion, indicating the presence of about 1% of spaces only large enough to admit molecules the size of water or smaller. Toward the surface is a dark, almost opaque, positively birefringent zone, calculated to contain 2 to 4% of larger spaces. The body or central zone of the lesion is negatively birefringent and contains from 5 to 25% of still larger spaces. The surface layer is still highly mineralized and radiopaque. Density measurements indicate an average volume loss of 1% mineral in the translucent zone, 6% in the dark zone, 24% in the body of the lesion, and 10% in the surface layer. The net effect is thinning, shortening, and eventual disappearance of crystallites, creating microcavities, mainly along the striae of Retzius, and enlargement of the interstices between rods. Eventually, such areas merge across adjacent rods. Deeper planes of enamel are attacked via the interstices between rods. Demineralization of rod cores proceeds from their peripheries inward. This whole process may extend as deep as a millimeter and even involve the dentin superficially, while the enamel surface remains grossly intact. Finally, however, this relatively untouched surface zone either demineralizes or collapses from loss of supporting structure. The classic cavity has now developed and bacterial invasion becomes evident. Commonly, demineralization of subjacent dentin has also begun.

The rate of caries development varies greatly. The median rate for occlusal surfaces (mostly fissure caries) is from 20 to 24 months in enamel, with a range from less than 3 to more than 48; the median time to mild dentinal involvement is 36 months. The median time from initial detection in enamel to dentinal involvement is about 4 years, but some lesions do not progress for several additional years or longer. White spot lesions which develop within 1½ years of eruption on free smooth surfaces have been followed to determine their fate. A small proportion soon progress to cavitation, but most remain unchanged for up to 8 years; and a small proportion even revert to "normalcy." These data indicate that remineralization of enamel by saliva is a real and clinically important phenomenon.

In dentin the carious process is characterized by primary bacterial invasion of the tubules; gram positive cocci predominate but gram positive bacilli and filaments are not infrequent. Demineralization proceeds in advance of bacterial growth. The lesion expands most rapidly laterally via cross-connections between tubules but also continues to penetrate inward toward the pulp on a relatively broad front. Further destruction of enamel mostly results from the lateral spread of the destructive process in dentin, which undermines the enamel. After demineralization, the collagenous dentinal matrix is usually lysed by bacterial proteases. Alternatively, in slow or arrested caries the dentin matrix remains as a tough leathery mass.

Unless halted by sclerosis (occlusion of tubules by mineralization), formation of reparative dentin, or reparative dentistry, bacterial invasion of the tubules eventually penetrates to the pulp, which becomes infected and inflamed, and ultimately undergoes necrosis. Subsequent infection, inflammation, and necrosis of the periapical tissue lead to formation of a periapical abscess which may expand into cancellous bone and eventually establish fistulas to a body cavity or to the outside.

Caries in cementum (root surface caries) is characterized by an overlying bacterial mat containing an abundance of filamentous forms. Underneath this mat there is a roughening and softening on a rather broad scale, and brownish discoloration. The lesion may encircle the tooth cervically without spreading apically, and adjacent enamel is often undermined. Demineralization far in advance of the bacteria is not common in cemental caries.

Chemistry of Caries

Acidity. The paramount chemical fact about the carious lesion is that its prevailing acidity is sufficient (pH 5.2 or lower) to account for demineralization. Numerous publications attest to the general acidity of caries in both enamel and dentin, determined both colorimetrically with pH indicators and electrometrically with antimony and glass electrodes. The range observed at different depths of clinically different types of cavities is exemplified by the data in table 16/1. Average acidity is greatest in cavities with small openings and deeper layers. In some cavities judged clinically to be inactive, the pH at the base of the cavity was between 3.5 and 4.8. A neutral or even slightly alkaline reaction in a minority of cavity layers presumably indicates temporary neutralization or a quiescent period.

Neutralization has only a temporary effect, suggesting either continual production of acid or a reservoir of acid in the deeper layers. Cavity acidity can persist for a long time without additional external substrate. The mean pH of an area of a carious lesion need not remain below the critical point for demineralization. The necessary acid condition need prevail only transiently in the hydration shell of the hydroxyapatite.

Associated Chemical Changes. Even superficial demineralization not only exposes the respective organic phases of enamel and dentin to chemical change but also strikingly increases the reactivity of the mineral phase. These changes imply that the close complexing between organic and inorganic phases in the sound tooth reduces the chemical reactivity of both and impedes their solubilization. They imply also the possibility of remineralization by uptake of calcium and phosphate from saliva or redeposition of calcium phosphate. Another possibility is increased resistance to progress of the lesion by increased uptake of fluoride. Fluoride also accelerates remineralization of enamel, for arrested lesions in dentin contain a fluoride-rich surface zone.

Caries removes calcium and phosphate from enamel and dentin in essentially the same proportion as they occur in the sound tissues. Magnesium and carbonate are lost preferentially, indicating that they are held by only weak bonds. Fluoride is not leached from enamel caries *in situ* by acid buffers. Thus, fluoride increases 5-fold in carious enamel and 10-fold in carious dentin.

The fate of the organic phase of enamel during caries is incompletely ascertained. Dentin undergoes proteolysis or turns yellow-to-brown, and undergoes marked change in composition: an average 25% reduction in the content of arginine, hydroxyproline, and proline, doubling of the phenylalanine, and tripling of the tyrosine. These changes result in a collagenase-resistant fraction that is deficient

Table 16/1
Mean pH of carious cavities at different depths[a,b]

Cavity Type[c]	No. of Cavities	Cavity Layers								
		Surface			Intermediate			Bottom		
		pH	S.D.	Range	pH	S.D.	Range	pH	S.D.	Range
I	31	4.9	0.75	3.5–6.6	4.2	0.51	3.2–5.7	3.9	0.40	3.2–4.9
II	42	5.8	0.74	4.0–7.7	4.9	0.74	3.3–7.2	4.5	0.77	3.3–6.8
III	16	6.3	0.63	5.2–7.3	—[d]	—	—	5.4	1.22	3.5–7.3

[a] Adapted from T. R. Dirksen, M. F. Little, and B. G. Bibby: The pH of Carious Cavities; II. The pH at Different Depths of Isolated Cavities. *Archives of Oral Biology*, **8**, 91, 1963.
[b] Isolated from saliva by rubber dam and excavated progressively; pH determined *in situ* by antimony microelectrode. Hours after eating, 1–15; median, 2.
[c] Type I, small clinical opening, thick layer of decay; Type II, large clinical opening, thick layer of decay; and Type III, large clinical opening, thin layer of decay; designated as "inactive" or "arrested."
[d] Thickness of decay insufficient for adequate measurements on intermediate layers.

in arginine but contains 14% carbohydrate. Sound dentin matrix is nearly carbohydrate-free. The resistant fraction results from reactions between demineralized matrix and such sugars as glucose and glucosamine, or intermediary products of their fermentation.

Chemically Induced Enamel Caries. If acids are the cause of dental caries, it should be possible to form a carious lesion simply by immersing a tooth in an acid solution. Actually, it was reported in 1926 that 8 weeks of exposure of teeth *in vitro* to a flow of carbon dioxide-free water etched the enamel surface, producing discernible opaque white spots. However, in most of the many studies of teeth exposed to acid solutions, the changes resembled erosive dissolution of the enamel and not dental caries. Since the mid-1950s, however, numerous investigators have reproduced the successive zones typical of enamel caries by acid demineralization in the pH range 3.4 to 5.5. Enamel was untouched by acidity as low as pH 3.5 if the buffer was initially saturated with calcium phosphate. White spot enamel caries occurs regularly in an organic acid buffer (usually lactate or acetate) in the pH range 3 to 6 (most often 4.5), with strict avoidance of agitation, and inclusion of a colloid. Unless agitation is avoided, simple surface dissolution results. The added colloid simulates the role played *in vivo* by acquired pellicle and overlying plaque.

The nature of the resistant surface layer of enamel is incompletely understood. The outer few micrometers of normal enamel are indeed harder and less soluble than the subjacent tissue. If this outer layer is polished off and the enamel then subjected to an *in vitro* caries test, a radiodense surface zone results nonetheless. There is a transient initial demineralization at the very surface, with regeneration of a seemingly sound surface. Calcium phosphate redeposits from a saturated solution, diffusing outward from the subsurface demineralized area. In natural caries both an inherently more resistant surface layer and redeposition of calcium phosphate are involved.

The entire sequence of events seen in dentinal caries cannot be reproduced by the action of acids alone. The collagenous matrix is resistant to the degree of acidity that prevails in dentinal caries. Changes in the organic phase must be attributed to bacterial invasion. However, the organic phase of dentin must be demineralized to be susceptible to degradative reactions. The abundant organic matter released from dentin and the invading bacteria may sequester calcium in soluble complexes and may be an important ancillary factor in dentinal caries.

Dynamics. Chemical kinetic analyses of physical models of dental caries show that the rate of solution of calcium and phosphate is diffusion controlled. It increases with increasing concentrations of hydrogen ion and of undissociated acid and, using different acids, with decreasing dissociation constants of the acids and of their anionic complex with calcium. Carious demineralization commences then after initial diffusion of undissociated acid (mainly lactic) through the resistant surface layer into subsurface enamel. The ambient concentration of hydrogen ions would be small relative to that of undissociated acid and they would be a minor component of the inward diffusion. Within the hydroxyapatite hydration shell, the acid would dissociate and convert hydroxyapatite into relatively soluble $CaHPO_4 \cdot 2H_2O$, $Ca(H_2PO_4)_2 \cdot H_2O$, and calcium lactate, plus their several cognate ionic species and complexes. The controlling solid surface phase on the enamel crystallite becomes $CaHPO_4 \cdot 2H_2O$. These solutes must diffuse outward to the oral environment, a process that is opposed by the concentrations of calcium and phosphate in plaque, and by the neutralizing action of the salivary bicarbonate system. Controlling diffusion in caries is the permeability of plaque matrix (calcium, phosphate, bicarbonate, bacterial nutrients, particularly sugars, and bacterial metabolic products, particularly acids). Also involved are the permeabilities of acquired pellicle, relatively intact surface layer, partially demineralized subsurface zones, sound portions of enamel, and, ultimately, of dentin.

Whether the outcome in enamel is demineralization, steady state, or remineralization depends on the relative concentrations of the products from a complex series of competing chemical reactions. Demineralization would be most active at the interface between sound enamel and organic acid and would tend toward an equilibrium value in intermediate zones. Remineralization would be most likely near the surface. The key variable is the external concentration of organic acid. The rates of the individual reactions are not critical determinants of the overall outcome, which is controlled by much slower diffusion processes. Mathematical formulations have been derived that describe reasonably well the dissolution rate of enamel during the formation of white spot caries in the experimental models. An important requirement is a correction factor for complex formation between calcium ion and the anion of the demineralizing acid.

ETIOLOGY OF CARIES

Dental caries has a multifactorial etiology. The now classic triad of host, microbial and substrate factors should probably be joined by a time factor since this parameter emphasizes the need for a simultaneous interaction of the various contributors to the disease (fig. 16/2).

A.

B.

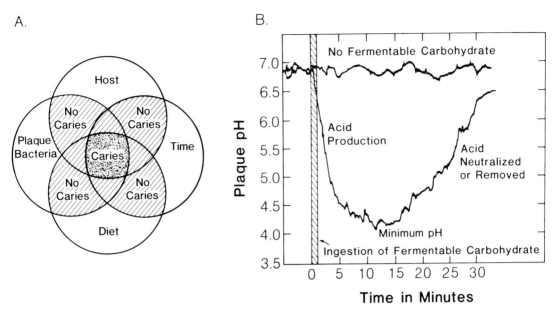

Figure 16/2. (*A*) Interaction of factors known to be involved in the etiology of human dental caries. (*B*) Stephan curve illustrating response observed following interaction of plaque bacteria on the surface of the tooth with dietary fermentable carbohydrate. The pH drops as acid is produced and returns towards neutrality with time.

Bacteria and Caries

One of the most fascinating and rapidly progressing areas of microbiology involves studies on the indigenous oral flora of man. The stimulus for interest in oral microbiology involved a series of discoveries that showed that caries was a transmissible disease dependent upon bacteria with unique properties. The discovery and analysis of *Streptococcus mutans* has led to an understanding of a bacterium which has essentially every feature that you could desire in a microorganism designed to cause the production of carious lesions. *S. mutans* lives only on the teeth, it can utilize sucrose in very clever ways to foster its colonization while using virtually every sugar in the diet for acid production. It can resist attempts at removal by most oral hygiene procedures and can be selected for amongst other plaque bacteria due to its ability to tolerate the presence of acids. Once the lesion is initiated other bacteria such as the acidogenic lactobacilli take over and this ensures that the destructive process progresses rapidly. *S. mutans* has to be given credit for stimulating research by oral microbiologists and although it is not the only cariogenic bacterium its control and eventual eradication will provide a model for means to alter the levels of other members of the indigenous oral flora.

Bacterial plaques develop on the tooth surface and under normal conditions the end products of its metabolism are not harmful. However, with time and under the right conditions plaque can develop enhanced cariogenic potential. This is reflected in

an elevation in the levels of the acidogenic bacteria described above and possibly changes in the physical nature of the plaque which restricts the diffusion of harmful acids away from the teeth and the penetration of buffers from saliva.

Carbohydrate and Caries

Although plaque can form under conditions where no food is ingested it is now known that food components can play a major role in converting plaque from an innocuous to a cariogenic state. Carbohydrates are the substrates which can force the production of harmful acids. It is not really the quantity of carbohydrate that is critical for disease development but the frequency with which it is presented and its physical form when it is presented to the dentition during ingestion. Many carbohydrates can contribute to caries formation.

Acid Dissolution

This phenomenon was discussed in detail when the carious process was analyzed. However, the actual cause of caries can be best visualized if the plaque bacteria are supplied *in situ* with fermentable carbohydrate and the pH of the plaque is monitored for a period of time. The data which are obtained allow the drawing of what has been termed a Stephan curve (fig. 16/2). Prior to carbohydrate ingestion the pH is at a level which is normally only slightly acidic or alkaline. Immediately after exposure to carbohydrate the plaque pH rapidly drops two or more pH units indicating an increase in hydrogen ion concentration of greater than 100-fold. It has been proposed from *in vitro* studies that when the pH drops below a "critical" value the tooth enamel is demineralized. Theoretically, the curve could be equated to the acidic attack on the teeth and the degree of the challenge calculated from some feature of the curve. The length of time that the curve stays at a low level may be critically related to the challenge to the tooth surface.

DENTAL PLAQUE AND CARIES

The oral environment and the nonmineralized coverings of the teeth play an essential role in the initiation and continuation of caries. As a tooth erupts into the oral environment, its coronal surface is covered by an inner acellular structure called the primary enamel cuticle. Covering it is a cellular structure, the reduced enamel epithelium. As the tooth erupts, the epithelium of the oral mucosa may also fuse with the reduced enamel epithelium. After the tooth erupts, its coronal surfaces may acquire a number of distinctive deposits that are categorized as acquired pellicle, dental plaque, dental calculus, food debris, or materia alba. Some of these structures play an important role in maintaining the integrity of the coronal enamel surface, while others are involved in both dental caries and periodontal disease.

The role of the primary enamel cuticle and reduced enamel epithelium in dental caries has not been clearly defined. Once the tooth has erupted they are rapidly lost from the enamel surfaces that are subject to abrasion during mastication. Due to their origin they cannot reform. The organic matrices of the enamel surface are quite resistant to enzymes and acids and alkalis, but they are permeable to organic acids and to microbial products formed in dental plaque. The primary enamel cuticle is involved in the attachment of the other dental integuments and deposits on the coronal surfaces. However, the one-time contribution of the primary enamel cuticle and reduced enamel epithelium to the formation of additional nonmineralized coatings of the teeth probably makes their role in caries formation inconsequential.

The Acquired Pellicle

External to the primary enamel cuticle and reduced epithelium, exposed coronal enamel is normally covered by an acquired pellicle that is generally described as acellular, structureless, bacteria-free and of salivary origin. This pellicle forms as the tooth erupts and when fully matured after several weeks is either colorless, light brown, or gray. It can be removed by vigorous brushing with an abrasive dentrifice, but when the enamel is re-exposed to saliva it rapidly reforms as an almost invisible film.

At maturity, when it is about 8 μm thick, it is sufficiently pigmented to be visible, and it is insoluble in acids. The acquired pellicle has been divided into surface, subsurface, colorless, and pigmented types. The subsurface type occurs when the enamel surface is partially decalcified, especially in interproximal areas, or when it is abraded. Colorless or pigmented pellicles have no particular significance, except that they seem to respectively represent young or older pellicles. The pellicle is primarily derived from salivary glycoproteins, and it contains carbohydrates, neutral polysaccharides complexed with protein, and some lipid; it is not collagenous and it is not keratinous. It is quite resistant to hydrolysis, stable at room or body temperature, and relatively insoluble. Even when freed from the enamel surface, it is resistant to proteolytic enzymes.

Initially, acquired pellicle is essentially bacteria-free. However, at maturity it often contains muramic acid that is indicative of bacterial cell walls. Oral microorganisms are not directly involved in pellicle formation. *In vitro* studies, where "experimental" pellicles have been created by suspending enamel in different glandular salivas, have shown that there are present in both submandibular and parotid salivas similar glycoproteins that are selectively deposited onto etched enamel as an initial pellicle.

Acquired pellicle is a diffusion barrier to most dietary acids, if it is not exposed to them for a long time, and to a certain extent to those formed by the glycolytic metabolism of oral acidogenic bacteria; hence, it serves as a deterrent to the initiation of dental caries. It may also impregnate minor defects in enamel and prevent cariogenic bacteria from entering and colonizing. If the subsurface pellicle can be mineralized, minor damage to the enamel surface may be repaired. Pellicle may also function as a lubricating medium between opposing enamel surfaces. A controversial function of pellicle involves its role in the utilization of fluoride as an anticaries agent. Normally, prior to topically applying fluoride the dentist requires a thorough prophylaxis with abrasives. Since the outer layer of enamel is known to contain the highest levels of fluoride it is possible that thorough cleaning with an abrasive is not the ideal preparation for the application of fluoride. Brushing and flossing prior to treatment may be adequate and preferred. Others have suggested that the pellicle can block ionic interactions of fluoride with the enamel and should be removed. There is also the possibility that the pellicle acts as a reservoir for fluoride and causes enhanced interactions with the enamel over an extended interval of time. More work on the role of pellicle in interactions with the enamel of various agents would be beneficial.

Plaque Formation

Dental plaques may be defined as dense, nonmineralized bacterial masses which are so firmly attached to the tooth surface that they are not removed by the flow of saliva or a gentle stream of water. After tooth cleaning plaque develops on the acquired pellicle as a number of distinct bacterial aggregates which form colonies which eventually grow and coalesce to form a continous layer of bacteria. The mass of the plaque grows until it is limited by the abrasive forces exerted by the surrounding oral tissues. One of the unique features of such plaques is their heterogeneity. The microbial composition of plaque not only varies between individuals but between different teeth in the same mouth and, more critically, between different sites on an individual tooth surface. This point will be dramatically emphasized when the oral ecology of S. mutans is discussed. It has been stated that "the microbial composition of a dental plaque on a single tooth, is unique to that site at that time." The consequences of this microbial heterogeneity are great. Differences in biochemical activity exist throughout plaque and this is reflected in the localized production of bacterial end products. With regard to dental caries the pattern of the disease in the dentition indicates that the production and accumulation of acid at localized sites is essential for lesion development. One of the most interesting, and not thoroughly understood, processes essential to caries formation involves the transition from what might be termed a plaque with minimal cariogenic potential to a cariogenic plaque.

Following initial formation, plaque matures through a series of phases involving growth of the original microorganisms, continued attachment of additional bacteria to the tooth and the early colonizers, changes in the flora, and accumulation of extracellular substances.

Various investigators have studied the development of plaque during its initial stages. The young developing plaque consists mostly of gram positive and gram negative cocci and short rods and some filaments in an amorphous or finely granular matrix. Socransky and co-workers divided plaque development into an initial phase, about 8 hours long, during which initial colonization occurred; a phase of rapid growth, lasting for an additional 16 hours, when the numbers of organisms increased rapidly; and a third phase where the numbers of bacteria remained constant but remodeling occurred. In this study *Streptococcus sanguis*, which was consistently present, made up 15 to 35% of the plaque isolates during the initial phase. *Streptococcus mitis* was present in some of the early samples but later disappeared, while *Streptococcus salivarius* was only transiently present. *Veillonella alcalescens* and peptostreptococci were irregularly present in early samples but were more frequently isolated after one day. Several unidentified gram positive cocci were also found in the early samples. Organisms considered to be corynebacteria were present during the first few hours, then disappeared. *Actinomyces viscosus* was present in proportions ranging from 15 to 50% through the initial phase.

Generally cocci increase rapidly within plaque and in a few days make up 80 to 90% of the resident flora. In the study cited above *S. sanguis* reached between 60 and 70% of the cultivated bacteria during the second phase. The proportion of *Actinomyces* decreased during this stage, most likely due to an increase in the number of other bacteria which grew more rapidly. By the end of the second phase other actinomycetes could be detected and their numbers increased to reach proportions of 10 to almost 30% of the total flora. After a week or so cocci are reduced to about 50% of the plaque flora, having been replaced by bacteria such as fusobacteria, nocardia, neisseriae, vibrios, and spirochetes. In older plaque, the total number of bacteria remains about the same, but again there are changes in relative proportions. The percentages of streptococci decrease but they remain prominent, along with actinomycetes and veillonellae. Some plaques have been shown to consist mostly of filamentous bacteria at the end of 2 weeks. In summary, these types of studies illustrate that plaque is a complex, dynamic system which can undergo relatively rapid changes. The nature of these changes will be regulated by the site where the plaque is forming and the local environment at the time of formation.

Adhesive Interactions. As illustrated in figure 16/3 there are three basic cell interactions which must be involved in plaque formation. The bacteria in saliva must interact with the tooth surface, cells of the same type can attach to each other (homotypic adherence), and different types of cells can attach to each other (heterotypic adherence). The first interaction in plaque formation involves the selective sorption of bacteria from saliva onto pellicle-coated enamel. This type of adherence is governed, in part, by the concentration of each bacterium in saliva. This will determine the relative frequency with which a bacterium comes in contact with the tooth surface. Another basic factor involves the relative affinity of each bacterium to binding sites on the pellicle. The greater the affinity of a bacterium for the surface the greater its chances for becoming irreversibly bound. We know that adherence to pellicle can be divided into two stages. The initial interaction is reversible and the bacterium can return to saliva. Some of the bacteria which interact with the pellicle become irreversibly bound through one of several mechanisms. This type of adherence and the homotypic and hetero-

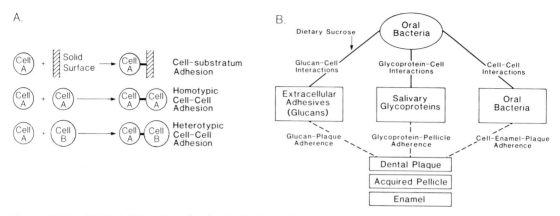

Figure 16/3. (A) Basic interactions involved in the formation of bacterial plaque on teeth. (B) Some of the factors known to be involved in the interactions which occur during dental plaque formation.

typic cell-to-cell interactions are all influenced by extracellular products produced by the bacteria, specific factors present in saliva, and specific binding sites on the surfaces of the various bacteria (fig. 16/3).

Extracellular Polymers. The most intensely studied example of the role of extracellular material in plaque formation involves the production of glucan from sucrose by S. mutans. Due to the intimate relationship between this phenomenon and the cariogenic potential of this bacterium this unique interaction will be discussed in detail later in this chapter.

It is important that extracellular glucan production from sucrose is not limited to S. mutans since other oral streptococci produce these types of polymers. However, the chemical bonds in the glucans and the degree of branching in the glucans formed by these other bacteria are different from those produced by S. mutans enzymes and the glucan is clearly not essential for their colonization of the tooth surface. For example, S. sanguis is one of the primary colonizers of human teeth and although this bacterium can produce glucan from sucrose the presence of this disaccharide in the diet is neither required for S. sanguis colonization nor does it stimulate accumulation of this organism on the tooth surface. S. sanguis does not have glucan specific binding sites on its cell surface, as does S. mutans, and this may be a partial explanation for these observations.

It has recently been demonstrated that additional plaque bacteria such as some of the Actinomyces can bind glucan and aggregate. The functioning of this interaction in human plaque formation is not known. As yet, there is no evidence that the level of these bacteria in plaque is markedly enhanced through elevations in the level of sucrose in the diet.

Certain oral bacteria appear to produce extracellular products which could enhance their ability to

participate in plaque formation. Strains of A. viscosus produce a polymer which is not a glucan and this material allows them to form in vitro plaque-like masses on solid surfaces. It is worth emphasizing that heterogeneous dental plaques can form on the teeth of subjects who receive their diet by nonoral means. Thus, most plaque bacteria have mechanisms to become a part of plaque which are unrelated to the presence of certain components in the diet. As we will see some bacteria, such as S. mutans, have mechanisms which allow them to take advantage of substrates in the diet to become dominant members of the plaque flora at specific sites.

Salivary Constituents. There is little question that various components in human saliva are critically involved in plaque formation. The chemical composition of the saliva components which form the acquired pellicle will govern the capacity of bacteria from saliva to be primary colonizers of a cleaned tooth surface. It has been demonstrated that strains of S. sanguis, S. mutans, S. mitior, and several Actinomyces aggregate when mixed with whole human saliva. Saliva glycoproteins and calcium ions appear to be involved in aggregate formation. It appears that there are separate agglutinins for the different streptococci and the interactions appear to be chemically specific. In one study it was demonstrated that a high molecular weight mucin glycoprotein agglutinated both S. sanguis and S. mutans. If the sialic acid residues were removed from the agglutinin the polymer would no longer cause the agglutination of S. sanguis but was still capable of agglutinating S. mutans. Other investigators have reported that oral bacteria can selectively bind lysozyme and blood group reactive mucins from saliva. The latter material appears to be present in some samples of acquired pellicle.

The specificity of the interaction between oral bacteria and saliva components which may be a part of the acquired pellicle can be demonstrated utilizing hydroxyapatite which has been treated with saliva to form a layer of pellicle-like material. By studying the adherence of bacteria to saliva-coated hydroxyapatite it has been demonstrated that lactose and *N*-acetylgalactosamine inhibit the attachment of *Leptotrichia buccalis*, hexosamines and other amines can block adherence of *S. mutans*, and various simple sugars are capable of blocking attachment of *Actinomyces naeslundii*. Thus, it appears that some of the components from saliva which adhere to the enamel tooth surface provide unique sites where specific oral bacteria can adhere. An analogy which supports this mechanism of plaque formation involves the "lectin-receptor" type of interaction where specific proteins can be shown to selectively bind to carbohydrate receptors. These types of interactions would partially explain the bacterial specificity of early plaque formation. It is important that the binding of salivary components to bacteria could also prevent adherence to teeth or plaque due to the masking of binding sites and/or enhancing their removal from the oral cavity via swallowing.

Cell-to-Cell Attachment. Under certain conditions plaque bacteria can be shown to undergo heterotypic interactions in the absence of exogenous factors. For example, strains of *A. viscosus* will aggregate with certain strains of *S. sanguis*, *Neisseria*, *Leptotrichia*, *Veillonella* and *Nocardia* when cell suspensions are mixed together. Direct visualization of interactions of this type may be obtained from visualization of plaque by appropriate microscopy although it is difficult to exclude participation of salivary components under these conditions. It is difficult to estimate the contribution of direct cell-to-cell interactions to *in situ* plaque formation.

THE MICROBIOLOGY OF DENTAL CARIES

Evidence for Bacterial Etiology

In spite of the fact that there was great precedence for the involvement of microorganisms in many diseases of animals and humans it was not until the 1880s that W. D. Miller performed a series of simple experiments which placed dental caries into the category of a bacterially dependent problem. In one experiment Miller exposed extracted human teeth to salivary bacteria in the presence of carbohydrate and was able to demonstrate demineralization of the tooth enamel. Based on his observations Miller postulated that bacteria were the etiologic agents of dental caries and that their acidic and proteolytic products caused destruction of the mineral and organic components of the teeth, respectively. This chemico-parasitic theory of caries formation eventually gained substantial support through a wide range of investigations, many of which are still being performed and expanded upon.

Orland and his colleagues made a series of observations in the 1950s which clearly demonstrated that in rodents the development of caries was absolutely dependent upon the presence of bacteria. Rats raised under conditions where they were free of living bacteria did not develop caries when supplied with a carbohydrate-containing diet capable of producing the disease in animals with a normal bacterial flora. When the germ-free animals were orally infected with selected bacteria they developed carious lesions.

In 1960 Keyes performed a series of experiments which established dental caries as an infectious disease (fig. 16/4). The offspring of caries active dams did not develop caries if the mothers were treated with antibiotics during pregnancy and lactation. Caries-inactive hamsters failed to develop extensive lesions unless they were caged with animals exhibiting rampant decay or unless they were supplied with fecal material from carious animals and consequently became orally infected due to coprophagous habits. Caries was shown to involve transmission of antibiotic-sensitive bacteria as has been demonstrated for many infectious diseases.

Specific Bacteria and Caries

During his investigations Miller isolated several types of bacteria capable of producing large amounts of acid. Consequently, he concluded from his studies that no single species was responsible for dental caries but that the process simply required any microorganism that could produce acid and degrade protein. This conclusion is still being evaluated today and a great deal of subsequent investigation has involved searches designed to determine the type and number of bacteria which contribute to caries formation in humans. It is known that plaques from both carious lesions and sound tooth surfaces are best described as variable and complex. However, significant differences in bacterial composition from such plaques have been demonstrated and further studies in this area are being performed in several institutions.

Based on the work of early investigators, such as Miller, several principles were formulated as a guide to investigators attempting to study the microbial etiology of human caries:

1. The causative organism should be the most acidogenic species that could be found in the oral cavity and in carious lesions.

2. The causative agent should be able to endure the acidity that it produced in the carious lesion.

3. The causative microorganism must be isolated from all stages of the carious lesion and grown in pure culture.

4. The pure culture of the microorganisms must

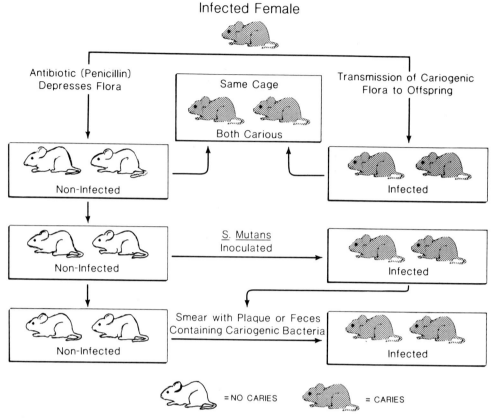

Figure 16/4. Schematic diagram illustrating caries formation due to passage of bacteria from rat dams to their pups, elimination of the disease by treatment of animals with antibiotics, and the occurrence of caries following various types of inoculations. The infection was reintroduced by contact with infected animals, inoculation with isolated strains of "caries-inducing" streptococci, and transfer of bacterial plaque or feces.

be able to produce caries when inoculated into the oral cavity or directly onto the tooth and no other organism should be able to do so.

5. The causative microorganism should be absent from the surfaces of teeth that do not undergo carious decalcification and from the saliva of "caries-free" individuals.

6. Other microorganisms that produce sufficient acid to decalcify enamel and dentin must not be present in any stage of the carious process. If they are present, it must be proved that they cannot produce a carious lesion.

These rather stringent principles had a reasonable basis at the time of their development. However, it is now clear that dental caries should probably be divided into a number of unique diseases or disease states defined by the site of microbial attack, the time at which the attack is occurring, and the nature of the dietary substrate being provided. By clearly defining the clinical parameters associated with the disease a clearer picture of the microbial etiology of caries can be developed.

Lactobacilli. These bacteria were thought to play an important role in caries etiology when it

was first found that early carious plaque contained elevated levels of lactobacilli when compared to plaque from noncarious surfaces. By exploiting the ability of lactobacilli to grow on acidified culture media it became possible to detect low numbers of these bacteria in oral samplings containing mixtures of bacteria. Consequently, lactobacilli were isolated from saliva, plaque and carious lesions, and it was possible to make a correlation between high lactobacillus numbers in saliva and caries activity in groups of subjects. For example, in a group of caries-free children the mean number of lactobacilli per ml of saliva could be shown to be in the hundreds while in caries-active children the mean number per ml was in the range of 100,000.

Further evidence for the role of lactobacilli in caries involved investigations where a rise in salivary lactobacilli could be shown to precede the formation of cavities by 3 to 6 months. Increases or decreases in the level of fermentable carbohydrate in the diet were also shown to cause corresponding changes in the level of salivary lactobacilli. Actually, the studies by Jay in 1947, where it was demonstrated that the level of oral lactobacilli could be reduced by restricting the intake of dietary carbohydrate, represent one of the first reports where a change in the level of an oral bacterium in the mouth could be associated with a shift in diet. Interestingly, it was also demonstrated that elimination of carious lesions in humans by placement of restorations caused a precipitous reduction in the level of salivary lactobacilli. In a study with 39 patients the mean number of lactobacilli was 138,000/ml prior to restorative work. One week after completion of the operative procedures the mean number of lactobacilli was 1,600/ml.

The early observations on changes in lactobacillus levels in the oral cavity led many dental scientists to consider these bacteria as the specific microbial etiologic factor in human caries. For example, Snyder and co-workers designed a simple laboratory test for the assessment of caries activity by monitoring salivary lactobacillus populations. The method is based on the rate of acid production in a glucose medium by oral acidogenic microorganisms that will grow at a pH from 4.7 to 5.0 (principally lactobacilli). From 0.1 to 0.2 ml of saliva is mixed thoroughly with 10 ml of melted medium in a test tube. During incubation at 37 C the production of acid is detected by an indicator, bromcresol green, which changes from blue-green (pH 4.7 to 5.0) to green (pH 4.2 to 4.6) to yellow (pH 4.0 or lower). Yellow indicates a positive test after incubation for 72 hours. Unfortunately, when attempts were made to utilize such tests for predicting future caries activity in a given individual the degree of correlation was not sufficient to allow these tests to be fully accepted. It is worth pointing out that lactobacillus counts might be useful as a diagnostic index under special circumstances. For example, practitioners should be able to use postoperative counts to assess completion of the case. If the lactobacillus counts remained high after restoration of the lesions it might be advisable to have the dentist look for undetected lesions or restorations with poor marginal adaptation. An additional situation where the bacterial counts might be useful is in the monitoring of a patient's dietary habits and ability to restrict the level of dietary carbohydrate. Such techniques have been used quite successfully on certain populations of patients in Sweden.

There are a number of reasons why the lactobacilli failed to qualify as an exclusive etiologic agent in human caries formation. Lactobacilli are found in saliva in proportions far exceeding those in dental plaque because they also colonize the dorsum of the tongue, vestibular mucosa and hard palate. The affinity of lactobacilli for tooth surfaces has been shown to be low and they represent less than 0.01% of the cultivable flora of plaque on intact tooth surfaces. Although elevated levels of lactobacilli tend to exist after caries has developed it has been demonstrated that caries can frequently be initiated in children in the absence of detectable lactobacilli. Loesche and Syed have reported that lactobacilli made up 0 to 11% (average 4%) of the flora in six samples of plaque from approximal lesions, indicating that lactobacilli in some, but not all, cases increased after decay had started. In corresponding samples of plaque from carious dentin the lactobacilli made up 0 to 85% (average 21%) of the flora. These types of data have supported the conclusion that the lactobacilli are secondary invaders in some carious lesions where they may contribute to the progression of decay due to their acidogenic and aciduric properties. The level of these bacteria in saliva may reflect spill-over from lesions which contain high concentrations of lactobacilli.

Attempts to produce caries in experimental animals by inoculation with lactobacilli have shown that when these bacteria have been established in rodents they produce caries less regularly and less extensively than several other microbial species. In the rat model caries development is normally associated with the molar fissures where this bacterium can most easily become established.

Streptococci. From the time that Miller found streptococci in the oral cavity and associated them with caries formation, these bacteria have received considerable attention from dental scientists. Initially, oral streptococci were implicated in caries due to their abundance in the mouth, their presence in deep dentinal carious lesions, and their consistent association with pulpitis accompanying dentinal caries where the pulp had not been exposed. Understanding of the role of streptococci in dental caries has been greatly advanced by studies with animal model systems, *in vitro* laboratory studies with defined strains, and epidemiologic studies with human subjects including analysis of plaque from various sites on the tooth surface.

Fitzgerald and Keyes in 1960 isolated certain streptococci from carious lesions in hamsters. When these bacteria were inoculated into the mouths of caries-inactive albino hamsters rampant decay developed. Subsequent testing of other bacteria including lactobacilli and acidogenic streptococci indicated that caries formation in the hamsters was very specifically related to the presence of strains of bacteria with characteristics similar to the isolates used in the initial studies. It is now known that the bacteria responsible for producing extensive smooth enamel decay in the hamster model belonged to a group of bacteria designated *S. mutans*. The hamster model is clearly a good system to evaluate the ability of a bacterium to colonize smooth tooth surfaces and initiate carious lesions. However, failure to cause caries in this model may partially reflect the fact that some strains of acidogenic oral bacteria are simply unable to colonize the hamster tooth surface under the conditions used and it is possible that changes in the diet or time and mode of infection might provide different results. Formation of adequate quantities of plaque is surely a prerequisite for significant lesion development.

When germ-free and conventional rats were used to evaluate the cariogenic potential of various oral bacteria the relationship was not nearly as specific as with the hamsters. As presented in table 16/2 a large number of bacteria were shown to be capable of causing caries in germ-free rats. Although the microbial specificity for attack on the smooth surfaces was retained it was demonstrated that fissure lesions could be initiated by a greater variety of streptococci and other bacterial types. In contrast to the hamster, the molar teeth of rats contain occlusal fissures similar in relative size to those of human molars. These stagnent areas foster accumulation of bacteria that are incapable of colonizing smooth nonretentive tooth surfaces. A wide range of acidogenic streptococci can consequently produce lesions in the occlusal fissures of rat teeth. It is worth noting that in all of these studies the animals were provided with a caries-promoting diet containing high concentrations of sucrose.

Several oral streptococci have been shown to produce root surface lesions in germ-free rats (table 16/2). It appears that strains of *S. mutans* are the more versatile bacteria since they cause caries on buccal and lingual smooth surfaces, in pits and fissures, and on root surfaces in the rat model.

In vitro studies with the oral streptococci have demonstrated many features which support their role as cariogenic agents:

1. They have a relatively rapid generation time and dense liquid cultures can be obtained in less than 12 hours following subculturing. Although the rate of growth of streptococci in the oral cavity is surely not this rapid, when these bacteria are compared with other oral bacteria, there is no doubt that they have the capacity to grow faster when provided with the appropriate environment.

2. They produce large quantities of acid during growth and the terminal pH in broth cultures is normally close to 4.0. Although the rate and extent of acid production is dependent on the growth conditions the high acidogenicity of the oral streptococci has been repeatedly observed.

3. The various oral streptococci do not appear to be as aciduric as the lactobacilli. Most oral streptococci do not grow well at pH 5.5 and die within 48 hours at pH 4.2. However, these *in vitro* observations may not be applicable to the situation in the oral cavity since these bacteria can clearly form large quantities of plaque on teeth under conditions where fermentable carbohydrate is being supplied in high concentrations. The buffering capacity of saliva, plaque and enamel are apparently adequate to protect the streptococci from their own acidic end products. A possible explanation for variations in the capacity of various strains of *S. mutans* to produce caries in model systems may reflect differences in acid tolerance.

4. The streptococci can utilize a wide range of fermentable carbohydrates including all of the predominant simple sugars found in the human diet. Selected strains can ferment mannitol and sorbitol.

5. They can store carbohydrate intracellularly for prolonged utilization as an energy or carbon source with the subsequent production of acid.

6. They can produce extracellular polysaccharides from sucrose. These polymers can function as storage polysaccharides and facilitate colonization of the streptococci on tooth surfaces.

7. They can be manipulated to form plaque on various surfaces under conditions simulating the *in vivo* situations which they normally encounter.

Each of these properties of the oral streptococci will be discussed in more detail when we analyze *S. mutans* as a cariogenic bacterium.

Studies on the ecology of oral streptococci have strengthened their relationship to dental caries formation. Plaques from human teeth can contain up to 10^{11} streptococci per gram of wet weight. Collectively, the various oral streptococci can make up 30 to 60% of the total bacterial populations which live at various sites in the human oral cavity. If the distribution of these bacteria in the mouth is examined (table 16/3) it is clear that the various strains have a predelection for particular sites within the oral cavity. The localization of *S. mutans* on the tooth surface indicates that this particular bacterium has a rather limited, but critically important ecological niche.

Evidence for the role of streptococci in human

Table 16/2
Bacteria capable of producing carious lesions at different sites in the dentition of germ free rats

Bacterium	Site		
	Smooth surfaces	Occlusal fissures	Root surfaces
Lactobacillus acidophilus	−	+	−
Lactobacillus casei	−	+	−
Streptococcus mutans	+	+	+
Streptococcus sanguis	−	+	−
Streptococcus salivarius	+	+	+
Streptococcus mitior	−	+	−
Streptococcus milleri	+	+	−
Streptococcus faecalis	−	+	−
Actinomyces viscosus	−	+	+
Actinomyces naeslundii	−	+	+
Actinomyces israelii	−	+	+
Rothia sp.	−	−	+

Table 16/3
Distribution of oral streptococci at various sites in the human oral cavity[a]

Streptococcus	Site			
	Plaque	Tongue	Saliva	Gingival crevice
S. mutans	0–50	0–1	0–1	0–30
S. sanguis	40–60	10–20	10–30	10–20
S. salivarius	0–1	40–60	40–60	0–1
S. mitior	20–40	10–30	30–50	10–20
S. milleri	3–25	0–1	0–1	14–56

[a] All values reported as a percentage of the total cultivable facultative streptococci.

dental caries formation can not be directly obtained due to practical, methodological and, maybe most importantly, ethical considerations. Consequently, epidemiologic approaches have been used where attempts have been made to correlate the presence of streptococci in samples of plaque and saliva with caries activity, to correlate the presence of streptococci in plaque from carious lesions with results with plaque from adjacent tooth surfaces, and to utilize longitudinal studies where periodic sampling at caries-prone sites is used in attempts to obtain an association between the presence of streptococci, or other bacteria, and the development of disease. Briefly, it appears that the streptococci capable of causing caries in the rodent models are also associated with human caries.

In conclusion, the oral streptococci represent a predominant group of bacteria in the human oral cavity. Selected species can be shown to cause caries at distinct sites in the dentition of rodents. These bacteria have a number of biochemical properties which can be directly related to their cariogenic potential. The oral streptococci represent likely candidates for primary involvement in dental caries formation in humans.

Other Cariogenic Bacteria. As indicated in table 16/2 caries formation in the rat model system is not restricted to the lactobacilli and streptococci. Animals infected with *A. viscosus* and *A. naeslundii* exhibit large plaque accumulations along the gingival margin rather than on the occlusal surfaces as observed with the streptococci. Under the appropriate conditions the accumulation of such plaque leads to breakdown of the periodontal tissues. Although these bacteria are not as acidogenic as the lactobacilli and streptococci they do produce enough acid to cause slight damage to enamel and much greater disruption to the less mineralized cementum. The *Actinomyces* species and other gram positive rods may be involved in the initiation of lesions on root surfaces of humans. In plaques over root surface lesions in humans it has been demonstrated that *S. mutans* may make up to 30% of the total flora or be absent. In the latter case *S.*

sanguis can make up approximately 48% of the total flora. In both cases *A. viscosus* was the dominant microorganism. It may be relevant that *A. viscosus* has been shown to be significantly more resistant to fluoride than other oral bacteria such as *S. mutans*. Whether this lack of sensitivity to fluoride by the *Actinomyces* is important for treatment plans involving root surface lesions is not known at this time.

The complexity of caries formation in humans is emphasized when the microbial content of deep dentinal lesions is analyzed. In these areas where a unique environment has developed the incidence of streptococci is often very low and lactobacilli are predominant. However, other bacteria frequently isolated from such sites include members of the following genera: *Actinomyces, Arachnia, Bacillus, Bifidobacterium, Eubacterium, Propionibacterium* and *Rothia*. Whether these bacteria contribute positively or negatively to lesion progression is not known.

There is precedence for the concept that certain bacterial strains could be antagonistic to caries production. Members of the genus *Veillonella* are obligate anaerobes and are found in significant numbers in dental plaque and saliva from humans. Members of this genera are asaccharolytic due to lesions in their glycolytic pathway but can readily metabolize a variety of short chain acids including lactic acid. Lactate is converted to propionate, acetate, CO_2, and H_2. Consequently, within plaque these bacteria have the capacity to utilize lactic acid as it is produced and to convert the acid to less harmful products. The production of weaker acids from lactate could cause a reduction in caries formation. Although a study in humans has not been performed where the level of caries has been compared to levels of *Veillonella* there is clear evidence from animal model studies that such an investigation might provide important data. If germ-free rats are provided with a high sucrose diet and infected with both *S. mutans* and *V. alcalescens* it can be demonstrated that less caries are formed in comparison to animals which are infected with *S. mutans* alone.

STREPTOCOCCUS MUTANS AND DENTAL CARIES

The great progress made in oral microbiology research during the past decade has been intimately tied to a series of discoveries involving a unique group of bacteria. The story which has evolved relating the formation of dental caries to these bacteria involves the uncovering of a fascinating relationship between a specific host tissue, the presence of sucrose and other fermentable carbohydrates in the diet, and a group of bacteria called *S. mutans*. There can be little doubt that *S. mutans* is intimately involved in caries formation in humans. The evidence for this will be presented in detail in order to illustrate the support for this conclusion. However, it is important that our discussion of S. *mutans* be placed in proper perspective. The oral cavity, and specifically dental plaque, contains a complex mixture of bacteria in an environment which is almost continuously changing. Oral biologists have documented many fluctuations which occur in the mouth as a consequence of almost every human activity. The complexity of the environment and the microbial community on the tooth surface combined with the impossibility for repeating in humans the infectivity studies done in germ-free rats makes it unlikely that one bacterium could ever be implicated as the sole etiologic agent in human caries formation. Indeed, when caries is looked at as a process involving lesion initiation and lesion extension, and when the microbial composition at the various sites at which caries occurs is analyzed, it begins to appear that the disease results from a concerted effort by specific bacteria who can be positively or negatively effected by their microbial neighbours.

It is important that focusing on S. *mutans* as a model to study the possibility of reducing or eliminating a specific bacterium from the oral cavity is reasonable. By utilizing the S. *mutans* model dental scientists are assessing the possibility of controlling a member of man's indigenous oral flora. The results of this work could open the door for the control of other odontopathic bacteria and possibly lead to reductions in the incidence of caries in humans. An interesting question which dental scientists are close to answering is what effect will the elimination of S. *mutans* from the human oral cavity have on the development of dental caries? To evaluate current attempts to answer this question we must understand the uniqueness of S. *mutans* as a cariogenic bacterium and why certain approaches are being pursued with great effort.

Historical Perspective

S. *mutans* is a bacterium whose rise to prominence required time and insight. In the early 1920s Clark was attempting to evaluate the etiology of caries by analyzing the microbial content of plaque from human carious lesions. A streptococcal bacterium was consistently isolated from the samples and its pleomorphic nature (ranging from cocci to rods, depending upon the culture conditions) caused it to be named *Streptococcus mutans*. After this initial report there were sporadic publications on bacteria with similar characteristics but it was not until nearly four decades later that intense investigations on S. *mutans* were initiated. The impetus for this work was mentioned previously and involved investigations performed at the Na-

tional Institute of Dental Research in the 1960s. In an expansion of the pioneering studies of Orland and his coworkers, who had conclusively demonstrated that microorganisms were required for the initiation of dental caries in rats, Keyes and Fitzgerald showed that in the rodent model caries is an infectious and transmissible disease and that specific streptococci from carious lesions in animals could induce extensive decay in hamsters. Streptococci which had characteristics very similar to the animal strains were subsequently isolated from human mouths and shown to be capable of causing caries when implanted in rodents. More recently it was demonstrated that the cariogenic potential of S. *mutans* from caries-active and caries-resistant adults is similar when tested in the hamster model system.

The bacteria used in many of the early studies were designated as S. *mutans* due to their expression of traits which we now use to identify these microorganisms. In general, S. *mutans* is recognized by its ability to: produce a distinctive colonial morphology when grown under standardized conditions on a sucrose-containing selective medium called mitis salivarius agar; synthesize extracellular polysaccharide from sucrose; undergo cell-to-cell aggregation when mixed with sucrose or the polymer of glucose called dextran; grow in the presence of the antibiotics sulfadimetine and bacitracin; and, ferment the polyols mannitol and/or sorbitol. Although the extent of the expression of these traits may vary from isolate to isolate it has been shown that in most cases these characteristics can be related to the cariogenic potential of this bacterium.

S. *mutans* and Human Caries

As mentioned previously the only feasible approaches to studying the association between a specific oral bacterium and caries formation in humans are epidemiologic. Unfortunately, causation in the epidemiologic sense can not provide unequivocal answers in defining the microbial etiology of dental caries. However, such investigations have greatly increased our understanding of the role of bacteria in caries formation in humans.

Based on the results from the rodent model systems, where S. *mutans* was shown to have great cariogenic potential, a large number of investigations have focused on relating this bacterium to disease. Initial studies revealed that S. *mutans* normally makes up 5 to 10% of the total bacteria present in pooled plaque samples obtained from caries-active subjects. In contrast, S. *mutans* represents less than 1% of the flora in pooled plaque from caries inactive individuals. Unfortunately, pooled plaque samples do not actually reflect the concentrations of S. *mutans* on specific sites of the teeth. Data from such samples present a significant underestimation of the levels of *S. mutans* due to the dilution of the samples with plaque from sites in the dentition which do not normally harbor high concentrations of *S. mutans*. It is now known that *S. mutans* is found mainly at retentive sites such as carious lesions, occlusal surface pits and fissures, and approximal areas.

When disease-prone or diseased sites are analyzed the association between *S. mutans* and caries becomes stronger. For example, plaque samples taken from a defined interproximal surface in 164 young adults revealed that *S. mutans* was present in 72% of the cases where radiographs subsequently revealed lesions (83 total lesions). A strong positive correlation was observed between early detectable lesions and *S. mutans*. In another large study where the areas of sampling included retentive sites a significant association between percentage levels of *S. mutans* and caries was found in plaques taken from a single occlusive fissure and pooled plaques from representative occlusal and approximal molar surfaces. It was important that in this study saliva samples were equivocal in demonstrating a relationship between *S. mutans* and decay.

In spite of the observation by many investigators that *S. mutans* can be associated with human decay in cross-sectional, association type studies such investigations fail to indicate whether the presence of these bacteria are the cause or the result of dental decay. Although some of the problems in these types of studies have been circumvented others still remain. Dental caries is a chronic disease where it may take months for the destruction to progress to a clinically detectable level. It is also very difficult to diagnose the incipient carious lesion. There is a real need for the development of more sensitive and selective caries detection techniques. The complex nature of the oral flora presents technical problems which are often difficult to avoid. Plaque samples should be analyzed immediately after collection since the levels of *S. mutans* and other bacteria can decrease during storage. *S. mutans* is usually reported as a percentage of the total streptococcal flora which grows on mitis-salivarius agar. This and other selective media may cause underestimation of the *S. mutans* counts. In addition, the results give a false impression of *S. mutans* relative to the total plaque flora. Finally, plaque sampling is a problem in that retentive areas are difficult if not impossible to examine and the ability of *S. mutans* to exist as dense polysaccharide-coated microcolonies close to the enamel may make their collection and dispersion difficult.

Longitudinal studies can be proposed as a means for demonstrating whether an increase in caries development coincides with an elevation of *S. mutans* counts. There are several inherent difficulties in performing such studies. They are expensive and labor intensive since a large number of subjects are needed to provide for patient loss and the likelihood of a given tooth surface becoming carious during the time of the study. Some of the additional factors which would complicate such studies involve changes in dietary habits, exposure to fluoride, utilization of medications, oral hygiene habits, composition and flow rate of saliva, microbial interactions within plaque, and the immunological state of the subjects. All of these factors have been shown to influence caries formation in man. The design of a longitudinal caries study in humans will probably always be less than ideal with many compromises being necessary.

In a very large longitudinal study performed in England some interesting findings were obtained. As a part of a much larger sample 19 subjects were followed for 2 years with bilateral plaque samples being taken from the distal surface of the upper first premolars at 6-month intervals. Radiographs were used to document caries development and extensive microbiological analyses were performed on each of 224 plaque samples. During the 2-year interval caries developed at 20% of the target sites. In general the microbial composition of plaque samples from caries free sites and from carious sites before and after radiographic detection of lesions was similar. In 2 of 15 sites *S. mutans* became numerically dominant before detection of a lesion. Pooled data from the sites that developed decay indicated a rise in the isolation frequency and mean numbers of *S. mutans* after detection of caries. It is of particular interest that in 2 of 15 instances no isolations of *S. mutans* were made from sites which developed caries. From this interim report it was concluded that no single species of bacteria was uniquely associated with the onset of dental caries. In this study an abrasive strip was used to obtain the plaque samples and it is possible that the level of cariogenic bacteria was diluted due to the presence of supragingival plaque from gingival margins.

In a longitudinal study of the role of *S. mutans* in human fissure decay, where great care was taken to define disease and sites, it was demonstrated that the proportions of *S. mutans* increased significantly at the time of caries diagnosis. Samples were obtained by scratching the tip of a needle along the entire fissure length. In a cross-sectional portion of the study it was found that the proportion of *S. mutans* in carious fissures was significantly higher than the proportions from caries-free fissures. More direct evidence for involvement of *S. mutans* has been obtained using a fissure sampling technique where the fissure is removed with a bur in a high speed handpiece under conditions where the entire microbial content of the fissure could be retained for analysis. In samples from 48 carious teeth the only bacterium found in every case was *S. mutans*.

Other bacteria present in some of the samples included *S. sanguis*, *A. viscosus* and lactobacilli. These studies indicate that *S. mutans* is significantly involved in occlusal fissure decay. This is important since decay in these sites normally occurs prior to caries development on smooth surfaces and represents the most prevalent form of tooth decay in children.

Ecology of *S. mutans*

In order to appreciate the focus of attempts to eradicate *S. mutans* from the oral cavity the ecology of this bacterium must be considered. In the broadest sense the distribution of *S. mutans* has been shown to be worldwide. More specifically, the only natural habitat of *S. mutans* appears to be the mouth of humans and some animals. It can be demonstrated that this bacterium requires a non-desquamating surface for colonization of the mouth and consequently is found primarily in plaque on the surfaces of teeth. *S. mutans* does not colonize the mouth of predentate infants but appears shortly after teeth have erupted. This bacterium disappears from the human mouth after the loss of teeth. The bacterium will remain or reappear if dentures are placed either immediately or at a later date. The explanation for these types of phenomena is that although the teeth are *S. mutans'* primary ecological niche this bacterium does not have a high affinity for the tooth surface. For example, it takes only about 1×10^3 *S. sanguis* cells in saliva to allow adherence of this bacterium to the tooth surface while with *S. mutans* approximately 5×10^4 cells are required before one might expect to see adherence to the teeth. Since *S. mutans* appears unable to colonize the mucosal surfaces of the oral cavity the reservoir for this microorganism is limited to the sites on the teeth which have been previously colonized. Removal of these sites can cause dramatic decreases in *S. mutans* levels in the mouth. It may be a consequence of this need for a stable surface in the mouth for colonization that *S. mutans* has developed mechanisms that allow it to become very firmly attached to the tooth surface. As will be discussed later the mechanisms for fixation involve a complex interaction between *S. mutans* and dietary sucrose.

Our current knowledge concerning acquisition of *S. mutans* by children indicates that maternal transfer is a likely possibility. Parental or sibling reservoirs of *S. mutans* are a potential source of bacterial infection for infants whose erupting teeth are being colonized for the first time. By using growth inhibitory bacteriocins to identify specific types of *S. mutans* the person providing the initial effective oral inoculum can sometimes be identified. Logically, this person is most likely to be someone who has close contact with the infant at the time of tooth arrival in the oral cavity. In adult subjects the situation appears to be much more complicated. It has been shown to be difficult to experimentally establish characterized strains of *S. mutans* in the mouths of individuals with a well established oral flora. Rinsing the mouth with cultures of *S. mutans* does not usually lead to implantation and the bacterium is quickly cleared from the oral cavity. Interestingly, one of the most effective ways to implant strains of *S. mutans* on human adult teeth is to place a drop of a culture of this bacterium onto a piece of dental floss and to work the floss at an approximal site. The procedure may need to be repeated on consecutive days. Intense localization of high densities of *S. mutans* at specific sites appears to overcome some of the suppressors of the colonization. The floss implantation technique has significant implications for the proper use of this material during an individual's routine hygiene procedures.

It is known that the factors which can regulate the interoral spreading of *S. mutans* include: the frequency and time of exposure to the bacterium; the dose received during each exposure; the nature and quantity of antibacterial substances present in saliva at the time of exposure; the flow rate of saliva; the nature of the indigenous flora at the sites of initial tooth contact; and other factors related to the specific adhrence mechanisms of *S. mutans*.

One of the key concepts related to *S. mutans* infections and caries involves the results which clearly indicate that this bacterium colonizes teeth in a very localized manner and that the sites which harbor high concentrations of *S. mutans* are those sites which most readily become diseased. In humans, *S. mutans* is isolated with greatest frequency from occlusal surface pits and fissures, approximal areas and close to the gingival margin. It is well documented that fissure decay is the most prevalent form of human dental caries and that the smooth surfaces of teeth are attacked less readily. A role for *S. mutans* in smooth surface decay has recently been supported with data obtained by taking small plaque samples from directly over and adjacent to incipient white spot lesions on buccal tooth surfaces in children. The proportions of *S. mutans* in samples from carious areas were significantly higher than those from the adjacent sound surface areas. It is important to point out that in the samples from the lesions lactobacilli were not detected. This supports the role of the lactobacilli as a secondary invader of carious lesions where the retentiveness and acidic environment are enhanced.

Another issue of concern related to the ecology of *S. mutans* is the intraoral spreading of this bacterium. In a normal infectious disease the invading pathogen will spread from an infected site until endogenous and/or exogenous forces suppress the infection. In the dental floss implantation study discussed previously it was noted that the established *S. mutans* strains could rarely be subsequently isolated from plaque obtained from teeth on the other side of the mouth. Confirmation of the limited intraoral movement of *S. mutans* has been obtained by the placement of *S. mutans* "seeded" artificial fissures into the mouths of human volunteers. In these studies streptomycin-resistant strains of *S. mutans* were shown to spread relatively slowly to the adjacent teeth and even more slowly to teeth in the opposing arch or on the other side of the mouth. It was shown that the intraoral establishment and spread of the implanted *S. mutans* was favored under conditions where the subject had high salivary concentrations of endogenous strains of *S. mutans* and high caries experience. There are clearly strong inhibitors which prevent *S. mutans* from spreading in a manner analogous to more rapidly disseminating bacterial infections. Elucidation of these factors would provide interesting information relative to ongoing attempts to prevent caries by suppressing *S. mutans* infections. The limited movement of *S. mutans* has direct implications for clinical dentistry when we consider the possible effects of various techniques routinely used by the practitioner. The most striking finding is the recent demonstration that by probing with a dental explorer one can transfer *S. mutans* from a fissure on one side of the mouth to a fissure on the other side and, most importantly, get establishment of the bacterium at the new site. The high frequency with which this transfer could be achieved emphasizes that alteration of the microbial content of caries-prone sites on human teeth with a dental explorer is an event whose incidence and significance is surely worthy of additional study.

S. mutans and Sucrose

One of the more unique features of *S. mutans* is the ability to utilize dietary sucrose to enhance its colonization of the oral cavity. In the rodent models sucrose has been shown to significantly enhance *S. mutans*-induced caries formation. In studies with humans it can be demonstrated that the level of *S. mutans* in the oral cavity can be raised or lowered by elevating or decreasing, respectively, the quantity of sucrose in the diet.

S. mutans has the ability to metabolize the disaccharide sucrose by several pathways. Two extracellular sucrose-dependent polysaccharide-forming enzymes are constitutively produced and excreted from the cell by *S. mutans* (fig. 16/5). By taking advantage of the energy in the bond between the glucosyl and fructosyl moieties of sucrose the *S. mutans* enzymes produce extracellular polysaccharides containing either fructose or glucose.

The fructans produced by *S. mutans* are predominantly made up of fructose moieties attached together through β (2→1)-fructofuranoside linkages. The quantities of fructan synthesized by the *S. mutans* fructosyltransferase varies from strain to strain depending upon the cultural conditions. Although there are no reports that *S. mutans* produces a fructan hydrolase there are many bacteria in plaque which produce such enzymes. The fructans may thus be classified as extracellular storage polysaccharides which may benefit the survival of *S. mutans* in the presence of other bacteria which can bring about the release of the metabolizable fructose.

The production of extracellular glucans by *S. mutans* is considered to be the critical reaction in the oral accumulation and cariogenicity of this bacterium. The reaction involves the conversion of sucrose to polyglucans with the release of free fructose (fig. 16/6). Dextransucrase or glucosyltransferase (GTF) is the enzyme responsible for glucan production. The importance of this enzyme is emphasized by the fact that mutants of *S. mutans* which produce elevated or reduced levels of the enzyme initiate correspondingly higher or lower

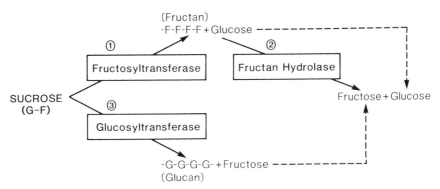

Figure 16/5. Extracellular sucrose metabolism by *Streptococcus mutans*. The disaccharide is cleaved releasing the hexoses glucose and fructose and forming the polysaccharides fructan (*Step 1*) and glucan (*Step 3*). The fructan can be degraded to free fructose (*Step 2*) which is available for cell metabolism. Formation of glucan enhances *S. mutans* ability to colonize human teeth.

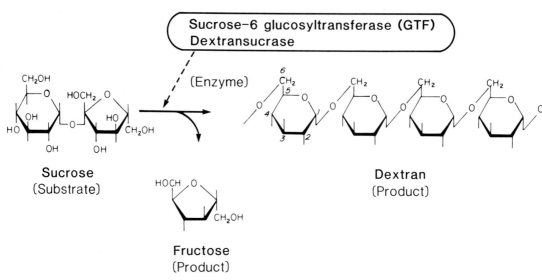

Figure 16/6. Schematic drawing of the conversion of the glucosyl moiety of sucrose to dextran by the enzyme glucosyltransferase (GTF, dextransucrase). This enzyme is essential for the production of extracellular glucans by *Streptococcus mutans* and is the prime candidate antigen for immunization against *S. mutans*-dependent dental caries.

levels of caries when tested in rodent model systems. The goal of several current approaches to reducing caries formation in humans involves attempts to inhibit GTF activity in the mouth with antibodies, enzyme active site inhibitors or enzymes capable of altering glucan synthesis by destruction of polymer as it is synthesized.

Great effort has been expended in attempts to purify the *S. mutans* GTF and to understand the mechanism of glucan formation. Several points related to the ongoing work in this area can be made:

1. The GTF is produced in several forms by *S. mutans* and the various enzyme activities appear to work together to produce complex glucan products.

2. Although many laboratories have partially purified various forms of GTF there is currently no convenient means to obtain large quantities of each of the enzymes sufficient to allow detailed chemical and immunologic analyses.

3. The activity of the GTF can be stimulated by various entities including dextran (an $\alpha(1\rightarrow6)$-linked glucan), phospholipids, and various surface active agents such as detergents.

4. When glucan is formed by GTF the products contain varying proportions of $\alpha(1\rightarrow6)$- and $\alpha(1\rightarrow3)$-linkages. The ratio of the linkages can vary greatly depending upon the enzyme source and reaction conditions. The $\alpha(1\rightarrow3)$-linkages are critically important in that as their proportion increases the glucan becomes less soluble in water. This water-insolubility may give unique properties to colonies of *S. mutans* on the tooth surface. Indeed, glucan-coated colonies of *S. mutans* adjacent to the tooth enamel surface may limit access to the site of

buffering or antibacterial entities from saliva and block diffusion of acid away from the teeth. In addition, aggregated compact colonies of *S. mutans* might be less suceptible to disruption and removal for analysis. This could affect the efficiency of certain oral hygiene procedures and complicate attempts to perform the longitudinal caries studies discussed previously. Greater problems can be envisioned when *S. mutans* colonizes retentive areas with limited accessibility.

5. Glucan production may be effected by the presence of enzymes which can degrade or modify the polysaccharide as it is being synthesized. *S. mutans* produces a dextranase activity which is capable of breaking the $\alpha(1\rightarrow6)$-bonds in the glucan. Interestingly, the enzyme is endohydrolytic which means it fragments the glucans into pieces. The fragments may interfere with glucan synthesis in several ways resulting in changes in the nature of the final polysaccharide product. In order for the fragments to be metabolized to fermentable glucose units they must be degraded by additional enzymes. The presence of significant numbers of dextranase-producing bacteria in human dental plaque has been demonstrated so that under certain conditions the extracellular glucans may function as an energy source. It is significant that the glucan remaining after such interactions would be highly enriched for $\alpha(1\rightarrow3)$-linkages.

Sugar Metabolism by *S. mutans*

The extracellular metabolism of sucrose by *S. mutans* involves utilization of only a small portion of the substrate which may be available to the bacterium. Most of the sucrose is directly transported into the *S. mutans* cell by a membrane-associated phosphoenolpyruvate (PEP)-dependent phosphotransferase system. The sucrose is phosphorylated by the PEP during transport and when inside the cell the molecule is cleaved by an enzyme called invertase (fig. 16/7). The products of this reaction can be readily incorporated into the glycolytic metabolic pathway. In addition to sucrose *S. mutans* can readily ferment essentially all of the simple sugars found in the normal human diet (fig. 16/7). The polyols sorbitol and mannitol can be utilized by certain strains of *S. mutans*.

After entering the cell the sugar molecules can go in either of two directions. Under conditions of sugar excess *S. mutans* is capable of storing glucose as an intracellular glycogen-like polysaccharide which can be metabolized after prolonged incubation. The ability to store glucose in this manner may be important for *S. mutans* survival under certain conditions and may also be related to its cariogenic potential. Plaques associated with high caries activity have been shown to contain significantly higher proportions of glycogen storing bacteria than plaques from sound enamel surfaces. Electron microscopic analyses of plaque overlying carious lesions have revealed the presence of large numbers of bacteria containing glycogen-like granules.

The other direction which sugars can take after entering the cell involves fermentation. *S. mutans* has been historically designated as a homofermentative lactic acid bacterium. However, under certain environmental conditions *S. mutans* may produce fermentation end products other than lactic acid. Both *in vitro* and *in vivo* studies have demonstrated that *S. mutans* can produce significant amounts of formate, acetate and ethanol. Glucose limitation caused these products to be formed in the *in vitro* studies. When excess glucose or sucrose is made available to *S. mutans* this bacterium is capable of producing mannitol.

S. mutans is capable of utilizing sucrose at a significantly faster rate than other oral bacteria

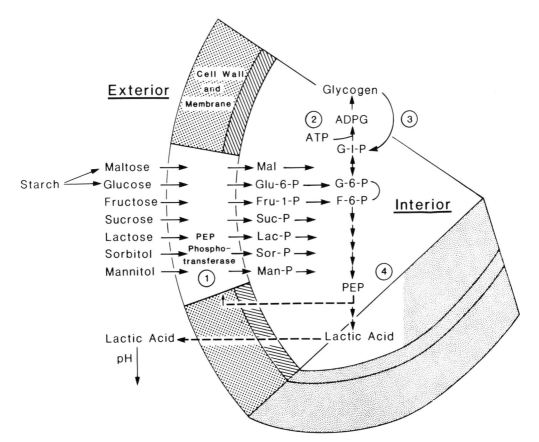

Figure 16/7. Schematic drawing of fermentable carbohydrate metabolism by *Streptococcus mutans*. Carbohydrates are transported into the cell by a PEP-dependent phosphotransferase system (*Step 1*) and can be stored in the form of glycogen (*Pathway 2*) which can be subsequently degraded (*Step 3*). Carbohydrates can also be metabolized to lactic acid (*Pathway 4*). Enolase is an enzyme in the glycolytic pathway which can be inhibited with fluoride. When this enzyme is inhibited carbohydrate transport is reduced due to a lack of PEP.

such as *S. sanguis*, *S. mitis* and *A. viscosus*. In a study where the pH of colonies of *S. mutans*, *S. sanguis* and *S. mitis* was determined it was demonstrated that under carefully controlled conditions *S. mutans* produced greater quantities of acid which could be measured in the agar directly below the bacterial colonies. Support for the high metabolic potential of *S. mutans* was obtained in a study where the utilization of sucrose to form various products was monitored in small plaque samples from carious lesions and samples from sound tooth surfaces. The plaque from the lesions metabolized significantly more sucrose and produced higher levels of metabolic end products. These results support the concept that *S. mutans* is metabolically dominant in plaque associated with carious lesions since this bacterium was, on the average, the numerically dominant species in the samples taken from the lesions.

Adherence of *S. mutans*

Another unique property of *S. mutans* is that when washed-cell suspensions of the bacterium are supplied with sucrose the cells become firmly attached to the walls of the container in which they are being held. This phenomenon has been shown to involve conversion of sucrose to glucan by GTF enzyme present on the bacterial cell surface. From these types of observations the term "adherent glucans" has evolved to describe the mode of cell attachment. Unfortunately, glucans with $\alpha(1{\rightarrow}6)$- and $\alpha(1{\rightarrow}3)$-linkages are not adherent by themselves and have little affinity for solid surfaces. The charge needed to achieve firm adherence to a surface by *S. mutans* must be supplied by some other bacterial molecule with glucan acting as a carrier and matrix former. Many cellular products could be involved in the *in vitro* adherence phenomenon with lipoteichoic acids and phospholipids being possible contributers.

An additional property displayed by *S. mutans* is that when washed cells are provided with dextran they undergo a clumping reaction. This dramatic demonstration of bacterial-polymer interaction is best explained by the presence of dextran-binding sites on the bacterial cell surface. Proteins capable of binding dextrans have been isolated from *S. mutans*. Several models have been proposed to explain the interactions between *S. mutans*, GTF, sucrose and glucans (fig. 16/8).

The relationship of the sucrose-dependent adherence reactions and dextran-induced cell clumping to *in vivo* adherence is not fully understood. Since dental plaque can accumulate on teeth in the absence of sucrose it is clear that the disaccharide is not involved in plaque formation by many plaque bacteria. Since *S. mutans* can grow well on a variety of carbohydrate sources the ability of sucrose to enhance accumulation of *S. mutans* on teeth appears to be due to the stimulation of cell-to-cell interactions. The studies where glucan synthesis was shown to enhance colonization of the teeth of rodents and the *in vitro* adherence and aggregation data led to the conclusion that glucan formation

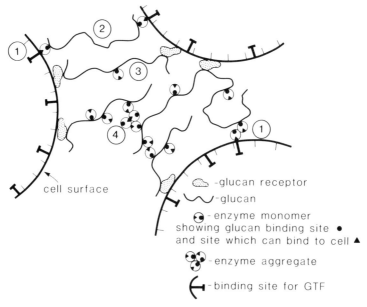

cell surface

⌒ -glucan receptor

〰 -glucan

◑ - enzyme monomer
showing glucan binding site ●
and site which can bind to cell ▲

✿ -enzyme aggregate

⊢ -binding site for GTF

Figure 16/8. Schematic representation of the association of GTF and glucan with the *Streptococcus mutans* cell and their participation in cellular aggregation. *1*, Binding of GTF to cell surface receptor; *2*, cell-to-cell attachment via glucan-enzyme interactions; *3*, cell-to-cell attachment via glucan-glucan receptor interactions; and *4*, enzyme aggregate involvement in glucan mediated cell aggregation.

was necessary for the initial attachment of *S. mutans* cells to the teeth. Evidence from a number of studies indicates that this conclusion is probably not valid and that sucrose is not required for the initial attachment of *S. mutans* to the tooth surface. It appears that the attachment of the bacterium to pellicle-coated enamel may involve a glycoprotein in the pellicle and a polysaccharide on the bacterial surface. However, the presence of the components could be reversed with the protein residing on the bacterial surface. It has recently been proposed that lectins are involved in the initial attachment of *S. mutans*. Such carbohydrate-binding proteins make reasonable candidates for causing some of the interactions which occur during dental plaque formation. Little is known about the adherence of *S. mutans* to preformed layers of dental plaque although it is very likely that such interactions are involved in colonization by this bacterium.

Classification of *S. mutans*

As demonstrated in table 16/4 the characterization of *S. mutans* isolates has become relatively sophisticated. There is no doubt that we are dealing with a group of bacteria which have a number of important phenotypic characteristics in common but which show significant heterogeneity when studied serologically, genetically and biochemically.

Various serotypes of *S. mutans* have been identified (*a* through *g*) and the specific antigen which allows the typing has been purified and characterized chemically. A biochemical scheme has been developed for separating strains of *S. mutans* into biotypes (I through V). Although the biotyping cannot be completely correlated with the serotypes the system has proved useful for many studies. Based on analysis of the deoxyribonucleic acid (DNA) from various strains it has been proposed

that the subspecies of *S. mutans* be given species names which would include *S. mutans*, *S. rattus*, *S. cricetus*, *S. sobrinus* and *S. ferus* (table 16/4). Although further work on these bacteria will be required before the taxonomy of *S. mutans*-like strains can really be set and accepted it is very clear that there are differences in these bacteria with regard to their cariogenic potential. For example strains of *S. ferus* form plaques on the teeth of rats but the plaques do not cover the surfaces of the teeth to the extent observed with other strains. Of importance was the observation that minimal caries developed in the *S. ferus* infected animals under conditions where other strains were highly cariogenic. This failure to initiate decay was attributed to a lack of copius plaque formation and production of less acid.

Immunological Aspects of *S. mutans*

The serotyping of *S. mutans* allowed investigations on the distribution of the various types of these bacteria in plaques from 14 different human populations. The primary finding from these studies was that the *c* serotype is most frequently found, 80% of total isolates, irrespective of the age of the subject, place of residence, site of plaque sampling, and the isolation and serotyping procedures used. Serotypes *d*, *e*, *f* and *g* have been detected in human plaques but *a* and *b* types are very rare. The dominance of the *c* serotype has been confirmed using the biochemical biotyping method. At this time it is not known why *c* strains dominate in human plaques. For some reason they are well suited to survive in the human oral cavity.

Antibodies raised against whole *S. mutans* or isolated fractions of this bacterium have provided a powerful tool for studying *S. mutans*. Sites involved in various cellular activities can be blocked

Table 16/4
Characteristics of the various types of *Streptococcus mutans*

Serotype	Biotype	Antigenic Determinants[a]	Guanine and Cytosine Content of DNA (%)	Distinguishing Biochemical Characteristics	Proposed Species Name
c, e, f	I	Glc-α(1,4)-Glc Glc-α(1,6)-Glc Glc-β(1,4)-Glc Glc-β(1,6)-Glc	36–38	—	*S. mutans*
b	II	α-Gal	41–43	Ammonia from arginine, grows at 45 C	*S. rattus*
a	III	Glc-β(1,6)-Glc	42–44	Bacitracin sensitive	*S. cricetus*
d, g	IV	Gal-β(1,6)-Glc	44–46	Fails to ferment raffinose, produces H_2O_2	*S. sobrinus*
c	—	Glc-α(1,4)-Glc	43–45	Fails to ferment raffinose, bacitracin sensitive	*S. ferus*
e	V	Glc-β(1,6)-Glc Glc-β(1,4)-Glc	—	—	—

[a] Glc, glucose; Gal, Galactose.

with different antibody preparations and this has allowed clarification of some of the reactions involved in *in vitro* sucrose-dependent adherence of *S. mutans*. For example, antibody specific for the a–d site of the serotype *a S. mutans* inhibits binding of GTF to the cell surface and subsequent sucrose-induced adherence. In addition, some cross reactions between the GTF from the various *S. mutans* groups have been observed with certain antibody preparations. These types of studies have supported the possibility that immunization against *S. mutans* might allow a reduction in the ability of this bacterium to colonize the oral cavity.

Genetics of *S. mutans*

With regard to *S. mutans* this area of investigation is in its infancy. However, advances in streptococcal genetic systems are being made very rapidly and many current findings may be applicable to *S. mutans*. Although a variety of mutants of *S. mutans* have been isolated and partially characterized at this time the technology to determine the type or degree of mutation is not available. The variants have been used in attempts to define certain "virulence factors" for *S. mutans* and have been helpful in understanding the production and role of extracellular glucans. Development of a system where *S. mutans* DNA could be analyzed in detail and a genetic map created would greatly facilitate work in this area. Until such a system is available studies with mutated strains of *S. mutans* must be evaluated with considerable caution. Recent reports have demonstrated that a few strains of *S. mutans* contain extrachromosomal elements known as plasmids. No function for these pieces of DNA have been determined although in many other bacterial systems they are known to contribute to a wide range of cell properties including fermentation of sugars, production of toxins, bacteriocins and antigens, and antibiotic resistance.

CARIES PREVENTION AND CONTROL

The formation of dental caries in humans may be completely prevented by the systematic application of measures currently available to the dental profession. Reductions in caries development can result from utilization of fluoride and occlusal surface sealants in a manner which optimizes their effectiveness, through application of appropriate oral hygiene procedures and via alterations in the patterns of ingestion of foodstuffs containing fermentable carbohydrate. Unfortunately, these control measures require either changes in individual habits, development of adequate dexterity and skills or strong motivation. Few individuals prescribe their lives in a manner which supports these types of measures, especially for control of a chronic

problem which is not life threatening. In addition, the disease primarily effects children and young adults whose concerns are usually directed to areas other than the oral cavity. In light of these problems dental scientists have attempted to develop means for caries prevention which require minimal effort and cooperation by the public. The current approaches to preventing caries formation in humans are all based on attempts to disrupt the interactions between the etiologic factors known to be responsible for the disease. In every case either directly or indirectly the attempts to prevent and control caries have a significant effect on the oral microbial flora.

Protecting the Teeth

One of the major approaches for caries prevention involves an attempt to protect the teeth from the acid attack which occurs due to metabolism of carbohydrate by the plaque flora. Without any doubt this approach has proven to be the most effective.

Fluoride. The cariostatic effects of the fluoride ion have been thoroughly documented. Water fluoridation, salt fluoridation and fluoride-containing tablets, dentifrices, mouthrinses and gels have all been shown to be capable of preventing caries in populations and/or selected subjects. It is now believed that there are three primary means by which fluoride exerts its cariostatic effect. First, by the conversion of hydroxyapatite to fluoroapatite the solubility of apatite is changed and it becomes more resistant to acid attack. Second, the fluoride ion fosters remineralization of carious lesions with deposition of a mixture of fluoride containing salts. Finally, fluoride can exert an antibacterial effect which decreases acid production by plaque bacteria.

The hydroxyl groups in hydroxyapatite are arranged in columns that are surrounded by channels formed by triangles of calcium ions. Fluoride ions become incorporated into this structure by substituting for hydroxyl groups. X-ray diffraction studies of fluoroapatite show that the fluoride ions, in contrast to the original hydroxyl groups, are situated in the planes of the calcium triangles equidistant from the three calcium ions. The fluoride substitution can exert several significant effects on the chemical and physical properties of hydroxyapatite. As a consequence of its position in the apatite the relatively small fluoride ion is able to form Coulomb interactions with the calcium ions which are stronger than the interactions of the hydroxyl ions with the calcium. It has been demonstrated that the calcium ions are actually pulled in closer to the fluoride due to the interactions. In addition, the substituting fluoride ions can establish hydrogen bonding interactions with neighboring hydroxyl groups. Consequently, the enamel structure is more stable and is less soluble in acid. Even trace quantities of fluoride can have profound effects on enamel solubility and in the normal oral environment fluoroapatite is relatively insoluble. Optimum utilization of fluoride can clearly make the tooth enamel more resistant to attack by bacterial acids.

One of the important effects of fluoride relative to caries involves the enhancement of remineralization of the enamel surface when the ion is present. The shifting of the demineralization-remineralization balance towards the latter process would retard the progression of incipient carious lesions. The exact mechanism of fluoride enhancement of remineralization is not fully known but it appears that fluoride salts can accumulate in the microspaces found in subsurface carious lesions. This mechanism of fluoride action emphasizes the importance of having optimum concentrations of the ion in the oral cavity when the teeth are undergoing acid attack and when they are being repaired through remineralization.

There is a good deal of information supporting the antimicrobial effects of fluoride. The principal mechanism of fluoride action on oral bacteria involves inhibition of acid production. In the streptococci fluoride inhibits the enzyme enolase (fig. 16/7) which converts 2-phosphoglycerate to PEP in the glycolytic pathway. Production of lactic acid is thus prevented. In addition, by decreasing the availability of PEP in the cell the transport of sugars into the bacterium is also suppressed. As illustrated in figure 16/7 PEP is involved in the transport of many of the sugars utilized by S. mutans. Due to the blockage of glucose 6-phosphate formation the storage of glucose in the form of intracellular glycogen-like polysaccharides will also be inhibited by fluoride.

There are some indications that fluoride may have a selective effect on certain members of the oral flora. For example, daily applications of acidulated phosphate fluoride has been shown to reduce S. mutans levels in plaque from the occlusal surfaces of human teeth. The effect appeared to be site specific in that there was little effect on S. mutans at approximal sites. The level of S. sanguis was unaffected at both of the sampling sites. In a study with rats consuming high levels of fluoride in their drinking water it was demonstrated that the levels of S. sanguis and A. viscosus actually increased due to the presence of the ion. It may be important that certain strains of the latter organism have been shown to be resistant to the presence of elevated levels of fluoride while S. sanguis is fluoride sensitive. No attempt was made to look for fluoride-resistant strains of S. sanguis although such bacteria have been induced by prolonged

growth in the presence of increasing concentrations of the ion. The issue of the development of fluoride-resistant oral bacteria has not been carefully addressed by oral microbiologists although many in vitro studies have demonstrated the phenomenon.

A very dramatic effect of fluoride on oral bacteria is observed during the treatment of patients with radiation-induced xerostomia. In this situation a marked change in the oral flora occurs concomitantly with the decrease in saliva flow. S. mutans shows a rapid increase in numbers which parallels the onset of rampant caries. Daily utilization of a 1% sodium fluoride gel as a topical treatment can significantly reduce the rate of increase of S. mutans while preventing lesion development. Since the fluoride regimen only delayed the increases in S. mutans the fluoride must have had additional effects in inhibiting caries formation. The ion was capable of blocking caries development in the presence of what would have to be considered a highly cariogenic flora.

It has been demonstrated that the presence of fluoride in drinking water or supplementation with fluoride from birth has little effect on the presence of S. mutans in human dental plaque. It has been proposed that fluoride may effect plaque formation by interfering with the binding of plaque components to the enamel surface and by altering the production of extracellular polysaccharides by oral streptococci. Further studies will be required to confirm that such effects can actually occur and consequently affect the formation of dental caries.

Three new approaches to delivering fluoride more effectively to the human oral cavity are being developed. The technology being used takes advantage of recent advances in controlled drug release. Uses of controlled delivery devices in human therapy include the supplying of pilocarpine to the eyes of glaucoma patients, progesterone delivery by an intrauterine device and the delivery of insulin to diabetics. This technology is based on the need to ensure that an agent gets to the correct site at a concentration and for a period of time which will allow it to exert its maximal effect. An agent can be delivered in vivo at a constant or slowly declining rate if it is encased in a protective polymeric sheath which allows release by either diffusion or erosion. Sodium fluoride has been incorporated into capsules which when chewed or sucked in the mouth release 10 to 15% of the encased ion. When the capsule is swallowed, the remaining fluoride is released in the gastrointestinal tract over a two day period. The net effect of the capsules is that fluoride is immediately available for local oral interactions and then for a prolonged interval through elevated levels in blood and saliva. A related approach involves attempts to develop an oral aerosal delivery system which would cause fluoride-containing microcapsules to adhere directly to the teeth. Sodium fluoride is encapsulated in carboxymethyl cellulose and mixed with guar gum as an adhesive. It is envisioned that the adherent capsules would enhance fluoride uptake by plaque and enamel over a prolonged interval. Probably the most advanced utilization of time-release technology is in the development of fluoride-containing "sandwiches." A very small trilaminate device consisting of an inner core of a fluoride-containing copolymer surrounded by a copolymer membrane can be made and attached on or near the teeth. Fluoride is slowly released from the biocompatible device at a constant predetermined linear rate for at least 6 months. It is envisioned that utilization of means to supply increased levels of fluoride to caries prone sites will reduce caries formation by suppressing fermentable sugar metabolism by cariogenic bacteria, by making the enamel more resistant to dissolution and by stimulating remineralization of the tooth surface. Recent attempts to stimulate the latter effect by utilization of "artificial saliva" containing fluoride and appropriate minerals have been successful in some clinical trials. This approach would appear to be promising in light of what is now known about the repair capacity of enamel due to interactions with saliva.

Sealants. It is important that fluoride is most effective in reducing caries on the smooth surfaces of teeth, *i.e.*, the approximal, buccal and lingual surfaces. Fluoride used at the concentration normally available is much less effective in reducing caries which develop on the occlusal surfaces. Unfortunately, occlusal caries accounts for approximately 40% of all carious surfaces in 6- and 7-year-old children. This probably reflects the normally inaccessible pits and fissures which are found on these surfaces and which can accumulate oral debris and bacteria. Consequently, efforts have been made to develop materials which can be used to seal and protect these surfaces. Excellent materials have become available and shown to firmly adhere to the enamel surfaces of teeth and block caries formation. Although the sealing of occlusal tooth surfaces is utilized as part of some preventive dentistry programs these materials are surely underused by the dental profession. In a study where human carious lesions were covered with a pit and fissure sealant for five years it was found that very few bacteria survived under the material and that they were not capable of continuing destruction of the teeth. If we consider our previous discussion on the oral ecology of S. *mutans* it becomes apparent that sealants will remove one of the niches in the mouth which can harbor high concentrations of this bacterium. One could predict that sealing decreases the overall cariogenic challenge to the teeth

by reducing the number of sites capable of harboring the infection.

Combatting Cariogenic Bacteria

Focus on S. *mutans*. We have emphasized that dental caries in humans is associated with S. *mutans*. Many dental scientists feel that great progress in caries control could be made by specifically reducing or blocking infections of tooth surfaces by this bacterium. Success in such endeavors would greatly clarify the microbial specificity of human caries and possibly open the door to disease eradication.

By accepting S. *mutans* as a target we are endorsing a concept that has been labeled the "specific plaque hypothesis." It is believed by most dental scientists that only certain plaques cause harmful infections due to the presence of elevated levels of certain indigenous plaque bacteria. Perturbation of the homeostatic state in the oral cavity has been shown to result in this exact type of detrimental change in the oral flora. Marked changes in the level and frequency of fermentable carbohydrate intake into the oral cavity, alterations in saliva flow due to the use of drugs capable of causing minor xerostomic effects, and the frequent utilization of topical fluorides all represent changes in the oral environment which have a marked effect on the oral flora. The first two situations can result in increases in the levels of S. *mutans* in plaque while the third situation can cause a decline in S. *mutans* levels. The resulting changes in bacterial concentrations will be reflected in an alteration in the cariogenic challenge to the teeth.

Attempts to sequester S. *mutans* from the complex plaque flora have met with varying success. As our understanding of the virulence factors of S. *mutans* grows more approaches become available for testing. There are now many effective tools and techniques available to the researcher which have not moved into the daily practice of dentistry. Hopefully, as with fluoride and sealants, many of the caries preventing techniques based on antimicrobial effects will become available to the practitioner. In several instances appropriate clinical trials are close to being completed. In other cases a significant amount of basic research needs to be performed.

Antimicrobial Agents

General Considerations. There are several advantages to treating dental caries as an infectious disease with a distinct microbial etiology. By focusing on specific microbial targets the problems involved in causing gross changes in the oral flora can be avoided. Superinfections by exogenous pathogens or marked increases in indigenous oral bacteria with latent pathogenic potential are less likely to occur if most of the indigenous flora remains intact. An obvious example of the problems which can occur when the indigenous flora is modified is the increase in yeast or fungi when certain antibiotics are utilized to treat oral bacterial infections.

The formation of dental plaque on teeth is a natural process which reflects the presence of a dense oral flora which does not normally cause disease. In fact there is evidence that the indigenous oral flora can contribute to our nutrition, induce the production of potentially protective antibodies, and influence the development of various organs and tissues. We are just beginning to appreciate the developmental and immunological consequences of the several grams of oral bacteria which humans swallow each day. The generation time of bacteria on the tooth surface has been estimated to be 8 to 12 hours. Great fluctuations in generation times are probably caused by changes in the quantity and quality of saliva, the periodic supplying of fermentable substrates, and the microbial content of the plaque in each microenvironment. Timing of the utilization of antimicrobial agents may be critical to their effectiveness and this will be governed by the properties of the agent and its mode of utilization.

The testing of potential anticaries agents is complex and, based on the nature of the drug, consideration must be given to the type of subjects which will be used, how long the study will continue, the means for delivery of the agent, the quantity of agent to be used, the frequency of utilization, and how the effectiveness of the agent will be assessed. Logically, each of these considerations can be determined through *in vitro* studies and animal models prior to human application. Selection of a drug for testing must take into account effects not only on the target bacteria but on the host as well. The ideal agent would by necessity have the following properties: safe for intraoral use in humans; rapid and effective killing to avoid selection of strains resistant to the agent; capable of penetrating into caries-prone sites; not be needed for the treatment of life-threatening diseases; not affect the intestinal flora; capable of being effectively distributed and utilized without loss of activity; and, have reasonable organoleptic properties to foster patient compliance.

The mode of application of an agent can be either topical or systemic with the former being the most reasonable. Agents have been tested using mouthrinses, dentifrices, gels, varnishes and, as discussed previously with fluoride, slow release delivery systems. The selection in this area is governed by the properties of the agent including its mechanism of action.

Antibiotics. Initial studies with antibiotics and dental caries were encouraging due to findings from animals supplied with antibiotics in their food and water and epidemiologic evidence from patients receiving penicillin each day for rheumatic fever or chronic respiratory diseases. In both instances reductions in caries development were observed. Frustration was encountered when broad spectrum antibiotics were used due to the creation of imbalances in the oral and intestinal flora with the overgrowth of resistant microorganisms and the development of allergic and anaphylactic reactions. An appreciation for the specific microbial etiology of caries has stimulated attempts to find antibiotics with a limited antimicrobial spectrum and properties amenable for utilization in the oral cavity.

The cariostatic effects of a large number of antibiotics have been studied including penicillin, kanamycin, vancomycin, Aureomycin, bacitracin, chloromycetin, streptomycin, Terramycin, Panthenol, tyrothricin, actinobolin, subtilin and spiramycin. Important observations have been made with several of the drugs. Penicillin can kill gram positive streptococci by inhibition of cell wall synthesis. When placed in the drinking water of rats the drug can almost completely block caries formation. However, when penicillin-containing dentifrices were tested in children few positive data were obtained. This was probably due to ineffective delivery at suboptimal concentrations. Although the effectiveness of penicillin in preventing caries in humans was demonstrated in the retrospective studies mentioned previously there is little justification for long term systemic administration of this important drug for dental caries prevention. Short term usage under defined conditions might be justified in cases of severe rampant caries where for some reason other preventive methods cannot be effectively utilized.

Vancomycin is another inhibitor of bacterial cell wall synthesis effective against gram positive bacteria. Since this drug is not absorbed into the body it has been tested as a topical anticaries agent. In a series of clinical studies the drug was shown to suppress the levels of S. *mutans* on occlusal surfaces but showed little effect on S. *mutans* on approximal surfaces. After daily application for prolonged intervals a reduction of caries by 20% could be achieved. Since it was most effective in retentive areas such as the occlusal pits and fissures it is possible that the antibiotic did not effectively inhibit bacteria on surfaces where the drug could not be retained for a prolonged interval. To be effective the drug may need to be retained at a site for a long time due to the slow growth rates of the bacteria in plaque. It is also possible that the drug did not get to the approximal surfaces at adequate concentrations due to the mode of delivery. In a study where subjects used a solution of vancomycin three times each day for five days a significant increase in the proportion of gram negative bacteria was observed. Due to the suspected role of such bacteria in human periodontal disease vancomycin may be considered unsuitable for further investigations on caries.

Utilization of kanamycin as an anticaries agent has provided insight into the functioning of drugs relative to bacterial specificity and the specific plaque hypothesis. Patients with significant active decay used a 5% kanamycin or placebo gel in an applicator tray twice a day for one week prior to placement of all necessary dental restorations. Treatment was continued for one additional week. Surprisingly, within ten months after treatment the number of new carious lesions in the kanamycin group was greater than in the control group. However, during the subsequent two years the kanamycin patients developed few new lesions while the control group continued to develop lesions to a level that exceeded the kanamycin patients. After the entire study was completed it was demonstrated that the kanamycin patients had a net caries reduction of 45% when compared to the placebo group. Based on these findings Loesche has formulated the "white spot hypothesis." Briefly, the incipient white spot lesion is considered as a reservoir for cariogenic bacteria. When the tooth is treated with an antimicrobial agent there is a nonspecific reduction in the entire flora. If the agent fails to penetrate the white spot lesion, either due to the agents structure or blockage by embedded bacterial cells, all of the cariogenic bacteria in the lesion are not killed. Consequently, when treatment ceases the cariogenic bacteria can rapidly grow and become dominant in the nascent plaques. This would accelerate decay. The reason for the long term reduction in caries at sites where no lesions were present would be due to a reduction in the overall level of cariogenic bacteria in the mouth due to the agent. As discussed previously establishment of a cariogenic plaque at the sites would require a significant time interval.

In a very interesting test of the white spot hypothesis relatively high concentrations of fluoride were used in an attempt to eradicate the bacteria in incipient lesions. The penetrability of fluoride presented in gels was shown to provide the desired effect via a reduction in caries in comparison to controls and application of the agent in a less effective vehicle, a mouthrinse. The consequences of these important studies are great since they confirm previous ideas and emphasize that treatment of caries by antimicrobial agents must be carried out under conditions which guarantee the complete destruction of the cariogenic bacterial flora. A challenge to investigators in this area is to develop agents which will penetrate and kill cariogenic bacteria in the depths of occlusal surface pits and fissures. If for some reason sealants can not be used on these surfaces such an agent would be extremely useful.

Topical Antiseptics

Chlorhexidine. Repeated clinical trials have shown that this compound is an effective antiplaque agent. The structure of this compound includes hydrophobic and hydrophilic groups with a net positive charge at neutral pH. Consequently it acts as a cationic detergent and can effectively kill a wide range of bacteria. Its antiplaque properties can be related to its retention in the mouth for long intervals due to extensive binding to various surfaces. Although chlorhexidine has been extensively studied and utilized in plaque control experiments in other countries it has yet to be approved by the Food and Drug Administration for use in the United States.

Chlorhexidine is capable of reducing S. mutans populations when applied topically although it has not been extensively employed as an anticaries agent. Under the proper conditions the compound would be expected to be markedly inhibitory to caries development. Negative aspects of chlorhexidine include its bitter taste, staining of enamel and the tongue and development of resistant microorganisms. However, the concept that antimicrobial agents with unique structures could be retained in the oral cavity for prolonged intervals is important and might be useful in the development of new agents and the designing of future studies.

Iodine. The utilization of iodine as an anticaries agent has recently been proposed as a way to take advantage of the specific plaque hypothesis and the limited capacity for interoral and intraoral transfer of S. mutans. Iodine has been used in medicine and dentistry for many years as an antiseptic and thus there is precedence and approval for its utilization in the oral cavity. Low toxicity and the ability to kill bacteria upon contact are attractive features. Several studies with humans have shown that iodine in the form of an I_2-KI solution can reduce S. mutans levels on smooth surfaces for prolonged intervals. Lack of iodine penetration of occlusal pits and fissures or rapid recolonization of these sites caused a less prolonged reduction of S. mutans at these sites. It is possible that this halogen will join fluoride as an effective means for reducing dental caries in humans.

Enzyme Preparations. A large number of enzymes believed to be capable of disrupting plaque have been tested. Due to the emphasis on the role of glucan in S. mutans colonization of teeth attempts to disrupt plaque with polysaccharide destroying enzymes have been performed in animals and human subjects. A dextranase preparation capable of hydrolyzing $\alpha(1 \rightarrow 6)$-linked glucans was tested as a mouthrinse in several groups of subjects with equivocal results being obtained. In retrospect, these studies were premature in that it is now known that the glucans in plaque have a high proportion of $\alpha(1 \rightarrow 3)$-linkages and are subsequently water-insoluble as well as resistant to $\alpha(1 \rightarrow 6)$-specific hydrolases. Subsequently, as discussed previously, it has been shown that there are dextranase-producing bacteria in plaque and endogenous levels of the enzyme may actually be higher than those used in the mouthrinse studies. Enzymes capable of hydrolyzing $\alpha(1 \rightarrow 3)$-linked glucans have been used in several studies with some promising results.

A unique combination of enzymes has recently been tested with a dentifrice as the vehicle. Amyloglucosidase and glucose oxidase are proposed to activate a naturally occurring antibacterial system which involves lactoperoxidase catalysed oxidation of thiocyanate with hydrogen peroxide with the formation of hypothiocyanite. The latter compound oxidizes thiol groups and interferes with bacterial sugar metabolism. Tests with a rat model have failed to support some of the conclusions made from the human trials. The dentifrice is marketed in Europe under the name Zendium.

Problems with the utilization of enzymes as antiplaque or anticaries agents include retaining the enzymes at the needed site for an adequate interval and getting the enzymes to penetrate into areas of the dentition which are difficult to reach by conventional hygiene techniques. Sensitization of the host to the protein enzymes must also be considered.

Immunization against Caries

An approach to caries prevention which has received considerable publicity and elicited great interest from the public is the development of an anticaries vaccine. The reason for much optimism in this area is our increased understanding of the microbial etiology of human caries and man's secretory immunologic system. Since enhanced colonization of teeth by S. mutans involves production of glucans from dietary sucrose, it is possible that inhibition by antibodies of the enzyme involved in glucan synthesis could prevent S. mutans-induced caries. Indeed, the S. mutans dextransucrase (fig. 16/6) is a primary candidate for the antigen to be used in a caries vaccine. When crude preparations of the enzyme are injected in the salivary gland region of rats and hamsters a local protective secretory immune response is induced. There are several groups of scientists using genetic engineering to isolate and manipulate the S. mutans DNA which codes for the production of dextransucrase. Large quantities of antigen will become available when this DNA is cloned into appropriate bacteria. Pure antigen will greatly accelerate studies on development of an effective vaccine.

Caries-immunization studies with rodents and primates have clearly suggested a role for secretory immunoglobulin A (sIgA) antibodies in protection against caries. The secretory immune system's role in regulating the human oral flora is being studied with increasing intensity. Briefly, the external secretions of the body, including saliva, contain sIgA as their predominant immunoglobulin. These fluids bathe the mucous membrane surfaces of the body and their immunoglobulins are involved in "first-line defenses" such as the trapping of microorganisms at mucous surfaces, coating of bacteria and inhibition of their adherence, viral and toxin neutralization, lysis of bacteria, and opsonization. With regard to caries it has been shown that local injection followed by direct instillation of S. mutans antigen into the parotid duct of monkeys induced the production of sIgA which reduced the levels of S. mutans on the animal's teeth. Recent excitement in caries immunization stems from the observation that oral or intragastric administration of antigens results in the appearance of sIgA antibodies in saliva and other external secretions. It has been proposed that antibody-producing lymphoid cells originate and are stimulated in the gut-associated lymphoid tissue. These cells can migrate through the lymphatics via the mesenteric lymph nodes into the blood stream. They may then home to secretory tissues located in various parts of the body. When they are in the environment of these tissues the lymphocytes differentiate into mature IgA-secreting plasma cells with antibody specificity directed to the ingested antigen. Local synthesis of antibody would result in enhanced levels in the corresponding secretion.

Our advancing knowledge of secretory immunity stimulated a pioneering study by investigators at the University of Alabama in Birmingham. Four adult volunteers ingested gelatin capsules filled with 100 mg of formalin-killed S. mutans cells for 14 consecutive days. Antibodies to the strain of S. mutans used in the capsules could be detected in samples of saliva and tears within one week of immunization. A second cycle of antigen ingestion in capsules produced a more rapid and pronounced increase in antibody levels. The immunoglobulins were shown to be sIgA and were not present in the subject's serum. The data are consistent with the concept that the ingested antigen stimulated precursor IgA cells in the gut-associated lymphoid tissue and that homing of cells to the salivary glands resulted in the localized production of specific antibodies. This approach to immunization eliminates some of the many problems previously encountered during attempts to immunize against caries by injections in the region of the salivary glands. An interesting point to be made here is that due to the swallowing of large numbers of oral bacteria each day it is likely that we are being continuously immunized against our indigenous oral flora. Indeed, when saliva from patients is analyzed antibody against various serotypes of *S. mutans* can be detected. Due to the low titers obtained in the *S. mutans* ingestion study it appears that a means to elevate the concentration of sIgA with a designated specificity is an essential next step in this work. A potential problem in this area involves studies which have demonstrated antigenic drift among bacteria residing in the oral cavity. This may reflect the selective pressure applied by the continuous production of secretory antibodies.

Another facet of caries immunization involves the passive transfer or direct supplying to the oral cavity of antibodies specific for *S. mutans*. It has been demonstrated that rat dams immunized by various methods to *S. mutans* have high levels of antibody to this bacterium in colostrum, milk and serum. When offspring suckling these dams were challenged with *S. mutans* it was observed that fewer carious lesions developed in the pups. Passive transfer and immunity could be important to man since caries primarily affects children at a time when they may be consuming large quantities of milk. It is not inconceivable that bovine milk supplemented with antibody or milk from cows immunized with the appropriate cariogenic bacteria could be used as part of a caries prevention program. What is exciting about this approach to suppression of *S. mutans* infections is that breakthroughs in the area of monoclonal antibody production will make available large quantities of human antibodies specific for *S. mutans*. The supplying of such molecules to the human oral cavity at appropriate times could markedly suppress *S. mutans* infections and possibly eliminate this bacterium as a member of the human oral flora. Sequestering of other oral bacteria with cariogenic potential might also be accomplished.

Modification of Cariogenic Bacteria

Evidence has been presented in several systems that certain bacterial infections may be controlled by allowing the host to be colonized with nonvirulent variants of bacteria with disease-producing potential. Mutants of *S. mutans* have been isolated which lack the enzyme lactate dehydrogenase. Although these isolates produce less acid from glucose than wild-type strains they appear to be capable of colonizing the oral cavity to high levels. Replacement therapy would involve supplying the mutants to the mouths of subjects either prior to colonization of the teeth by cariogenic strains of *S. mutans* or after reduction in the levels of *S. mutans* by various methods (*i.e.*, iodine application). It is possible that the mutant strains could occupy the sites normally colonized by *S. mutans* and consequently there would be a reduction in the cariogenic challenge to the teeth. The mutants would be expected to reduce the ability of superinfecting acid-producing strains of *S. mutans* to become established in the oral cavity.

An additional and related approach would involve the creation of unique oral bacteria using recently developed genetic engineering techniques. Gene splicing with recombinant DNA methods could be used to selectively remove from or add to oral bacteria specific genetic traits which would alter the microorganisms' cariogenic or anticariogenic properties. Due to the amazing progress being made in this area of science and our increasing knowledge of oral bacteria, it seems reasonable that new approaches to caries prevention will evolve in the near future.

Diet Modification

General Considerations. Based on the etiology of dental caries it seems reasonable to attempt to prevent disease development by either reducing the availability of fermentable carbohydrate or by supplying agents which could minimize the consequences of bacterial acid production at the time of food ingestion. Such attempts need to consider the nutritional status of the oral bacterial flora and the host as well as the interactions which occur when various substrates for acid production are made available in the diet.

If we compare the oral cavity to other microbial niches in nature it would appear that the mouth is a nutritionally rich environment. Substrates capable of supporting a complex and fastidious mixture of bacteria are obtained from the host, other oral bacteria and the diet. The localized entry into the mouth of various host fluids has a significant influence on the composition and metabolic activity of bacteria at different sites in the oral cavity. Saliva and gingival crevicular fluid contain many potential bacterial substrates and *in vitro* growth in these fluids has been demonstrated. Support for the nutritional contribution of the host is obtained from the data which show that a complex bacterial flora exists and plaque accumulates on the teeth of human subjects who receive all of their food by stomach tube. It is important that the plaque which accumulates under such conditions has diminished acid-producing potential when supplied with fermentable carbohydrate. These types of experiments emphasize the observation that exogenous carbohydrate causes the development of an acidogenic flora through the acid killing mechanism discussed previously. Although diet may affect the oral flora by altering the ability of the host to supply a homeostatic environment, at this time we are primarily concerned with local effects which can occur when substrates are directly supplied as foodstuffs. Surprisingly, with one exceptional case, this is an area which has received minimal attention. Little information is available on the effect of diets with varying levels of nutrients on the oral flora. Dental researchers have obviously missed ideal opportunities to collaborate with investigators involved in past human nutrition studies where diet control was carefully maintained.

Role of Fermentable Carbohydrate. Research with animals and epidemiological analyses have strongly implicated fermentable carbohydrate, and simple sugars in particular, in human dental caries formation. It has been concluded that decay in humans is associated with both the frequency of ingestion of readily fermentable carbohydrate and the duration of time the substrate is retained in the mouth. It is known that alterations in the ingested levels of carbohydrate can dramatically influence the oral concentrations of certain types of bacteria. Specifically, we know that the *S. mutans* levels in the mouth can be markedly elevated by increasing the quantity of sucrose in the diet. Reduced ingestion of sucrose or replacement of this disaccharide with other carbohydrates causes a decrease in the numbers of *S. mutans* on the teeth. Similar results have been observed with the lactobacilli relative to the presence of total fermentable carbohydrate and retentive sites in the dentition. These observations on the response of acidogenic bacteria to dietary carbohydrate have been discussed by many scientists and clinicians and are the focal point for much of the controversy concerning the role of dietary components in caries etiology.

Few clinical trials designed to determine the cariogenicity of different sugars in humans have been performed. One of the most significant studies was reported from Turku, Finland. One group of subjects was supplied with a diet containing a "normal" level of sucrose. Another group received a diet which consisted of similar products made with fructose in place of the sucrose. A third group consumed a similar diet with xylitol in place of the sucrose. In spite of some criticisms it is acknowledged that this study provided unequivocal support for the role of fermentable sugar in human caries formation. After two years on the various diets it was determined that the group consuming sucrose had a mean increment in the number of decayed, missing and filled tooth surfaces (DMFS) of 7.2. The DMFS index of the group consuming the fructose diet was 3.8 while the xylitol group had an index of 0.0.

Sucrose Replacement. It has been proposed that caries could be prevented by altering the diet through replacement of sucrose with a less cariogenic substrate. However, replacement of sucrose by some acceptable sweetener has proven to be difficult and expensive for a number of reasons. Briefly, sucrose has many properties which have caused it to be used in many foodstuffs. In addition to considerations such as cost, sucrose increases the sweetness, osmotic pressure, viscosity, boiling point and moisture retention of foods. Sucrose also enhances flavor and appearance by improving clarity, luster and gloss. Finally, the disaccharide provides calories, affects the solubility of other ingredients, imparts plasticity, provides bulk and body, and assists emulsification and color development. These properties make attempts to substitute other agents extremely difficult. In order to select an appropriate sucrose substitute we have to consider such things as the absorption, metabolism and safety of the compound, practical problems in using the sweetener in various foodstuffs, and the legal and regulatory aspects of its utilization. Evaluation of the cariogenic potential of a possible substitute is in many instances upstaged by an evaluation of its carcinogenicity. This subject may be viewed by some as a reasonable approach to caries control but the scientific problems which are many, may actually be irrelevant when compared to regulatory and acceptance complications.

Sorbitol is a sugar alcohol which meets many of the criteria for a sugar substitute. Although there are problems with its utilization in a wide range of foodstuffs, it has been generally accepted in chewing gums and a significant portion of the gum sold in this country is of the sugarless type. Some producers have labeled their gums as noncariogenic. In animal model studies where sorbitol and sucrose are compared the latter is clearly more cariogenic. Supplying sorbitol to dental plaque either *in vivo* or *in vitro* causes a minimal pH drop due to limited production of acid. There are few bacteria in the oral cavity capable of utilizing sorbitol for growth. However, as illustrated in figure 16/7, *S. mutans* has the ability to transport sorbitol and metabolize it for energy and possibly to produce acid. Due to the complexity of the oral flora and competition between oral bacteria for substrates the possibility that polyols give *S. mutans* a selective advantage over other bacteria in the oral cavity should be considered. Since individuals chewing sorbitol-containing gum or ingesting this compound in other forms are probably also obtaining sucrose in their diet *S. mutans* colonization might be enhanced under these conditions. The enzymes to metabolize sorbitol may need to be induced for production by the bacterium and this would reduce the utilization of sorbitol by *S. mutans* within plaque. However, the metabolic capabilities of this bacterium when it is in the mouth are not known and it may be derepressed to metabolize sorbitol under conditions where more readily fermentable carbohydrates are not available. Although end products other than acid may be produced from sorbitol the supplying of this substrate between meals might be aiding a bacterium with documented cariogenic potential.

Aspartame is a methyl ester of a dipeptide consisting of the amino acids aspartate and phenylalanine. The compound is 150 to 200 times sweeter than sucrose and has recently been approved by the Food and Drug Administration for utilization in cold cereals, sugarless gums, drink mixes, instant coffees and teas, gelatins, puddings and fillings. Aspartame would be expected to be noncariogenic and preliminary data indicate that this is true. In addition, the dipeptide has been shown to reduce sucrose-dependent *in vitro* plaque formation by *S. mutans* and reduce the production of lactic acid from glucose by the bacteria in whole human saliva. The compound may eventually be shown to be slightly anticariogenic.

Decreasing Sucrose in the Diet. One of the recently proposed dietary guidelines for people in the United States suggests a reduction in the consumption of refined and other processed sugars including foods high in sugars such as soft drinks, cereal and bakery products and confections. If this goal were achieved it would reduce simple sugar consumption from about 13 million tons to 6 million tons per year in the United States. This decrease might have some helpful effects on the population. However, with regard to dental caries it is difficult to project any change in disease level. There is no experimental support for a direct correlation between the total intake of sugar and the incidence of dental caries. It has been demonstrated with dose-response studies in rats that very low levels of sucrose (1%) can support significant *S. mutans*-induced caries. The frequency of ingestion and the form of the carbohydrate are the most critical parameters regarding caries enhancement by food consumption.

A strong controversy exists concerning the relative cariogenicity of different carbohydrates. In general, monosaccharides and disaccharides are more cariogenic than starch, and sucrose is considered the most cariogenic sugar. However, there are conflicting data on this subject and some animal studies indicate that there is little difference in the cariogenicity of sucrose, glucose and fructose. It should be emphasized that monitoring which surfaces of the teeth are being attacked in such studies and the type of bacterial flora present on the teeth before, during and at the termination of the experiment is very important. The level of *S. mutans* in the subjects under study is important since high levels of this bacterium have been associated with ele-

vated decay on the smooth surfaces of teeth. As illustrated in figure 16/7 *S. mutans* can readily transport the predominant sugars found in the typical human diet. Thus, a great deal of caution should be used when attempting to evaluate studies where multiple types of fermentable carbohydrate are available. Another problem would be in diet shifting studies. A subject with high or moderate levels of *S. mutans* might develop significant caries after changing to a diet free of sucrose if the new diet contained quantities of a carbohydrate that this bacterium could readily ferment. There are no simple answers when discussing the cariogenicity of various fermentable carbohydrates.

Anticariogenic Additives. An ideal way to prevent caries would involve the adding of a substance to cariogenic foods which would either prevent the production or block the activity of the lactic acid responsible for the disease.

Phosphate containing agents have been proposed to have cariostatic effects when added to foods containing fermentable carbohydrate. Approximately 200 studies with rats have demonstrated caries inhibition with a wide range of phosphates present in the diet at low levels. Data from human caries studies can best be described as inconsistent and relatively discouraging in comparison to the rat studies. In one positive study sodium trimetaphosphate was used in a chewing gum supplied to children and a reduction in caries was observed along with a reduction in *S. mutans* levels in plaque. More studies specifically designed to test the effect of phosphate containing compounds on human caries may be justified.

There are many mechanisms through which phosphates could have an anticariogenic effect. Excluding the obvious effect on the tooth enamel, which could be very significant, phosphates could buffer acid produced by plaque bacteria, affect bacterial metabolism, modify adsorption of proteins to enamel, and alter the adherence capacity of plaque bacteria. Hopefully, further work will allow confirmation of one or more of these mechanisms as a reasonable explanation for some of the phosphate data.

Some investigators have seriously questioned the utilization of phosphate as an anticaries agent by suggesting that the human diet already contains levels of phosphate that would provide maximum protection against caries. Other problems involve the rat model which for a number of reasons may have been ideally suited to maximize the anticariogenic potential of phosphate.

Trace elements may have the potential to affect caries if added to the diet at specific levels and times. Some of the elements could act synergistically with fluoride and enhance protection against caries. Elements suggested to have an anticariogenic effect include boron, lithium, molybdenum, strontium, and vanadium. There is a clear need for additional investigations on trace elements especially with regard to their ability to affect cariogenic microorganisms.

Cariogenicity of Foods

Current interest in the relationship between diet and dental caries has placed the dental profession in a difficult situation. Ideally, the clinician should recommend to patients a diet which is compatible with both oral and total health. Unfortunately, due to the complex interactions involved in human caries formation this is very difficult. For example, based on our increased understanding of the etiology of dental caries the practitioner might suggest a reduction or elimination of between meal snacking. Unfortunately, in modern societies snacking is becoming more prevalent and recommendations contrary to this trend are unlikely to be effective. Consequently, there is increased pressure on the clinician to recommend foods which might be eaten with minimum risk to the teeth. Since there are problems with pinpointing the contribution of specific carbohydrates to caries and difficulties in-

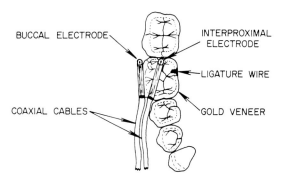

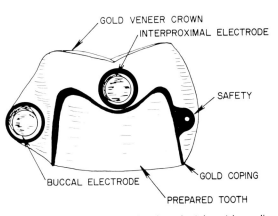

Figure 16/9. Schematic drawing of a telemetric appliance used to monitor plaque pH. Plaque is allowed to accumulate on the electrode and the response is to fermentable carbohydrate. (Reproduced with permission from C. F. Schachtele and M. E. Jensen: *Cereal Foods World*, **26**, 14, 1981.)

Table 16/5

Factors capable of influencing the cariogenic potential of a food at the time of ingestion

Host factors:
  Buffering capacity of saliva
  Calcium and phosphate concentration of saliva
  Flow rate and viscosity of saliva
  Presence and age of plaque at caries-prone sites
  Composition of the plaque matrix
  Anatomy of the dentition
  Microstructure of the enamel
  Fluoride content of enamel and plaque
  Pattern of mastication, sucking, rinsing, swallowing
  Breathing by mouth
  Frequency of food ingestion

Microbial factors:
  Concentration of acidogenic bacteria at specific sites on the teeth
  Acidogenic potential of bacteria on mucosal surfaces and in saliva
  Concentration of acid-utilizing bacteria in plaque

Substrate factors:
  Total fermentable carbohydrate
  Concentration of mono-, di-, oligo-, and polysaccharides
  Concentration and types of proteins and fats
  Physical form including factors that effect oral retention
  Presence of fluoride, calcium, phosphate and trace elements
  Total buffering capacity
  Presence and quantity of sialogogues, metabolic inhibitors, flavors and organic phosphates
  Acidity of the food
  Sequences of ingestion relative to other foods

volved in altering the carbohydrate content of foods it is important to consider the status of attempts to evaluate the cariogenicity of individual foodstuffs.

Table 16/5 presents a brief summary of the various factors which may contribute to the cariogenic potential of a food when it is ingested. Since the relative contribution of each of the factors could vary depending on the food in question it is clear that a formidable task confronts the scientist attempting to study food cariogenicity. Practical and ethical considerations have limited researchers' capacity to evaluate the cariogenicity of individual foods through human clinical trials. A variety of procedures have been used to obtain data on particular food items relative to their cariogenic potential. These procedures include chemical analysis of foods, measurement of oral retention, quantitation of buffering capacity, evaluation of enamel decalcification potential, plaque pH responses and *in vitro* caries formation. Although all of these procedures provide useful data attempts to correlate results between the procedures has not proven very meaningful. The primary problem here is in assigning a relative weight to the results from any one method. For example, is buffering capacity more important than oral retention with regard to smooth surface decay?

Although there are many approaches to this complex problem emphasis in recent years has focused on two major methods for evaluating a food's cariogenic potential. Studies with rats where actual disease can be measured and studies on plaque pH changes following food ingestion by humans have both provided data of considerable importance. The goal of this work is to compare the two models with regard to their ability to assess, with various foods, caries and *in situ* acid production. Agreement between the models would allow the evolution of a testing system which could be standardized and used to estimate the cariogenic potential of foods in humans. Such a test would provide a means for evaluating the effect of changes in food composition relative to caries and hopefully allow the production of noncariogenic foods.

In the rat model animals are handled under carefully controlled conditions to ensure reproducible results. Standardized inoculums of *S. mutans* are used to infect the animals at a defined age to cause maximum lesion production. The animals are supplied with a defined diet by one of two methods which minimize contact with the teeth. In one case gastric intubation of the food through a tube is performed at certain intervals during the day. In the other method the food is packaged in a gel which prevents caries formation since the carbohydrate is not available to the oral flora. The test food can be presented in several ways but utilization of a programmed feeding machine seems to provide the most consistent results. This machine supplies the test foods on a carousel which is programmed to move at certain intervals and provide a known quantity of food. Up to 17 nocturnal feedings are frequently used to maximize caries formation. Although the rat models have several important limitations they have been used to compare foods and a Cariogenic Potential Index has been created using sucrose as a standard.

Various methods have been used to measure

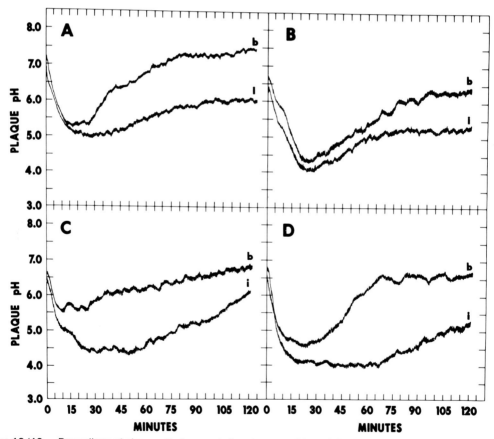

Figure 16/10.   Recordings of plaque pH changes in four human subjects following rinsing with a sucrose solution. Data was obtained from plaque-coated microelectrodes positioned at buccal and interproximal sites as illustrated in figure 16/9. In each case the upper curve represents the buccal (*b*) electrode and the lower curve the interproximal (*i*) electrode. The caries-prone interproximal site retains greater quantites of acid for a longer period of time. (Reproduced with permission from M. E. Jensen, C. F. Schachtele, and P. J. Polansky: *Foods, Nutrition and Dental Health*, Vol. 3, Pathotox Publishers, Inc., Park Forest South, Ill.)

plaque pH. A technique usually referred to as "plaque sampling" has been used with considerable success by a number of investigators. In this method, plaque is removed from the teeth at intervals following test food ingestion, and the pH is measured after dispersion of the sample in diluent. Some of the limitations of this technique are that the plaque is disturbed each time a sample is collected, the sample represents a pooling of plaque from different sites, and intermittent rather than continuous measurements are made.

In a second method, microelectrodes are placed within plaque on the tooth surface at intervals after food ingestion. Such "touch electrode" techniques allow direct readings of pH on the plaque surface. Investigations with both antimony and glass electrodes have provided useful data. In general, this method provides information similar to that obtained by plaque sampling.

In a more complex technique, plaque is allowed to accumulate on glass electrodes that have been fixed within the dentition (fig. 16/9). After food ingestion, pH readings can be made continuously from the "indwelling electrode" by either wire or radio telemetry.

Graf and Mühlemann pioneered work in this area and a wealth of information has resulted from subsequent studies. Indeed, the Swiss Health Authorities issued regulations that sweets could be advertised as "zahnschonend" (i.e., friendly to teeth) when studies showed that telemetric measurements did not drop below 5.7 within 30 minutes after ingestion.

Because an electrode used in telemetry is normally placed so that its pH-sensitive tip is on a proximal surface between abutting teeth, it is not surprising that this method shows greater levels of acid production than other methods, such as plaque sampling. A compelling argument in favor of telemetry is that it allows pH measurements at sites in the dentition that are known to be prone to caries development and permits continuous rather than intermittent measurements (fig. 16/10).

The primary finding at this time relative to the acidogenic potential of foods is that most foods with a measurable content of fermentable carbohydrate cause a significant drop in pH at caries-prone interproximal sites. Foods which do not show this response include some meats, some cheeses, eggs, peanuts and various confections containing sugar substitutes.

In addition, many foods can cause prolonged drops in plaque pH probably due to their retention at the interproximal site. These data emphasize the importance of using adequate oral hygiene techniques such as flossing after eating most foods.

In summary, progress is being made in evaluating the cariogenic potential of individual foods. By focusing on dietary components which are known to have anticariogenic properties such as lipids, phosphates and proteins it should be possible to develop products with minimal cariogenic potential. Achieving this goal may eventually lead to a reduction in the formation of dental caries in humans.

ADDITIONAL READINGS

BIBBY, B. G., AND SHERN, R. J. (Eds.) 1978 Proceedings "Methods of Caries Prediction," Special Supplement, Microbiology Abstracts, Information Retrieval Inc., Washington, D.C.

BOWDEN, G. H. W., ELLWOOD, D. C., AND HAMILTON, I. R. 1979 Microbial Ecology of the Oral Cavity. In *Advances in Microbial Ecology*, Vol. 3, p. 135. Plenum Press, New York.

BOWEN, W. H., AMSBAUGH, S. M., MONELL-TORRENS, S., BRUNELLE, J., KUZMIAK-JONES, H., AND COLE, M. F. 1980 A Method to Assess Cariogenic Potential of Foodstuffs. J Am Dent Assoc, **100,** 677.

BOWEN, W. H., GENCO, R. J., AND O'BRIEN, T. C. 1976 "Immunologic Aspects of Dental Caries," Special Supplement, Immunology Abstracts, Information Retrieval Inc., Washington, D.C.

BOWEN, W. H., AND GUGGENHEIM, B. 1978 Therapeutics of Caries Prevention-Concepts and Prospects. Acta Odontol Scand, **36,** 185.

CAUFIELD, P. W., AND GIBBONS, R. J. 1979 Suppression of *Streptococcus mutans* in the Mouths of Humans by a Dental Prophylaxis and Topically-applied Iodine. J Dent Res, **58,** 1317.

CLARK, J. K. 1924 On the Bacterial Factor in the Aetiology of Dental Caries. Br J Exp Pathol, **5,** 141.

COHEN, S. N. 1975 The Manipulation of Genes. Sci Am, **233,** 24.

COYKENDALL, A. L. 1977 Proposal to Elevate the Subspecies of *Streptococcus mutans* to Species Status, Based on Their Molecular Composition. Int J Syst Bacteriol, **27,** 26.

DAWES, C. 1968 The Nature of Dental Plaque, Films, and Calcareous Deposits. Ann NY Acad Sci, **153,** 102.

DUCHIN, S., AND VAN HOUTE, J. 1978 Relationship of *Streptococcus mutans* and Lactobacilli to Incipient Smooth Surface Dental Caries in Man. Arch Oral Biol, **23,** 779.

EDMAN, D. C., KEENE, H. J., SHKLAIR, I. L., AND HOERMAN, K. C. 1975 Dental Floss for Implantation and Sampling of *Streptococcus mutans* from Approximal Surfaces of Human Teeth. Arch Oral Biol, **20,** 145.

ELLEN, R. P. 1976 Microbiological Assays for Dental Caries and Periodontal Disease Susceptibility. Oral Sci Rev, **8,** 3.

ENGLANDER, H. R., AND KEYES, P. H. 1970 Effect of Phosphate Supplements on Cavitation in Hamsters Infected with Caries-conducive Streptococci. J Dent Res, **49,** 140.

FITZGERALD, R. J. 1972 Inhibition of Experimental Dental Caries by Antibiotics. Antimicrob Agents Chemother, **1,** 296.

FITZGERALD, R. J., AND KEYES, P. H. 1960 Demonstration of the Etiologic Role of Streptococci in Experimental Caries in the Hamster. J Am Dent Assoc, **61,** 1960.

GERMAINE, G. R., AND SCHACHTELE, C. F. 1976 *Streptococcus mutans* Dextransucrase: Mode of Interaction with High Molecular Weight Dextran and Role in Cellular Aggregation. Infect Immun, **13,** 356.

GERMAINE, G. R., HARLANDER, S. K., AND SCHACHTELE,

C. F. 1977 *Streptococcus mutans* Dextransucrase: Functioning of Primer Dextran and Endogenous Dextranase in Water-soluble and Water-insoluble Product Formation. Infect Immun, **16**, 637.

GIBBONS, R. J., AND VAN HOUTE, J. 1973 On the Formation of Dental Plaques. J Periodontol, **44**, 347.

GIBBONS, R. J., AND VAN HOUTE, J. 1975 Dental Caries. Ann Rev Med, **26**, 121.

GIBBONS, R. J., AND VAN HOUTE, J. 1975 Bacterial Adherence in Oral Microbial Ecology. Ann Rev Microbiol, **29**, 19.

GUGGENHEIM, B. 1970 Extracellular Polysaccharides and Microbial Plaque. Int Dent J, **20**, 657.

GUGGENHEIM, B. 1979 *Health and Sugar Substitutes.* S. Karger, Basal, Switzerland.

HAMADA, S., AND SLADE, H. D. 1980 Biology, Immunology, and Cariogenicity of *Streptococcus mutans*. Microbiol Rev, **44**, 331.

HARDIE, J. M., THOMSON, P. L., SOUTH, R. J., MARSH, P. D., BOWDEN, G. H., McKEE, A. S., FILLERY, E. D., AND SLACK, G. L. 1977 A Longitudinal Epidemiological Study on Dental Plaque and the Development of Dental Caries-Interim Results after Two Years. J Dent Res, **56**, C90.

HARLANDER, S. K., AND SCHACHTELE, C. F. 1978 *Streptococcus mutans* Dextransucrase: Stimulation of Glucan Formation by Phosphoglycerides. Infect Immun, **19**, 450.

HEFFERREN, J. J., AND KOEHLER, H. M. 1981 *Foods, Nutrition and Dental Health*, Vol. 1. Pathotox Publishers, Inc., Park Forest South, Ill.

HEFFERREN, J. J., AYER, W. A., AND H. M. KOEHLER. 1981 *Foods, Nutrition and Dental Health*, Vol. 3. Pathotox Publishers, Inc., Park Forest South, Ill.

HILLMAN, J. D. 1978 Lactate Dehydrogenase Mutants of *Streptococcus mutans*: Isolation and Preliminary Characterization. Infect Immun, **21**, 206.

JAY, P. 1947 The Reduction of Oral *Lactobacillus acidophilus* Counts by the Periodic Restriction of Carbohydrate. Am J Orthod Oral Surg, **33**, 162.

JOHNSON, C. P., GROSS, S. M., AND HILLMAN, J. D. 1980 Cariogenic Potential *in Vitro* in Man and *in Vivo* in the Rat of Lactate Dehydrogenase Mutants of *Streptococcus mutans*. Arch Oral Biol, **25**, 707.

KLEINBERG, I. 1978 Prevention and Dental Caries. J Prev Dent, **5**, 9.

KLEINBERG, I. (Ed.) 1979 Proceedings "Saliva and Dental Caries," Special Supplement, Microbiology Abstracts, Information Retrieval Inc., Washington, D.C.

KEYES, P. H. 1960 The Infectious and Transmittable Nature of Experimental Dental Caries. Arch Oral Biol, **13**, 304.

LAZZARI, E. P. 1976 *Dental Biochemistry*. Lea & Fibiger, Philadelphia.

LEACH, S. A. (Ed.) 1980 Proceedings "Dental Plaque and Surface Interactions in the Oral Cavity," Information Retrieval Ltd., London.

LEHNER, T. 1977 *The Borderland between Caries and Periodontal Disease*. Academic Press, London.

LEVINE, M. J., HERZBERG, M. C., LEVINE, M. S., ELLISON, S. A., STINSON, M. W., LI, H. C., AND VAN DYKE, T. 1978 Specificity of Salivary-Bacterial Interactions: Role of Terminal Sialic Acid Residues in the Interaction of Salivary Glycoproteins with *Streptococcus sanguis* and *Streptococcus mutans*. Infect Immun, **19**, 107.

LEWIS, D. W., AND HARGREAVES, J. A. 1975 Epidemiology of Dental Caries in Relation to Pits and Fissures. Br Dent J, **138**, 345.

LISTGARTEN, M. A. 1976 Structure of Surface Coatings on Teeth. A Review. J Periodontol, **47**, 139.

LOE, H. 1971 The Control of Dental Plaque by Chemical Means. Int Dent J, **21**, 41.

LOESCHE, W. J. 1975 Chemotherapy of Dental Plaque Infections. Oral Sci Rev, **9**, 65.

LOESCHE, W. J., AND STRAFFON, L. H. 1979 Longitudinal Investigation of the Role of *Streptococcus mutans* in Human Fissure Decay. Infect Immun, **26**, 498.

LOESCHE, W. J., AND SYED, S. A. 1973 The Predominant Cultivable Flora of Carious Plaque and Carious Dentine. Caries Res, **7**, 201.

LOESCHE, W. J., SVANBERG, M. L., AND PAPE, H. R. 1979 Intraoral Transmission of *Streptococcus mutans* by a Dental Explorer. J Dent Res, **58**, 1765.

McGHEE, J. R., AND MICHALEK, S. M. 1981 Immunobiology of Dental Caries: Microbial Aspects and Local Immunity. Annu Rev Microbiol, **35**, 595.

McGHEE, J. R., MESTECKY, J., AND BABB, J. L. (Eds.) 1977 *Secretory Immunity and Infection*. Plenum Press, New York.

McHUGH, W. D. (Ed.) 1970 *Dental Plaque*. E. & S. Livingstone Ltd. London.

MEIERS, J. C., WIRTHLIN, M. R., AND SHKLAIR, I. L. 1982 A Microbiological Analysis of Human Early Carious and Non-carious Fissures. J Dent Res, **61**, 460.

MENAKER, L. (Ed.) 1980 *The Biologic Basis of Dental Caries*. Harper & Row, Hagerstown, Md.

MERGENHAGEN, S. E., AND SCHERP, H. W. (Eds.) 1973 Comparative Immunology of the Oral Cavity, DHEW Publication No. (NIH) 73-438, U.S. Government Printing Office, Washington, D.C.

MICHALEK, S. M., AND McGHEE, J. R. 1977 Effective Immunity to Dental Caries: Passive Transfer to Rats of Antibodies to *Streptococcus mutans* Elicits Protection. Infect Immun, **17**, 644.

MICHELICH, V. J., SCHUSTER, G. S., AND PASHLEY, D. H. 1980 Bacterial Penetration of Human Dentin *in Vitro*. J Dent Res, **59**, 1398.

MIKX, F. H. M., VAN DER HOEVEN, J. S., KONIG, K. G., PLASSEHAERT, M., AND GUGGENHEIM, B. 1972 Establishment of Defined Ecosystems in Germ-Free Rats; I. The Effect of the Interaction of *Streptococcus mutans* or *Streptococcus sanguis* with *Veillonella alcalescens* on Plaque Formation and Caries Activity. Caries Res, **6**, 211.

MILLER, W. D. 1890 *The Microorganisms of the Human Mouth*. S. S. White Dental Manufacturing Company, Philadelphia.

MILSTEIN, C. 1980 Monoclonal Antibodies. Sci Am, **243**, 66.

MINAH, G. E., AND LOESCHE, W. J. 1977 Sucrose Metabolism in Resting-cell Suspensions of Caries-associated and Non-caries-associated Dental Plaque. Infect Immun, **17**, 43.

MJÖR, I. A., AND PINDBORG, J. J. (Eds.) 1973 *Histology of the Human Tooth*. Munksgaard, Copenhagen.

NAVIA, J. M. 1977 *Animal Models in Dental Research*. The University of Alabama Press, Birmingham, Ala.

NEWBRUN, E. (Ed.) 1975 *Fluorides and Dental Caries*. Charles C Thomas, Springfield, Ill.

NEWBRUN, E. 1978 *Cariology*. Williams & Wilkins, Baltimore.

NEWMAN, H. N. 1980 *Dental Plaque. The Ecology of the Flora on Human Teeth*. Charles C Thomas, Springfield, Ill.

ONOSE, H., AND SANDHAM, H. J. 1976 pH Changes during Culture of Human Dental Plaque Streptococci on Mitis-Salivarius Agar. Arch Oral Biol, **21**, 291.

ROIT, I. M., AND LEHNER, T. 1980 *Immunology of Oral Diseases*. Blackwell Scientific Pub., London.

RØLLA, G., SØNJU, T., AND EMBERY, G. (Eds.) 1981 Tooth

Surface Interactions and Preventive Dentistry, Information Retrieval Ltd., London.

SAXTON, C. H. 1973 Scanning Electron Microscopic Study of the Formation of Dental Plaque. Caries Res, **7,** 102.

SCHACHTELE, C. F., AND MAYO, J. A. 1973 Phosphoenolpyruvate-dependent Glucose Transport by Oral Streptococci. J Dent Res, **52,** 1209.

SHAW, J. H., AND ROUSSOS, G. G. (Eds.) 1978 Sweeteners and Dental Caries, Information Retrieval Inc., Washington, D.C.

SHAW, J. H., SWEENEY, E. A., CAPPUCCINO, C. C., AND MELLER, S. M. 1978 *Textbook of Oral Biology.* W. B. Saunders, Philadelphia.

SIMS, W. 1968 A Modified Snyder Test for Caries Activity in Humans. Arch Oral Biol, **13,** 853.

SILVERSTONE, L. M. 1978 *Preventive Dentistry.* Update Books, Fort Lee, N.J.

SILVERSTONE, L. M., JOHNSON, N. W., HARDIE, J. M., AND WILLIAMS, R. A. D. 1981 *Dental Caries Aetiology, Pathology and Prevention.* Macmillan, London.

SOCRANSKY, S. S., AND MANGANIELLO, A. D. 1971 The Oral Microbiota from Birth to Senility. J Periodontol, **42,** 485.

SOCRANSKY, S. S., MANGANIELLO, A. D., PROPAS, D., ORAM, V., AND VAN HOUTE, J. 1977 Bacteriological Studies of Developing Supragingival Dental Plaque. J Periodont Res, **12,** 90.

STAAT, R. H., AND SCHACHTELE, C. F. 1974 Evaluation of Dextranase Production by the Cariogenic Bacterium *Streptococcus mutans.* Infect Immun, **9,** 467.

STAAT, R. H., GAWRONSKI, T. H., CRESSEY, D. E., HARRIS, R. S., AND FOLKE, L. E. A. 1975 Effects of Dietary Sucrose Levels on the Quantity and Microbial Composition of Human Dental Plaque. J Dent Res, **54,** 872.

STAAT, R. H., GAWRONSKI, T. H., AND SCHACHTELE, C. F. 1973 Detection and Preliminary Studies on Dextranase-producing Microorganisms from Human Dental Plaque. Infect Immun, **8,** 1009.

STILES, H. M., LOESCHE, W. J., AND O'BRIEN, T. C. (Eds.) 1976 Proceedings "Microbial Aspects of Dental Caries," Special Supplement, Microbiology Abstracts, Vol. I, II, III, Information Retrieval, Washington, D.C.

SVANBERG, M. L., AND LOESCHE, W. J. 1978 Implantation of *Streptococcus mutans* on Tooth Surfaces in Man. Arch Oral Biol, **23,** 551.

SVANBERG, M. L., AND LOESCHE, W. J. 1978 Intraoral Spread of *Streptococcus mutans* in Man. Arch Oral Biol, **23,** 557.

SYED, S. A., LOESCHE, W. J., PAPE, H. L., AND GRENIER, E. 1975 Predominant Cultivable Flora Isolated from Human Root Surface Caries Plaque. Infect Immun, **11,** 727.

TANZER, J. M. (Ed.) 1981 Animal Models in Cariology, Information Retrieval Inc., Washington, D.C.

TOMASI, T. B. 1976 *The Immune System of Secretions.* Prentice-Hall, Englewood Cliffs, N.J.

VAN HOUTE, J., AND GREEN, D. B. 1974 Relationship between the Concentrations of Bacteria in Saliva and the Colonization of Teeth in Humans. Infect Immun, **9,** 624.

VAN HOUTE, J., AND UPESLACIS, V. N. 1976 Studies of the Mechanism of Sucrose-Associated Colonization of *Streptococcus mutans* on Teeth of Conventional Rats. J Dent Res, **55,** 216.

WEI, S. H. Y. (Ed.) 1979 National Symposium on Dental Nutrition, The University of Iowa, Iowa City, Iowa.

chapter 17

Periodontal Disease

Mark R. Patters

INTRODUCTION

Diseases of the periodontium are among the most common afflictions of mankind. In fact, bone resorption consistent with periodontitis has been observed in the fossil remains of Neanderthal man, and detailed descriptions of periodontal disease in Chinese and Egyptian writings predate this chapter by more than 4000 years. Epidemiological surveys conducted during this century suggest that essentially all the world's populations have experienced some form of periodontal disease. This chapter will present the current status of our understanding of factors involved in the etiology and progression of inflammatory periodontal disease in man.

Four structures, termed collectively the periodontium, invest the teeth and support them in functional relationship to each other. These are 1) the alveolar bone, which is formed around the root of the developing tooth; 2) the cementum, a calcified matrix laid down on the root of the tooth by differentiated cells of the periodontal ligament (or membrane); 3) the periodontal ligament proper, which has transverse collagen fibers anchoring the tooth by embedment in alveolar bone and cementum; and 4) the gingiva, which in health forms a tight cuff about the neck of the tooth.

The periodontium is subject to a variety of pathoses, collectively but loosely termed periodontal disease. The unmodified term periodontal disease usually means a chronic, slowly progressive and destructive inflammatory process affecting one or more of the four components of the periodontium—literally, chronic periodontitis. The term "gingivitis" is used for readily reversible inflammation involving marginal gingiva, and "periodontitis" for inflammation extending deeper into the periodontium.

The principal features of inflammatory periodontal disease are 1) occurrence most frequently in otherwise healthy persons; 2) accumulation of bacterial plaque at the gingival margin, which may mineralize to form subgingival calculus; 3) chronic inflammation of the gingiva and periodontal ligament, with degeneration of connective tissue ground substance and collagen fibers; 4) apical migration of epithelium with formation of periodontal pockets in which additional bacterial debris accumulates, often accompanied by purulent exudate; and 5) resorption of alveolar bone and to a lesser extent cementum, with loss of anchoring of the periodontal collagen fibers and consequent mobility and eventual exfoliation of the teeth. Fundamentally, periodontal disease is a pathosis of connective tissue.

Research has defined many of the microbial and host factors involved in periodontal disease. The early phases may involve the action of cytotoxic substances and histolytic enzymes from plaque bacteria on cells and intercellular substance of gingival junctional epithelium. Later destruction of periodontal tissues and alveolar bone may result from excessive and continued host inflammatory response that is sustained by chemotactic and toxic bacterial products, and by hypersensitivity. Host factors predisposing to increased or decreased resistance of the periodontium are summarized in figure 17/1.

Periodontal disease is a major global public health problem. Nearly all adults have gingival inflammation or periodontitis. After age 35 years, this syndrome causes two to three times as many extractions as dental caries.

EPIDEMIOLOGY OF CHRONIC INFLAMMATORY PERIODONTAL DISEASE

Surveys made during the past 40 years indicate that nearly every adult in North America has some periodontal disease. About half of those who still retain some teeth at age 50 have extensive periodontal tissue destruction. As a consequence of caries before age 35 years and mostly of periodontal disease thereafter, between 20 and 30 million adults in the United States have lost all of their teeth; the eventual total loss from each disease is about the same.

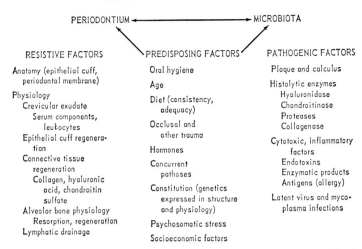

PERIODONTIUM ⟷ MICROBIOTA

RESISTIVE FACTORS — PREDISPOSING FACTORS — PATHOGENIC FACTORS

RESISTIVE FACTORS

Anatomy (epithelial cuff, periodontal membrane)

Physiology
Crevicular exudate
Serum components, leukocytes
Epithelial cuff regeneration
Connective tissue regeneration
Collagen, hyaluronic acid, chondroitin sulfate
Alveolar bone physiology
Resorption, regeneration
Lymphatic drainage

PREDISPOSING FACTORS

Oral hygiene

Age

Diet (consistency, adequacy)

Occlusal and other trauma

Hormones

Concurrent pathoses

Constitution (genetics expressed in structure and physiology)

Psychosomatic stress

Socioeconomic factors

PATHOGENIC FACTORS

Plaque and calculus

Histolytic enzymes
Hyaluronidase
Chondroitinase
Proteases
Collagenase

Cytotoxic, inflammatory factors
Endotoxins
Enzymatic products
Antigens (allergy)

Latent virus and mycoplasma infections

Figure 17/1. Status of the periodontium is the resultant of numerous interactions with the sulcal microbiota, conditioned by many predisposing factors. (Adapted from H. W. Scherp: Current Concepts in Periodontal Disease Research: Epidemiological Contributions. *Journal of the American Dental Association*, **68**, 667, 1964.)

Periodontal and Oral Hygiene Indexes

Critical quantitative data on a scale sufficient to substantiate the relative importance of various etiological factors have become available only recently as adequate indices have been developed. Operational necessity has limited a large fraction of periodontal studies to scoring the reversible inflammatory involvements of the gingiva. In the PMA (papillary, marginal, attached) gingival index, the P and M components score increasing involvement about each tooth on a scale of 5, culminating with atrophy and loss of papillae and recession of marginal gingiva below the cementoenamel junction; the A component allows scoring of periodontitis with pocket formation.

Many recent studies have used the gingival index (GI) which scores the mesial, distal, buccal, and lingual gingival areas around each tooth from 0 (no inflammation) to 3 (severe inflammation, ulceration, spontaneous bleeding).

The periodontal index (PI), which enables quantitative assessment of the more advanced stages of tissue destruction, has been widely used to assess the periodontal status of populations. In determining the PI, each tooth is scored as follows: 0, health; 1, mild gingivitis in a discrete region; 2, marginal gingivitis circumscribing the tooth without pocket formation; 6, gingivitis with pocket formation; and 8, advanced periodontal destruction with loss of masticatory function. The PI for a given mouth is the sum of the scores of individual teeth divided by the number of teeth examined.

An alternative periodontal index (PDI) depends on assessment of gingivitis and measurement of the distance by which the bottom of the gingival sulcus extends apically beyond the cementoenamel junc-

tion. The recommended clinical examination also provides data for indices of occlusal and incisal attrition, tooth mobility, lack of contact, plaque, and calculus.

Oral hygiene indices of unmineralized debris plus calculus have been described. For the oral hygiene index-simplified (OHI-S), the condition of each of six tooth surfaces is scored according to the fraction of exposed tooth surface covered by loose soft debris and calculus, respectively; 0, none; 1, up to one-third; 2, between one- and two-thirds; 3, more than two-thirds, or a continuous heavy band of subgingival calculus around the cervical portion of the tooth. Ordinarily, the buccal surfaces of the upper first molars, the lingual surfaces of the lower first molars, and the labial surfaces of the upper right and lower left central incisors are scored. The mean debris index score (DI-S) plus the mean calculus index score (CI) gives the OHI-S; the maximum possible score.

The plaque index measures the thickness of plaque at the gingival margin on the buccal, lingual, mesial and distal of each tooth. The scores used are 0, none; 1, plaque which is not visible to the eye but can be seen on an instrument when scraped along the gingival margin of the tooth surface; 2, plaque can be seen with the unaided eye; and 3, gross accumulation of plaque. In conjunction with the gingival index, the plaque index has been used extensively in research to yield the current knowledge of the relationship of plaque accumulation to gingival inflammation.

Other plaque indices have been developed which measure the surface area of tooth covered with plaque after staining the teeth with a dye which reveals plaque. These indices usually do not correlate well with gingival inflammation because they measure plaque distant from the area of the gingival margin which has little effect on inflammation.

Epidemiological Findings and Their Significance

Gingivitis is negligible during the first 5 years of life. However, by age 7 it affects at least two-thirds of suburban children. Prevalence remains at about this level through the 3rd decade. The PMA score rises with increasing age, but is not correlated with prevalence of caries.

Gingivitis increases rapidly to a peak at the onset of puberty, presumably due to hormonal factors and decreases somewhat to reach a plateau from age 16 to age 25 years, when a very slow, long-term rise begins.

Periodontal disease has often been considered to be antagonistic to dental caries, in the sense that the oral environment associated with periodontal disease is not conducive to the development of caries, and vice versa. Epidemiological analysis does not support this concept.

Surveys measuring the prevalence and severity of periodontal disease, without exception, indicate a correlation of increasing oral uncleanliness and age with increasing prevalence and severity of periodontal disease. When the group data have been equalized for oral hygiene and age by statistical analysis, no correlation has yet been established between periodontal index and geography, water fluoride levels, race, ABO blood groupings, sex, molar attrition, total serum protein, hemoglobulin, socioeconomic factors, or nutritional status with respect to vitamin A, ascorbic acid, thiamine, riboflavin, or nicotinamide.

The rising prevalence of periodontal disease with age and the correlated onset of periodontitis are illustrated in figure 17/2. In this study, signs of periodontal disease were common in childhood, and the fraction of persons having obvious disease reached 60% in the 20- to 24-year age group, but only 9% of these had pockets. In the next 5-year period, the diseased fraction increased only to 68%, but the proportion of those with pockets rose sharply to 23%. This increase continued steadily thereafter, reaching 68% after age 45 years. Evidence of periodontal destruction generally does not appear until the 3rd decade of life.

Figure 17/3 illustrates the correlation of periodontal index, debris index, calculus index, and age group. The group periodontal index and the group oral hygiene index increase roughly in parallel with increasing age. When the two components of the oral hygiene index are considered separately, the debris index reaches a high level early in life and increases only slightly with time. The cumulative rise in the oral hygiene index is caused mostly by a steady rise in the calculus index with age. Progressive accumulation of calculus is recognized repeat-

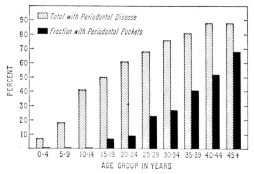

Figure 17/2. Periodontal inflammation is widely prevalent early in life but pocket formation remains infrequent until the third decade. *Hatched bars*: percent distribution by age group of persons with manifest periodontal disease, periodontal index score greater than zero. *Solid bars*: percent of those periodontally diseased who had developed periodontal pockets. Data for 1877 subjects. (Reproduced with permission from L. Barros and C. J. Witkop, Jr.: Oral and Genetic Study of Chileans 1960; III. Periodontal Disease and Nutritional Factors. *Archives of Oral Biology*, **8**, 195, 1963.)

edly as a close correlate of increasing severity of periodontitis.

In a given oral hygiene score group, the severity of periodontal disease increases progressively with age, especially after 25 years (fig. 17/4). Evidently throughout the teen years one can have an extraordinarily dirty mouth (OHI-S score of 4.1 or greater) with an average risk of developing nothing worse than gingivitis (PI score of about 1.0 or less).

Periodontitis is uncommon before 25 years, but rises rapidly thereafter. If one maintains only moderately good oral hygiene (OHI-S of 2.1 to 3.0), eventually one is likely to develop severe periodontitis. If one maintains good oral hygiene (OHI-S of 2.0 or below) from age 5 to age 50 years, one has a good chance of avoiding periodontitis.

Structure and Physiology of the Periodontium

The anatomic relationships of the periodontium are shown diagrammatically in figure 17/5. The term sulcus applies to the proportionately long (1.5 to 2.5 mm) area of contact between the junctional epithelium and the enamel; and the term *periodontal pocket* designates the clinically patent gingival pouch that develops under pathological conditions.

Mucous membrane entirely lines the oral cavity except for the erupted teeth. The gingiva is that part of the mucosa that is attached to the teeth and alveolar bone. It consists of keratinized surface epithelium overlying dense connective tissue. A well-differentiated submucosa cannot be recognized in the gingiva. "Oral epithelium" extends from the alveolar mucosa over the tip of the marginal gingiva into the sulcus, where the superficial cells become

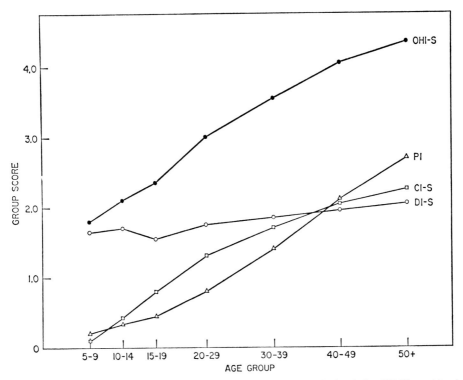

Figure 17/3. Correlation of periodontal index (*PI*), debris index (*DI-S*), calculus index (*CI-S*), oral hygiene index (*OHI-S* = DI-S + CI-S), and age group. Combined data for civilians in Ecuador (1959) and Montana (1961). (Reproduced with permission from J. C. Greene: Oral Hygiene and Periodontal Disease. *American Journal of Public Health*, **53**, 913, 1963, copyright by the American Journal of Public Health, Inc.)

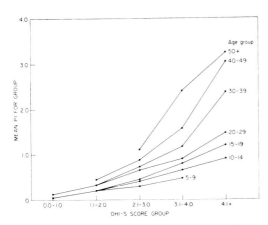

Figure 17/4. In a given oral hygiene index score (*OHI-S*) group, the severity of periodontitis increases with age. Combined data for civilians in Ecuador (1959) and Montana (1961). (Reproduced with permission from J. C. Greene: Oral Hygiene and Periodontal Disease. *American Journal of Public Health*, **53**, 913, 1963, copyright by the American Journal of Public Health, Inc.)

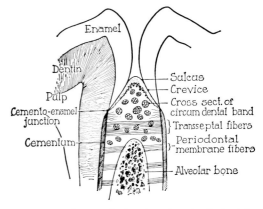

Figure 17/5. Schematic drawing of anatomical relationships of the periodontium.

less keratinized. Apically, sulcular epithelium merges with so-called junctional epithelium, which interposes between gingival connective tissue and tooth surface from the bottom of the sulcus where it ranges from 15 to 30 cells thick. Throughout this area the junctional epithelium normally adheres to the enamel of the fully erupted tooth as far as the cementoenamel junction. The attachment between epithelium and tooth is maintained by hemidesmosomes and is termed the epithelial attachment. In man, monkey, and dog, junctional epithelium does not keratinize.

The marginal gingiva surrounding one tooth joins the marginal gingiva of an adjacent tooth to form interdental papillae. The papillae seen at the oral and vestibular aspects do not necessarily extend across the interproximal space. Particularly between recently erupted teeth, the interproximal gingiva falls off to form a "col" between the two peaks. The sulcus may be correspondingly short in the col area. With newly erupted teeth in apposition, the col is covered by reduced enamel epithelium, a not very dynamic vestigial tissue, which ordinarily is gradually undergrown and replaced by stratified squamous epithelium from the adjacent papillae.

The lamina propria underlies and supports the gingival epithelium, with which it forms an undulating margin (epithelial ridges). The lamina propria is typical dense connective tissue. In this tissue many of the collagenous bundles are disordered but others are embedded at one end in the cementum (dentogingival fibers) or alveolar bone (alveogingival fibers), thereby anchoring the attached gingiva. Other functional groups are the circumdental fibers, which form interlacing bands around the tooth, and the transeptal fibers, which run interproximally between adjacent teeth and are embedded in cementum at the ends.

Connective tissues consist largely of collagens, a family of fibrous proteins produced by fibroblasts and characterized by several unique chemical and physical properties. As extruded from fibroblasts, a collagen molecule ("tropocollagen") is comprised of three polypeptide chains, each of about 1000 amino acids and molecular weight 120,000, held together by hydrogen bonds in a triple helix about 300 nm long and 1.4 nm in diameter. Under physiological conditions of salinity, pH, and temperature, collagen molecules aggregate spontaneously in an overlapping manner with their axes parallel to form submicroscopic collagen fibrils, held together by labile noncovalent bonds. Extracellularly, specific amino groups on lysine and hydroxylysine residues are oxidized enzymatically to aldehyde groups which react nonenzymatically to form covalent intermolecular cross-links either by aldol condensation of two aldehyde groups or by Schiff base formation between an aldehyde group and a residual ϵ-amino group on lysine or hydroxylysine. Thus, fibrils are united into the collagen fibers of tissue. Cross-links via glycosaminoglycans may also be involved. Such mature collagens are variably insoluble in aqueous media and, unless denatured, resist proteases other than specific collagenases. Mature collagens tend to be metabolically inert but vary widely; tendon collagen turns over minimally, whereas periodontal ligament collagen is quite dynamic.

The ground substance of connective tissue consists of a colloid-rich, water-poor, viscid gel matrix, enclosing submicroscopic vacuoles (0.05 to 0.2 μm) with protein-rich walls, and containing chiefly water. The gel phase consists primarily of complexes of proteins and the acid mucopolysaccharides hyaluronic acid, chondroitin, chondroitin sulfates (A, B, C), and keratosulfate. Glycoproteins, plasma proteins, and other soluble components of plasma are also present.

The acid mucopolysaccharides are products of fibroblasts and perhaps mast cells, with molecular weights of many millions. Hyaluronic acid and chondroitin sulfates have been demonstrated in human gingiva. Also present is sialic acid. So-called neutral heteropolysaccharides have been found in ground substance glycoprotein.

The ground substance is the medium through which water, salts, gases, nutrients, metabolic products, and internal secretions are exchanged selectively between blood and parenchymal cells. It functions as a selectively permeable barrier, controlling the distribution of solutes in part by Donnan equilibrium. Because of its net excess of acidic groups, the ground substance acts also like a cation-exchange resin. Its permeability is readily altered by a variety of physiological and pathological factors that alter its degree of polymerization. Ground substance is subject to disaggregation by mucopolysaccharases (hyaluronidase, chondroitinase, chondrosulfatase) and proteases. The production of such enzymes by oral bacteria and their possible pathogenic role in periodontal disease is discussed later in this chapter.

Alveolar bone, which serves as the rigid support of the periodontium, closely resembles ordinary bone. The principal fiber bundles of the periodontal ligament continue as Sharpey's fibers into the adjacent layer of alveolar bone, therefore called "bundle bone." The outer portion of alveolar bone consists of periosteum covering cortical plates. The cortical plate invaginates into the interstitial bone, forming the sockets in which the teeth are held by the principal fibers of the periodontal ligament.

By its nature alveolar bone is regularly subjected to asymmetrical forces and therefore the bone must be highly adaptable. Normally, alveolar bone is constantly in a state of remodeling. The failure of reconstruction to match resorption of alveolar bone is one of the most serious and least understood features of chronic periodontitis.

The periodontal ligament consists of a sheet of connective tissue between the root of the tooth and the alveolar bone, from 0.15 to 0.38 mm thick and continuous with the gingival lamina propria. Its principal collagenous fibers attach tooth to bone. Failure of these fibers to regenerate, or to be reembedded in newly formed alveolar bone or cementum is an important feature of periodontal disease.

Cementum is the specialized calcified connective tissue that covers the anatomical root of the tooth to a depth of 0.02 to 0.2 mm and attaches it to the principal fibers of the periodontal membrane. Cementoblasts induce disordered collagen fibrils, ground substance, and hydroxyapatite crystals to be laid down on the dentin of the root. Cementum apposition continues throughout life by gradual mineralization of the periodontal ligament. Cementum closely resembles bone in chemical composition but is considerably less hard than dentin. It has not been found to be softened on periodontally-involved teeth.

Gingival Sulcus

A clinically normal marginal gingiva is held in close apposition to enamel by its turgor, by the native firmness of its lamina propria, by circumdental bands of connective tissue, and by adhesion of junctional epithelium through hemidesmosomes and by a basement lamina. This adhesion is quite tenuous. The marginal gingiva can be detached from the enamel by careful insertion of thin strips of metal or plastic. However, adhesive contact reestablishes promptly after removal of the separating element. Frequently, junctional epithelial cells do not directly contact enamel or cementum. Instead, they abut the "secondary" dental cuticle, an acellular coat from 2 to 10 μm thick composed of acidophilic protein, carbohydrate, and some protein-bound lipid. Its origin remains uncertain. The junctional epithelium seems to adhere to this cuticle on the tooth surface by means of extracellular protein-polysaccharide complexes.

The junctional epithelium is constantly in an active state of renewal and possesses great powers of repair and adaptation. In fact, junctional epithelium renews itself in approximately 3 to 6 days, compared with 8 to 12 days for oral epithelium.

Sulcular exudate can be collected readily on strips of filter paper or in micropipettes inserted in the sulcus. With clinically normal gingiva the flow is negligible. However, it increases in chronic gingivitis, approximately in proportion to the severity of inflammation. This gingival exudate contains globulins, albumin, fibrinogen, and other plasma proteins. The potassium-sodium ratio of this fluid is from 3 to 7 times that of plasma. Its composition indicates that gingival fluid is not a simple filtration product but in part an inflammatory exudate.

The gingival sulcus seems to be the principal source of oral leukocytes. In stained sections of gingiva, neutrophilic granulocytes abound interstitially in junctional epithelium. They constitute from 20 to 80% of the tissue cells in scrapings from the gingival sulcus, compared to 1.6% obtained from six other areas of the oral mucosa. Leukocytes constitute 79% (range, 67 to 95%) of the cells in sulcular exudate from clinically normal gingiva, compared to 92% (range, 81 to 99%) in those with chronic gingivitis. In edentulous mouths without gingival sulci, the salivary leukocyte count is very low. Using a special technique to protect leukocytes from saliva, it has been found that at least 100,000 leukocytes enter the oral cavity every second. This steady supply of phagocytic cells and the resulting increase in lysozyme in gingival fluid, plus antibodies in the exudate, contribute to the oral defenses against bacteria.

CLASSIFICATION OF INFLAMMATORY PERIODONTAL DISEASE

No universally recognized classification of inflammatory periodontal diseases currently exists. Prior to the systematic study of the microbiology and host-response associated with periodontal diseases, the range of gingivitis through severe periodontitis was thought to be a continuum of the same disease process. Recently, evidence suggests that these may be separate disease entities characterized by differing clinical, microbiological and host-response parameters. The following classification is arbitrary but serves as a guide for later discussions of the bacteriology and immunologic considerations of each disease.

Gingivitis

Chronic gingivitis, which ranges in degree from mild to severe, is characterized by inflammation confined to the gingival tissue which does not involve the alveolar bone or periodontal ligament. Clinically, the gingiva may appear erythematous and swollen, with a tendency to bleed on mild provocation. Plaque is always present and calculus may sometimes be observed. Gingivitis occurs in all age groups.

Acute necrotizing ulcerative gingivitis (ANUG) (Vincent's infection) is distinguished by necrosis and ulceration of the interdental gingiva, with marked soreness and bleeding tendency. A gray pseudomembranous slough forms superficially. Oral fetor is pronounced. If neglected, the infection may spread to the fauces (Vincent's angina). Prodromal episodes of debilitating disease, physical and emotional stress, dietary irregularity, excessive smoking of tobacco, and gross neglect of oral hygiene have been related to the onset of this condition. This infection is not communicable. Epidemic outbreaks in populations living under uniform conditions should be attributed to a common traumatic experience.

Periodontitis

Chronic adult periodontitis is characterized by gingival inflammation, loss of connective tissue attachment to cementum of the tooth, alveolar bone loss, and apical migration of the junctional epithelium leading to pocket formation. The tissue-destructive processes proceed slowly, usually beginning in early adulthood and culminating in complete loss of tooth support in 20 or more years. Plaque is always present and both supragingival and subgingival calculus are usually abundant. Suppuration exuding from the periodontal pocket may be seen.

Rapidly progressive or aggressive adult periodontitis differs from chronic adult periodontitis primarily in rate of progression. Severe bone loss affecting many teeth in an individual usually between 20 and 35 years of age is characteristic of this disease process. Suppuration is usually present though plaque may be minimal. Abundant calculus is rarely found.

Localized juvenile periodontitis (periodontosis) is seen in adolescents and is characterized by rapid vertical bone loss affecting the first molar and incisor teeth. Plaque is usually minimal and calculus is absent. When other teeth are affected besides the first molars and incisors, the term *generalized juvenile periodontitis* is more descriptive. Individuals affected by these diseases are usually in good systemic health.

PROGRESSION OF PERIODONTAL DISEASE

Current concepts of the pathogenesis of inflammatory gingival and periodontal diseases are based to a large extent upon histopathologic and ultrastructural analysis of the lesion. Recently, understanding of progression of the periodontal lesion from health through periodontal breakdown has been facilitated by subdivision of the lesion into four histopathologic classifications: the initial, early, established and advanced stages.

Initial Lesion

In experimental situations with teeth maintained plaque-free by mechanical and/or antimicrobial means, absolute gingival health can be established. Under histological examination, small numbers of neutrophils can be seen migrating toward the gingival sulcus and within the junctional epithelium (fig. 17/6A). Few lymphocytes and plasma cells may be observed within the connective tissue, and no pathologic tissue alterations can be seen. If plaque is then allowed to accumulate, the initial lesion develops within 2 to 4 days.

The initial lesion remains localized to the junctional epithelium and the most coronal aspect of the connective tissue. The vessels of the gingival plexus become engorged and dilated and large numbers of emigrating neutrophils can be observed. Perivascular collagen disappears and serum proteins, especially fibrin, are seen extravascularly in addition to an exudation of fluid from the gingival sulcus. The initial lesion is characteristic of an acute exudative inflammatory response.

Early Lesion

After 4 to 7 days of plaque accumulation, the early lesion develops. It is characterized by the formation of a dense lymphoid cell infiltration. Immunoblasts are frequently seen. Within the infiltrated tissue greater than 60% of the collagen is lost and the remaining fibroblasts show significant alterations (fig. 18/6B). The exudative response expands and increased migration of leukocytes and gingival fluid flow is evident. The lesion appears characteristic of cellular hypersensitivity reactions.

Established Lesion

This lesion develops within 2 to 3 weeks of plaque accumulation and is consistent with the clinical features of chronic gingivitis. The distinguishing characteristic of the established lesion is the predominance of plasma cells within the connective tissue prior to significant bone loss (fig. 17/6C). Most of the plasma cells produce IgG, a lesser number IgA, and a few IgM. Immunoglobulins are present extravascularly in the connective tissue and junctional epithelium, and there is evidence for deposition of antigen-antibody complexes and complement around blood vessels. Loss of connective tissue substance continues and the junctional epithelium proliferates laterally and apically. It is not presently known if the established lesion is reversible and under what circumstances it progresses to the advanced lesion.

Advanced Lesion

The advanced lesion represents overt periodontitis. There is loss of alveolar bone, fibrosis and scarring of the gingiva, and widespread manifestation of inflammatory and immunopathologic tissue damage. The inflammatory infiltrate of plasma cells, lymphocytes, and macrophages extends into the alveolar bone and the periodontal ligament (fig. 17/6D). Periods of acute exacerbation, with pus and abscess formation, occur, but can be followed by periods of quiescence.

Currently, it is impossible to distinguish between established lesions which remain stable and those which become aggressive. Whether a progressively destructive lesion results from activation of additional destructive-host mechanisms or from a change to a more pathologic bacterial flora is also unknown. Studies of the natural history of periodontitis in human populations demonstrate that in those who receive regular dental care and maintain fairly good plaque control, the average rate of attachment loss is less than 0.1 mm per year. However, in populations with limited access to dental care and poor plaque control, the rate of attachment loss occurs at least 3 times more rapidly. From these results it is clear that, in the presence of plaque, chronic destructive periodontitis will occur in a population. However, on an individual basis, it remains unclear as to which mechanisms are responsible for the conversion of the stable established lesion into the advanced destructive lesion.

MICROBIOLOGY OF INFLAMMATORY PERIODONTAL DISEASE

Nonspecific Plaque Hypothesis of Periodontal Disease

During this century, there has been continuing evidence to establish the bacterial etiology of inflammatory periodontal disease. A direct relationship between the accumulation of oral debris and periodontal destruction has been recognized for some time. In the late 1950s, careful epidemiologic studies found a strong association between the effectiveness of oral cleaning methods and the amount of alveolar bone loss. During the early 1960s, elegant experiments clearly demonstrated that the accumulation of dental plaque along the gingival margin caused gingival inflammation. When this plaque was removed on a daily basis, the gingival tissues quickly returned to a state of health. Further evidence to establish the microbial etiology of inflammatory periodontal disease was provided by observing the effect of antimicrobial agents. Both oral antiseptics and antibiotics prevented the establishment of gingivitis in animal models which received no mechanical cleansing. Germ-free rodents exhibited little periodontal breakdown, but showed rapid periodontal bone loss when mono-infected with certain oral microorganisms. Based on the above evidence, bacterial plaque appears to be the only factor which can initiate inflammatory periodontal disease.

Until the 1970s, it was generally accepted that dental plaque had a relatively complex but constant composition of microorganisms and their products. Although microscopic studies during the 1940s and 1950s showed an increased percentage of gram negative organisms and spirochetes in inflamed sites when compared to healthy sites, the differences were unimpressive. When plaque from healthy and diseased sites was injected subcutaneously in guinea pigs, similar inflammatory reactions developed suggesting equal pathogenic potentials. The first comprehensive cultural studies of bacterial plaque conducted in the early 1960s tended to confirm the notion that dental plaque had a consistent composition. When pooled supra- and subgingival plaque samples from healthy and periodontally diseased sites were studied, marked differences in composition were not found. Other studies have shown that the accumulation of plaque at a previously healthy site always caused gingivitis, and that the bacterial composition of the plaque shifted to one with more gram negative and motile organisms with

time. However, this change in bacterial composition could not be related to the onset of inflammation (fig. 17/7).

From this information, it was assumed that a quantitative increase in plaque rather than a qualitative change in microorganisms, was the major cause of periodontal disease. However, this nonspecific plaque hypothesis failed to explain the fact that individuals with large plaque accumulations often have little destruction, while some individuals with little plaque had severe periodontitis. This hypothesis also could not account for the localized nature of periodontal destruction. Frequently individuals with an equal distribution of plaque throughout the mouth have destruction localized to only a few teeth.

In the 1970s, improvements in technique led to new findings. Difficulties which had plagued previous studies, such as inadequate sampling methods, poor dispersion of plaque, inadequate techniques to prevent loss of oxygen sensitive organisms and incomplete media for growth of fastidious organisms, have been substantially overcome. Now considerable evidence supports the conclusion that certain microbial species are associated with different types and severities of periodontal disease.

Specific Plaque Hypothesis

Following various improvements in technique, a clearer understanding of the composition of dental plaque is now available. Although technical difficulties remain and present knowledge is incomplete, some conclusions about the nature of the bacteria associated with periodontal disease can be made. However, it has not been proven that any specific organism causes periodontal disease, only that its presence is associated with a given type or severity of disease. To date, the specific organism or group of organisms which actually initiates periodontal tissue destruction remains unknown.

Microbial Flora Associated with Periodontal Health

Electron microscope studies of *in situ* plaque at healthy gingival sites reveal a thin layer of gram positive coccal bacteria. In culture, streptococci, mainly *Streptococcus sanguis*, and species of *Actinomyces* predominate. Few motile forms or spirochetes are seen. Little difference between the subgingival and supragingival plaque is evident.

Microbial Flora Associated with Gingivitis

Sites of gingivitis contain 10 to 20 times more organisms than healthy sites. All of the species present in healthy sites seem to be present in gingivitis. *Actinomyces* and streptococci each constitute one-fourth of the flora. Gram negative anaerobic rods now comprise another 25% of the flora.

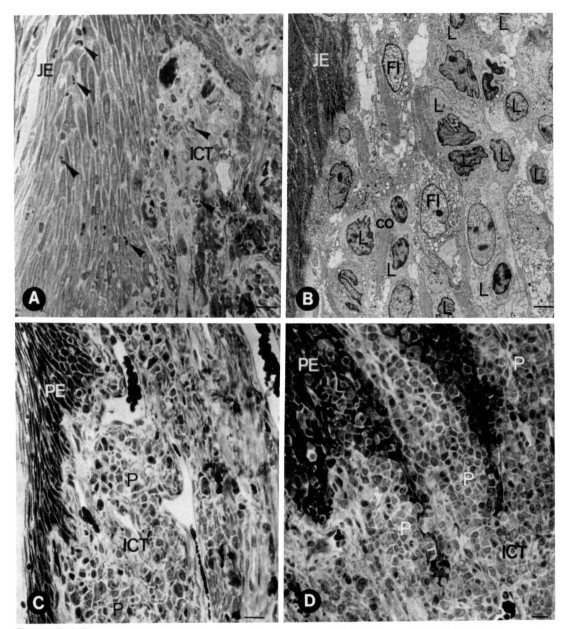

Figure 17/6. Electron micrographs of the progressive stages of periodontal disease. (*A*) The initial lesion seen in a beagle dog with experimentally induced gingivitis. Note the presence of neutrophils (*arrows*) in the infiltrated connective tissue (*ICT*) and junctional epithelium (*JE*). (*B*) The early lesion in a human biopsy. Pathologically altered fibroblasts (*FI*), numerous lymphocytes (*L*) and remnants of collagen (*CO*) can be seen. (*C*) The established lesion in a human biopsy. Note pocket epithelium (*PE*) and numerous plasma cells (*P*). (*D*) The advanced lesion in a human biopsy. The infiltrated connective tissue (*ICT*) adjacent to the pocked eipthelium (*PE*) consists primarily of plasma cells (*P*). The *bar* represents 10 μm in *A*, *C*, and *D*, and 1 μm in *B*. (Reproduced with permission from R. C. Page and H. E. Schroeder: Pathogenesis of Inflammatory Periodontal Disease. A Summary of Current Work. *Laboratory Investigation*, **34**, 235, 1976.)

The majority of these species include *Bacteroides melaninogenicus* subsp. *intermedius, Fusobacterium nucleatum* and other *Bacteroides* species. *Veillonella* species are present in low numbers and spirochetes can be found.

Microbial Flora Associated with Chronic Adult Periodontitis

Gram negative anaerobic rods (mostly asaccharolytic) constitute 75% of the subgingival flora in

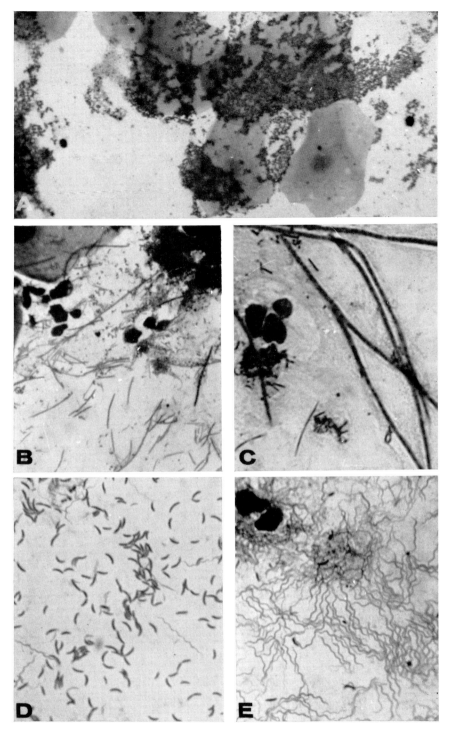

Figure 17/7. The changing microbiota at the gingival margin during a period of no oral hygiene. Impression preparations, crystal violet stain. (*A*) Predominantly coccoid bacteria and desquamated epithelial cells in early phase (×460). (*B*) Filamentous organisms and leukocyte accumulations after 7 days of no oral hygiene (×730). (*C*) Higher magnification of filaments and fusobacteria from preparation shown in *B* (×1150). (*D*) Concentration of vibrios in same preparation as *E*. (*E*) Spirochetes and vibrios predominate after 2 weeks of no oral hygiene and 3 days before gingivitis could be diagnosed clinically (×1150). (Reproduced with permission from H. Löe, E. Theilade, and S. B. Jensen: Experimental Gingivitis in Man. *Journal of Periodontology*, **36**, 177, 1965.)

adult periodontitis. The most common isolate is *Bacteroides gingivalis* (formerly called *Bacteroides asaccharolyticus* and *B. melaninogenicus* subspecies *asaccharolyticus*). *F. nucleatum, Selenomonas sputigena, Eikenella corrodens* and *Capnocytophaga* species are usually seen. *Actinomyces* constitute the majority of the gram positive isolates.

Microbial Flora Associated with Adult Aggressive Periodontitis

Although few patients with rapidly progressive adult periodontitis have been studied, *B. gingivalis* and *Actinobacillus actinomycetemcomitans* are often recovered in large numbers. However, more saccharolytic gram negative anaerobic rods are found than in chronic adult periodontitis.

Microbial Flora Associated with Juvenile Periodontitis (Periodontosis)

Little plaque is seen attached to the tooth in juvenile periodontitis. Many unclassified saccharolytic organisms have been recovered. The most common identifiable species are *Capnocytophaga* and *A. actinomycetemcomitans*. *B. gingivalis* is rarely found.

The above discussion of those organisms associated with periodontal disease does not do justice to the complexities of the subgingival microflora. As techniques improve, new species of bacteria are being isolated and classified. The information available is based on a small number of patients who have been completely studied. However, the evidence suggests several conclusions. Information is available to show that as periodontal disease increases in severity, a shift from gram positive aerobic bacteria to gram negative anaerobic bacteria occurs (table 17/1). The microflora of adult periodontitis differs enough from gingivitis and from juvenile periodontitis to suggest that these are separate disease entities. *B. gingivalis* is associated with destructive disease in adults while *A. actinomycetemcomitans* is linked with destructive disease in juveniles. Even with this leap in knowledge, it must be emphasized again that no cause and effect relationship can be established for any specific microbial species.

PATHOGENIC POTENTIAL OF SPECIFIC PERIODONTAL PATHOGENS

Bacteroides gingivalis

Sufficient microbiological evidence exists to state that *B. gingivalis* is associated with destructive periodontitis in humans. In monkeys, when a silk ligature is placed subgingivally, *B. gingivalis* increases from a few percent to nearly ⅓ of the flora (table 17/2). This increase in *B. gingivalis* parallels loss of periodontal attachment and pocket forma-

Table 17/1
Prominant cultivable microorganisms associated with various periodontal conditions[a]

Periodontal Condition	No. of Samples	% Gram Negative Anaerobic Rods	% Gram Negative Facultatively Anaerobic Rods	% Gram Negative Anaerobic Cocci	% Gram Negative Facultatively Anaerobic Cocci	% Gram Positive Anaerobic Rods	% Gram Positive Facultatively Anaerobic Rods	% Gram Positive Anaerobic Cocci	% Gram Positive Facultatively Anaerobic Cocci
Healthy periodontium	7	12.7	Not detected	2.0	0.3	9.5	35.1	0.8	39.6
Gingivitis	9	25.0	14.8	4.3	Not detected	9.2	16.9	3.0	26.8
Advanced periodontitis	8	74.3	Not detected	0.6	Not detected	15.1	3.9	Not detected	6.2
Juvenile periodontitis:									
Deep pockets	8	59.3	4.5	1.8	Not detected	15.3	3.1	6.1	10.2
Normal pockets	8	27.4	8.4	2.9	0.7	7.3	11.8	4.3	37.2

[a] From J. Slots: *Journal of Clinical Periodontology*, **6**, 351, 1979.

Table 17/2
Change in cultivable subgingival flora during ligature-induced periodontitis in monkeys[a,b]

	Stage I (Time = 0)	Stage II (1–3 weeks)	Stage III (4–7 weeks)
N[c]	7	4	7
Total count (×10^6)[d]	7.78	11.05	5.48
	(2.6 − 73.6)	(0.5 − 27.6)	(0.8 − 11.4)
G + cocci[e]	25.9 ± 7.7	14.9 ± 11.8	7.1 ± 7.1
Anaerobic	12.3 ± 12.7	6.9 ± 7.4	3.0 ± 5.1
Facultative	13.6 ± 10.9	8.0 ± 7.1	4.1 ± 3.2
G + Rods	17.8 ± 12.7	18.9 ± 5.8	5.3 ± 6.3
Anaerobic	4.3 ± 10.5	7.2 ± 12.5	3.9 ± 6.4
Facultative	13.5 ± 10.1	11.7 ± 11.4	1.4 ± 3.4
G − cocci	2.2 ± 3.8	3.2 ± 3.6	4.1 ± 10.0
G − rods	49.0 ± 14.6	56.8 ± 30.7	77.1 ± 14.2
Anaerobic	31.4 ± 7.5	28.8 ± 9.1	61.9 ± 15.3
B. melaninogenicus ss. intermedius	17.2 ± 9.5	6.8 ± 10.1	0.9 ± 1.3
B. asaccharolyticus (B. gingivalis)	1.3 ± 3.5	5.3 ± 9.2	34.2 ± 15.7
Fusobacterium species	8.2 ± 6.4	8.3 ± 3.5	14.8 ± 5.0
Facultative	17.6 ± 8.2	28.1 ± 5.2	15.2 ± 14.6
Motile and surface translocating G − rods	6.6 ± 2.9	20.0 ± 3.5	14.3 ± 20.9

[a] From K. S. Kornman, S. C. Holt, and P. B. Robertson: *Journal of Periodontal Research,* **16**, 363, 1981.
[b] Stage I represents spontaneously occurring gingivitis prior to ligature placement, while Stage III represents periodontitis and Stage II represents a transitional phase. G = Gram stain reaction.
[c] Number of sample sites.
[d] Mean total colony-forming units with range of counts in parentheses.
[e] Mean percentage of total cultivable flora ± standard deviation.
Values within box are significantly different ($p < 0.01$, Student t test) from Stage I values in row.

tion. These longitudinal studies in monkeys support the role of *B. gingivalis* as an important pathogen in periodontitis.

Other findings substantiate the pathogenicity of *B. gingivalis.* This organism is required in the transmission of mixed anaerobic infections and will cause significant bone loss when inoculated into germ free animals. Some strains of *B. gingivalis* are encapsulated and resist phagocytosis and killing by neutrophils. *B. gingivalis* also elaborates various cytotoxic and proteolytic substances including a potent collagenase. Endotoxin from this species will stimulate bone resorption *in vitro.* This organism can affect the phagocytic function of neutrophils in mixed infections.

In addition, *B. gingivalis* stimulates a potent immune response in the host. Both high antibody titers and significant numbers of sensitized T cells reactive with antigens of this organism are found in patients with severe periodontitis.

Actinobacillus actinomycetemcomitans

A. actinomycetemcomitans is found in high numbers in patients with juvenile and aggressive adult periodontitis. This species causes severe bone loss when inoculated into gnotobiotic rats. Both whole organisms and sonic extracts of this organism are directly toxic to neutrophils (polymorphonuclear leukocytes, (PMNs). This toxin, termed a leukotoxin, is not lethal to most other cell types. This effect on local PMNs at the site of the lesion coupled with a systemic PMN defect in juvenile periodontitis may cause loss of protective neutrophil function at the disease site. Antibody which neutralizes the leukotoxin has been found in the serum of localized juvenile periodontitis patients but not in those with generalized juvenile periodontitis. It has been hypothesized that the disease does not go beyond involvement of the first molars and incisors in individuals who can respond with significant antibodies. In those who do not make antibodies, however, localized disease may become generalized.

DIRECT EFFECTS OF BACTERIAL PRODUCTS ON HOST TISSUES

Bacteria damage tissue directly by exotoxins, endotoxins, and histolytic enzymes. They also harm the tissue indirectly by triggering excessive inflammatory reaction of the tissue itself in response to toxins, to products of tissue breakdown, or as a result of specific hypersensitivity to bacterial antigens. Several reports show that gingival accumulations contain filterable, relatively heat-stable factors toxic to man and animals. Cytotoxicity of plaque is indicated by the degenerative changes induced in cultured mammalian cells by debris, or bacteria-free filtrates of debris, from either normal sulci or periodontal pockets. No oral microorganisms have been shown to produce significant exotoxins, but a number of them contain endotoxins, liberate histolytic enzymes, and initiate the inflammatory process.

Endotoxins

Glycolipid endotoxins have been isolated by a conventional two-phase, phenol-water extraction procedure from representative strains of the principal bacteria that have been implicated in periodontitis, namely, *F. nucleatum, B. melaninogenicus, Treponema vincentii, Treponema buccale*, small oral treponema (*Treponema microdentium*), *Selenomonas sputigena, Veillonella* species, and *Leptotrichia buccalis*, but not from an oral viridans streptococcus. They have also been obtained in solution by autolysis or tryptic digestion of fusobacteria and veillonellae but not of oral diphtheroids or anaerobic streptococci. Toxicity was demonstrated by production of intracutaneous inflammatory necrotic lesions, preparation of cutaneous and oral mucosal sites for the local Shwartzman phenomenon, enhancement of cutaneous reactivity to epinephrine, pyrogenicity in rabbits, and lethality for mice. Applied to superficially denuded human skin beneath coverslips, single doses induce an acute inflammatory response persisting for as long as 16 hours with increased migration of neutrophils into the area. A similar result can be induced by repeated application of 0.2-μg doses every second hour. Presumably under the influence of the endotoxin, the mobilized neutrophils exhibit increased phagocytic activity. Additionally, endotoxin activates the alternate pathway of complement which generates inflammatory mediators.

Histolytic Enzymes

Among the many enzymes produced by oral bacteria, hyaluronidase, chondrosulfatase (chondroitinase), neuraminidase, miscellaneous proteases, and collagenase attack substrates that form structural elements of the periodontium. Coagulase and streptokinase affect the fluid portion of blood; lysins attack the cellular components of blood; deoxyribonuclease and lecithinase disrupt component parts of cells.

Hyaluronidase is present in most human salivas, and its concentration is greater in subjects with gingivitis and poor oral hygiene. When injected into monkey interdental papillae, it produces histological changes resembling some of those seen in human gingivitis. The instillation of hyaluronidase into the gingival sulcus of humans caused a loss of intercellular substance from the junctional epithelium, with dilatation of vessels, vacuolization, and disorganization of subjacent connective tissue. However, the hyaluronidase content per milligram of gingival accumulations has been found to be identical in normal and periodontitis subjects.

Hyaluronidase is produced by some pure cultures of viridans streptococci, enterococci, peptostreptococci, staphylococci, and diphtheroids isolated from dental plaque, but not by fusobacteria and spirochetes. The main source of oral bacterial hyaluronidase is the streptococci. Chondrosulfatase is present regularly in mixed cultures of sulcal contents. Neuraminidase, which hydrolyzes sialic acid polymers, is usually found in broth cultures inoculated with human subgingival plaque.

Gingival debris, salivary sediment, and pure cultures of various oral bacteria attack a variety of proteinaceous substrates, including collagen preparations. Ground substance of connective tissue is disaggregated by proteases, as well as by mucopolysaccharases. A majority of broth cultures inoculated with human gingival plaque digest reconstituted, presumably undenatured, collagen gel. *B. melaninogenicus* is known to produce collagenase. In view of the abundance of this organism in the gingival sulcus and of its indispensability in certain experimental mixed anaerobic infections, its role may be particularly significant in the pathogenesis of periodontitis. In addition, *B. melaninogenicus* digests proteins other than collagen and, in exudates of experimental infections, produces ammonia to the extraordinarily high and possibly toxic concentration of 0.1 M.

Cytotoxic Substances

Soluble materials can be extracted from dental plaque which are toxic to cells both *in vivo* and *in vitro*. The specific bacteria which elaborate these substances are unknown as is their role in periodontal tissue destruction.

ROLE OF THE IMMUNE MECHANISM IN PERIODONTAL DISEASE

The components and products of the microbiota of dental plaque are major factors in the pathogenesis of periodontal disease. Some of these components contribute to the development of periodontal disease by direct action on appropriate substrates in periodontal tissues. On the other hand, as the plaque microbiota products often penetrate the epithelium of the gingival sulcus and even the deeper tissues of the periodontium, they stimulate the immune mechanism of the host and elicit immunological responses that are involved in the pathogenesis of periodontal disease (fig. 17/8).

Human Immune Mechanism

The human immune mechanism consists of a recognition system and an effector system (fig. 17/9). The recognition system involves macrophages and lymphocytes that interact with appropriate foreign antigens. One lymphocyte that accepts such antigens is the immunocompetent, nonsensitized type that is thymic-derived and is termed thymic-dependent or the T lymphocyte. The other lymphocytes are derived from bone marrow and are termed the B lymphocytes. Other lymphoid tissues, such as those associated with the intestinal tract, may also influence the differentiation of B lymphocytes.

During differentiation, T and B lymphocytes become sensitive to antigens. When an antigen is initially introduced into the body it enters the lymphatics, passes to adjacent lymph nodes, and is then absorbed on the surface of cortical dendritic macrophages. The absorbed antigen is presented to

the B and T lymphocytes perhaps by the lymphocytes binding to the antigen while it is attached to the surface of a macrophage. In response to antigenic stimuli, the small lymphocytes undergo blastogenesis and become large lymphoblasts. After numerous cell divisions, the short-lived lymphoblasts localize in the lung, intestinal tract, and other sites of antigen localization, where they become plasma cells.

The effector systems then amplify the host response by eliciting inflammatory and immune reactions. Components of the effector systems that are involved are complement, kinin formation, and the clotting system. Biologically active molecules are also involved, including vasoactive amines derived from basophils, mast cells and platelets, and lymphokines derived from the sensitized T lymphocytes. Also, several other effector cells are involved, including: T cells that are directly lymphocytotoxic, antibody-killer cells that are T lymphocyte-dependent, B lymphocytes that produce antibodies and plasma cells that produce antibodies. The differentiated small lymphocytes (sensitized T cells) are

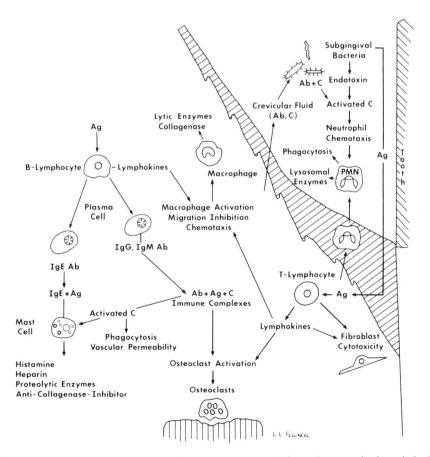

Figure 17/8. Schematic representation of host-mediated mechanisms which may be operative in periodontal disease. (Reproduced with permission from R. J. Nisengard: The Role of Immunology in Periodontal Disease. *Journal of Periodontology*, **48**, 505, 1977.)

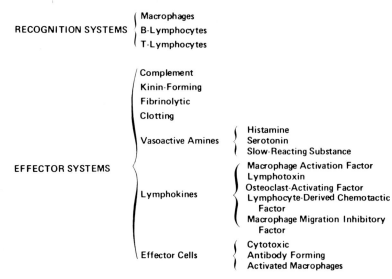

Figure 17/9. Recognition and effector systems involved in the human immune mechanism. (Reproduced with permission from J. E. Horton, J. J. Oppenheim, and S. E. Mergenhagen: A Role of Cell-mediated Immunity in the Pathogenesis of Periodontal Disease. *Journal of Periodontology*, **45**, 351, 1974.)

essentially responsible for cell-mediated immunity (delayed hypersensitivity). Some of the plasma cells derived from the large lymphoblasts localize in the intestinal tract or lung and locally produce antibodies that are involved in immune reactions in tissues. Plasma cells that inhabit the lymph nodes produce most of the circulating antibodies involved in humoral immunity. Both types of immunity elicit the acute inflammatory response and maintain it, and both may operate in acute and chronic periodontal diseases.

Humoral Immunity in Periodontal Disease

There is considerable evidence that soluble substances applied to the gingiva can stimulate specific antibody production by the host. When cotton pellets containing the antigen egg albumin were inserted into the gingival sulcus of rabbits, antibody reactive with the antigen was evident in 2 weeks after initial gingival immunization. Upon repeated challenge, gingival inflammation developed at the gingival challenge site, while little change occurred in rabbits similarly treated with saline. Similar results were seen in monkeys challenged with antigen soaked threads placed in the gingival sulcus after systemic immunization with the same antigen. These and other similar studies clearly show that immunization can be attained through the gingiva and inflammation develops upon challenge with antigen when specific antibody titers exist.

Antibodies. Using several assays to measure specific antibodies such as immunofluorescence, hemagglutination, and precipitation in gel, antibodies to many periodontal microorganisms have been observed in humans. Antibodies in human serum have been detected to *L. bucalis, Fusobacterium, T. microdentum, Actinomyces, Veillonella,* and *B. melaninogenicus.* While some studies have found a relationship between antibody titer and disease, others have not. Recently, using a sensitive enzyme-linked immunosorbent assay, subjects with chronic adult periodontitis were found to have significantly higher antibody titers reactive with *B. gingivalis* than subjects with gingivitis or juvenile periodontitis (fig. 17/10). On the other hand, higher antibody titers to *A. actinomycetemcomitans* were seen in juvenile periodontitis patients than subjects with chronic adult periodontitis. It is not surprising that these findings correlate with the microbiologic findings in these disease states.

Evidence exists that microbial antigens enter the gingival tissue. Therefore, interaction of these foreign substances with specific antibody may occur in the gingiva. Immunofluorescent studies of inflamed gingiva have demonstrated the presence of antigen-antibody complexes and C3 deposition in the gingival tissue. These interactions could activate complement as well as stimulate other tissue destructive mechanisms described in table 17/3. On the other hand, antibodies may exert a protective effect by neutralizing bacterial toxins or enzymes as well as by enhancing the phagocytosis and killing of plaque microorganisms (table 17/3).

Complement and Periodontal Disease. Recent evidence suggests that complement (C') activation may be an important mechanism in the local inflammatory process occurring in periodontal disease. Activation of the classical pathway by antigen-antibody complexes or the alternative pathway by such substances as endotoxin leads to the gen-

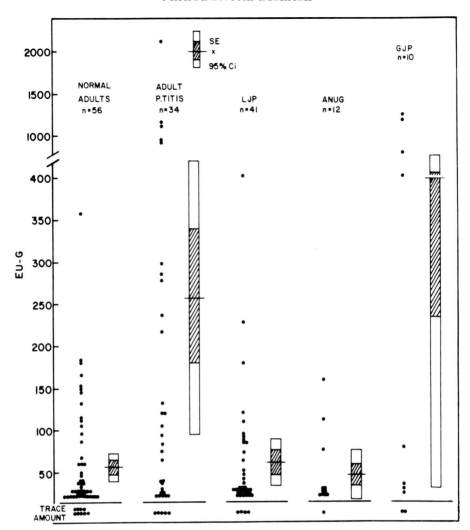

Figure 17/10. Levels of IgG specific for oral *Bacterioides asaccharolyticus* (*B gingivalis*) in various periodontal conditions. Each point represents the antibody activity level of an individual serum sample. Shown for each group is the mean ± standard error (*SE:*□) and ± the 95% confidence interval (*Cl:*□). *ANUG*, acute necrotizing ulcerative gingivitis; *P.TITIS*, periodontiis; *LJP*, localized juvenile periodontitis; *GJP*, generalized juvenile periodontiis. (Reproduced with permission from C. Mouton *et al.*: Serum Antibodies in Oral *Bacteroides asaccharolyticus* (*Bacteroides gingivalis*): Relationshipe to Age and Periodontal Disease. *Infection and Immunity*, **31**, 182, 1981.)

Table 17/3
Possible role of gingival antibodies in periodontal disease[a]

Reaction or Process	Effects
1. Activation of C' by Ag-Ab complexes	Protective early changes in inflammation
2. Phagocytosis of Ag-Ab complexes by PMNL with release of lysozomes	Destructive
3. Enhanced lymphocyte stimulation by Ag-Ab complexes	Release of lymphokines with protective and destructive effects
4. Blocking of lymphocytes by free antibody or by Ag-Ab complexes	Suppression of cell-mediated immune reactions
5. Neutralization of bacterial allergens, toxins, or histolytic enzymes	Protective
6. Enhanced opsonization or bacteriolysis of plaque bacteria	Protective

[a] From R. Genco *et al.*: *Journal of Periodontology*, **45**, 330, 1974.

eration of complement fragments with potent biologic activity. Activation of either pathway produces C3a and C5a, which have been shown to increase vascular permeability and are chemotactic for neutrophils and monocytes. Other tissue destructive mechanisms in which complement components may play a significant role include the release of lytic enzymes from neutrophils, stimulation of lymphokine release by B lymphocytes and activation of prostaglandin-mediated bone resorption. The generation of these inflammatory mediators, as well as others reviewed in table 17/4, may contribute significantly to the chronic inflammation and tissue destruction associated with periodontal disease.

The potential for complement activation to occur in the periodontal lesion by the classical pathway is associated with the presence of antigen and specific antibody of the IgG or IgM class. It is clear that foreign substances of potent antigenicity can enter the gingival tissue and sensitize the host to produce specific antibodies. Bacterial antigens have been shown to be present in inflamed periodontal tissues. There is also considerable evidence that humans have significant titers of antibody to many bacterial antigens derived from the periodontal microflora. Interaction between these specific antibodies and bacterial antigens either within the gingival tissue or in the periodontal pocket may cause activation of the classical complement pathway and the elaboration of inflammatory mediators.

Activation of the alternative pathway may also occur in periodontal disease. Gram negative bacteria, which predominate in lesions of periodontitis, contain endotoxins in their outer membrane. Endotoxins have been shown to be potent activators of the alternative pathway. Products of certain gram positive organisms, including actinomyces and streptococci, can also activate complement in the absence of specific antibody. Activation by the alternative pathway will generate similar inflammatory mediators as those produced from classical pathway activation including C3a and C5a.

Much of the direct evidence concerning the role of C′ in periodontal inflammation has been gathered in the study of the local exudate of the periodontal lesion, gingival fluid. Gingival fluid arises from the gingival capillaries as a transudate of serum and is modified by the inflammatory process as it exists into the oral cavity through the orifice of the gingival sulcus or pocket. Studies of the cellular, protein, carbohydrate, and enzymatic constituents of gingival fluid from inflamed periodontal lesions show it to be an altered inflammatory exudate. Although there is controversy as to whether gingival fluid flow occurs in periodontal health, it is known that the rate of fluid flow increases with inflammation. Analyses of the protein constituents of gingival fluid have shown that gingival fluid represents a 15 to 30% dilution of serum. However, native C3 has been shown to be reduced to 25% of the serum level suggesting the possibility of its utilization by complement activation. Further studies confirmed that C3 is cleaved in gingival fluid derived from severe periodontal lesions, as the terminal cleavage products C3c and C3d are present (fig. 17/11). To determine if components of the classical and/or alternative complement pathways were also utilized in gingival fluid, both C4 (classical pathway component) and Factor B (alternative pathway component) were assessed for cleavage. Cleavage of Factor B to the active enzyme Factor Bb has been uniformly found in all fluids from lesions of both adult and juvenile periodontitis. However, activation of C4 has been found to occur rarely in adult periodontitis. C4 cleavage was commonly seen in gingival fluid from juvenile periodontitis lesions.

These alterations in C′ components in gingival fluid might occur due to the action of nonspecific bacterial proteases rather than classical or alternative pathway activation. However, the available direct and indirect evidence suggests that activation of the complement system may play an important role in periodontal inflammation.

Immediate Hypersensitivity and Periodontal Disease

As described above, one of the immunological responses to the entrance of the bacterial antigens of dental plaque into the tissues of the periodontium is the development of cell-mediated immunity or delayed hypersensitivity, an important factor in the pathogenesis of periodontal disease. Depending on the nature of the bacterial antigen, however, the host may develop another immunological response that results in the formation of humoral antibodies and an immediate hypersensitivity, which is also

Table 17/4
Biological effects of components of the complement system[a]

Activity	Complement Components
Cytolytic and cytotoxic damage to cells	C1–9
Chemotactic activity for leukocytes	C3a, C5a, C567
Histamine release from mast cells	C3a, C5a
Increased vascular permeability	C3a, C5a
Kinin activity	C2, C3a
Lysosomal enzyme release from leukocytes	C5a
Promotion of phagocytosis	C3, C5
Enhancement of blood clotting	C6
Promotion of clot lysis	C3, C4
Inactivation of bacterial lipopolysaccharides from endotoxin	C5, C6

[a] From R. J. Nisengard: *Journal of Periodontology,* **48,** 505, 1977.

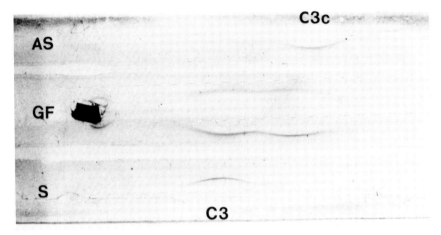

Figure 17/11. Immunoelectrophoretic pattern obtained when anti-human C3/C3c is reacted with zymosan-activated serum (*AS*, positive control with C3c, *top*), gingival fluid (*GF*) from a lesion of gingivitis (C3 + C3c, *middle*), and fresh serum (*S*, negative control, C3 only). The gingival fluid shows a pattern indicative of a complement activation. (Adapted from M. R. Patters, H. A. Schenkein, and A. Weinstein: A Method for Detection of Complement Cleavage in Gingival Fluid. *Journal of Dental Research*, **58**, 1620, 1979.)

called atopic allergy, anaphylactic reaction, or re-agin-dependent allergy. Even a single pathogenic bacterial species, *e.g.*, *Mycobacterium tuberculosis*, will induce both delayed and immediate types of hypersensitivity, with the delayed hypersensitivity predominating over immediate hypersensitivity. All the elements necessary for the formation of an immediate type of hypersensitivity are present in the tissues of the oral cavity of a human host. Though its exact role has not been entirely defined, this mechanism undoubtedly functions in the pathogenesis of periodontal disease.

The mediator of immediate type hypersensitivity is the reaginic or humoral antibody designated as IgE. The plasma cells that form IgE are found principally in respiratory and gastrointestinal mucosa and in regional lymph nodes. They are also present in the gingiva. IgE is formed in tissues and, even though it is present in low concentrations, its participation in the allergic reactions is critical. IgE does not ordinarily activate complement by the classical pathway. It does react with specific receptor sites in the membranes of tissue cells. Mast cells and basophilic leukocytes have specific receptor sites for IgE on their cell membranes and IgE is homocytotropic for these cells. These cells are a source of the inflammatory agents histamine, serotonin, and heparin when properly stimulated by bacterial antigens.

Immediate hypersensitivity is mediated by the interaction of a specific antigen with IgE fixed to tissue cells. In this interaction, alterations occur in the Fc portion of the IgE antibodies. This reaction activates energy-dependent reactions that release histamine, bradykinin, and slow-reacting substance of anaphylaxis (SRS-A). While serotonin is involved in this type of hypersensitivity in animals, it has not been found to be released in human immediate hypersensitivity reactions. Histamine's pharmacologic action increases capillary permeability, contracts smooth muscle, stimulates exocrine glands, causes dilatation of blood vessels, and increases venule permeability. In the skin it causes a wheal and erythema response. SRS-A causes smooth muscle contraction and increases vascular permeability. Bradykinin is involved with smooth muscle contraction, vasodilation, capillary permeability, migration of leukocytes, and also causes pain.

The mast cells seen in biopsies of inflamed gingiva have a similar ultrastructural appearance as mast cells in immediate hypersensitivity. Following an immediate hypersensitivity reaction or as seen in gingival inflammation, the granules of mast cells are enlarged and their perigranular membranes are ruptured; the contents of the ruptured granules tend to mix together in the cytoplasm.

Other changes in inflamed gingival tissue also indicate that immediate hypersensitivity may be involved in the pathogenesis of periodontal disease. The histamine levels are increased in inflamed gingival tissues in comparison to normal gingiva, as indicated by analysis of biopsied tissues. One of the clinical responses indicative of immediate hypersensitivity is the wheal and flare reaction when a susceptible individual is challenged with an antigen. A significant correlation exists between the incidence of immediate hypersensitivity to plaque bacterial antigens and the severity of periodontal disease.

Cell-mediated Immunity and Periodontal Disease

Cell-mediated immunity seems to be an important factor in the pathogenesis of periodontal disease. In the early gingival lesions, the cellular response is characterized by a predominance of small or medium-sized lymphocytes, together with blastogenic lymphocytes. This cellular response is typical of delayed hypersensitivity. In chronic periodontal lesions, antibody-producing plasma cells predominate and T lymphocytes are also present.

Cell-mediated immunity is initiated by component T lymphocytes. When immunocompetent lymphocytes are initially exposed to an appropriate antigen, it sensitizes them and they transform and replicate. The transformed T cells continuously recirculate in lymphatic and vascular channels to other tissues and organs. If transformed cells intercept their specific antigen, they produce substances called lymphokines that can directly destroy tissues. The lymphokines may also activate other monocyte-derived cells to destroy tissues (table 17/5). Host cells that have antigens on their surface may be subject to direct cell-mediated lymphocytotoxic reactions.

Cell-mediated immunity has been studied by culturing lymphocytes from peripheral blood, spleen, or lymph nodes. An appropriate antigen stimulates these cultured lymphocytes to transform and proliferate if such lymphocytes were sensitized before culturing. In periodontal disease, bacterial antigens which have entered through the gingiva interact with immunocompetent lymphocytes and this clone of specifically sensitized cells expands by cell division and circulates throughout the body (fig. 17/12). When these specifically sensitized lymphocytes are cultured in vitro with specific antigen, these cells synthesize and release lymphokines and then proliferate. In vitro assays to determine if an individual shows significant sensitization to a specific antigen generally measure either lymphokine release or subsequent cell division. Assessment of

Table 17/5
Some of the biological activities of mediators of cell-mediated immunity (lymphokines)[a]

Inhibition of macrophage migration (MIF)
Chemotactic for macrophages
Activation of macrophages
Inhibition of leukocyte migration
Chemotactic for neutrophils, basophils and eosinophils
Act as mitogens inducing blast formation of nonsensitized lymphocytes
Transfer cell-mediated immunity
Cytotoxic for fibroblasts
Osteoclast activating factor (OAF)

[a] From R. J. Nisengard: *Journal of Periodontology*, **48**, 505, 1977.

lymphokine release requires an assay to measure the biologic activity of these substances, such as fibroblast killing by lymphotoxin (LT) or macrophage migration inhibition by migration inhibition factor (MIF). Measures of cell division are generally easier, as de novo synthesis of DNA can be assessed by incorporation of radio-labelled thymidine. Measurement of in vitro lymphocyte proliferation stimulated by specific antigen is termed "lymphocyte transformation" or "lymphocyte blastogenesis." These assays of cell-mediated immunity provide information similar to in vivo skin tests such as the tuberculin skin test for tuberculosis. If an individual has been significantly sensitized by previous exposure to a specific antigen, re-exposure to this antigen either in vivo by skin injection or in vitro by culturing lymphocytes with the specific antigen, will cause lymphokine release and proliferation. In vivo, these reactions cause a delayed (48 to 72 hours) skin reaction. In vitro, lymphocyte blastogenesis or lymphokine assays provide quantitative data as to the magnitude of sensitization of the individual to the antigen.

Studies of cell-mediated immunity by measurement of lymphokine release clearly show that lymphocytes from individuals with periodontal disease release lymphokines when cultured with plaque-related antigens. If this lymphokine release occurs in the gingival tissue when antigen and sensitized lymphocyte interact, the potential exists for cellular infiltration and tissue destruction. Lymphokines have many deleterious effects on tissue including destruction of fibroblasts, dissolution of collagenous fibers, and stimulation of bone resorption. Lymphocytes produce a macrophage-migration inhibitory factor (MIF) that inhibits the migration of macrophages. Lymphotoxin is produced by sensitized lymphocytes from persons with periodontal disease and is cytotoxic for cultured human gingival fibroblasts. LT is not produced by plaque-stimulated lymphocytes from persons without periodontal disease or from unstimulated lymphocytes from persons with periodontal disease (fig. 17/13).

Another lymphokine, termed osteoclast activating factor (OAF), has been found in the culture fluid of leukocytes from persons with periodontal disease when such cultures were stimulated with human dental plaque. OAF induces osteoclastic activity in tissue cultures containing bone. OAF action is distinguishable from parathormone, an active metabolite of vitamin D, and from prostaglandins.

During the 1970s, considerable research into cell-mediated immunity and its role in periodontal disease has provided a better but incomplete understanding. It is clear that the ability of dental plaque to stimulate lymphocyte transformation relates to a specific antigenic component rather than to a

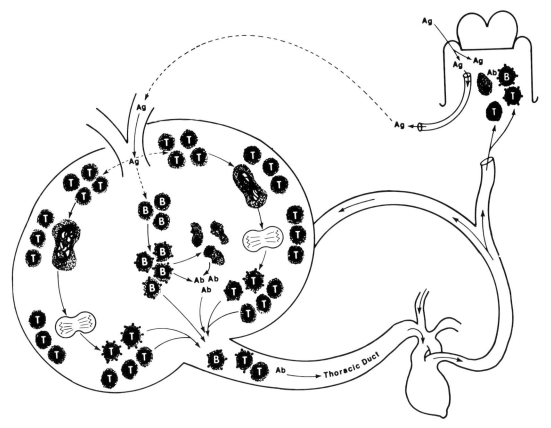

Figure 17/12. Diagrammatic representation of lymphocyte recirculation from peripheral lymphoid tissues to organs and tissues via the vascular and blood channels. The initial exposure of immunocompetent lymphocytes to antigen (*Ag*) at the gingiva (or in other peripheral lymphoid tissue) results in sensitization of T lymphocytes (*T*) which induces them to undergo transformation and replication. During this time the B lymphocytes synthesize antibodies (*Ab*). (Reproduced with permission from J. E. Horton, J. J. Oppenheim, and S. E. Mergenhagen: A Role of Cell-mediated Immunity in Pathogenesis of Periodontal Disease. *Journal of Periodontology*, **45**, 351, 1974.)

generalized reaction. At birth, lymphocytes obtained from cord blood are immunologically competent but do not respond to dental plaque antigens, indicating little or no previous exposure to them. Initial studies suggested that antigens from dental plaque stimulate lymphocytes to transform in proportion to the clinical severity of periodontal disease of the individual from which the cultured lymphocytes were derived. It was hypothesized that they became increasingly sensitized by exposure to the plaque antigens after birth, particularly if periodontal disease is present; the more severe the disease the more lymphocytes become sensitized. However, more recent studies have shown a specificity in the cell-mediated response which varies according to the specific organism from which these antigens are derived. As certain microorganisms are associated with different severities and types of periodontal disease, it would follow that individuals with mild gingivitis might be sensitized to different bacterial antigens than individuals with severe periodontitis. Although only certain organisms have

been tested for their ability to stimulate cell-mediated immunity reactions of individuals with varying severities of disease, certain patterns have emerged. Figure 17/14 shows the response of individuals with varying severities of periodontal disease (including edentulous subjects with a history of tooth loss due to periodontitis) to four different microorganisms. The first pattern is represented by the response to *Actinomyces*. This organism proved to be a potent stimulator of lymphocytes in most patients tested. Although this response pattern might appear to be similar to the response to a nonspecific mitogen, this preparation stimulates very few human fetal cord lymphocytes and therefore does not appear to be a nonspecific mitogen to human peripheral lymphocytes. This response pattern appears to reflect host sensitization caused by the ubiquitous presence of this organism in the oral cavities of humans.

Microbiological evidence suggests that *Actinomyces* are present in all dentulous subjects and that their numbers correlate with the presence of periodontal disease. This agrees with the lower blasto-

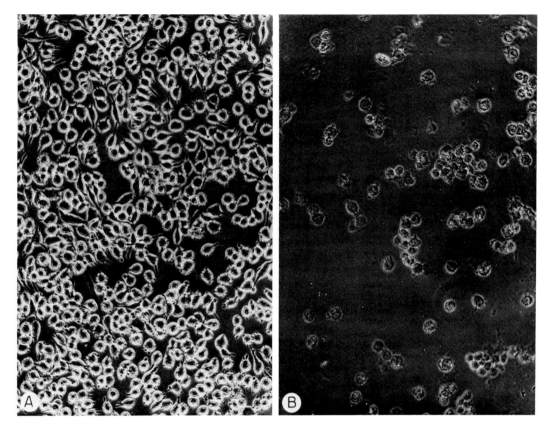

Figure 17/13. Effect of lymphotoxin on cultured human gingival fibroblasts. (A) Normal appearing fibroblasts exposed to cell-free supernatant from plaque-stimulated nonreactive leukocyte cultures from a clinically normal subject (×160). (B) Damaged fibroblasts exposed to cell-free supernatant from plaque-stimulated reactive leukocyte cultures from a subject with periodontal disease (×160). (Reproduced with permission from J. E. Horton, J. J. Oppenheim, and S. E. Mergenhagen: A Role of Cell-mediated Immunity in the Pathogenesis of Periodontal Disease. *Journal of Periodontology*, **45**, 31, 1974.)

genic responses obtained from normal subjects who harbor fewer organisms than diseased subjects. The edentulous subjects who responded strongly may have been continually sensitized due to the presence of *Actinomyces* on artificial dentures. Therefore, the measured response to *Actinomyces* appears to represent a naturally occurring cell-mediated immune response to a commensal organism which sensitizes the host primarily through the oral tissues.

In contrast to the *Actinomyces* response, all groups responded weakly to *Streptococcus sanguis*. Although a commensal organism, this bacterium appears to be unable to stimulate a strong cellular immune response and has not been associated with periodontal disease in humans.

Finally, a different pattern of reactivity is shown by the blastogenic response to *Treponema denticola*, a spirochete and *B. gingivalis*. Although these organisms appear to be capable of eliciting strong cellular immune responses, these responses seem to be limited to those individuals with destructive periodontitis. Recently, microbiological findings

have related the presence of these organisms in subgingival plaque to destructive periodontitis in both humans and monkeys.

Although it is not clear that the magnitude of the cellular immunity response to plaque microorganisms correlates with the severity of periodontal disease, the fact that individuals have sensitized lymphocytes to plaque microorganisms suggests a potential role for cell-mediated immunity in local tissue destruction. The understanding of this mechanism in the pathogenesis of peridontal disease might allow for the prevention of the development and continuation of the destructive phases of the inflammatory response.

BONE DESTRUCTION IN PERIODONTAL DISEASE

Destruction or resorption of alveolar bone is characteristic of the more advanced stages of periodontal disease. While a definite relationship has been established between alveolar bone resorption and dental plaque, the manner in which the bone

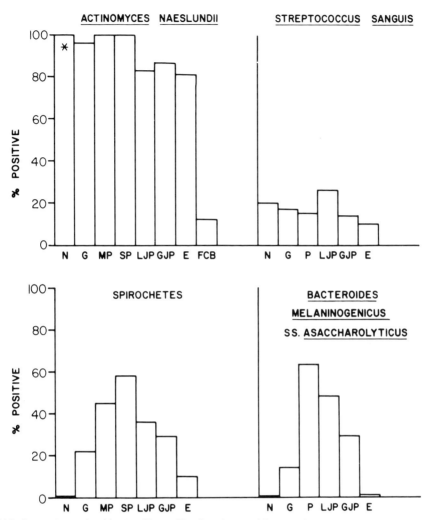

Figure 17/14. Percentage of subjects with positive lymphocyte blastogenic response to four oral organisms. *N*, normal; *G*, gingivitis; *MP*, moderate periodontitis; *SP*, severe periodontitis; *LJP*, localized juvenile periodontitis; *GJP*, generalized juvenile periodontitis; *P*, periodontitis; *E*, edentulous; *FCB*, fetal cord blood. (*) Although all normal patients were reactive to *Actinomyces naeslundii*, they responded at a significantly lower level than the other patient groups. *B. melaninogenicus* ss. *asaccharolyticus* is now called *B. gingivalis*.

is resorbed has not been completely elucidated. While it is clear that plaque bacteria do not usually penetrate intact gingiva, their products do and are involved in the pathogenesis of even the earlier stages of periodontal disease. In later stages, when there is pocket formation, plaque agents would more readily penetrate the tissues and cause bone resorption.

Several possible pathways have been described by which the products of the dental plaque could gain access to the alveolar bone and cause its resorption. Plaque products could stimulate progenitor cells in the periodontium to differentiate into osteoclasts. Complexing agents and hydrolytic enzymes from the plaque could act directly to decalcify bone and to hydrolyze its organic matrix. The products of the plaque could stimulate gingival cells

to produce mediators which, in turn, would stimulate progenitor cells to form osteoclasts which destroy bone. Plaque products could stimulate gingival cells to produce substances that serve as cofactors to potentiate otherwise inactive bone resorptive agents, or gingival cell products could destroy bone by a direct action.

Using a model system of fetal bone in tissue culture, investigations of the various postulations for alveolar bone resorption have been made. Endotoxins from gram negative bacteria, lipoteichoic acid (a glycolipid plus a glycerophosphate polymer) from gram positive bacteria, such as lactobacilli, and a factor from *Actinomyces viscosus* stimulate osteoclastic destruction of bone. However, the soluble products of plaque from both adults with gingivitis and children without evident destructive periodontal disease also stimulate bone resorption by osteoclastic activity. Endotoxins, lipoteichoic acid, and extracts of dental plaque cause no release of calcium if the osteoclasts in the test bone have been heat-devitalized. This indicates that these agents act by a direct action on osteoclasts rather than by a direct action on bone.

There is no question that gingival cells release or activate soluble mediators into periodontal tissues. Gingival mast cells release heparin and histamine. Heparin can act as a cofactor to potentiate bone resorption, but histamine has no demonstrable action on bone resorption. While kinins are released into inflamed periodontal tissues, they have no action on bone resorption. Antigen-antibody complexes activate some component(s) of the complement system which stimulate prostaglandin mediated bone resorption. Sensitized leukocytes release a factor (osteoclast activating factor, fig. 17/15) that stimulates bone resorption; prostaglandins also trigger bone resorption. Lysosomes, which contain many hydrolytic enzymes, have no known direct action on bone tissues. From such findings it is evident that alveolar bone resorption in periodontal disease is multifactoral, involving interactions between components of dental plaque and mediators in the periodontal tissues.

ROLE OF NEUTROPHILS

In response to chemotactic factors present in the gingival area, neutrophils constantly migrate from the gingival capillaries, through the connective tissue, epithelium, and gingival sulcus, and subsequently into the mouth. Several studies have revealed that the major source of oral leukocytes is the gingival sulcus, as few leukocytes can be recovered from the mouth when the orifices of the gingival sulcus are closed off with a plastic splint. Significantly more neutrophils are recovered from the mouth of individuals with inflamed gingiva when compared to a healthy mouth. In histologic examinations of inflamed periodontal tissues, neutrophils are seen as one of the major cell popula-

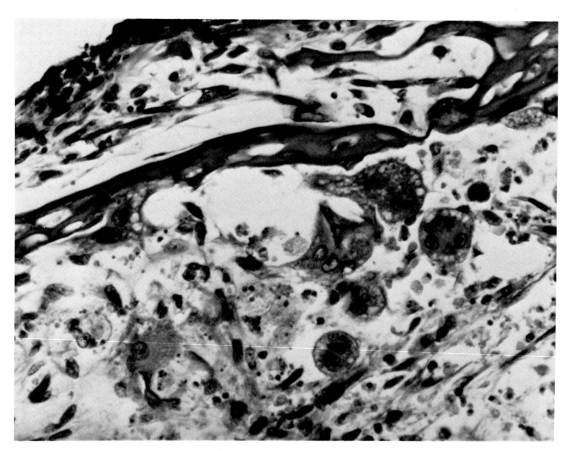

Figure 17/15. Histologic appearance of a resorbing rat fetal bone shaft cultured for 96 hours with supernatant fluid from dental plaque-stimulated leukocyte cultures. Note the presence of numerous active osteoclasts as well as the loss of bone matrix (×400). (Reproduced with permission from J. E. Horton, J. J. Oppenheim, and S. E. Mergenhagen: A Role of Cell-mediated Immunity in the Pathogenesis of Periodontal Disease. *Journal of Periodontology*, **45**, 31, 1974.)

tions in the inflammatory infiltrate. Within the periodontal pocket, neutrophils appear to be associated with the tissue surface of the plaque mass and often contain phagocytized bacteria.

Numerous endogenous and exogenous chemical attractants (chemotactic factors) for neutrophils are present in the periodontal lesion. Many plaque microorganisms are known to produce low molecular weight substances which are strongly chemotactic for neutrophils. Additionally, activation of the alternative pathway of complement by bacterial endotoxin or other bacterial products generates chemotactic complement fragments such as C5a. Complement activation may also occur by the classical pathway following interaction of specific host antibodies with plaque bacterial antigens. Lymphocyte-derived chemotactic factors (lymphokines) may be elaborated by lymphocytes after interaction with specific bacterial antigens. These and other chemotactic factors probably account for the presence of significant numbers of neutrophils in the periodontal tissues.

Neutrophils may also contribute to tissue damage. These cells contain lysosomal enzymes with which they digest phagocytized matter. Upon the ingestion of bacteria or other debris, these enzymes often leak into the surrounding tissue. Also, interaction of neutrophils with many bacterial products, including endotoxin and products of *Actinomyces*, can cause release of these tissue destructive enzymes. Neutrophils contain collagenase which will degrade collagen and thus lead to loss of integrity of the connective tissue. Also present in neutrophils are other histolytic and proteolytic enzymes which can digest host tissue substance. The tissue destructive capacity of neutrophils has been demonstrated in leukopenic animals which fail to develop the usual abcesses seen in normal animals after injection of plaque into skin sites.

Although the tissue destructive capacity of neutrophils has received considerable attention, recent research has focused on the host-protective aspects of neutrophil function. It has been known for many years that the neutrophil is the first line of defense against infection. It is therefore not surprising that the neutrophil might play an important role in protection from periodontal infection. In the last 50 years, numerous case reports have been published describing patients with systemic neutrophil disorders including such conditions as agranulocytosis, cyclic neutropenia, "lazy leukocyte syndrome," Chediak-Higashi syndrome, etc. A consistent clinical finding in these cases has been exfoliation of permanent teeth, erythematous lesions of the gingiva, and spontaneous gingival bleeding. Careful clinical study of these patients revealed that many had extremely severe periodontitis occurring at a very young age, often in childhood. Additional evidence that impaired systemic neutrophil function is associated with severe periodontitis is seen in the study of juvenile diabetes. Young diabetic patients often have unusually severe periodontitis. Often these patients have systemic neutrophil disorders as well. Although the relationships between juvenile diabetes and periodontitis remains unclear, neutrophil disorders in some of these patients may be the link between these disorders.

The relationships between systemic neutrophil dysfunction and unusually severe periodontitis has led researchers to study neutrophil function in patients with an unusually severe periodontal disease, juvenile periodontitis (periodontosis). As discussed earlier, juvenile periodontitis is characterized by rapidly progressive bone loss affecting the first molars and incisors of otherwise healthy, young individuals. Although inflammation is present, large quantities of bacterial plaque or calculus are not consistently seen. Recent evidence shows that the microflora associated with juvenile periodontitis lesions differs markedly from chronic periodontitis. Nevertheless there has been no clear understanding of this disease process.

The possibility that this severe form of periodontitis might be associated with a neutrophil disorder has been the object of intense investigation. It is clear that if a systemic neutrophil disorder exists, it would have to be mild as these patients have no systemic disease. Using an *in vitro* assay of neutrophil chemotaxis, it has been demonstrated that peripheral blood neutrophils of subjects with juvenile periodontitis often have reduced neutrophil chemotaxis when compared to periodontally healthy subjects or subjects with chronic adult periodontitis. An example of such data is presented in figure 17/16, where reduced chemotaxis was observed when neutrophils from juvenile periodontitis subjects migrated towards a bacterial factor derived from *Escherichia coli*, the chemotactic factor released by mitogen-stimulated lymphocytes (LDCF) and the chemotactic factors generated by activation of complement. Current evidence suggests that this defect is not associated with serum inhibitors of chemotaxis but appears to be a cell defect. A recent report suggests that this cell defect is associated with a reduced number of membrane receptor sites for chemotactic molecules rather than a defect in locomotion. Also evidence suggests that this systemic neutrophil dysfunction may be pre-existing rather than induced by the disease process, and does not recover after the patients are successfully treated. A genetic cause of neutrophil dysfunction may explain the familial tendency of juvenile periodontitis.

Although the presence of a subtle systemic neutrophil defect in chemotaxis in patients with juvenile periodontitis is now well documented, no evi-

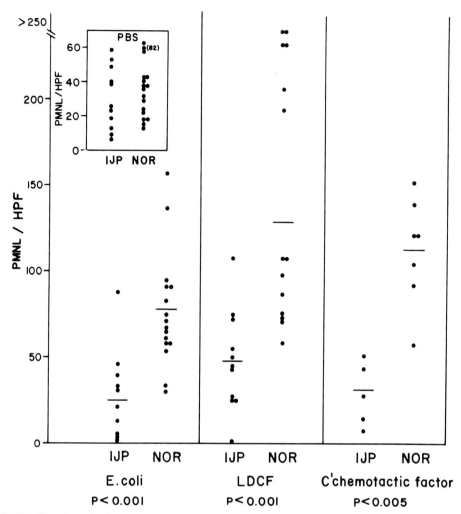

Figure 17/16. The chemotactic response of peripheral neutrophils (PMNL, polymorphonuclear leukocytes) from individuals with idiopathic juvenile periodontitis (*IJP*) and normal subjects (*NOR*) to (a) filtrate of a culture of *Escherichia coli*, (b) leukocyte-derived chemotactic factor (LDCF), and (c) (*C′*) chemotactic factor and buffer control. HPF, high power field; PBS, phosphate buffered saline. Reduced response is seen in the IJP population. (Reproduced with permission from L. J. Cianciola *et al.*: Defective Polymorphonuclear Leukocyte Function in a Human Periodontal Disease. *Nature*, **265**, 445, 1977.)

dence exists to suggest that systemic cell defects occur in other forms of rapidly progressive periodontitis. However, information has been obtained to support the concept of locally induced neutrophil dysfunction within the periodontal lesion. When neutrophils recovered from the gingival sulcus of rapidly progressing lesions were compared with cells recovered from chronic long-standing lesions, impaired phagocytosis was seen in the former. No differences in number, viability or percentage neutrophils in the recovered cells were noted (table 17/6). This reduction in phagocytosis was also evident when gingival neutrophils from progressive lesions were compared with noninvolved sites in the same mouth (table 17/7) suggesting that this functional abnormality was the result of factors operating within the periodontal pocket. A hypothesis to ex-

plain these findings is that healthy neutrophils are exposed to products from specific microorganisms associated with progressive disease and are rendered dysfunctionate by these substances. There is evidence that *Capnocytophaga* species and *A. actinomycetemcomitans* (organisms associated with juvenile periodontitis) and *B. melaninogenicus* (associated with adult periodontitis) produced substances which can seriously affect neutrophil function. The loss of function of these protective cells within the periodontal pocket may alter the environment of the pocket such that pathogenic bacteria may be able to become established leading to rapidly progressive disease.

The current body of evidence suggests both a possible tissue destructive as well as a protective role of neutrophils. However, it appears that the

Table 17/6
Number, viability, and phagocytic capacity of gingival neutrophils recovered from lesions of gingivitis, chronic adult periodontitis, and rapidly progressive periodontitis[a]

	Age range	Cells/Site[b]	% Viable[b]	% PMN[b]	% Phagocytosis[b]
Gingivitis ($N = 9$)	21–30	$7.3 \pm 1.7 \times 10^{3c}$	82 ± 2	90.0 ± 1.5	74.8 ± 2.6
Chronic periodontitis ($N = 8$)	49–62	$3.7 \pm 0.9 \times 10^4$	84 ± 2	86.0 ± 1.0	83.7 ± 4.8
Rapidly progressive periodonitis ($N = 14$)[d]	13–34	$3.1 \pm 0.2 \times 10^4$	79 ± 3.4	88.5 ± 1.5	12.9 ± 2.1^e

[a] From P. A. Murray and M. R. Patters: *Journal of Periodontal Research,* **15,** 463, 1980. PMN = polymorphonuclear leukocyte.
[b] Mean ± standard error.
[c] Significantly different from periodontitis groups ($p < 0.01$).
[d] A marked reduction in phagocytic capacity is seen in cells recovered from rapidly progressive lesions.
[e] Significantly different from gingivitis and chronic periodontitis groups ($p < 0.001$).

Table 17/7
Comparison of gingival polymorphonuclear leukocytes from periodontally involved and uninvolved sites in eight patients with localized periodontitis[a]

Site	Cell/site[b]	% Viable[b]	% Phagocytosis[b]
Diseased	$3.6 \pm 0.3 \times 10^{4c}$	77.1 ± 2.8	10.9 ± 1.9^c
Nondiseased	$4.0 \pm 0.3 \times 10^3$	84.3 ± 2.0	72.2 ± 3.3

[a] From P. A. Murray and M. R. Patters: *Journal of Periodontal Research,* **15,** 463, 1980.
[b] Mean ± standard error.
[c] Significantly different ($p < 0.001$).

protective aspects of neutrophil function have major consequences in the progression of periodontal disease.

DENTAL CALCULUS

Dental calculus is the concretion that accumulates on the teeth and on associated prostheses and restorations by calcification of dental plaque. It normally occurs infrequently or scantily in children under 10 years of age and is steadily more prevalent thereafter. The calculus index correlates closely with the periodontal disease index, but an etiological relationship is not clearly defined.

Calculus occurs in two main clinical types; supragingival, above the free margin, and subgingival, below the free margin of the gingiva, especially in the periodontal pockets. Though discrete foci of the two types are not uncommon, dental calculus seems to originate most often in plaque in cervical areas of the teeth and to form a continuum coronally and apically. Physical differences in color, texture, hardness, and adhesiveness have engendered the persistent but probably not very consequential designation of supragingival calculus as salivary in origin and subgingival calculus as serumal in origin. Supragingival calculus undoubtedly derives its inorganic and probably some of its organic matter constituents from saliva. The sulcular exudate almost certainly contributes similarly to subgingival calculus which to some degree is kept from contact with saliva by its protected position in the gingival pocket. The final result, however, is essentially the same, an organic matrix consisting mostly of microorganisms with granular intermicrobial material, all mineralized predominantly with calcium and phosphate. Mineralization seems to be spotty, since the hardness index may very 3-fold in different areas of a single specimen. The mean index is about twice that of cementum.

Mature calculus contains from 1.5 to 20% water and about 20% organic material. It contains, on the average, about 30% calcium and 16% phosphorus, with ratios ranging from 1.66 to 2.31. Calculus also contains, on the average, 1% magnesium, 2% sodium, and up to 5.3% carbonate. The inorganic part of calculus is a mixture of calcium phosphates (hydroxyapatite, $Ca_{10}(PO_4)_6 \cdot (OH)_2$; octacalcium phosphate, $Ca_8H_2(PO_4)_6 \cdot 5H_2O$; whitlockite, $Ca_3(PO_4)_2$; and brushite, $CaHPO_4 \cdot (2H_2O)$. The organic matrix of calculus contains mucopolysaccharide and a variety of sugars and protein in addition to the remains of bacterial cell walls.

Rates of calculus accumulation vary from person to person and in the same person in successive periods. In those who form calculus rapidly, plaque becomes as thick as 0.1 mm and begins to calcify within 3 days and mineralization is maximal (80% ash) in 2 weeks. Apatite crystals generally appear first between and on surfaces of the bacteria nearest the teeth. Later, the crystals appear inside them until the matrix is uniformly mineralized. Meanwhile, fresh bacterial growth accumulates on the surface. Mature calculus attaches to the tooth in four ways: to a cuticle layer on enamel or cementum, to minute irregularities in cementum, by penetration of plaque organsims into cementum, and by mechanical locking in undercut areas of cementum resorption. Plaque is considered to play an active role in calculus formation by providing nucleation sites where calcium, phosphate, and ancillary ions accumulate in the configuration of hydroxyapatite, thus initiating crystal growth. Such crystal nucleation by foreign substances is known as epitaxy.

Although bacteria are normally integral to dental calculus, they are not indispensable. The familiar calculi occurring in salivary glands and ducts are apparently bacteria-free. Also, calculus forms on the teeth of germ-free animals. Generally, however, dental calculus forms more abundantly in conventional rats, particularly in those on soft, sticky diets conducive to plaque accumulation. Even though bacteria are not essential to formation of dental calculus, they evidently enhance it under normal conditions.

Diet influences calculus formation in certain strains of experimental animals. Coarse, rough, abrasive diets are preventive, whereas fine, sticky, tenacious diets are conducive. The nutritional effects of varying the kinds and amounts of protein and carbohydrate in the diet are difficult to dissociate from their effects on dietary consistency. Certain altered calcium-phosphorus ratios and increased bicarbonate in the diet favor calculus formation in experimental animals. Variations in ordinary dietary factors have not convincingly shown an effect on calculus formation in man.

Calculus prevention has been attempted, without much success, by several mechanisms: 1) preventing attachment of plaque by repellent coatings on the teeth; 2) altering the nature of plaque or reducing its accumulation by antibacterial agents, hydrolytic enzymes, or detergents; and 3) dissolving the mineral salts of calculus by decalcifying or complexing agents. Regular, efficient toothbrushing and interdental hygiene to remove plaque before it mineralizes remain the only effective regimen.

The opinion has been accepted that subgingival calculus irritates the gingiva by its roughness. If it is sufficiently jagged, calculus can traumatize the tissue mechanically during mastication and toothbrushing. On the other hand, the junctional epithelium adapts readily and forms a normal contact with roughened enamel and various artifacts, *provided that bacteria are excluded*. The principal contribution of calculus to the progress of chronic periodontitis seems, therefore, to be due to its bacterial components.

PREDISPOSING FACTORS

A wide variety of factors has been implicated to predispose or aggravate the degree to which periodontitis develops. Such factors are classified as local or systemic, but this distinction is not very meaningful. Predisposing factors may also be grouped according to their modes of action. Many simply worsen the oral hygiene and augment bacterial plaque accumulations. A second group consists of some nutritional deficiencies, hormonal imbalances, and systemic disorders, which may either lower local tissue resistance or modify the oral microflora. A third group, including vitamin C deficiency and heavy metal or drug intoxications, induce distinct periodontal pathoses which might lower the resistance of the periodontium to infection. Owing to the preponderant effect of bad oral hygiene, the significance of other predisposing factors unfortunately is not clear.

Oral Hygiene

It is difficult to distinguish effects mediated by worsened oral hygiene from effects seemingly due to other mechansims. Even the age effect may be attributable in part to the concomitant rapid and progressive increase in the fraction of persons having extremely bad oral hygiene (fig. 17/4). The increased severity of periodontal disease associated with unfavorable socioeconomic conditions or psychosomatic disturbances is so closely correlated with poorer oral hygiene that concomitant lowering of local tissue resistance has not been ascertained.

Age

The reason periodontitis becomes more prevalent and destructive with increasing age, even in a given oral hygiene group (fig. 17/3) remains unclear. It might be simply the consequence of prolonged exposure to plaque. Pocket formation, the first clinical evidence of destructive change, is normally rare before age 25, but becomes more frequent after age 30. Similarly, gingival and alveolar bone recession are only moderately prevalent before age 30 regardless of the degree of plaque control, even in a population practicing little oral hygiene. Recession remains moderate until age 40 in those with only slight plaque and calculus, but increases markedly thereafter in proportion to the amount of plaque. The accumulated evidence strongly indicates that bacterial plaque is responsible for the degeneration of the periodontium with age.

Since calculus is uncommon during childhood despite an abundance of plaque, some change of oral physiology may occur during puberty that favors calcification of plaque. Conceivably, oral physiology in the older person also favors increased bacterial accumulations.

Whatever the factors adverse to the periodontium that develop with age may be, their consequences seem to be secondary to those of oral uncleanliness. Most persons can reasonably expect to keep a healthy functioning periodontium if they always maintain good oral hygiene.

Diet

Modern civilized diets have been implicated as predisposing to periodontal disease, partly because they lack detergency and partly because their consumption does not entail sufficient masticatory stimulation. Contemporary peoples subsisting on primitive diets comprised of raw, fibrous, coarse foods seem to have no better periodontal health. Some investigators concluded from a study of stain removal that vigorous mastication of coarse foods could *not* be expected to prevent accumulation of plaque in cervical areas of the teeth except in the maxillary palatal gingiva.

Persons with extreme deficiencies of vitamins and probably deficiencies in protein exhibit severe periodontal pathosis, part of which is independent of local infection. Available data are insufficient to determine if borderline dietary deficiencies prevailing in large areas of the world predispose to inflammatory periodontal disease.

Consequences of pronounced vitamin A deficiency include keratinizing metaplasia of epithelium, xerosis, disturbed osteogenesis, and lowered resistance to infection. A variety of periodontal abnormalities in epithelium, connective tissue, and bone have been discerned in vitamin A-deficient rats. Inflammation and pocket formation occur only in the presence of local irritation, such as that caused by bacteria and calculus. Associated deficiency of lysozyme may contribute to reduced resistance to infection.

Glossitis, glossodynia, cheilosis, gingivitis, and generalized stomatitis have been attributed to deficiency of the vitamin B complex (thiamine, riboflavin, niacin, pantothenic acid, pyridoxine, biotin, *p*-aminobenzoic acid, inositol, choline, folic acid, and cyanocobalamin). Individual deficiency of riboflavin or niacin produces such symptoms in humans. Riboflavin or niacin therapy has been reported to cure or alleviate Vincent's infection. Severe gingivitis develops in animals deficient in folic acid.

Lack of vitamin C (ascorbic acid) impairs a variety of biochemical functions, most notably synthesis of collagen and metabolism of mucopolysaccharides. Important consequences include loss of intercellular substance, edema, degeneration of collagen fibers, decreased osteoblastic function, increased osteoclastic function, and structural weakness and loss of contractility of peripheral blood vessels. Particularly in stressed areas, tissue integrity fails. The clinical result is known as scurvy, characterized by edema, marked tendency to perivenular hemorrhage, retarded wound healing, increased susceptibility to infection, and asthenia. The oral manifestations of edema, hemorrhage, "gangrene" of gingiva, and exfoliation of teeth, seem to be rare today. A local irritant, such as bacterial accumulation, seems to be necessary in addition to the ascorbate deficiency for the fully developed pathosis. The severe periodontal symptoms historically associated with scurvy nevertheless have fostered widespread suspicion that chronic borderline ascorbate deficiency might be a frequent predisposing factor. The majority of modern clinical trials, however, have *not* found significant benefit from vitamin C therapy of periodontal patients.

Occlusal and Other Trauma

Adequate mechanical stimulation from mastication is thought to be necessary for structural maintenance of the periodontal ligament and alveolar bone. Clinical experience indicates that in individual cases or in particular sites, occlusal forces may exceed the adaptive capacity of the periodontium. The resulting "trauma from occlusion" may act synergistically with coexisting inflammation to increase destruction of the periodontium. Such trauma may result from innate malocclusion, disharmony from missing teeth, high restorations, bruxism, and clenching. On the other hand, it is clear that trauma from occlusion in the absence of bacterial plaque *cannot* initiate periodontitis.

Other sources of trauma implicated as secondary factors in periodontal disease include dental calculus (see above), a wide variety of dental procedures, mouth breathing, tongue thrusting, excessive smoking of tobacco, betelnut chewing in large regions of Asia, chemical irritation as from strong mouth washes, too vigorous toothbrushing, and allergic reactions of the oral mucosa.

Hormones

An excess or deficiency of hormones has been considered responsible for an exaggerated reactivity of the periodontium to local irritation in a minor fraction of persons. Familiar examples are gingivitis associated with puberty, menstruation, or pregnancy. A chronic desquamative type of gingivitis occurs occasionally during and after menopause. For pregnancy only, the data are adequate to validate an exacerbation of gingivitis not attributable to increased plaque accumulation. Recent studies have found a qualitative change in plaque during pregnancy: a large increase in *Bacteroides melaninogenicus* ss. *intermedius*. This subsides postpartum leaving no permanent alteration.

It is a prevalent clinical impression that diabetes predisposes to periodontal disease, but careful clinical investigations have not always established a correlation between these two disorders. In animal diabetes induced by alloxan, no distinctive periodontal changes have been reported. On the other hand, a hereditarily diabetic strain of Chinese hamster develops severe periodontal disease with pocket formation, inflammation, and alveolar bone resorption. Calculus is reported to be abnormally abundant in human diabetics. The extensive periodontal destruction seen in many diabetic children also indicates that uncontrolled diabetes does have some direct or indirect action on the periodontium probably by affecting the protective function of neutrophils.

Large doses of corticosteroids depress resistance to infection. Smaller, but significantly increased, amounts of corticosteroids are secreted during emotional stress and may aggravate periodontal lesions. Stress results also in production of epinephrine from adrenals and norepinephrine from sympathetic nerve endings. Since both of these hormones produce severe necrotic hemorrhagic lesions when injected into tissues sensitized by minute amounts of endotoxins, they might exacerbate periodontal lesions in emotionally disturbed persons.

Concurrent Pathoses

Blood dyscrasias, such as leukemia, neutropenias, purpuras, and anemias, are frequently accompanied by characteristic and rather extensive changes in the periodontium often alleviated by control of the dyscrasia. In most instances the periodontal changes are associated with a lowering of the resistance of the periodontal tissues to infection.

Intoxication by heavy metals and a variety of drugs seems to lower the resistance of mucous membranes to infection, leading to gingival disturbances in some cases. Arsenic, bismuth, and mercury may be derived from drugs containing them or, like lead and other heavy metals, may be acquired by occupational exposure. Bismuth, lead, and mercury are deposited particularly around the blood vessels beneath the epithelium and can be seen as darkly pigmented gingival areas. Mercury is also secreted in the saliva and may then act upon the gingival mucosa. Dilantin sodium, used to control epilepsy, promotes gingival hyperplasia in a fraction of cases, sometimes complicated by secondary inflammatory changes.

Noma (cancrum oris) is essentially a gangrenous extension of Vincent's infection with destruction of facial soft tissues and bone, and usually a fatal outcome if untreated. Penicillin terminates this infection dramatically. Noma seems to be associated with severe general nutritional deficiency, particularly of protein. There is frequently a history of prodromal infection; measles, herpes simplex, smallpox, diptheria, scarlet fever, typhoid fever, whooping cough, kala azar, and malaria have been cited.

Genetics

Epidemiologic surveys have revealed no differences in periodontal experience attributable to racial characteristics. Inbred strains of mice, however, vary distinctively in the type and severity of the spontaneous periodontal pathosis they develop. In one study, gingivitis was shown to be slightly but significantly more frequent in inbred children in two Japanese cities, possibly due to greater susceptibility to infection. Acatalasemia, hypophosphatasia, and cyclic neutropenia, rare human syndromes attributable to respective single mutant genes, are regularly accompanied by severe periodontal disease in all environments. Down's syndrome individuals, whose condition results from an extra chromosome, experience abnormally high incidence and severity of periodontitis.

The accumulated evidence suggests that some factors of genetic origin predispose to periodontal disease. Under present conditions their influence is very subordinate to that of poor oral hygiene and age.

RELATIONSHIP OF PERIODONTAL DISEASE TO FOCAL INFECTION

The concept of focal infection means simply that microorganisms or their toxic products disseminate from a primary localized infection and initiate secondary loci of infection or tissue damage in distant parts of the body. For many years, an astonishing variety of ailments, mostly inflammatory, were attributed to such oral foci as periapical abscesses, chronic pulpitis and periodontitis, and tonsillitis. Tonsillectomy and extraction of periapically involved or pulpless teeth enjoyed a great vogue, whether infection at these foci was proved or only suspected. These practices were considered justifiable because 1) typical oral bacteria could be isolated regularly from certain nonoral lesions, where they undoubtedly were etiologic, 2) inoculation of animals with bacteria from oral foci was reported to produce systemic conditions seen in humans, 3) eradication of real or suspected oral foci was widely reported to alleviate presumably associated systemic ailments, and 4) it was reported that operative trauma at primary oral sites exacerbated secondary lesions. Microorganisms derived from the periodontium have been implicated etiologically in lung abscesses, subacute bacterial endocarditis, rheumatic fever, rheumatoid arthritis, neuritis, gastrointestinal disease, ocular diseases, skin diseases, prostatic diseases, and general malaise. Definitive evidence of a regular direct connection between oral infections and such systemic ailments is still lacking, and today clinical management of the oral phase is generally less drastic. This does not mean unconcern with oral infections; rather it accords with the realization that these infections do not often have the momentous systemic consequences once attributed to them.

ADDITIONAL READING

Attström, R. 1970 Presence of Leucocytes in Crevices of Healthy and Chronically Inflamed Gingiva in Humans. J. Periodont Res, **5,** 42.

Attström, R., Laurell, A. B., Larsson, U., and Sjöhölm, A. 1975 Complement Factors in Gingival Crevice Material from Healthy and Inflamed Gingiva in Humans. J Periodont Res, **10**, 19.

Baehni, P., Tsai, C. C., McArthur, W. P., Hammond, B. F., and Taichman, N. S. 1979 Interaction of Inflammatory Cells and Oral Microorganisms; VIII. Detection of Leukotoxic Activity of a Plaque-derived Gram Negative Microorganisms. Infect Immun, **24**, 233.

Cianciola, L. J., Genco, R. J., Patters, M. R., McKenna, J., and Van Oss, C. J. 1977 Defective Polymorphonuclear Leukocyte Function in Human Periodontal Disease. Nature, **265**, 445.

Clark, H., Page, R. C., and Wilde, G. 1977 Defective Neutrophil Chemotaxis in Juvenile Periodontitis. Infect Immun, **18**, 694.

Ebersole, J. L., Frey, D. E., Taubman, M. A., and Smith, D. J. 1980 An ELISA for Measuring Serum Antibodies to *Actinobacillus actinomycetemcomitans*. J Periodont Res, **15**, 621.

Fearon, D. T., and Austen, K. F. 1980 Alternative Pathway of Complement—a System for Host Resistance to Microbial Infection. N. Engl J Med, **303**, 259.

Forster, O. 1972 Nature and Origin of Proteases in the Immunologically Induced Inflammatory Reaction. J Dent Res, **51**, 257.

Genco, R. J., and Krygier, G. 1973 Localization of Immunoglobulins, Immune Cells and Complement in Human Gingiva. J Periodont Res. Suppl, **10**, 30.

Genco, R., Mashino, P. A., Krygier, G., and Ellison, S. A. 1974 Antibody-mediated Effects on the Periodontium. J Periodontol, **45**, 330.

Gibbons, R. J., Socarnsky, S. S., DeAranjo, W. C., and Van Houte, J. 1964 Studies of the Cultivable Microbiota of the Plaque. Arch Oral Biol, **9**, 365.

Gibbons, R. J., Socransky, S. S., Sawyer, S., Kapsimalis, B., and MacDonald, J. B. 1963 The Microbiota of the Gingival Crevice Area of Man; II. The Predominant Cultivable Organisms. Arch Oral Biol, **8**, 281.

Hellden, L., Lindhe, J., Attstrom, R., and Sundin, Y. 1973 Neutrophil Chemotactic Factors in Gingival Crevice Material. Helv Odontol Acta, **17**, 1.

Horton, J. E., Leikin, S., and Oppenheim, J. J. 1972 Human Lymphoproliferative Reaction to Saliva and Dental Plaque Deposits; an *in Vitro* Correlation with Periodontal Disease. J Periodontol, **43**, 522.

Horton, J. E., Raisz, L. G., Simmons, H. A., Oppenheim, J. J., and Mergenhage, S. E. 1972 Bone Resorbing Activity in Supernatant Fluid from Cultured Human Peripheral Blood Leukocytes. Science, **177**, 793.

Horton, J. E., Oppenheim, J. J., and Mergenhagen, S. E. 1973 Elaboration of Lymphotoxin by Cultured Human Peripheral Blood Leukocytes Stimulated with Dental Plaque Deposits. Clin Exp Immunol, **13**, 383.

Horton, J. E., Oppenheim, J. J., and Mergenhagen, S. E. 1974 A Role for Cell-mediated Immunity in the Pathogenesis of Periodontal Disease. J Periodontol, **45**, 351.

Ingham, M. R., Sisson, P. R., Tharagounet, D., Selkon, J. B., and Codd, A. A. 1977 Inhibition of Phagocysotis *in Vitro* by Obligate Anaerobes. Lancet, **2**, 1252.

Ishikawa, I., Cimasoni, G., and Ahmad-Zadeh, C. 1972 Possible Role of Lysosomal Enzymes in the Pathogenesis of Periodontitis; a Study on Cathepsin D in Human Gingival Fluid. Arch Oral Biol, **17**, 111.

Ivanyi, L., and Lehner, T. 1970 Stimulation of Lymphocyte Transformation by Bacterial Antigens in Patients with Periodontal Disease. Arch Oral Biol, **15**, 1089.

Karring, T. 1973 Mitotic Activity in the Oral Epithelium.

J Periodont Res, **8**, Suppl 13.

Kelstrup, J., and Theilade, E. 1974 Microbes and Periodontal Disease. J Clin Periodontol, **1**, 15.

Kornman, K. S., Holt, S. C., and Robertson, P. B. 1981 The Microbiology of Ligature-induced Periodontitis in the Cynomolgus Monkey. J Periodontol Res, **16**, 363.

Lang, N. P., and Smith, F. N. 1977 Lymphocyte Blastogenesis to Plaque Antigens in Human Periodontal Disease; I. Populations of Varying Severity of Disease. J Periodontol Res, **12**, 298.

Lindhe, J., and Hellden, L. 1972 Neutrophil Chemotactic Activity Elaborated by Human Dental Plaque. J. Periodontol Res, **7**, 297.

Listgarten, M. A. 1976 Structure of the Microbial Flora Associated with Periodontal Health and Disease in Man; a Light and Electron Microscopic Study. J Periodontol, **47**, 1.

Löe, H., and Silness, J. 1963 Periodontal Disease in Pregnancy; I. Prevalence and Severity. Acta Odontol Scand, **21**, 533.

Löe, H., Theilade, E., and Jensen, S. B. 1965 Experimental Gingivitis in Man. J Periodontol, **36**, 177.

Manson, J. D., and Lehner, T. 1974 Clinical Features of Juvenile Periodontitis (Periodontosis). J Periodontol, **45**, 636.

Mouton, C., Hammond, P. G., Slots, J., and Genco, R. J. 1981 Serum Antibodies to Oral *Bacteroides asaccharolyticus* (*Bacteroides gingivalis*): Relationship to Age in Periodontal Disease. Infect Immun, **31**, 182.

Murray, P. A., and Patters, M. R. 1980 Gingival Crevice Neutrophil Function in Periodontal Lesions. J Periodont Res, **15**, 463.

Newman, M. G., and Socransky, S. S. 1977 Predominant Cultivable Microbiota in Periodontosis. J Periodont Res, **12**, 120.

Nisengard, R. J. 1977 The Role of Immunology in Periodontal Disease. J Periodontol, **48**, 505.

Page, R. C., and Schroeder, H. E. 1976 Pathogenesis of Inflammatory Periodontal Disease; a Summary of Current Work. Lab Invest, **33**, 235.

Patters, M. R., Genco, R. J., Reed, M. J., and Mashimo, P. A. 1976 Blastogenic Response of Human Lymphocytes to Oral Bacterial Antigens; Comparison of Individuals with Periodontal Disease to Normal and Edentulous Subjects. Infect Immun, **14**, 1213.

Patters, M. R., Sedransk, R. N., and Genco, R. J. 1977 Lymphoproliferative Response during Resolution and Recurrence of Naturally Occurring Gingivitis. J Periodontol, **48**, 373.

Patters, M. R., Schenkein, H. A., and Weinstein, A. 1979 A Method for Detection of Complement Cleavage in Gingival Fluid. J Dent Res, **58**, 1620.

Patters, M. R., Chen, P., McKenna, J., and Genco, R. J. 1980 Lymphoproliferative Responses to Oral Bacteria in Humans with Varying Severities of Periodontal Disease. Infect Immun, **28**, 777.

Payne, W., Page, R. C., Ogilvie, A. L., and Hall, W. B. 1975 Histopathologic Features of the Initial and Early Stages of Experimental Gingivitis in Man. J Periodont Res, **10**, 51.

Polson, A. M., Meitner, S. W., and Zander, H. A. 1976 Trauma and Progression of Marginal Periodontitis in Squirrel Monkeys; IV. Reversibility of Bone Loss Due to Trauma Alone and Trauma Superimposed upon Periodontitis. J Periodont Res, **11**, 290.

Raisz, L. G., Sandberg, A. L., Goodson, J. M., Simmons, H. A., and Mergenhagen, S. E. 1974 Complement-dependent Stimulation of Prostaglandin Synthesis of Bone Resorption. Science, **185**, 789.

RANNEY, R. R., AND ZANDER, H. A. 1970 Allergic Periodontal Disease in Sensitized Squirrel Monkeys. J Periodontol, **41,** 12.

RANNEY, R. R. 1978 Immunofluorescent Localization of Soluble Dental Plaque Components in Human Gingiva Affected by Periodontitis. J Periodont Res, **13,** 99.

RIZZO, A. A., AND MITCHELL, C. H. 1966 Chronic Allergic Inflammation Induced by Repeated Deposition of Antigen in Rabbit Gingival Pockets. Periodontics, **4,** 5.

RUSSELL, A. L. 1956 System of Classification and Scoring for Prevalence Surveys of Periodontal Disease. J Dent Res, **35,** 350.

SCHENKEIN, H. A., AND GENCO, R. J. 1977 Gingival Fluid in Serum in Periodontal Diseases; I. Quantitative Study of Immunoglobulins, Complement Components, and Other Plasma Proteins. J Periodontol, **48,** 772.

SCHENKEIN, H. A., AND GENCO, R. J. 1977 Gingival Fluid in Serum in Periodontal Diseases; II. Evidence for Cleavage of Complement Components C3, C3 Proactivator (Factor B) and C4 in Gingival Fluid. J Periodontol, **48,** 778.

SCHROEDER, H. E. 1970 The Structure and Relationship of Plaque to the Hard and Soft Tissues; Electron Microscopic Interpretation. Int Dental J **20,** 353.

SHURIN, S. B., SOCRANSKY, S. S., SWEENEY, E., AND STOSSEL, T. P. 1979 A Neutrophil Disorder Induced by *Capnocytophaga*, a Dental Microorganism. N Engl J Med, **301,** 849.

SILNESS, J., AND LÖE, H. 1964 Periodontal Disease in Pregnancy; II. Correlation between Oral Hygiene and Periodontal Condition. Acta Odontol Scand, **22,** 121.

SLOTS, J. 1976 The Predominant Cultivable Organisms in Juvenile Periodontitis. Scand J Dent Res, **85,** 1.

SLOTS, J. 1977 The Predominant Cultivable Microflora of Advanced Periodontitis. Scand J Dent Res, **85,** 114.

SLOTS, J. 1977 Microflora in the Healthy Gingival Sulcus in Man. Scand J Dent Res, **85,** 247.

SLOTS, J., MOENBO, D., LANGEBAEK, J., AND ERANDSEN, A. 1978 Microbiota of Gingivitis in Man. Scand J Dent Res, **86,** 174.

SLOTS, J. 1979 Subgingival Microflora and Periodontal Disease. J Clin Periodontol **6,** 351.

SLOTS, J., AND HAUSMANN, E. 1979 Longitudinal Study of Experimentally Induced Periodontal Disease in *Macaca arctoides*; Relationship between Microflora and Alveolar Bone Loss. Infect Immun, **23,** 260.

SOCRANSKY, S. S., GIBBONS, R. J., DALE, A. C., BORTNICK, L., ROSENTHAL, E., AND MACDONALD, J. B. 1963 The Microbiota of the Gingival Crevice Area of Man; I. Total Microscopic and Viable Counts and Counts of Specific Organisms. Arch Oral Biol, **8,** 275.

SOCRANSKY, S. S. 1970 Relationship of Bacteria to the Etiology of Periodontal Disease. (In Conference on Specific Questions Related to Periodontal Diseases, edited by H. M. Fullmer). J Dent Res, **49,** 191.

SOCRANSKY, S. S. 1977 Microbiology of Periodontal Disease—Present Status and Future Considerations. J Periodontol, **48,** 497.

SUOMI, J. D., AND DOYLE, J. 1972 Oral Hygiene and Periodontal Disease in an Adult Population in the United States. J Periodontol, **43,** 677.

TAICHMAN, N. 1970 Mediation of Inflammation by the Polymorphonuclear Leukocytes as a Sequela of Immune Reactions. J Periodontol, **41,** 228.

TANNER, A. C. R., HOFFER, C., BRATTHAL, G. T., VISCONTI, R. A., AND SOCRANSKY, S. S. 1979 A Study of the Bacteria Associated with Advancing Periodontitis in Man. J Clin Periodontol **6,** 278.

THEILADE, E., WRIGHT, W. H., JENSEN, S. B., AND LÖE, H. 1966 Experimental Gingivitis in Man; II. A Longitudinal Clinical and Bacteriological Investigation. J Periodont Res, **1,** 1.

VAN DYKE, T. E., HOROSZEWICZ, H. U., CIANCIOLA, L. J., AND GENCO, R. J. 1980 Neutrophil Chemotaxis Dysfunction in Human Periodontitis. Infect Immun, **27,** 124.

chapter 18

Infections of the Tooth Pulp, Periapical Tissues, and Contiguous Structures

George S. Schuster and Keith R. Volkmann

INTRODUCTION

Within the confines of the tooth and about its periapical regions are tissues and structures that are often subject to infection. These tissues and the morphology of the structures they form are unique in the body, as is the response of the region to infection. Localized infection of this region is common and can constitute a site from which infection spreads to other parts of the body. For a complete understanding of the course of infection of these structures a knowledge of their gross and microscopic anatomy is essential. For this the reader is referred to the various texts on anatomy and histology of the teeth and supporting structures.

ETIOLOGY OF PULPAL AND PERIAPICAL DISTURBANCES

Following eruption of the tooth into the oral environment, the enamel and dentin protect the pulp by acting as a physical barrier to harmful solutions and as insulators against temperature changes so long as they remain intact. At the same time, enclosure of the pulp in any unyielding space is sometimes detrimental, for changes in pressure within the area, caused for instance by inflammation, are transmitted directly to the tissues, with some interference to blood circulation. Thus, while the pulp is protected by dentin and enamel, the arrangement of these tissues may have a decided influence upon its response to irritation. Most changes in the pulp are caused by irritation. The chief irritants to the pulp are microbial, mechanical, thermal, chemical, and electrical. We will only be concerned with the effects of microorganisms on the pulp.

Microbial Action on Pulp. Microorganisms are a principal source of irritation to the pulp, which they invade if given the opportunity. Enamel and dentin are ordinarily sufficient to protect the pulp from infection by the oral microbiota but any action that breaches this barrier will allow bacteria to invade the pulp. The principal pathways by which they may gain entrance into the pulp or periapical areas are: 1) through an open cavity caused by trauma such as fracture of the crown or root, operative dental procedures, or dental caries; 2) through the tubules of cut or carious dentin; 3) via the gingival crevice and by invasion along the periodontal ligament in several forms of periodontal disease; 4) by extension of periapical infection from adjacent infected teeth; and 5) through the bloodstream during bacteremia or septicemia.

The fracture of crown or root with pulpal exposure almost always allows the oral bacteria to invade and infect pulp. Operative procedures that accidentally expose the pulp usually allow ingress of the oral microbiota, unless carefully controlled by prior isolation of the tooth. Similarly, progression of dental caries sufficient to expose the pulp physically allows large numbers of the oral microbiota to invade the pulp.

In the cutting of teeth during operative dental procedures, the cut dentinal tubules are exposed to the oral cavity. If the dentinal cavity is exposed to saliva, oral microorganisms have access to exposed tubules. There is some question as to how often such bacteria subsequently gain entrance to the pulp or, if they do so, how often they infect it. This is probably not a common occurrence, considering the untold numbers of cavities prepared daily from which there is no subsequent clinically discernible infection of the pulp.

A more important route of bacterial invasion of the pulp is through the tubules of carious dentin. Such an invasion may occur even before the pulp is exposed directly to the oral environment by cavitation. The bacteria that penetrate the dentin before cavitation has exposed the pulp are undoubtedly some of those involved in the carious process. Streptococci, staphylococci, lactobacilli, and filamentous microorganisms have been isolated from the advancing carious lesion deep within the dentin. Of this group, streptococci have been found most consistently as the causative agent of pulpitis arising from deep dentin caries that has not exposed the pulp. In such circumstances, staphylococci and filamentous microorganisms are also sometimes the cause of pulpitis.

In periodontal disease, microorganisms often invade along the periodontal ligament and in large numbers inhabit areas closer to the periapical regions than they do when they are confined to the normal gingival sulcus. As the periodontal lesions progress toward the apex, lateral or accessory canals may be exposed to the oral environment, also providing access to the pulp. These bacteria, perhaps because of the interlacing nature of the blood and lymph systems of the periodontal ligament and the pulp, are often able to reach the pulp where they may infect. While bacteria are, at times, found in pulps of teeth in which there is no caries and no disturbance in the periodontium, in the case of caries or a pocket in the periodontium, bacteria have been found in more than 40% of such pulps, and more than half of the bacteria found were nonhemolytic streptococci. Although the method of obtaining bacterial samples from pulps is usually conducive to contamination, such studies do indicate relative differences in the access of bacteria to periapical areas and to the pulp.

Microorganisms infecting a pulp or periapical areas of one tooth may find their way to adjacent noninfected pulp or periapical regions of sound teeth by the interlacing of blood and lymph systems or by physical extension, under pressure, of the periapical infection from one tooth to another. Bacteria in the bloodstream may localize and infect in these areas by anachoresis (literally, convocation or refuge) if there is a circumscribed area of inflammation. The fixation of bacteria in the process of anachoresis has been attributed to their mechanical obstruction by a fibrin network and by thrombosis of efferent lymphatics, to the osmotic pressure in transuded material, to the electrostatic condition of the tissue, to phagocytes, and to their agglutination, but none of these concepts adequately explains the process. Circulating microorganisms are more often present in apparently healthy persons than had been previously supposed, for studies now indicate that their average incidence is about 5%. The incidence of bacteremias in persons with foci of infection presumably would be much higher: in fact, an

average of 20% of individuals with periodontitis were found to have bacteremias. Operations on, or other manipulations of the teeth or gingivae further increase the incidence of bacteremias. Thus, transient bacteremias do exist in considerable numbers of individuals, depending upon the circumstances, and these bacteria may be localized and fixed in sufficient quantities to produce infection in periapical areas or the pulp if for any reason these tissues are irritated and inflamed. Cavity preparation and medication are often sufficient irritation to cause anachoresis, though the more severe the irritation, whatever its nature, the more likely the bacteria are to be attracted to the area. Experimental studies of the influence of pulpal irritation on anachoresis indicate that deep cavity preparation and subsequent placement of irritating medication are much more likely to attract bacteria to the pulp than is the preparation of a shallow cavity, followed by nonirritating medication. Thus, it is likely that the result of pulpal or periapical irritation during cavity preparation, with a simultaneous transient bacteremia, is an accumulation of bacteria in the affected area, resulting in infection and the production of a postoperative "idiopathic" pulpitis or periapical infection.

Microorganisms Involved in Pulpal Disorders. The primary causative microorganism of pulpitis is difficult to determine, partially because of the technical difficulties associated with obtaining valid samples for culturing and partially because the exact time of the initial infection is difficult to ascertain. Bacteria with fairly high pathogenic potential are found with some regularity in tooth pulps that do not show clinically demonstrable reactions to them. On the other hand, it is not always possible to demonstrate bacteria even where there is a clinically obvious pulpitis, which is also not easily attributable to other forms of irritation than bacteria.

Table 18/1 is a compilation of the microorganisms obtained from nonvital teeth. Streptococci were the most common, especially the α-hemolytic strains (about one-half of the teeth examined), although nonhemolytic strains were also present. Enterococci and group D (nonenterococci) streptococci were present in about 35% of teeth sampled. Enterococci are apt to be difficult to eliminate from root canals, particularly when antibiotics are used, as are yeasts and gram negative bacteria, especially gram negative rods. While staphylococci are found with some degree of regularity in samples, many feel that they are contaminants resulting from sampling technique. A recent study demonstrated that in endodontic infections there were large numbers of bacteria present, both in total numbers and in number of species. The mean concentration of bac-

Table 18/1
Microorganisms isolated from infected root canals

Aerobic or Facultative Microorganisms	Anaerobic Microorganisms
α-Hemolytic streptococci	Lactobacillus species
Nonhemolytic streptococci	Bacteroides species
Enterococci	Peptococcus species
Group D streptococci (nonenterococcus)	Peptostreptococcus anaerobius
Corynebacterium species	Bifidobacterium species
Bacillus species	Eubacterium species
Staphylococcus epidermidis	Propionibacterium acnes
Proteus species	Veillonella species
Escherichia coli	Actinomyces species
Candida albicans	
Unidentified gram positive rods and cocci	
Unidentified gram negative bacteria	

teria was almost 10^8 per gram of sample, with anaerobes accounting for nearly two-thirds of all isolates. Furthermore, these investigators showed that there was an average of six distinctive species per specimen. The significance of lactobacilli in root canals is not known but since they are not pathogenic in soft tissues they may be contaminants of the canal.

Microorganisms that can produce gas, mostly from the degradation of organic materials in the root canals include streptococci, diphtheroids, coliform bacteria, and several of the anaerobic bacteria. This may be an important source of pain, and perhaps sinus tract formation in teeth so infected.

In addition, a variety of microorganisms have been isolated from nonvital, infected teeth that had intact pulp chambers and no apparent communication with the oral environment. These include: Actinomyces species, Bacteroides species, Fusobacterium species, Campylobacter sputorum, Eubacterium species, Peptococcus species, and several unidentified anaerobic and facultative microorganisms.

One wonders how many of the bacteria isolated from pulp canals under various conditions are actual residents and how many are contaminants resulting from the various mechanical procedures, including the sampling procedures.

The persistence of microorganisms in pulps during treatment has also been investigated, and here again, chance contamination in sampling procedures may greatly influence the data which indicate that microorganisms found at initial treatment tend to persist during subsequent root canal treatment. In general, however, streptococci persist more abundantly in root canals than do other organisms.

Studies of the overall frequency distribution of microorganisms in root canals as obtained by various investigators have shown that streptococci are the predominant microorganisms found in root ca-

nals, whatever the clinical history. Other microorganisms such as staphylococci, diphtheroids, spirochetes, fusiform bacteria, filamentous forms, and other miscellaneous microorganisms have been found in varying numbers by the different investigators. Many species of microorganisms, while perhaps infecting at the time they were isolated from the root canal, are really opportunists which must be regarded as secondary invaders to initial infection.

Somewhat the same situation exists with regard to the bacteria involved in periapical infection, except that perhaps there is a greater likelihood of contamination in sampling. Nevertheless streptococci are the most prevalent microorganisms isolated from periapical infections. Staphylococci are also relatively abundant in such areas, usually as a mixed infection with streptococci.

CLINICAL COURSE OF PULPAL AND PERIAPICAL DISTURBANCES

The basic tissue reactions of the pulp to stimuli or irritants of varying intensity are mitosis, inflammation, repair, formation of secondary dentin, and necrosis. However, it must be remembered that different conditions may coexist in various parts of the same pulp. The clinical responses are either acute or chronic pulpitis, and pulp death (necrosis).

Periapical Infections. At some point in the progress of the pulp toward degeneration is the involvement of the periapical regions. During the course of pulpitis, the infecting bacteria, their products, and the products of tissue disintegration may find egress through cavitation of the crown, if such exists. It is more likely that they are carried to the periapical regions by the circulatory system of the pulp, eliciting a series of reactions. One of the structures involved is the periodontal ligament which, at first, thickens in response to irritation about the apex of the tooth arising from disturbances of the pulp by bacteria. According to the type and duration of bacterial irritation, the periapical tissue respond in several different ways.

An acute inflammatory reaction may result in acute periapical periodontitis. The inflammation and thickening of the apical periodontal ligament, together with serous exudate, extrudes the tooth. Such a reaction may resolve if conditions are favorable, or if not, and if the irritation is severe and continued, it may progress by breaking down alveolar bone and result in the next developmental stage, which is an alveolar abscess.

The alveolar or apical abscess may be either acute or chronic, according to circumstances. The acute alveolar abscess is the extension of a pulp infection into the periapical area, causing necrosis of the bone and tissue in the affected area and the accumulation of pus. Virulent bacteria may move from the root canal into the apical regions. Toxic products from the pulp may also play a pathogenic role in these responses. The subsequent course of such reactions will be discussed later.

A chronic alveolar abscess may develop from extension into the periapical area of long-standing, low-grade infection of the pulp of an affected tooth. It may develop also as a result of the unsatisfactory treatment of a root canal. As with the acute alveolar abscess, there is degradation of tissue and the accumulation of pus. This may result in a fistulous tract that drains to a surface intraorally or extraorally. Sometimes the pus does not reach the exterior but is absorbed by the blood and lymph systems almost as rapidly as it is formed. Thus, a chronic alveolar abscess differs from an acute one principally in the degree of infection. In an acute abscess the microorganisms cause rapid and extensive tissue reaction and damage. In a chronic abscess the microorganisms cause less tissue damage more slowly, and an equilibrium between the organisms and the tissue is occasionally established during the course of the infection.

Immunopathology of Pulpal and Periapical Infections. It is likely that in addition to the direct actions of microorganisms and their products on the pulpal and periapical tissues, and the direct response of the tissues to these factors, there is an immunological component to the response to odontogenic infections.

Antigenic components from root canals, be they microbial in origin or components of necrotic pulp, can trigger immune responses both of the humoral and cell-mediated variety. Immunoglobulins of the classes IgG, IgA and IgM, specific for intraoral antigens, have been found in longstanding periapical lesions in humans. These have been observed both extracellularly and in plasma cells. IgE containing cells also have been identified in inflamed

pulp tissue. In addition the C3 component of complement has been demonstrated to be present on endothelial lined structures in the region: these structures appeared to be blood vessels. Whether the C3 attachment to these structures is or is not immunologic is not clear at this time. Furthermore, endotoxin has been demonstrated to be present in endodontically involved teeth. Its antigenicity is variable but when it reacts with antibodies the complex can trigger a complement reaction. Endotoxin also may activate the alternate complement pathway. In either instance the release of biologically active fragments may result in inflammatory changes. Arthus-like reactions have been demonstrated in periapical areas. With the attendant influx of polymorphonuclear leukocytes and mononuclear cells there is a release of tissue damaging enzymes and other side reactions resulting in production of lesions characterized by bone and collagen loss in the periapical region. If the challenge continues, the response can become prolonged and produce chronic disease.

Similarly, cell-mediated immunity may play a role in the pathogenesis of periapical disease as it responds to antigens originating in the root canal. It has been shown that there are macrophages and T lymphocytes present in periapical lesions, and patients with pulp pathology have circulating lymphocytes that are sensitized to antigens derived from necrotic homologous pulp. When the presence of the sensitized lymphocytes was determined by *in vitro* production of a lymphokine, leukocyte migration inhibition factor, the patients with periapical pathosis had a greater response to soluble antigens derived from the necrotic pulp than did normal subjects. If microbial antigens sensitize a patient then later enter the periapical tissues via an infected pulp, sensitized cells may be available to initiate periapical pathosis. Thus, like humoral immunity, cell-mediated immunity may be involved in pathology of the pulpal and periapical tissues.

COMPLICATIONS OF PULPAL AND PERIAPICAL INFECTIONS

Fatal complications from periapical infections are relatively rare, considering the enormous numbers of infected teeth that exist in the world today, from which a wide variety of microorganisms pour regularly into the rest of the body. However, complications from periapical infection are not unknown for in some cases the infection spreads to tissues in other areas of the oral cavity, causing submandibular or superficial sublingual abscesses; abscesses may be produced also in the submaxillary triangle or in the parapharyngeal or submasseteric space. From these areas the infection can spread by the fascial planes of the neck to areas where it may become more serious. For example, extension of a periapical infection may produce Ludwig's angina, an infection of the throat and neck involving such severe swelling as to sometimes block the air passages and produce asphyxiation.

In the maxilla, periapical infection may affect only the soft tissues of the face where it is not so serious but it may extend to the infratemporal space, and then to the meninges where the infection is often fatal.

The dental profession has developed treatment procedures which prevent the development of any large number of teeth with pulpal pathosis and has also developed satisfactory endodontic treatment procedures. Nevertheless, for many years there has been controversy about periapical infection acting as a focus of infection. In many acute periapical infections, there can be little doubt of the effect of dissemination of bacteria and various toxic substances from the affected area, for the patient is ill, and by the application of proper techniques it can be demonstrated that a bacteremia or septicemia exists. There is some question, however, as to whether bacteria are disseminated from some of the more chronic periapical infections, for it is often difficult to demonstrate significant numbers of bacteria in them. Furthermore, it is not always possible to determine whether bacteria present in an area are being disseminated, or if so, that they are producing an infection in some other area of the body. It may be that bacteria are simply attracted to a site by the process of anachoresis.

Microorganisms Involved in Odontogenic Soft Tissue Infections. The microorganisms found in soft tissue infections of odontogenic origin may be the same as those causing the pulpal infections. A change in the primary isolate may be a result of a change in the proportion of organisms following spread of the infection. If multiple bacterial types were originally present, the pulp could favor one type while the soft tissues may favor a coinfecting organism. Alternatively, the pulpal infection could have favored infection by the second type.

Many infections of the periapical regions or originating in the pulp are of the mixed variety and include both aerobic and anaerobic bacteria. It has been estimated that 25 to 35% of isolates are anaerobes; other estimates are as high as 50%. Several studies have examined the incidence of various microorganisms isolated from infected pulp and periapical tissues and although the ranges vary, the averages are similar (table 18/2). The most common bacteria are nonhemolytic and α-hemolytic streptococci, although other streptococci may be found. Gram negative species, especially the rods, may be difficult to eliminate from infections and if they degrade tissue proteins and produce gas, pain can result.

Table 18/2

Average incidence of bacterial isolates from periapical infections

Microorganism	Percent
Facultative streptococci	50
Enterococci	3
Peptostreptococci	18
Staphylococci	16
Actinomyces species	4
Diphtheroids	4
Propionibacterium acnes	20
Bacteroides species	15
Veillonellae	30
Fusobacteria	5
Neisseriae	5
Lactobacilli	5
Enterobacteria	4

Although most infections involve a mixture of either aerobic or facultative organisms in conjunction with an anaerobic flora, some studies have shown the number of infections by purely anaerobic organisms to be as high as 33%. Almost one-half of the anaerobes isolated were gram negative. Some infections contained one species, others contain several.

The organisms listed were found in the majority of cases while others have been found in lesser numbers but with some degree of regularity. Also, there are occasional reports of infections involving uncommon pathogens, for example, *Serratia marcescens*; or *Klebsiella pneumoniae*, an organism that, while pathogenic, usually causes respiratory tract infections.

One must also be cognizant of the fact that infections of the head and neck region may be nonodontogenic in origin, but once initiated, the appearance and outcome may be similar to those of odontogenic origin. Indeed, in situations where the teeth or periodontium have undergone breakdown it may be difficult to identify the source of the infection.

As in other sites, in infections of the pulp and periapical tissues and contiguous structures, the infection will progress and cellulitis or an abscess may result if the invading organisms overcome the host's defenses and conditions are favorable for microbial proliferation.

Abscesses. Abscesses that occur in the oral tissues most frequently are in or originate in periapical regions. The abscess is composed mainly of a central area of organisms and disintegrating polymorphonuclear leukocytes, surrounded by viable leukocytes and some lymphocytes. The clinical features of pain, swelling, and sometimes regional lymphadenitis are usually confined to the immediate region of the source of infection (fig. 18/1). However, microbial by-products and tissue break-

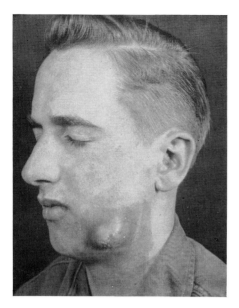

Figure 18/1. Cellulitis arising from an abscessed pulp and periapical infection. (AFIP 0-7744.)

down products may produce systemic illness. A periapical abscess may remain limited to the osseous structures, or burrow through the bone until it reaches the surface and invades the soft tissues. During abscess formation there may be a regional cellulitis. The infection then becomes well circumscribed, producing the localized collection of pus in a cavity which is the true abscess.

Abscesses of the head and neck are caused by aerobic and anaerobic microorganisms, and similar appearing lesions may be found in single or mixed infections. The facultative staphylococci and streptococci are commonly associated with such lesions. Various studies differ as to which organism is most frequently associated with such infections. Some have indicated that α-hemolytic streptococci were more common where only one type of organism was isolated with the remaining infections due to *Staphylococcus aureus* or *Staphylococcus epidermidis* in about equal proportions. Other studies reported that staphylococcal infections were more common. Other single organism infections have been attributed to *Actinomyces* species; enterococci, *Proteus* species; *Branhamella catarrhalis*; and pleomorphic gram positive, irregularly arranged organisms classified as *Corynebacterium* species.

In mixed culture infections the α-hemolytic streptococci and staphylococci were the predominant isolates. Other contributors to such infections included *Pseudomonas aeruginosa*, enterococci, *Streptococcus pyogenes*, and *Branhamella*. In most instances, two or three organisms were involved, with streptococci usually being one of them. Reported combinations include α-hemolytic strepto-

cocci and staphylococci (the most frequent combination); α-hemolytic streptococci, β-hemolytic streptococci and staphylococci; α-hemolytic streptococci and pseudomonas; α-hemolytic streptococci or enterococci and *Branhamella*; and enterococci and α-hemolytic streptococci or *Staphylococcus aureus*.

Gram positive and gram negative anaerobes have been isolated from head and neck abscesses. The gram positive anaerobes most frequently isolated include *Peptostreptococcus* species, *Peptococcus* species, and *Eubacterium* species. The gram negative anaerobes were *Bacteroides* species, some *Fusobacterium* species, and *Veillonella* species. In addition many studies show high percentages of unidentified anaerobic gram negative rods. Several studies indicated that the anaerobic infections tended to be a mixture of organisms. Indeed, some investigators have suggested the possibility that many of the species isolated are incapable of producing abscesses by themselves.

Although there is disagreement as to the role of various bacteria in abscesses of the head and neck region, it is apparent that the streptococci are predominant in infections at the tooth apex secondary to dental caries. Some of the differences may be due to sampling procedures, such as how soon after the infection began, how far it had progressed, and what other factors were superimposed (*e.g.*, therapeutic attempts) at the time of sampling. Also there may be a shift in the type of microorganisms most frequently isolated due to our increased ability to recognize and isolate the others.

Cellulitis. Cellulitis is a diffuse inflammatory reaction in which the host defenses are unable to contain the infection to one area. Instead, it progresses through the surrounding tissues and along fascial planes to areas away from the original site of infection. Cellulitis of the face and neck most commonly results from periapical infection or following periodontal infection. The tissues involved show separation of muscle or connective tissue and nonspecific acute inflammation. Clinically there is firm, painful swelling of the involved tissues and usually a regional lymphadenitis. If superficial tissues are involved, the overlying skin appears inflammed, or even purple in color. The diffuse spread of the infection may involve considerable areas of the face and neck. Streptococci and some strains of staphylococci are the more common causes of cellulitis in the orofacial region.

Cellulitis readily resolves with treatment. If it persists, it can become localized, forming an abscess that may break through to a surface and drain spontaneously (fig. 18/2).

A particularly severe form of cellulitis is Ludwig's angina, which frequently begins in the submandibular space then invades other tissue spaces bilat-

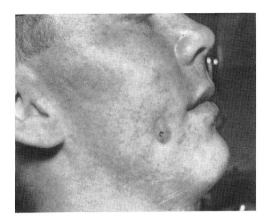

Figure 18/2. Periapical abscess with draining fistula of the face. (AFIP 56-12889.)

erally. The source of infection is often a mandibular tooth but it may result from a fracture or penetrating injury. The clinical features of Ludwig's angina are rapid development of a board-like swelling in the floor of the mouth which is elevated. The tongue protrudes and swallowing and respiration are difficult. The swelling does not localize and it continues to involve the neck, the parapharyngeal spaces and other regions. If the larynx becomes edematous, the patient may suffocate. Streptococci are commonly involved in Ludwig's angina but usually it is a mixed infection. A variety of gram positive and gram negative aerobic and anaerobic bacteria have been implicated including fusiforms, spirochetes, diphtheroids, staphylococci, *Bacteroides*, *Klebsiella*, *Escherichia coli*, *Pseudomonas aeruginosa*, *Haemophilus influenzae*, and *Branhamella catarrhalis*.

Osteomyelitis. Osteomyelitis is an acute, subacute or chronic inflammation of bone and bone marrow which may develop as a result of odontogenic or other infections. Acute osteomyelitis often results in a diffuse spread of infection throughout the medullary spaces, with necrosis of bone. A variety of bacteria have been associated with osteomyelitis. Staphylococci and a few strains of *Streptococcus* are the most common, although actinomycetes and anaerobic bacteria are not uncommon. Other infections, such as tuberculosis or syphilis also may produce osteomyelitis.

ROLE OF BACTERIOLOGICAL CONTROL IN TREATMENT OF PULPAL AND PERIAPICAL DISORDERS

When the tooth pulp is exposed to the environment under some circumstances it can be successfully treated by capping, *e.g.*, if the area of exposure is not too large. If the area of exposure of a young pulp is large or exposure has led to the death of a portion of the coronal pulp, pulpotomy can be accomplished before using one of the capping materials to fill the coronal pulp chamber.

The purpose of these procedures is to maintain the pulp tissue intact and protect it from the oral microbiota with a tissue-tolerant material that will stimulate the pulp to establish a hard-tissue pulpal seal. Several factors interact to determine the success or failure of pulp capping or pulpotomy. It is most likely, however, that the oral microbiota is the most important factor contributing to breaking down the integrity of the pulp tissue. It has been shown that the exposure of tooth pulps of rats to their oral microbiota invariably leads to complete pulpal necrosis with granulomas and abscess formation. In contrast, the exposed pulps of germ-free animals were never devitalized and no apical granulomas or abscesses were ever produced in such pulps. In the germ-free animals, a dentinal bridge began to form in about 2 weeks and was complete by the 3rd or 4th week, in spite of gross food impactions.

When a pulp is infected and pulp capping or pulpotomy are not indicated, pulpectomy must be performed. This involves removing the pulp in its entirety and filling the chamber with some inert, innocuous material which will seal the chamber sufficiently to prevent further contamination by bacteria. As part of the procedure for controlling bacteria in an infected root canal before filling, it is necessary to remove the proteinaceous material that may serve as a nutrient source for microorganisms and to eliminate (or to reduce to negligible numbers) the bacteria from the pulp canal and from the apical-periapical tissues. It is also necessary to decrease the likelihood that bacteria may survive in the apical-periapical tissues and to prevent soluble products of such bacteria from entering into the circulatory system in quantities that may be harmful. Finally, it is necessary to leave the periapical tissues in a state in which their resistance is not significantly compromised; otherwise they cannot be expected to remain healthy and to successfully resist subsequent bacterial infection. The achievement of such goals is facilitated by excluding external contamination by the use of rubber dam to isolate the tooth being operated on, by sterilizing all instruments used in the operation to treat the root canal, by eliminating or reducing to a minimum all microorganisms in the pulp chambers and root canals by thorough biomechanical debridement and by treating with antiseptics or chemotherapeutic agents.

The most reliable method by which sterility of the area can be determined is by bacteriological culture, although this practice is not universally accepted. Various systems of endodontic therapy follow different procedures for culture. These are discussed in the standard endodontic texts. In recent years a wide variety of broth and agar media have been used with the expectation of sustaining the growth of as many aerobic and anaerobic bacterial species as possible. Failure to detect bacteria by culture techniques is related to the nature of the species concerned, to the number of microorganisms present, to the efficacy of the sampling techniques, and to the culture technique. With some bacterial species only a few bacteria need be present in the sample to obtain a positive culture, while others, such as some *Treponema* species, are difficult or impossible to culture. Also, while it has been suggested that the number of canal microorganisms is a decisive factor in initiating an infection, few data are available to indicate the actual numbers of bacteria in root canals, nor the relationship of numbers present at the time of filling to clinical success or failure. Similarly, it has been suggested, though not definitely proven, that the virulence of the root canal flora is a critical factor in successful endodontic therapy.

Because of these variables, the culture procedure must be placed in its proper perspective. Negative cultures are no more of a guarantee of a successful outcome of endodontic therapy than positive cultures are a guarantee of failure. Instead, the procedure may serve as an additional control for determining the thoroughness of the steps related to the removal of bacteria and their nutrient sources from the root canals. However, the proper use of bacteriological culture techniques apparently does enhance the chances of successful endodontic therapy.

ADDITIONAL READING

ADAMKIEWICZ, V. W., PEKOVIC, D. D., AND MASCRES, C. 1978 Allergies of the Dental Pulp. Oral Surg, **46**, 843.

AKPATA, E. S. 1974 Total Viable Count of Microorganisms in the Infected Dental Pulp. J Dent Res, **53**, 1330.

BAUME, L. J. 1970 Diagnosis of Diseases of the Pulp. Oral Surg, **29**, 102.

BROWN, J. I. 1972 An Evaluation of the Antimicrobial Effectiveness of Intracanal Medicaments. J SC Dent Assoc, **40**, 845.

BROWN, L. R., AND RUDOLPH, C. E., JR. 1957 Isolation and Identification of Microorganisms from Unexposed Canals of Pulp-involved Teeth. Oral Surg, **10**, 1094.

COTTON, W. R. 1974 Bacterial Contamination as a Factor in Healing of Pulp Exposures. Oral Surg, **38**, 441.

DWYER, T. G., AND TORABINEJAD, M. 1981 Radiographic and Histologic Evaluation of the Effect of Endotoxin on Periapical Tissues of the Cat. J Endodontol, **7**, 31.

GROSSMAN, L. I. 1972 Sterilization of Infected Root Canals. J Am Dent Assoc, **85**, 900.

GROSSMAN, L. I., LEE, E., AND DEMP, S. 1962 Isolation of Gas-producing Organisms from Root Canals. J Dent Res, **41**, 495.

JACKSON, F. L., AND HALDER, A. R. 1963 Incidence of Yeasts in Root Canals During Therapy. Br Dent J **115**, 459.

KAKEHASHI, S., STANLEY, H. R., AND FITZGERALD, R. J. 1965 The Effects of Surgical Exposures of Dental Pulps in Germ-free and Conventional Laboratory Rats. Oral Surg, **20**, 340.

KALMAN, M. I. 1964 The Microbial Status of the Root Canal During Endodontic Treatment. NY State Dent J, **30**, 419.

KANTZ, W. E., AND HENRY, C. A. 1974 Isolation and Classification of Anaerobic Bacteria from Intact Pulp Chambers of Non-vital Teeth. Arch Oral Biol, **19**, 91.

KORZEN, B. H., KRAKOW, A. A., AND GREEN, D. B. 1974 Pulpal and Periapical Tissue Responses in Conventional and Monoinfected Gnotobiotic Rats. Oral Surg, **37**, 783.

KUNTZ, D. D., GENCO, R. J., GUTTOSO, J., AND NATRELLA, J. R. 1977 Localization of Immunoglobulins and the Third Component of Complement in Dental Periapical Lesions. J Endodontol, **3**, 68.

LANGELAND, K., RODRIGUES, H., AND DOWDEN, W. 1974 Periodontal Disease, Bacteria, and Pulpal Histopathology. Oral Surg, **37**, 257.

MJÖR, I. A., AND TRONSTAD, L. 1972 Experimentally Induced Pulpitis. Oral Surg, **34**, 102.

MJÖR, I. A., AND TRONSTAD, L. 1974 The Healing of Experimentally Induced Pulpitis. Oral Surg, **38**, 115.

NAIDORF, I. J. 1974 Clinical Microbiology in Endodontics. Dent Clin North Am, **18**, 329.

NAIDORF, I. J. 1977 Correlation of the Inflammatory Response with Immunopathological and Clinical Events. J Endodontol, **3**, 223.

OLIET, S. 1962 Evaluation of Culturing in Endodontic Therapy. Oral Surg, **15**, 727.

ROANE, J. B., AND MARSHALL, F. J. 1972 Osteomyelitis: A Complication of Pulpless Teeth. Oral Surg, **34**, 257.

ROBINSON, H. B. G., AND BOLING, L. R. 1941 The Anachoretic Effect in Pulpitis; I. Bacteriologic Studies. J Am Dent Assoc, **28**, 268.

ROGERS, A. H. 1976 The Oral Cavity as a Source of Potential Pathogens in Focal Infection. Oral Surg, **42**, 245.

ROSENGREN, L., AND WINBLAD, B. 1975 Periapical Destructions Caused by Experimental Pulpal Inoculation of *Streptococcus mutans* in Rats. Oral Surg, **39**, 479.

SABISTON, C. B., JR., GRIGSBY, W. R., AND SEGERSTROM, N. 1976 Bacterial Study of Pyogenic Infections of Dental Origin. Oral Surg, **41**, 430.

STABHOLZ, A., AND MCARTHUR, W. P. 1978 Cellular Immune Response of Patients with Periapical Pathosis to Necrotic Dental Pulp Antigens Determined by Release of LIF. J Endodontol, **4**, 282.

TORABINEJAD, M., AND BAKLAND, L. K. 1978 Immunopathogenesis of Chronic Periapical Lesions. Oral Surg, **46**, 685.

TRONSTAD, L., AND MJÖR, I. A. 1972 Capping of the Inflamed Pulp. Oral Surg, **34**, 477.

WEINE, F. S., HEALEY, H. J., AND THEISS, E. P. 1975 Endodontic Emergency Dilemma: Leave Tooth Open or Keep It Closed? Oral Surg, **40**, 531.

WINKLER, K. C., AND VAN AMERONGEN, J. 1959 Bacteriologic Results from 4,000 Root Canal Cultures. Oral Surg, **12**, 857.

WINKLER, T. F., MITCHELL, F. D., AND HEALEY, H. J. 1972 A Bacterial Study of Human Periapical Pathosis Employing a Modified Gram Tissue Stain. Oral Surg, **34**, 109.

WITTGOW, W. C., JR., AND SABISTON, C. E., JR. 1975 Microorganisms from Pulpal Chambers of Intact Teeth with Necrotic Pulps. J Endodontol, **1**, 168.

ZAVISTOSKI, J., DZINK, J., ONDERDONK, A., AND BARTLETT, J. 1980 Quantitative Bacteriology of Endodontic Infections. Oral Surg, **49**, 171.

PART 6

BACTERIAL INFECTIONS

---

chapter 19

Staphylococci and Staphylococcal Infections

George S. Schuster

Staphylococci are responsible for a significant portion of suppurative diseases encountered in practice. Besides causing infections of the skin they may invade and produce severe infections in other parts of the body. Three species of staphylococci are currently recognized, *Staphylococcus aureus*, *Staphylococcus epidermidis*, and *Staphylococcus saprophyticus*. Of these, *S. aureus* is the most significant pathogen for man. *S. epidermidis*, a common inhabitant of the skin and mucous membranes, may produce abscesses, while *S. saprophyticus* is generally regarded as nonpathogenic.

CELL AND COLONIAL MORPHOLOGY

Staphylococci are gram positive, facultatively anaerobic, spherical bacteria that are widely distributed in the environment and on man and animals. They range from 0.5 to 1.5 μm in diameter. They seldom form chains but more often appear as irregular grape-like clusters of cells, are nonmotile, and do not form spores (fig. 19/1). Colonial variants of the staphylococci are mucoid, smooth, and rough. Many strains of *S. aureus* freshly isolated from staphylococcal disease produce golden-yellow pigment, while the colonies of *S. epidermidis* are usually chalky or porcelain white; some staphylococcal colonies are lemon-yellow in color. However, pigment production is a variable trait of staphylococci and not reliable for differentiation.

CULTURE

Staphylococci grow well on most extract and infusion media and in sweat, urine, and tissue and plant extracts. Their metabolism is respiratory and fermentative and they utilize a wide variety of carbohydrates. Aerobically they can obtain energy and nitrogen from peptones, but anaerobically they seem to prefer glycolysis. Staphylococci grow on several differential media that restrict other microorganisms, often tolerating as much as 15% NaCl and 40% bile. Growth occurs over a wide range of temperature and pH, with optima of 30 to 37 C and pH 7.0 to 7.5, respectively.

ENZYMATIC ACTIVITY

Proteolytic Activity. Staphylococci produce enzymes that are active on fibrin (clotted blood), inspissated serum, egg white, or gelatin. Collagenase is not produced by staphylococci.

Coagulase Activity. Pathogenic staphylococci produce an extracellular staphylocoagulase that acts on citrated or oxalated rabbit or human plasma. Nonpathogenic staphylococci are unable to coagulate plasma but coagulase-negative staphylococci may be pathogenic. Staphylocoagulase clots fibrinogen in the presence of a coagulase-reacting factor (CRF), an apparent derivative of prothrombin. There are multiple antigenic types of coagulase, but there is no evidence that the antibodies are

273

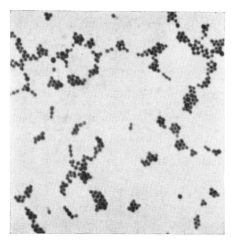

Figure 19/1. *Staphylococcus aureus.*

important in resistance to staphylococcal infections.

Staphylokinase. Most staphylococci pathogenic for man can dissolve fibrin clots from man and a variety of animals. The lytic factor is produced as a kinase which activates serum or plasma protease. The active protease then lyses the fibrin of the clot. Staphylokinase has no relationship to staphylococcal virulence.

Lipases. Both pathogenic (99%) and nonpathogenic (30%) staphylococci produce lipases (phospholipases, lipoprotein-lipases, esterases). Lipases may assist *S. epidermidis* in being a consistent resident of the skin.

Hyaluronidase. Most pathogenic staphylococci produce hyaluronidase, which breaks down hyaluronic acid in connective tissue. It has a reputation as a "spreading factor" in bacterial infections, but its importance is limited to early stages of the infection because inflammation antagonizes the spreading action.

Phosphatase. Acid phosphatase is generally produced by pathogenic staphylococci. It could be used as a reasonably reliable indicator of staphylococcal virulence.

Lysozyme. Most coagulase-positive strains produce lysozyme, but the staphylococci are not sensitive to it.

Penicillinase. Staphylococci readily become resistant to penicillin by the production of penicillinase or β-lactamase. Penicillinase inactivates penicillin by breaking its β-lactam ring.

TOXINS

The pathogenic staphylococci produce immunologically distinct toxins that are designated as alpha (α), beta (β), gamma (γ), and delta (δ). Commonly these toxins lyse erythrocytes, although they may be dermonecrotic, lethal, or leukocidic.

α-Toxin (Hemolysin). α-Toxin is a staphylococcal protein exotoxin that hemolyzes some animal erythrocytes, but not those of humans. It disrupts lysosomes and is cytotoxic for a variety of tissue culture cells, and can damage human macrophages and platelets but not monocytes. It is also dermonecrotic, lethal, causes spasm of smooth muscle, aggregates blood platelets, injures renal cortex, and causes death by ventricular fibrillation. Current evidence suggests that α-toxin acts together with other virulence factors to play a role in development of staphylococcal disease.

β-Toxin (Sphingomyelinase). Staphylococci of animal origin produce a β-toxin that lyses goat, ox, and sheep erythrocytes, but it has only a slight activity on human erythrocytes. It acts on cell membrane sphingomyelin and on lysophosphatidyl choline, is lethal for rabbits and mice, and it aggregates platelets.

β-Toxin produces hot-cold lysis of erythrocytes. When allowed to act on blood agar at 37 C, it produces only a darkened zone and no hemolysis. If the culture is refrigerated overnight, lysis of the erythrocytes occurs.

δ-Toxin. Staphylococci produce an antigenically distinct δ-toxin. It acts on phosphatidylserine but not sphingomyelin. δ-Lysin is slightly dermonecrotic and damages erythrocytes, macrophages, lymphocytes, neutrophils and platelets.

γ-Toxin. Staphylococci produce a hemolysin, termed γ-toxin. It is cytolytic for human and some animal erythrocytes: its precise mode of action is unknown. The presence of specific neutralizing antibodies in human staphylococcal bone disease suggests the possible contribution of this toxin to the disease state.

Leukocidin. The nonhemolytic Panton-Valentine (P-V) leukocidin produced by most pathogenic staphylococci attacks only macrophages and polymorphonuclear leukocytes. It produces a primary effect of altered permeability to cations. Other changes are secondary to this event. Although the leukocidin alone is not responsible for the pathogenicity of the staphylococci, it protects the organisms from host leukocytes.

Exfoliative Toxin (Epidermolytic Toxin). Strains of staphylococci belonging to phage group II are etiologic agents of a spectrum of dermatologic conditions that are termed staphylococcal scalded-skin syndrome. The causative strains of staphylococci produce an exotoxin, exfoliative toxin, that is responsible for the clinical manifestations of this condition. There is an intraepidermal cleavage plane at the stratum granulosum inducing intraepidermal separation. This results in severe exfoliation characteristic of these diseases.

Enterotoxin Action. Some coagulase-positive staphylococci produce heat-resistant, diffusible enterotoxins that are a common cause of food poisoning in man and have been implicated in enterocolitis seen in patients following antibiotic therapy. Such enterotoxins are produced in foods contaminated with toxogenic staphylococci. Food poisoning, which is an intoxication, occurs when the preformed toxins are ingested in such foods. The mechanism of action of the enterotoxins is unknown. The diarrhea has been attributed to inhibited water absorption and increased fluid flux into the lumen. The receptor for the emetic effect is the abdominal viscera from which sitc thc stimulus reaches the vomiting center via vagus and sympathetic nerves.

ANTIGENIC STRUCTURE

Polysaccharides A and B. Staphylococci contain two phosphorus-containing polysaccharide antigens, designated A and B. The serologic determinants of both are techoic acids, but of differing composition. Polysaccharide A is found in the cell wall of *S. aureus*, while polysaccharide B is present in the cell wall of *S. epidermidis*.

Protein A. Most strains of *S. aureus* possess a surface protein that is designated as protein A. It is a group-specific antigen present only in *S. aureus*. Protein A elicits a hypersensitivity reaction in guinea pigs and rabbits. It precipitates normal γ-globulin and is antiphagocytic, anticomplementary, and elicits platelet injury.

Capsular Antigens. Mucoid strains of staphylococci produce capsular antigens. One antigen is a polypeptide. Another capsular antigen, a polymer of glucuronic acid, is antiphagocytic.

BACTERIOPHAGE TYPING

While some 30 type-specific agglutinogens have been identified, serological typing of staphylococci has not been useful in epidemiological studies.

A better method of typing coagulase-positive *S. aureus* is by determining the patterns of sensitivity shown by the various strains to bacteriophages. The phage patterns of the strains fall essentially into four large groups. Phage typing is particularly useful in epidemiological studies, but it is not used for classifying staphylococci. The correlation of phage types with other properties of staphylococci has not been precise.

GENETIC VARIATION

Genetic variation occurs readily in staphylococci. Loss of pigment is common and may occur independently of coagulase production. Staphylococci commonly undergo smooth-rough dissociation and loss of capsule. They mutate reversibly to form minute G colonies whose cells are relatively avirulent. Other variations include changes in suscepti-

bility to bacteriophages, hemolytic abilities, toxin formation, and coagulase formation.

The development of resistance to drugs and antibiotics, both *in vivo* and *in vitro*, is a most important variation of staphylococci. Most antibiotic resistance appears to be plasmid-mediated. Penicillin resistance is accomplished by the production of penicillinase. Staphylococci may become resistant to "synthetic" penicillins that are not susceptible to penicillinase by means of lysogenic conversion. The facility with which the staphylococci become resistant to one or more antibiotics greatly complicates patient care in hospitals.

STAPHYLOCOCCAL INFECTIONS

Staphylococci cause a wide variety of diseases in man (boils, abscesses, furuncles, pyemia, meningitis, osteomyelitis, infection of wounds, and food poisoning). Such infections depend on type, number, and route of introduction of the organisms, their toxic products, and previous exposure to staphylococci. In the human host, mediating factors are trauma, general health, nutritional status of the individual, toxemias, allergic reactions, and uncontrolled diabetes. Locally, mediating factors are changes in the capillary bed, the biochemical environment, and the inflammatory response.

Skin Infections. Skin, the most common site of staphylococcal infection, is affected by furuncles, boils, carbuncles, complication of wounds, paronychia, and the generalized skin infection known as impetigo (figs. 19/2–19/4). The furuncle is a circumscribed area of swelling that softens in the center and discharges pus. With a carbuncle the ulcera-

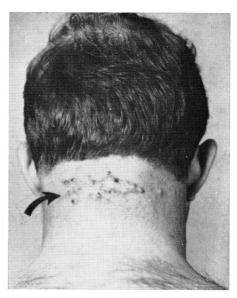

Figure 19/2. Chronic furunculosis, folliculitis, and keloidosis due to staphylococcal infection. (AFIP 53-12335.)

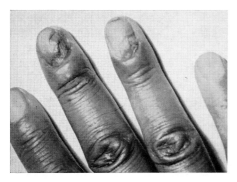

Figure 19/3. Chronic staphylococcal paronychia. (AFIP 58-13966-13.)

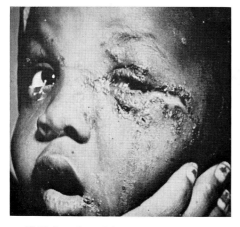

Figure 19/4. Impetigo of the face and lips due to staphylococci. (AFIP 13966-6.)

tions are deep and involve wide areas of the skin, and it is accompanied by fever and general malaise. Septicemias sometimes develop from severe carbuncles and may result in production of metastatic abscesses throughout the body. Infections of the upper lip and nose are particularly dangerous, for staphylococci can easily invade the regional veins, causing cavernous sinus thrombosis, septicemia, and death.

In acne, staphylococci, together with diphtheroid bacilli, complicate and aggravate the changes that occur in the skin, and together they mediate the persistence and severity of the lesions.

It has recently been shown that *Staphylococcus aureus* is a significant cause of angular cheilitis, an eroded and erythematous nonvesicular lesion radiating from the angle of the mouth. The staphylococcal disease often can be recognized by a yellow crust. *S. aureus* may be the sole infecting agent, or act in combination with streptococci or *Candida albicans*.

Coagulase-positive staphylococci of phage group II produce exfoliative toxin that has been associated

with a dermatitis characterized by intraepidermal separation known as Ritter's disease in newborn infants and as toxic epidermal necrolysis in older individuals. In addition, these staphylococci may produce a scarlatiniform eruption. These diseases, together with bullous impetigo, have been termed staphylococcal scalded skin syndrome because of their resemblance to skin lesions produced by scalding. The syndrome usually is seen in infants and young children. The exfoliative disease generally presents with tenderness of the skin and abrupt onset of a diffuse erythema over most of the body. Mild edema of the face may be seen. Within a day or two the upper layers of epidermis appear wrinkled or have peeled off, producing the Nikolsky sign. There may be appearance of flacid, fluid-filled bullae followed by separation of the epithelium leaving a moist, red, glistening surface. The exfoliated areas then dry yielding large flakes. The secondary desquamation may last 3 to 5 days. Exfoliative lesions on the face and mucous membranes of the oral cavity, lips and pharynx may be present. In addition, there may be purulent lip lesions and fissures about the mouth.

Staphylococci may produce a scalatiniform rash with skin tenderness but without significant exfoliation. It resembles that produced by streptococci but there is no palatal exanthema or strawberry tongue. It resolves differently also. After 1 or 2 days of erythema, cracks appear in the creases of the skin particularly around the eyes and mouth. After a few days epidermal flakes desquamate, revealing healing skin beneath. In all cases, the individuals are febrile, irritable and anorectic during the exofoliative stage of disease.

Osteomyelitis. Staphylococci are commonly involved in osteomyelitis. They enter the bloodstream from a cutaneous lesion and are carried to one of the long bones where an abscess develops, causing tenderness and pain. Staphylococcal osteomyelitis is often chronic, with periods of regression and renewed activity continuing for years.

Respiratory Infections. Staphylococcal infections of the lower respiratory tract range from chronic bronchitis to acute bronchopneumonia. Staphylococcal infections of the lower respiratory tract occur more often in influenza epidemics, at which time they may reach epidemic proportions. Staphylococcal pneumonia is particularly serious because of the tendency of the organism to produce abscesses and parenchymal destruction. Staphylococcal pneumonia is also likely to occur in young children, debilitated individuals, and hospitalized individuals taking antibiotics.

Food Poisoning. Some strains of *S. aureus* produce an enterotoxin when they grow in foods held for some hours at a warm temperature. The foods appear normal in odor, taste and appearance but when such food is eaten, vomiting, diarrhea, and prostration result within 1 to 6 hours, and last for several hours. Recovery is usually complete within a day or two.

Enterocolitis. Broad spectrum antibiotic therapy may upset the intestinal microbiota sufficiently for drug resistant staphylococci to become the predominant intestinal bacteria, causing an enterocolitis. The manifestations include cramps, fever, diarrhea, dehydration, and electrolyte imbalance.

Hospital Infections. Staphylococcal infections in hospitals are of considerable concern because of their severity and incidence. Hospital patients and personnel are the principal reservoirs of the causative staphylococci. Of all microorganisms encountered in hospitals, staphylococci are most likely to cause wound infections. Other staphylococcal hospital infections involve burns, bronchopneumonia, bacteremia (*e.g.*, from a cellulitis arising from venipuncture or intravenous catheters), diarrhea, and enterocolitis. Even at best, all aseptic precautions, as well as sterilization and filtration of the air in the hospital environment, can do no more than reduce the numbers of staphylococci to a noncritical point. Prophylactic treatment of the staff to reduce the staphylococci in the hospital environment is a doubtful control measure.

PATHOGENESIS

The pathogenesis of staphylococcal disease relates to resistance to phagocytosis, to the action of several staphylococcal enzymes, to the development of delayed hypersensitivity and to the activities of the toxins. Man is constantly exposed to staphylococci from birth until death. Even so, the most virulent staphylococci seldom cause serious infections in a human host unless resistance is drastically lowered by such things as severe burns, trauma or surgery.

An important factor is the resistance of the virulent *S. aureus* to phagocytosis. The nature of the antiphagocytic action relates mostly to the *in vivo* formation of a capsule. Very few virulent staphylococci produce a detectable capsule *in vitro*, but anticapsular antibodies are present in most adults and particularly in those who have recently had a staphylococcal infection. Staphylococcal protein A may also be antiphagocytic.

In spite of its role as an indicator of staphylococcal virulence, coagulase seems to have only a coincidental relationship to pathogenesis. A coagulase-negative mutant of a virulent, coagulase-positive staphylococcus is just as virulent as the original staphylococcus. The mutant is able to elicit a lesion, surrounded by a fibrin barrier, that is identical with that produced by the coagulase-positive strain.

Staphylococcal lipase seems to relate to the production of boils and carbuncles. Lipase-positive staphylococci predominate in skin infections and they seldom escape from the localized lesion.

α-Toxin is likely involved in the pathogenesis of staphylococcal infection through its hemolytic, dermonecrotic, leukocidal, and lethal actions. Leukocidins other than α-toxin, also contribute to the pathogenesis of staphylococcal infections.

Delayed hypersensitivity is also a factor in the pathogenesis of staphylococcal infections. Repeated bouts of staphylococcal infections in experimental animals increase the severity of their skin lesions.

The enteritis caused by staphylococci is essentially a toxemia resulting from the ingestion of the enterotoxin released by staphylococci growing in contaminated food. Similarly exfoliative skin disease is a result of the production and dissemination of a soluble toxin.

IMMUNITY

The more severe systemic staphylococcal infections induce both antibacterial and antitoxic antibodies and a moderate degree of immunity develops in response to such infections. This produces two types of immunity. One type increases the rate at which staphylococci are cleared from the bloodstream. The other type, apparently antitoxic, decreases the severity of local lesions.

LABORATORY DIAGNOSIS

The laboratory diagnosis of staphylococcal infections involves their detection in purulent exudates and their culture on blood agar. Smears of purulent exudate are stained with gram stains. The detection of gram positive cocci, not in chains, in such smears is presumptive of a staphylococcal infection. Blood agar is most useful in cultural diagnosis. Selective media which are useful for the detection of staphylococci in heavily contaminated specimens are tellurite glycine agar, phenylethyl agar, or media containing 7.5% sodium chloride. The virulence of an isolated colony can be established by demonstration of coagulase production. Enterotoxin in suspected food is demonstrated by immunological tests.

TREATMENT

Staphylococci are sensitive to penicillin, macrolide antibiotics, novobiocin, chloramphenicol, and tetracyclines. Nevertheless, staphylococci infections pose many problems in treatment. Because of the prevalence of antibiotic resistant staphylococci, especially in hospital populations, and the ability of any of the pathogenic staphylococci to rapidly develop resistance to one or more antibiotics during treatment, it is essential that drug sensitivity of the infecting staphylococcus be established as soon as possible. Whatever the antibiotic used in treatment, the establishment of adequate drainage greatly facilitates treatment.

EPIDEMIOLOGY AND CONTROL

Man is the principal reservoir of pathogenic staphylococci. Most infants become carriers soon after birth, and while the number of carriers fluctuates during the first few years of life, 50 to 60% of adults are continual or intermittent carriers. The anterior nares are the primary nidus for pathogenic staphylococci in the human body, but the skin is the residence of the other staphylococci. In hospitals, many of the personnel are nasal carriers of pathogenic and often antibiotic-resistant staphylococci. Such carriers widely dispense their staphylococci. The exclusion of nasal carriers from operating rooms, surgical wards, the burn ward, and infants wards and nurseries certainly lowers the rate of staphylococcal infection in hospitals. In addition, all surgical procedures and instrumentation should be performed with close attention to aseptic techniques.

ADDITIONAL READING

BADDOUR, H. M., DURST, N. L., AND TILSON, H. B. 1979 Frontal Lobe Abscess of Dental Origin. Oral Surg, **47,** 303.

BAUGHN, R. E., AND BONVENTRE, P. F. 1975 Phagocytosis and Intracellular Killing of *Staphylococcus aureus* by Normal Mouse Peritoneal Macrophages. Infect Immun, **12,** 346.

CERUTE, E., CONTRERAS, J., AND NEIRA, M. 1971 Staphylococcal Pneumonia in Childhood. Am J Dis Child, **22,** 386.

DOIG, C. M. 1971 Nasal Carriage of *Staphylococcus aureus* in a General Surgical Unit. Br J Surg, **58,** 113.

FACKLAM, R. R., AND SMITH, P. B. 1976 The Gram Positive Cocci. Hum Pathol, **7,** 187.

FADEN, H. S., BURKE, J. P., GLASGOW, L. A., AND EVERETT, J. R., III. 1976 Nursery Outbreak of Scalded-Skin Syndrome. Scarlatiniform Rash Due to Phage Group I *Staphylococcus aureus.* Am J Dis Child, **130,** 265.

HAMBRAEUS, A. 1973 Dispersal and Transfer of *Staphylococcus aureus* in an Isolation Ward for Burned Patients. J Hyg, **71,** 787.

HARRIS, D. M. 1973 Staphylococcal Infection in an Intensive Care Unit and Its Relation to Infection in the Remainder of the Hospital. J Hyg, **71,** 341.

HARTMAN, A. A. 1978 Staphylococci of the Normal Human Skin Flora. Arch Dermatol Res, **261,** 295.

JELJASZEWICZ, J. (Ed.) Staphylococci and Staphylococcal Disease. In *Proceedings of III International Sympo-* *sium on Staphylococci and Staphylococcal Infections.* New York, Gustav Fischer-Verlag, 1976.

KLOOS, W. E., AND SCHLEIFER, K. H. 1975 Simplified Scheme for Routine Identification of Human *Staphylococcus* Species. J Clin Microbiol, **1,** 82.

LACEY, R. W. 1975 Antibiotic Resistance Plasmids of *Staphylococcus aureus* and Their Clinical Importance. Bacteriol Rev, **39,** 1.

LACEY, R. W., AND STOKES, A. 1977 Susceptibility of the "Penicillinase-resistant" Penicillin and Cephalosporin to Penicillinase of *Staphylococcus aureus.* J Clin Pathol, **30,** 35.

MANNERS, B. T. B., GROB, P. R., BEYNON, G. P. J., AND GIBBS, F. J. 1976 An Investigation of Antibiotic Resistance of *Staphylococcus aureus* in General Practice. Practitioner, **216,** 439.

MEDOFF, G. 1975 Current Concepts in the Treatment of Osteomyelitis. Postgrad Med, **58,** 157.

MELISH, M., AND GLASGOW, L. A. 1971 Staphylococcal Scalded-Skin Syndrome: The Expanded Clinical Syndrome. J Pediatr, **78,** 958.

MILLER, T. E. 1974 *Staphylococcus epidermidis* as a Cause of Liver Abscess: A Case Report. NZ Med J, **79,** 692.

MINSHEW, B. H., AND ROSENBLUM, E. D. 1972 Transduction of Tetracycline Resistance in *Staphylococcus epidermidis.* Antimicrob Agents Chemother, **1,** 508.

MUDD, S. 1972 Resistance against *Staphylococcus aureus.* JAMA, **218,** 1671.

NELSON, K. E., BISNO, A. L., WAYTZ, P., BRUNT, J., MOSES, V. K., AND HAQUE, R. U. 1976 The Epidemiology and Natural History of Streptococcal Pyoderma: An Endemic Disease of the Rural Southern United States. Am J Epidemiol, **103,** 270.

NOBLE, W. C. 1977 Variation in the Prevalence of Antibiotic Resistance of *Staphylococcus aureus* from Human Skin and Nares. J Gen Microbiol, **98,** 125.

NOLAN, C. M., AND BEATY, H. N. 1976 *Staphylococcus aureus* Bacteremia. Am J Med, **60,** 495.

NYSTRÖM, B., AND MOLIN, L. 1972 Colonization with Staphylococci in Dermatology Wards with Different Designs and Practices. Br J Dermatol, **86** (Suppl 8), 21.

OSSOFF, R., AND GIUNTA, J. L. 1975 The Staphylococcal Scalded-Skin Syndrome versus Erythema Multiforme. Oral Surg, **40,** 126.

ROGOLSKY, M. 1979 Nonenteric Toxins of *Staphylococcus aureus.* Microbiol Rev, **43,** 320.

SABATH, L. D., WHEELER, N., LAVERDIERE, M., BLAZEVIC, D., AND WILKINSON, B. I. 1977 A New Type of Penicillin Resistance of *Staphylococcus aureus.* Lancet, **1,** 443.

VAN DER VIJVER, J. C. M., VAN ES-BOON, M. M., AND MICHEL, M. F. 1975 A Study of Virulence Factors with Induced Mutants of *Staphylococcus aureus.* J Med Microbiol, **8,** 279.

VERHOEF, J., AND VERBRUGH, H. A. 1981 Host Determinants in Staphylococcal Disease. Ann Rev Med, **32,** 107.

WISE, R. I. 1973 Modern Management of Severe Staphylococcal Disease. Medicine (Baltimore), **52,** 295.

WISEMAN, G. M. 1976 The Hemolysins of *Staphylococcus aureus.* Bacteriol Rev, **39,** 317.

chapter 20

Streptococci and Streptococcal Infections

George S. Schuster

STREPTOCOCCAL GROUPS

Streptococci are a group of spherical or ovoid, generally nonmotile, nonsporing, gram positive bacteria that may occur either singly, in pairs, in short chains, and in chains of 8 to 10 cocci when grown in appropriate media (fig. 20/1). The cells average 1 μm and are less than 2 μm in diameter. Capsules are difficult to demonstrate in other than *Streptococcus pneumoniae*, but occur in young cultures of many strains. Some capsules are polysaccharides, especially *S. pneumoniae*, while others are hyaluronic acid.

Classification by Hemolytic Action. By their hemolytic action on whole blood in an agar medium streptococci can be divided into:

1. Alpha (α)-hemolytic streptococci, which cause an inner zone of green discoloration and an outer zone of complete hemolysis. Such streptococci are also called the viridans group after the Latin, *viridis*, for green. *Streptococcus salivarius* is the most common α-hemolytic streptococcus.

2. Beta (β)-hemolytic streptococci, which produce a clear zone of complete hemolysis about the colony (fig. 20/2). The most common β-hemolytic streptococcus is *Streptococcus pyogenes*. However, some of the streptococci assigned to the β-hemolytic and immunologically related groups that are actually nonhemolytic include some members of Lancefield groups B, C, D, H, K, and O. All of group N are nonhemolytic.

3. Gamma (γ)-hemolytic streptococci produce no hemolysis on or in the medium. The most common γ-hemolytic streptococcus is *Streptococcus faecalis*.

Immunological Classification. Streptococci that produce a group-specific carbohydrate (C substance) were divided after 1930 into 13 groups, designated by the letters A through O. Type antigens of the species, the diseases produced, and the primary habitats of these groups are shown in table 20/1.

Anaerobic streptococci are generally nonhemolytic, but they are not grouped with the γ-hemolytic streptococci. They have been placed in a separate genus, *Peptostreptococcus*.

MORPHOLOGY OF GROUP A STREPTOCOCCI

β-Hemolytic, group A streptococci are gram positive cocci that form long chains *in vitro*, especially in an unfavorable environment such as unsuitable media. In tissues they form diplococci or occur singly.

The colonial forms of β-hemolytic streptococci are mucoid, matt, and glossy. Mucoid colonies are formed by streptococci that produce hyaluronic acid capsules. Matt colonies appear to be dried-out mucoid colonies. Small, glossy colonies are formed by streptococci that do not produce or retain a hyaluronic acid capsule. Group A streptococci also form L forms and protoplasts.

STREPTOCOCCAL METABOLISM

Facultatively anaerobic streptococci, when grown either aerobically or anaerobically, ferment carbohydrates, particularly glucose, forming lactic as well as formic and acetic acids and ethanol. They can be grown on complicated synthetic media. They grow well on beef-infusion or other common media if it contains blood or serum. Potassium tellurite selectively permits the grown of nonhemolytic streptococci by inhibiting other bacteria; crystal violet (1:25,000) and sodium azide (1:1,000) inhibit most of the oral and respiratory microbial flora, permitting the growth of streptococci.

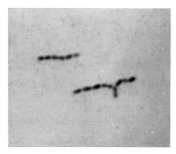

Figure 20/1. Cellular form of streptococci.

ANTIGENIC STRUCTURE OF STREPTOCOCCI

The antigenic components of group A streptococci and some of their characteristics are shown in table 20/2. The principal streptococcal antigens are hyaluronic acid, group-specific C antigens, type-specific M antigen, T antigens, R antigens, P antigens, glycerol teichoic acids, mucopeptide, and antigens of the cytoplasmic membrane.

Hyaluronic Acid. Group A streptococci produce hyaluronic acid that is nonimmunogenic probably because it is indistinguishable from the hyaluronate of ground substance. It is somewhat labile and readily diffuses away from the streptococcal cell. It is an important antiphagocytic factor.

Group-specific C Antigen. Hemolytic streptococci produce specific somatic antigenic polysaccharides, designated by the letter "C," that are utilized to divide the β-hemolytic streptococci into 13 groups, designated as A through O. C antigen is a component of the cell wall, making up about 10% of the dry weight of the organism. In the case of groups A and C the antigen is composed of rhamnose and hexosamine. Its specificity depends mainly on the nature of the terminal sugar of the rhamnose side chain. It is not related to the development of streptococcal immunity.

Type-specific M Antigens. Group A streptococci are divided into some 55 immunological types by cell wall protein antigens, designated M. Division is usually accomplished by precipitin tests although other immunological reactions can be used. M protein is attached to fimbriae on the cell surface and is readily accessible to anti-M antibodies. Such antibodies are protective. M proteins also are antiphagocytic.

Other Streptococcal Antigens. There are a number of other streptococcal antigens, none of which is particularly related to virulence. Streptococcal T antigens are several immunologically distinct proteins that are resistant to proteolytic enzymes. T antigens are not related to virulence and their specific antibodies do not offer protection against streptococcal infection. R proteins, two of

which are immunologically distinct, are present in streptococci as surface antigens. P, or nucleoprotein, antigen is present in both hemolytic and nonhemolytic streptococci in which it is antigenically similar. Glyceroltechoic acid is a group-specific antigen for groups D and N. A glycosaminoglycan is present in streptococci that is somewhat similar antigenically to that of other bacteria. It causes reactions in humans similar to those produced by the endotoxin of gram negative bacteria.

EXTRACELLULAR TOXINS AND ENZYMES

Immunoelectrophoretic analysis indicates that there are at least 20 extracellular antigens which are released when streptococci grow in human tissue. These substances include streptokinases, deoxyribonucleases (DNAses) or streptodornase, streptolysins S and O, erythrogenic toxin, proteinases, hyaluronidase, diphosphopyridine nucleotidase, amylase, and esterase. All but streptolysin S, amylase, and esterase are immunogenic.

Streptokinases. Streptococci rapidly lyse fibrin clots of normal human blood by an agent that was found to be a kinase and was named streptokinase. It is an activator of plasminogen in serum, converting it into plasmin. Streptokinase can be divided into two types, designated A and B. Streptokinases are produced by some strains of the groups A, C, G, and a few streptococci of B and F groups, as well as by some staphylococci and clostridia.

Deoxyribonucleases. Group A and some group C streptococci produce DNAses that are specifically active against highly viscous, extracellular DNA of purulent exudates. They do not penetrate into cells and have no action on intracellular DNA of living cells.

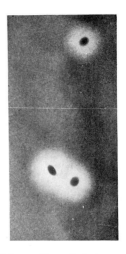

Figure 20/2. β-type of hemolysis by appropriate streptococci growing in rabbit's blood agar.

Table 20/1
Immunological groups of streptococci and their usual habitats

Group Antigen Designation	Type Antigen Designation	Chemical Nature Type Antigen	Species Designation	Location Type Antigen	Principal Type of Infection	Usual Habitat
A	M, R, T	Protein	S. pyogenes	Envelope	Acute pharyngitis, pneumonia, peritonitis, meningitis, peritonsillar abscesses, mastoiditis, otitis media, cervical adenitis, scarlet fever, rheumatic fever, acute nephritis, puerperal fever, erysipelas, acute hemorrhagic glomerulonephritis	Man
B	S(5 types)	Polysaccharide	S. agalactiae	Envelope	Mastitis	Cattle
C	(8 types)	Protein	S. equisimilis		Strangles and other animal diseases and human respiratory disease	Horse, man, lower animals
C	(8 types)	Protein	S. zooepidemicus			
C	(1 type)	Protein	S. equinus			
C	(3 types)	Protein	S. dysgalactiae			
D	(11 types)	Polysaccharide	S. faecalis	Cell wall	Human infection (urinary and wound) and food poisoning	Man, animals, dairy products
D	(19 types)		S. faecium			
D			S. avium			
D	(many types)	Carbohydrate	S. bovis	Capsule		
D	(1 type)	Carbohydrate	S. equinus	Capsule		
D			S. suis			
E	I-V	Polysaccharide	Streptococcus spp.		Pharyngeal abscess in swine	Milk, swine
F	I-V	Carbohydrate	S. anginosus		Occasional human infection	Man
G	(3 types)	Carbohydrates	Streptococcus spp.		Human and dog infection	Man, dog
H	(5 types)		S. sanguis		Occasional human infection	Man
K	I, II	Carbohydrates	S. salivarius		Occasional human infection	Man
L					Dog respiratory infection	Dog
M					Occasional dog infection	Dog
N					None	Milk, cream
O	(many types)				Occasional human respiratory tract infections, endocarditis	Man
None	(80 types)	Carbohydrates	S. pneumoniae	Capsule	Pneumonia	Man

Table 20/2

Cellular constituents of group A streptococci involved in antigenicity and virulence[a]

Constituent	Serological Reactions	Chemical Composition	Certain Distinctive Properties
C	Group-specific	Polysaccharide	Structural component of cell wall; composed of N-acetylglucosamine and rhamnose
M	Type-specific	Protein	Alcohol soluble; resistant to heart at pH 2; destroyed by proteolytic enzymes; important factor in virulence; M antibodies confer protection
T	Usually common to several types; occasionally type-specific	Protein	Resistant to proteolytic enzymes; destroyed by heating at pH 2; resists heating at slightly alkaline reactions
R	Occurs in type 28 strains and in certain strains of groups A, B, C, and G	Protein	Resistant to proteolytic enzymes except pepsin; destroyed by heating at pH 2; resists heating at alkaline reactions
Mucoid capsular substance	Nonantigenic	Hyaluronic acid	Occurs in groups A and C streptococci and animal tissues. Composed of N-acetylglucosamine and glucuronic acid; depolymerized by hyaluronidase (probably two enzymes involved; some relation to virulence)

[a] From R. C. Lancefield: Cellular Constitutents of Group A Streptococci Concerned in Antigenicity and Virulence. In *Streptococcal Infections*, Chapter 1, p. 3, edited by M. McCarty. Columbia University Press, New York, 1954.

Soluble Hemolysins. Group A streptococci and a few of group G and C of human origin produce distinct soluble hemolysins, O and S, which injure the cell membranes of erythrocytes and some tissue cells.

O hemolysin is an oxygen-labile, antigenic protein that is lethal for many laboratory animals, and is cardiotoxic for some. Its hemolytic activity can be neutralized by specific antibodies.

S hemolysin is bound to bacterial cells but it can be extracted with serum. It is not antigenic, is not sensitive to oxygen, but it is inhibited by serum lipoproteins. It causes contraction of smooth muscle, and is lethal for mice or rabbits. It is an important leukotoxic factor. Once streptococci are phagocytized their leukotoxic factor acts on the leukocyte's cytoplasmic granules, releasing potent hydrolytic enzymes that cause irreversible damage, death, and disintegration of leukocytes. In turn, hydrolytic enzymes released from the disintegrated leukocytes damage host tissues.

Erythrogenic Toxins. Group A and some strains of C and G groups produce soluble erythrogenic toxins that cause the rash in scarlet fever and elicit headache, fever, and vomiting. Such toxigenic strains are lysogenic. The erythrogenic toxins can be used to determine susceptibility or resistance to scarlet fever by the Dick test, in which erythrogenic toxin is injected intracutaneously. If an erythematous area, 10 to 30 mm in diameter, develops within 6 to 24 hours, the individual is susceptible to the toxin. If antitoxin to the erythrogenic toxin is injected into the erythematous skin of a suspected case, local blanching indicates that the individual

has scarlet fever. The blanching phenomenon is known as the Schultz-Charlton reaction.

Proteinase. Some streptococci produce proteinases (or a proteinase) that hydrolyze gelatin, cooked meat, casein, M protein, streptokinase, hyaluronidase, and human γ-globulin. The proteinase that is active against M antigen reduces the immunogenicity of M antigen and interferes with streptokinase production or inactivates it. Immunization with proteinases affords no protection against streptococcal infection.

Hyaluronidase. Some streptococci produce hyaluronidase, an enzyme which breaks down hyaluronic acid and has been thought to facilitate spread of streptococcal infections through tissues or interfere with localization of organisms in tissue. However, hyaluronidase is not essential to virulence, for some pathogenic group A streptococci do not produce it. The enzyme may remove the capsules of group A streptococci, increasing their susceptibility to phagocytosis.

DPNase. Most streptococci that are nephritogenic produce diphosphopyridine nucleotidase (DPNase), also termed nicotinamide adenine dinucleotidase (NADase), which releases nicotinamide from NAD. NADase has no proven relation to the pathogenesis of streptococcal infections.

Genotypic Variations. Streptococci undergo a smooth (mucoid) to rough (glossy) colonial variation, concurrent with the loss of capsules and virulence. Subcultured mucoid colonies lose capsules and emerge as glossy colonies. These will revert to a mucoid type by repeated animal passage. M protein, a virulence related cell wall component, may be lost from strains carried in the throat after an attack of streptococcal pharyngitis. Repeated animal passage will restore this component to the cell.

Hemolytic streptococci readily develop resistance to sulfonamides but not to penicillin, even after long clinical use. Streptococci that develop antibiotic resistance *in vitro* lose some of their virulence.

Streptococci also vary in hemolysin production and in their capacity to form cell wall antigens other than M protein.

STREPTOCOCCAL DISEASES

Streptococci cause both suppurative diseases and nonsuppurative sequelae-type diseases. Suppurative diseases include pharyngitis, either accompanied or not accompanied by scarlet fever; cervical adenitis; otitis media, mastoiditis; peritonsillar abscesses; meningitis; peritonitis; pneumonia; puerperal sepsis; cellulitis of skin and mucous membranes; impetigo contagiosa; and erysipelas. The principal nonsuppurative sequelae are acute glomerulonephritis, rheumatic fever, and erythema nodosum.

Pathogenesis and Pathology of Streptococcal Diseases. The source of pyogenic streptococci is principally the human carrier. A streptococcal infection requires transmission of virulent, antiphagocytic streptococci to a susceptible host. The antiphagocytic properties relate to presence of M protein and a capsule. The nature of the lesion and clinical manifestations also relate to the previous experience of the host with streptococci and streptococcal diseases.

The usual streptococcal infection in children from birth to about 12 years of age is an acute, purulent pharyngitis. This may be associated with various gradations of a syndrome composed of sore throat, fever, chills, headache, nausea, and vomiting. Such infections may be followed by complications such as rheumatic fever, scarlet fever, infection of tissues or organs adjacent to the pharynx (cervical adenitis, otitis media, mastoiditis, peritonsillar abscesses), and more generalized infections such as meningitis, peritonitis, and pneumonia. Nonsuppurative sequelae such as acute glomerulonephritis, rheumatic fever, and erythema nodosum also may result.

Pharyngitis and Tonsillitis. Group A β-hemolytic streptococci often cause pharyngitis and tonsillitis. Acute pharyngitis generally has a sudden onset with redness in the tonsillar area and on the mucous membranes of the pharynx and palate. Petechiae frequently appear on the soft palate, and in some patients elevated areas consisting of a normal colored center surrounded by an erythematous border may be present on the palate. The

mucous membranes and uvula often are edematous. The patients often have enlarged cervical lymph nodes that are sore to the touch and other regional lymph nodes may be involved. Group A streptococci can readily be isolated from the mucosa in these patients.

Scarlet Fever. Scarlet fever, a highly contagious disease of childhood has an incubation period of several days to a week. Onset is marked by a sore throat, fever, and vomiting, and in the early phase the cheeks become reddened. The throat becomes red and an exudate commonly develops. Within several days a rash appears, first on the trunk then on the limbs and face. In the latter instance the chin, nose and lips are not involved. The oral mucosa often develops an enanthema that appears earlier and is more marked than the skin reactions. The mucosa is congested and red punctate mottling is present on the hard palate. The palate and uvula are frequently edematous and the latter structure may become elongated, inducing coughing and regurgitation of fluids.

The tongue is also involved in scarlet fever. At first it has a milky white or gray appearance. The fungiform papillae become enlarged and swollen, projecting through the coat to appear as reddish protuberances, producing the so-called strawberry tongue. The tongue lesions subside after a time, followed by desquamation beginning at the tip and sides. The tongue eventually returns to normal size and appearance. Ulcerative glossitis also has been reported, as have other oral complications of scarlet fever.

Erysipelas. Erysipelas is an acute febrile disease that occurs most commonly in the elderly, although newborn infants are susceptible. It consists of an inflammatory reaction followed by invasion of the lymphatics by hemolytic streptococci, usually of group A. A minor lesion or abrasion often provides the initial entry site. However, this lesion often has healed by the end of the 3- to 7-day incubation period so the initial portal is not evident. At the outset the skin around the initial site becomes red and swollen but as the infection spreads outward the central point tends to clear. Organisms are found only toward the margins of the lesion and they may be readily isolated by excision of tissue. Although erysipelas may develop on any part of the body surface, the face is the most common site. It may extend into the mucous membranes or, infrequently, originate in these tissues, particularly those of the pharynx or nose.

Facial erysipelas begins abruptly with a short period of malaise, headache, fever, and vomiting. After a few hours a local itching or burning sensation occurs at the affected area. Skin lesions appear around the nose or mouth as irregular, bright red, slightly raised areas. Lymphadenitis is a character-

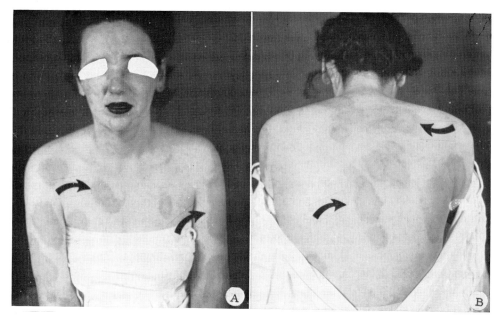

Figure 20/3. Erysipelas caused by streptococci. (AFIP 58-6180.)

istic feature as the submaxillary lymph nodes become enlarged. If untreated, the disease spreads at the periphery, extending over the face to produce a butterfly pattern (fig. 20/3). Due to the swelling, the lips become thick, the eyelids may become swollen and the nose broadens, producing facial distortion. As the disease progresses a toxemia occurs accompanied by fever and restlessness.

Erysipelas occasionally extends from the facial skin into the oral cavity producing redness, pain and swelling of the tongue. Infection initiating in the upper respiratory tract results in pain in the throat, submaxillary lymphadenitis, and possible edema of the uvula and epiglottis. Although it may be fatal, erysipelas usually resolves after several days, leaving a dry desquamating skin.

Sequelae-type Diseases. Acute glomerulonephritis, caused by only a few strains of streptococci, is preceded by an acute purulent infection of the pharynx or skin. The disease is believed to have an autoimmune component in which antigens of certain streptococcal strains trigger an autoimmune mechanism that induces antibodies to cross react with glomerular basement membrane. There also appears to be a reaction to an immune complex. These produce the characteristic symptoms of hematuria, edema, and hypertension about a week after onset of the acute pyogenic infection.

Rheumatic fever is also a sequelae-type disease caused by streptococci. It develops 2 or 3 weeks after an acute pharyngeal infection in about 3% of patients involved in streptococcal epidemics. Such individuals have a higher antibody titer than pa-

tients who do not develop rheumatic disease, but it is not clear how immunological reactions to streptococcal products produce the recurring joint, cardiac, and skin lesions characteristic of this illness. Rheumatic fever patients may develop an eruption of the throat and mouth. The lesions appear as dark red spots of variable size, up to 2 mm in diameter, most often on the buccal mucosa, soft palate, sides of the tongue, and uvula.

Erythema nodosum is associated with diseases such as tuberculosis or coccidioidomycosis, and probably with streptococcal infections. It has been produced experimentally in rabbits in a form that may resemble the human disease. The toxic factor appears to be the peptidoglycan component of streptococcal cell walls.

Immunity. Only anti-M antibodies protect significantly against streptococcal infections. Detectable anti-M antibodies develop after several weeks to months and may persist for years. There are at least 55 serological types in the group A streptococci, and it is likely that no single individual ever becomes immune to all streptococcal types. Since only a few streptococci cause acute glomerulonephritis, a single infection decreases the chances of a recurring infection. Most group A streptococci can produce rheumatic fever, however, so that even multiple attacks do not greatly decrease the chances of subsequent rheumatic fever attacks. There are at least three immunologic groups of the erythrogenic toxin associated with scarlet fever. The presence of antibodies to one type will protect against infection with only that type. Recurrences of scarlet fever do occur with the other antigenic types.

Laboratory Diagnosis. Laboratory diagnosis of streptococcal infections requires culture and isolation, a description of cell and colonial morphology and action on blood. Diagnosis may also be reinforced by group A being more susceptible to bacitracin than are other groups. Serological reactions (complement fixation, agglutination) have been widely used in identification, but are not too reliable. More useful is the measurement of anti-M antibodies by bactericidal and mouse protection tests, the measurement of antistreptolysin antibodies, and the measurement of antibodies against other enzyme antigens.

Treatment. Sulfonamides, penicillin, and broad spectrum antibiotics have been used to treat streptococcal infections. Streptococci develop resistance to sulfonamides and they will not eliminate streptococci from the upper respiratory tract in acute pharyngitis. Penicillins are the drugs of choice, and erythromycin also is useful for treatment. Many streptococci are resistant to tetracycline.

α-Hemolytic Streptococci. The α-hemolytic streptococci, or viridans group, normally inhabit the oral cavity and upper respiratory tract of humans. *S. salivarius* is a common representative of this group. They seem to belong to several different immunological groups, but only a few fit into groups A to O. While relatively avirulent, they do cause disease in humans, chiefly subacute bacterial endocarditis. As inhabitants of the oral cavity, they cause repeated transient bacteremias which sometimes induce subacute bacterial endocarditis. The disease results from infection of an endocardial surface, such as on the heart valves, already damaged by congenital heart disease or rheumatic fever.

Nonhemolytic Streptococci. All streptococci that are not β-hemolytic are sometimes referred to as nonhemolytic. In this instance, however, nonhemolytic streptococci refer to those which have no action on blood. The most notable nonhemolytic streptococcus is *Streptococcus faecalis*, a normal inhabitant of the gastrointestinal tract. Of the other enteric streptococci (enterococci), most are nonhemolytic but a few strains do produce β-hemolysis. Enterococci sometimes cause endocarditis. They are apt to be resistant to antibiotics making treatment of such infections difficult.

OBLIGATORILY ANAEROBIC STREPTOCOCCI

The eighth edition of *Bergy's Manual of Determinative Bacteriology* recognizes five species of obligately anaerobic streptococci: *Peptostreptococcus anaerobius*, *Peptostreptococcus productus*, *Peptostreptococcus lanceolatus*, *Peptostreptococ-*

cus micros, and *Peptostreptococcus parvulus*. Anaerobic streptococci have been isolated from Ludwig's angina, pleurisy, sinusitis, pelvic cellulitis, pulmonary abscesses, pleural empyema, cerebrospinal meningitis, from the uterus and bloodstream in puerperal infections, and from wound infections. They seem to prefer necrotic or gangrenous lesions. Most of the recognized species are a part of the normal flora of the mouth, intestine, and perhaps more consistently of the female genital tract. They cannot be demonstrated regularly in the upper respiratory and intestinal tracts.

Anaerobic streptococci include small chain-forming cocci that vary widely in function and activity, except for their anaerobic nature. Colonial forms range from coal black to translucent and grayish white colonies. Some anaerobic streptococci disintegrate fresh fibrin, blood, and fresh organs, causing green or black discoloration and fetid odors. It has been impossible to classify the anaerobic streptococci by serological methods but some antigenic relationship exists between anaerobic streptococci and groups A, B, and C hemolytic streptococci.

STREPTOCOCCUS PNEUMONIAE

Morphology. *S. pneumoniae* are fairly large, ovoid, spherical, or lanceolate bacteria that are nonmotile, nonsporing, aerobic, and facultatively anaerobic, actively fermentative, and catalase-negative (fig. 20/4). Pneumococci are generally gram positive but become mostly gram negative and autolyze in older cultures. Pathogenic pneumococci are encapsulated with immunogenic, highly polymerized polysaccharides which serve as the basis for their subdivision into different types, and for their pathogenicity. Heavily encapsulated types form mucoid colonies. Pneumococci cause α-hemolysis aerobically and β-hemolysis anaerobically.

Antigenic Structure. *S. pneumoniae* has distinctive polysaccharide capsular antigens and somatic antigens, R antigens, C substance, and M antigen similar to other streptococci. Pneumococcal capsules are polysaccharide polymers that apparently are chemically distinct. They are used to divide the pneumococci into more than 80 serological types. When the capsule is lost or not produced, pneumococci remain viable but become avirulent and easily phagocytized. Capsular polysaccharides are the basis for the Quellung reaction (fig. 20/5). When a given type of pneumococcus is exposed to its homologous type-specific antibody, the capsule appears to swell and becomes refractile. The test is a basis for the serological identification of pneumococcal types.

Pneumococci contain a somatic C substance (teichoic acid polymer) distinct from their capsular polysaccharide and antigenically distinct from the C substance of other streptococci.

Rough pneumococci have a protein antigen that is on or near the surface of the cell. They also possess type-specific somatic M antigens that are not antiphagocytic.

Genotypic Variations. If an encapsulated, virulent pneumococcus is cultured serially in the presence of its specific antipolysaccharide, it retains its

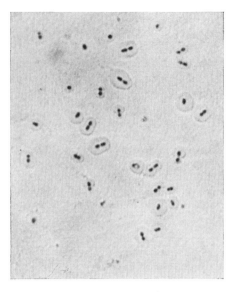

Figure 20/5. Quellung reaction of encapsulated type III pneumococci (×1100). (Reproduced with permission from R. Austrian: Morphologic Variation in Pneumococcus. *Journal of Experimental Medicine,* **98,** 21, 1953.)

viability but loses its capsule and becomes noncapsulated, nonvirulent, and nonspecific as to type. It also changes its colonial form from smooth to rough. If a rough colonial strain is grown in the presence of its homologous anti-R serum, a smooth type of pneumococcus is soon derived whose type-specificity is identical with that from which the rough strain was originally derived. The mechanism involved seems to be a selective process.

Pneumococcal Transformation. In culture, smooth virulent pneumococci mutate at a low but definite rate, lose their capsule and become rough and avirulent. By transfer of DNA a virulent pneumococcus can be transformed into another smooth type by way of the rough form. It can take place either *in vivo* or *in vitro.*

Toxins. No significant soluble toxin has been described for *S. pneumoniae* which could be related to their invasiveness or virulence. Two toxins are produced *in vitro.* Pneumolysin is an oxygen-labile endotoxin. Another endotoxin produces purpura when inoculated into experimental animals. Leukocidin and hyaluronidase are produced in small quantities.

PNEUMOCOCCAL INFECTION

The predominant pneumococcal infection is pneumonia. Pneumococci also cause a primary infection in sinusitis, otitis media, osteomyelitis, arthritis, peritonitis, meningitis, and possibly gingivitis. Pneumococcal septicemia, empyema, endocarditis, pericarditis, meningitis, and arthritis occur

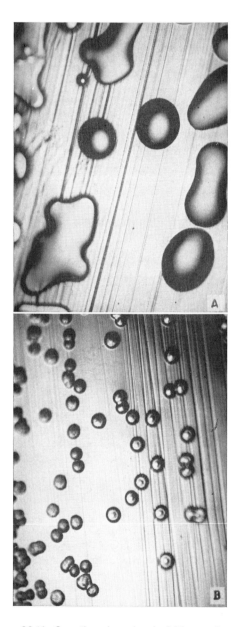

Figure 20/4. Smooth and rough colonial forms of pneumococci. (*A*) Smooth, capsulated type III pneumococci in blood agar (×14). (*B*) Rough, noncapsulated pneumococci in blood agar (×12). (Reproduced with permission from R. Austrian: Morphologic Variation in Pneumococcus. *Journal of Experimental Medicine,* **98,** 21, 1953.)

as secondary complications of pneumococcal pneumonia.

Pneumococcal Pneumonia. Pneumococcal pneumonia is characterized by its sudden onset and even early in the disease by both local manifestations (acute inflammation of the lungs, pleurisy), and systemic manifestations (general constitutional symptoms, chills, high fever, and frequently a bacteremia). Untreated cases of pneumococcal pneumonia that run an uncomplicated course are acutely ill for 7 to 10 days. Then circulating antibodies increase and there is a "crisis," after which the temperature and symptoms abate, usually quite rapidly. The symptoms of pneumococcal pneumonia patients treated with antibiotics abate within several days but all signs of pneumonia usually do not disappear for three or four weeks.

Pneumococcal Bacteremia. Pneumococcal bacteremia has been associated with the appearance of gingival lesions in infants. In these instances the children develop fever, leukocytosis, and lesions in the posterior maxillary tuberosity area, the buccal surface of the alveolar ridge and the posterior area of the hard palate. The lesions initially appear as a "boggy" fluid filled-erythematous area. These later become ulcerative and necrotic in appearance, then the swelling subsides and the lesions resolve. The relationship between the pneumococcal bacteremia and gingival lesions is not clear, but the lesions are characteristic enough that pneumococcal bacteremia should be suspected in infants with unexplained fever and leukocytosis in association with a gingival lesion like that described.

Pathogenesis. The pneumococci are strict parasites that are found in the human nasopharynx. They are disseminated in droplets of the nasopharyngeal secretions. Infection depends considerably on whether an individual is a carrier of a particular pathogenic pneumococcus at a given time and on some concurrent factor which sufficiently lowers resistance. Most epidemics of pneumococcal pneumonia occur in concurrence with other epidemics (*e.g.*, common cold or influenza), or in relatively closed communities such as hospitals, asylums, prisons, and military installations when resistance is low and carrier and contact rates are high.

Factors Affecting Mortality. Mortality in pneumonia is influenced by age, concomitant disease, the type of causal pneumococcus, the extent of lung involvement, and the presence of bacteremia. Concomitant diseases of special importance in mortality in pneumococcal pneumonia are circulatory disturbances, chronic chest diseases, diabetes mellitus, cirrhosis of the liver, and leukemia.

Complications. Complications of pneumococcal pneumonia are concerned either directly with the disease in the chest or with an extension of the infection to other organs or areas of the body. Complications of the disease in the chest are a prolonged febrile course in spite of treatment (alcoholics and debilitated individuals), pleural effusion, empyema, superinfection, delayed resolution, and relapse.

Pneumococcal meningitis sometimes occurs in individuals with pneumonia who develop a bacteremia. Pneumococcal endocarditis can be expected to occur in as many as one-third of all patients with pneumococcal meningitis, and it occurs more frequently in elderly individuals.

In addition to meningitis and endocarditis, other complications of pneumococcal pneumonia caused by bacteremia are metastatic localization in the peritoneal or synovial cavities and direct extension of the original infection to cause sinusitis, otitis media, pericarditis, or empyema.

Laboratory Diagnosis. Laboratory diagnosis is important in the treatment of pneumococcal infection. Sputum is stained by the gram method to determine if lanceolate diplococci are present, then cultured on blood agar for isolation and more positive identification. A blood culture should be made prior to antibiotic therapy. Serous and spinal fluids should also be examined for diplococci and cultured on adequate media. Diagnosis may also be made by injecting sputum or saliva intraperitoneally in mice. If pathogenic pneumococci are present, the mice will usually die within 48 hours.

Treatment. Pneumococci are most sensitive to penicillin and erythromycin, moderately susceptible to carbomycin, chlortetracycline, oxytetracycline, and tetracycline, less susceptible to chloramphenicol, bacitracin, and streptomycin, and relatively insusceptible to neomycin and polymyxin B. In treatment, penicillin, the tetracyclines, and erythromycin are the antibiotics of choice. Antibiotic therapy has reduced mortality in pneumococcal pneumonia from about 30% to about 5% or less.

ADDITIONAL READING

AYOUB, E. M., ANTHONY, B. F., MAUCERI, A. A., AND SANDERS, W. E., JR. 1975 Asymptomatic Epidemic Acquisition of Group A Streptococcus: Antibody Response to Extracellular and Type-specific Antigens. J Infect Dis, **132,** 20.

BECKER, C. G., RESNICK, G. D., AND SHUSTAK, S. 1973 On the Virulence of Group A Streptococci. Am J Pathol, **44,** 51.

BISNO, A. L., PEARCE, I. A., WALL, H. P., MOODY, M. D., AND STOLLERMAN, G. H. 1970 Epidemiology of Acute Rheumatic Fever and Glomerulonephritis. N Engl J Med, **283,** 561.

COLCHER, I. S., AND BASS, J. W. 1972 Penicillin Treatment of Streptococcal Pharyngitis. JAMA, **222,** 657.

COMMITTEE ON RHEUMATIC FEVER, COUNCIL ON RHEUMATIC FEVER AND CONGENITAL HEART DISEASE, AMERICAN HEART ASSOCIATION. 1972 House Officers' Knowledge of Group A Streptococcal Pharyngitis and Its Management. Am J Dis Child, **124,** 47.

DURACK, D. T., GILLILAND, B. C., AND PETERSDORF, R. G. 1978 Effect of Immunization on Susceptibility to Experimental *Streptococcus mutans* and *Streptococcus sanguis* Endocarditis. Infect Immun, **22,** 52.

FACKLAM, R. R. 1977 Physiological Differentiation of Viridans Streptococci. J Clin Microbiol, **5,** 184.

FEINSTEIN, A. R., AND LEVITT, M. 1970 The Role of Tonsils in Predisposing to Streptococcal Infections and Recurrences of Rheumatic Fever. N Engl J Med, **282,** 285.

FOX, E. N. 1974 M Proteins of Group A Streptococci. Bacteriol Rev, **38,** 57.

GHARAGOZLOO, R. A., MARGOLIS, E., MARCUS, H., ALAN, A. P., JAFARI, R., AND NEZAM, H. 1972 Streptococcal Infection, Rheumatic Fever and Rheumatic Heart Disease. Isr J Med Sci, **8,** 18.

HAUSMAN, D., HEATHERBELL, G., START, J., DEVITT, L., AND DOUGLAS, R. 1971 Increased Resistance to Penicillin of Pneumococci Isolated from Man. N Engl J Med, **284,** 175.

HUGHES, M., MOCHARDY, S. M., SHEPPARD, A. J., AND WOODS, N. C. 1980 Evidence for an Immunological Relationship between *Streptococcus mutans* and Human Cardiac Tissue. Infect Immun, **27,** 576.

JACKSON, H. 1976 Streptococcal Control in Grade Schools. Am J Dis Child, **130,** 273.

KAPLAN, M. H. 1979 Rheumatic Fever, Rheumatic Heart Disease and the Streptococcal Connection: The Role of Streptococcal Antigens Cross-Reactive with Heart Tissue. Rev Infect Dis, **1,** 988.

KAPLAN, O., HALFON, S. T., EVER-HADANI, P., AND DAVIES, A. M. 1974 Sensitivity of Serological Tests and the Diagnosis of Streptococcal Sore Throat in Children. Health Lab Sci, **11,** 178.

LERNER, P. I. 1975 Meningitis Caused by *Streptococcus* in Adults. J Infect Dis, **131,** 59.

LOCKWOOD, W. R., LAWSON, L. A., SMITH, D. L., MCNEILL, K. M., AND MORRISON, F. S. 1974 *Streptococcus mutans* Endocarditis. Ann Intern Med, **80,** 369.

LORIAN, V., WALUSCHKA, A., AND POPOOLA, F. 1973 Pneumococcal Beta Hemolysin Produced under the Effect of Antibiotics. Appl Microbiol, **25,** 290.

MATANOSKI, G. M. 1972 The Role of Tonsils in Streptococcal Infections. A Comparison of Tonsillectomized Children and Sibling Controls. Am J Epidemiol, **95,** 278.

MCCARTY, M. 1971 The Streptococcal Cell Wall. Harvey Lect, **65,** 73.

MCHENRY, M. C., ALFIDI, R. J., DEODHAR, S. D., BRAUN, W. E., AND POPOWNIAK, K. L. 1974 Hospital-acquired Pneumonias. Med Clin North Am, **58,** 565.

MERENSTEIN, J. H., AND ROGERS, K. D. 1974 Streptococcal Pharyngitis. JAMA, **227,** 1278.

MERRILL, C. W., GWALTNEY, J. M., JR., HENDLEY, J. O., AND SANDE, M. A. 1973 Rapid Identification of Pneumococci. N Engl J Med, **288,** 510.

MITSUHASHI, S., INOUE, N., FUSE, A., KANEKO, Y., AND OBA, T. 1974 Drug Resistance in *Streptococcus pyogenes.* Jpn J Microbiol, **18,** 98.

MOHR, D. N., FEIST, D. J., WASHINGTON, J. A., AND HERMANS, P. E. 1979 Infections Due to Group C Streptococci in Man. Am J Med, **66,** 450.

PATTERSON, M. J., AND HAFEEZ, A. E. B. 1976 Group B Streptococci in Human Disease. Bacteriol Rev, **40,** 774.

PELLETRER, L. L., JR., COYLE, N., AND PETERSDORF, R. 1978 Dextran Production as a Possible Virulence Factor in Streptococcal Endocarditis. Proc Soc Exp Biol Med, **158,** 415.

PERCH, B., KJEMS, E., AND RAVN, T. 1974 Biochemical and Serological Properties of *Streptococcus mutans* from Various Animal and Human Sources. Acta Pathol Microbiol Scand, **82,** 357.

PETERS, G., AND SMITH, A. L. 1977 Group A Streptococcal Infections of the Skin and Pharynx. N Engl J Med, **297,** 311.

RAMIREZ-RONDA, C. H. 1978 Adherence of Glucan-positive and Glucan-negative Streptococcal Strains to Normal and Damaged Heart Valves. J Clin Invest, **62,** 805.

REED, W. P., DRACH, G. W., AND WILLIAMS, R. C., JR. 1974 Antigens Common to Human and Bacterial Cells; IV. Studies of Human Pneumococcal Disease. J Lab Clin Med, **83,** 599.

ROBBINS, N., SZILAGYI, G., TANOWITZ, H. B., LUFTSCHEIN, S., AND BAUM, S. G. 1977 Infective Endocarditis Caused by *Streptococcus mutans.* Arch Intern Med, **137,** 1171.

STARKEBAUM, M., DURACK, D., AND BEESON, P. 1977 The "Incubation Period" of Subacute Bacterial Endocarditis. Yale J Biol Med, **50,** 49.

TORANTA, A., AND MOODY, M. D. 1971 Diagnosis of Streptococcal Pharyngitis and Rheumatic Fever. Pediatr Clin North Am, **18,** 125.

WALSH, B. T., BROOKHEIM, W. W., JOHNSON, R. C., AND TOMPKINS, R. K. 1975 Recognition of Streptococcal Pharyngitis in Adults. Arch Intern Med, **135,** 1493.

WANNAMAKER, L. W. 1970 Differences between Streptococcal Infections of the Throat and of the Skin. N Engl J Med, **282,** 23.

chapter 21

Neisseria: Gonorrhea and Meningitis

George S. Schuster

NEISSERIA GONORRHOEAE

General Characteristics. *N. gonorrhoeae* (commonly gonococci) are gram negative, nonmotile, aerobic, or facultatively anaerobic, nonsporing cocci that occur singly in culture, but in body exudates and phagocytes are diplococci with adjacent sides flattened. Individual cells range from 0.6 to 1.0 μm in diameter. They may possess a capsule of unknown composition. Gonococci may have pili and these have been related to their virulence.

The colonies of gonococci, which usually develop after 48 hours of incubation, are at first small and transparent, but after incubating for several days become grayish-white and have a lobate margin.

Cultivation and Metabolism. Gonococci grow best on enriched media containing heated blood or defined media. Typical media contain fatty acids and trace elements that are inhibitory to growth. Carbon dioxide is an absolute requirement for growth. Cultures are difficult to maintain even under the most favorable conditions.

The formation of indophenol oxidase by gonococci is useful for their detection in primary, mixed cultures. Agar plates on which the organisms have grown are treated with a 1% solution of tetramethyl- or dimethyl-*p*-phenylenediamine by flooding or spraying; alternately, single colonies can be tested with a drop of the reagent. Colonies that produce indophenol oxidase become pink, then black. However, many other bacterial species from the genital tract also produce indophenol oxidase.

Glucose is the only carbohydrate ordinarily fermented by gonococci, with the production of acid and no gas.

Antigenic Composition. There are at least 16 serotypes of gonococci, based upon differences in the principal outer membrane proteins. By immunofluorescence involving the intact cell surface, the gonococci have been classified into eight types and subtypes. The pili that have been isolated consist primarily of a single kind of protein subunit. Several serologically distinct types have been found. Also, it appears that there are several serologically heterogenous determinants of the gonococcal lipopolysaccharide. Tests for these are important in epidemiological studies of gonorrhea. Gonococcal lipopolysaccharide also has endotoxic activity.

Clinical Course of Gonorrhea. Gonococci have a predilection for mucous membranes of the genital tract. Very shortly after contact with the mucosal surface they attach by pili to the surface cells, thus establishing the infection. They penetrate between cells of the mucous membrane to subepithelial connective tissue within a few days, where they cause an inflammatory reaction of varying severity consisting of a dense infiltration of polymorphonuclear leukocytes. This produces the characteristic mucopurulent discharge. The incubation period is usually 3 to 5 days, but may range from 1 to 30 days. In men, the onset is typically sudden with a purulent discharge from the urethra (fig. 21/1) and painful urination; the patient may be febrile. Approximately 10% of cases are asymptomatic although such individuals may transmit the disease.

In females, infection is not as evident since a high proportion are asymptomatic. Also they are not as easily diagnosed. Signs of the disease include burning and frequency of urination, vaginal discharge, and fever. Infection of the fallopian tubes may produce pelvic inflammatory disease that produces blocking of the tubes resulting in sterility and fluid accumulation. Gonococcal infection of the birth canal is transmitted also to the eyes of newborn infants, producing ophthalmia neonatorum, which very frequently results in blindness if untreated.

Gonococcal infection of the oral cavity occurs in adults as a primary infection from oral sex or as a secondary infection brought about by the hands carrying the gonococci from infected genitalia to the oral cavity or from gonococcemia. In the oral cavity, the incubation period varies from 1 or 2 days to a week or more. Several types of lesions may

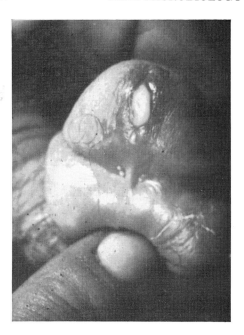

Figure 21/1. Acute gonorrhea. (AFIP 218663.)

subsequently develop. They range from sharply localized whitish or yellowish white patches to a more generalized lesion covering a large area of the oral mucosa with a grayish adherent membrane which eventually sloughs off, leaving bright areas with numerous bleeding points. The gingivae are usually inflamed and swollen. Pain in the area is a prominent symptom. Areas of the oral cavity most often affected are the gingivae, tongue, and soft palate. Patients with oral gonococcal infection are ill, sometimes seriously so, usually with a temperature above 100 F.

Local lesions and symptoms of oral gonococcal infection may simulate those of Vincent's infection, and pharyngeal streptococcal infection or pharyngeal diphtheria may have a similar superficial appearance. Without a concurrent genital infection, differential diagnosis may be quite difficult and depend finally upon isolation of gonococci from the area.

Gonococci invade tissues and the circulatory system during gonorrheal infections, establishing metastatic infections involving the heart (endocarditis); joints (arthritis); skin (dermatitis), especially on the elbows and dorsal surfaces of the wrists; salivary glands (parotitis); central nervous system (meningitis); and reproductive glands (sterility). Other complications include conjunctivitis.

Diagnosis. The diagnosis of gonorrhea requires the isolation of gram negative diplococci from pus or other exudate and their identification as gonococci by sugar fermentation tests (fig. 21/2). Microscopic observations of polymorphonuclear leuko-

cytes and intracellular gram negative diplococci in exudates are valuable but may be misleading in females due to presence of similar appearing saprophytes in cervical materials. Culture on Thayer-Martin medium or chocolate agar is useful for growing and recognizing neisseriae from clinical specimens, for subculture, and for performing an oxidase test. Distinction between species of *Neisseria* is usually based upon sugar fermentation: *N. gonorrhea* produces acid from glucose but not maltose, sucrose or lactose. Immunofluorescent staining of exudates and other serological tests are valuable adjuncts to the cultural demonstration of gonococci. The most significant clinical manifestation for diagnosis is a purulent urethral discharge.

Treatment. Uncomplicated gonococcal infections are best treated by intramuscular aqueous procaine penicillin G together with Probenecid by mouth. Alternatively ampicillin by mouth together with Probenecid may be used but this seems to have a slightly lower cure rate than penicillin. For patients who are allergic to penicillin, tetracycline by mouth or spectinomycin intramuscularly are alternative therapies.

Penicillinase-producing gonococci have been recognized in the United States. Patients infected with these strains do not respond to penicillin therapy. If such organisms are isolated, alternate therapies must be used.

NEISSERIA MENINGITIDIS

General Characteristics. Meningococci are aerobic, gram negative, nonmotile, nonsporing cocci or diplococci, ordinarily 0.8 μm or less in diameter. Fresh isolates of most serogroups are encapsulated. As are the other neisseriae, meningococci are very susceptible to adverse environmental conditions such as drying or unfavorable pH. Isolates should

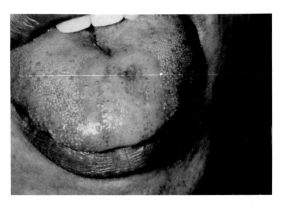

Figure 21/2. Lesion of the tongue in a 25-year-old male. The localized white patch resembled a lesion caused by *Neisseria gonorrhoeae* but by fermentation reactions the causative organism was identified as *Neisseria sicca*.

be put in culture without delay. *N. meningitidis* is difficult to grow, primarily because of toxic components in ordinary media and complex nutritional requirements. The addition of starch or albumin to media reduces toxicity. From normally sterile sites the organisms can be grown on chocolate agar but if other organisms are present the selective Thayer-Martin medium should be used. Like the gonococci, meningococci are oxidase positive.

Antigenic Composition. Virulent meningococci have been divided into groups on the basis of their capsular antigens. Some groups have distinctive protein antigens in the outer membrane that may contribute to induction of host immunity. The somatic antigens are closely related to other *Neisseria* species. These include nucleoprotein, a somatic carbohydrate, and an endotoxin. Meningococci and gonococci also share at least six other heat-stable somatic antigens.

Genetic Variations. Meningococci undergo genetic variation, producing strains that are highly resistant to sulfonamides, and to a lesser degree to penicillin. Penicillin-resistant strains revert to penicillin-sensitive strains when cultured in a penicillin-free medium. When grown in the presence of streptomycin, streptomycin-dependent strains develop whose virulence in experimental animals is enhanced by the presence of streptomycin. Meningococci go quickly from a virulent, smooth form to an avirulent, rough-colony form with loss of the surface antigens.

MENINGOCOCCAL INFECTION

Pathogenicity. The pathogenicity of the meningococcus relates to antiphagocytic and endotoxic mechanisms. The antiphagocytic activity of *N. meningitidis* relates to capsular polysaccharides that inhibit phagocytosis. Meningococci are extracellular parasites and in the presence of specific antibody they are phagocytized and destroyed. If they are to produce disease they must be able to resist phagocytosis.

The other virulence factor is the meningococcal endotoxin. This can produce vascular damage. Successive injections of endotoxin elicit the local Shwartzman phenomenon, while single injections produce venous thrombi in bone marrow and lungs and degenerative changes in heart, liver, and spleen.

Epidemiology. The primary habitat of the meningococcus is the nasopharynx of symptomless human carriers. One to two percent of the population are chronic carriers; an additional 5 to 20% are intermittent carriers. Preceding and during epidemics carrier rates rise 70 to 90%. Less than 0.1% of an exposed population develops overt disease, indicating that a high carrier rate is not the only determinant.

Meningococcal disease occurs mostly in the young and in the aged. The rate in men is double than that in women. In children infection is related to a high carrier rate but not to the seasons or to a social class. Meningococcal infection is not one of the effective "immunizing infections of childhood."

Clinical Types of Meningococcal Disease. The nasopharynx is the point of entry for the meningococci and this precedes hematogenous spread. A local infection occurs in capillaries of the skin and other organs from which the bacteria are carried to the central nervous system.

Dissemination via the bloodstream results in lesions in various areas such as the skin, meninges, joints and lungs. Clinical manifestations depend upon the site of localization. These can include a mild febrile illness accompanied by pharyngitis. Systemic disease is characterized by fever and prostration. An erythematous, macular rash may be observed, followed by appearance of a petechial eruption that leads to ecchymosis. This is characteristic of fulminant meningococcal disease. Meningoccemia may be accompanied by meningitis, pericarditis or arthritis. There may be a suppurative infection of the membranes surrounding the brain and spinal cord. Surviving patients may have permanent sequelae, especially of the nervous system. Pharyngeal lesions due to meningococci but resembling those produced in gonococcal infection have been described. Thus, infections produced by neisseriae must be diagnosed with special care due to possible social and legal implications.

Diagnosis. Laboratory diagnosis of meningococcal infections consists of the demonstration of meningococci in stained smears from the fluid of the petechial lesions in the skin or by cultures of blood, spinal fluid, and nasopharyngeal secretions on Thayer-Martin medium, chocolate agar, or other appropriate media.

Immunity. Man is inherently resistant to meningococcal disease. Newborns rarely contract the disease but become susceptible to it as they lose their maternal antibodies. It is likely that they then develop resistance from repeated exposure to subinfective doses of meningococci, or to a nonencapsulated strain, or to an encapsulated strain of low virulence. Recovery from meningococcal disease or the development of a carrier state is accompanied by the appearance of antibodies against both the capsular group-specific polysaccharide and the endotoxin.

Prevention. Introduction of sulfonamides in 1939 provided a successful prophylactic measure for both civilian and military populations. In time, however, sufficient numbers of the virulent meningococci became resistant to the sulfonamides that they were rendered useless. No other chemotherapeutic agent has emerged for widespread prophylaxis. If it is deemed necessary, rifampin may be used.

Treatment. Penicillin is the drug of choice for therapy. In the event of penicillin sensitivity, chloramphenicol is an effective alternative. In systemic infections, supportive therapy is important to the patient's care.

ADDITIONAL READING

ALTMANN, G., EGOZ, N., AND GOBOKOVSKY, B. 1973 Observations on Asymptomatic Infections with *Neisseria meningitidis*. Am J Epidemiol, **98,** 446.

ANDERSON, K. F. 1973 The Diagnosis and Treatment of Meningitis. Med J Aust, **1,** 897.

ANNUNZIATO, D. 1974 Gonorrheal Ophthalmia: Diagnosis and Treatment. NY State J Med, **74,** 1470.

APICELLA, M. A. 1974 Identification of a Subgroup Antigen on the *Neisseria meningitidis* Group C Capsular Polysaccharide. J Infect Dis, **129,** 147.

ARKO, R. J., DUNCAN, W. P., BROWN, W. J., PEACOCK, W. L., AND TOMIZAWA, T. 1976 Immunity in Infection with *Neisseria gonorrhoeae*: Duration and Serological Response in the Chimpanzee. J Infect Dis, **133,** 441.

BARR, J., AND DANIELSSON, D. 1971 Gonococcal Sepsis and Arthritis. Calif Med, **114,** 18.

BERGER, G. S., KEITH, L., AND MOSS, W. 1975 Prevalence of Gonorrhoea among Women Using Various Methods of Contraception. Br J Vener Dis, **51,** 307.

BHATTACHARYYA, M. N., JEPHCOTT, A. E., AND MORTON, R. S. 1973 Diagnosis of Gonorrhoea: A Comparison of Sampling Sites. Br Med J, **1,** 748.

BLANKENSHIP, R. M., HOLMES, R. K., AND SANFORD, J. P. 1974 Treatment of Disseminated Gonococcal Infection. N Engl J Med, **290,** 267.

BRO-JØRGENSEN, A., AND JENSEN, T. 1971 Gonococcal Tonsillar Infections. Br Med J, **4,** 660.

BRO-JØRGENSEN, A., AND JENSEN, T. 1973 Gonococcal Pharyngeal Infections. Br J Vener Dis, **49,** 491.

BROWN, W. J. 1975 A Comparison of Three Fermentation Methods for the Confirmation of *Neisseria gonorrhoeae*. Health Lab Sci, **13,** 54.

COOKE, C. L., OWEN, D. S., JR., AND IRBY, R. 1971 Gonococcal Arthritis. JAMA, **217,** 204.

COPPING, A. A. 1954 Stomatitis Caused by Gonococcus. J Am Dent Assoc, **49,** 567.

CORNELIUS, C. E., III. 1971 Seasonality of Gonorrhea in the United States. Health Serv Rep, **86,** 157.

DANS, P. E. 1975 Treatment of Gonorrhea and Syphilis; Part I. Gonorrhea. South Med J, **68,** 1287.

DEVINE, L. F., HAGERMAN, C. R., HANNAH, J. M., RHODE, S. L., III, AND PECKINPAUGH, R. D. 1973 Minocycline and Rifampin: Proposed Treatment Regimen for the Elimination of Meningococci from the Nasopharynges of Healthy Carriers. Milit Med, **138,** 20.

EISENSTEIN, B. I., SOX, T., BISWAS, G. BLACKMAN, E., AND SPARLING, P. F. 1977 Conjugal Transfer of the Gonococcal Penicillinase Plasmid. Science, **195,** 998.

FASS, R. J., AND SASLOW, S. 1972 Chronic Meningococcemia. JAMA, **130,** 943.

FAUR, Y. C., WEISBURD, M. H., AND WILSON, M. E. 1975 Isolation of *Neisseria meningitidis* from the Genito-Urinary Tract and Anal Canal. J Clin Microbiol, **2,** 178.

FIUMARA, N. J. 1972 The Diagnosis and Treatment of Gonorrhea. Med Clin North Am, **56,** 1105.

FRASER, P. K., BAILEY, G. K., ABBOTT, J. D., GILL, J. B., AND WALKER, D. J. C. 1973 The Meningococcal Carrier Rate. Lancet, **2,** 1235.

GAFFAR, H. A., AND D'ARCANGELIS, D. C. 1976 Fluores-cent Antibody Test for the Serological Diagnosis of Gonorrhea. J Clin Microbiol, **3,** 438.

HANDSFIELD, H. H., HODSON, W. A., AND HOLMES, K. K. 1973 Neonatal Gonococcal Infections. JAMA, **225,** 697.

HANDSFIELD, H. H., LIPMAN, T. O., HARNISCH, J. P., TRONCA E., AND HOLMES, K. K. 1974 Asymptomatic Gonorrhea in Men: Diagnosis, Natural Course and Prevalence. N Engl J Med, **290,** 117.

HARE, M. J. 1974 Comparative Assessment of Microbiological Methods for the Diagnosis of Gonorrhoea in Women. Br J Vener Dis, **50,** 437.

HYSLOP, N. E., JR., AND SWARTZ, M. N. 1975 Bacterial Meningitis. Postgrad Med, **58,** 120.

JACOBS, S. A., AND NORDEN, C. W. 1974 Pneumonia Caused by *Neisseria meningitidis*. JAMA, **227,** 67.

JAFFE, H. W., BIDDLE, J. W., THORNSBERRY, C., JOHNSON, R. H., KAUFMAN, R. E., REYNOLDS, G. H., AND WIESNER, P. J. 1976 National Gonorrhea Therapy Monitoring Study. N Engl J Med, **294,** 5.

KHURI-BULOS, N. 1973 Meningococcal Meningitis following Rifampin Prophylaxis. Am J Dis Child, **126,** 689.

KRAUS, S. J. 1972 Complications of Gonococcal Infection. Med Clin North Am, **56,** 1115.

LAMBERT, P. M. 1973 Recent Trends in Meningococcal Infection. Community Med, **129,** 279.

LEWIS, J. F., ARNOLD, C., AND ALEXANDER, J. 1973 Meningococcal Pneumonia. J Clin Pathol, **59,** 388.

LIGHTFOOT, R. W., JR., AND GOTSCHLICH, E. C. 1974 Gonococcal Disease. Am J Med, **56,** 347.

McGEE, Z. A., GROSS, J., DOURMASHKIN, R. R., AND TAYLOR-ROBINSON, D. 1976 Nonpilar Surface Appendages of Colony Type I and Colony Type 4 Gonococci. Infect Immun, **14,** 266.

MENDELSON, J., PORTNOY, J., ABEL, T., AND STEINMAN, R. 1975 Disseminated Gonorrhea: Diagnosis through Contact Tracing. Can Med Assoc J, **112,** 864.

MERCHANT, H. W., AND SCHUSTER, G. S. 1977 Oral Gonococcal Infection. J Am Dent Assoc **95,** 807.

MORSE, S. A., AND BARTENSTEIN, L. 1976 Adaptation of the Minitek System for the Rapid Identification of *Neisseria gonorrhea*. J Clin Microbiol, **3,** 8.

NANKERVIS, G. A. 1974 Bacterial Meningitis. Med Clin North Am, **58,** 581.

NOBLE, R. C., AND COOPER, R. M. 1979 Meningococcal Colonization Misdiagnosed as Gonococcal Pharyngeal Infection. Br J Vener Dis, **55,** 336.

O'BRIEN, N. G., AND O'CONNELL, E. 1972 Gonococcal Ophthalmia. J Ir Med Assoc, **65,** 320.

OFEK, I., BEACHEY, E. H., AND BISNO, A. L. 1974 Resistance of *Neisseria gonorrhoeae* to Phagocytosis: Relationship to Colonial Morphology and Surface Pili. J Infect Dis, **129,** 310.

PANIKABUTRA, K. 1973 Clinical Aspects of Uncomplicated Gonorrhoea in the Female. Br J Vener Dis, **49,** 213.

PARISER, H. 1972 Asymptomatic Gonorrhea. Med Clin North Am **56,** 1127.

PIEROG, S., NIGAM, S., MARASIGAN, D. C., AND DUBE, S. K. 1975 Gonococcal Ophthalmia Neonatorum. Relationship of Maternal Factors and Delivery Room Practices to Effective Control Measures. J Obstet Gynecol, **122,** 589.

POLLOCK, H. M. 1976 Evaluation of Methods for the Rapid Identification of *Neisseria gonorrhoeae* in a Routine Clinical Laboratory. J Clin Microbiol, **4,** 19.

PUNSALANG, A. P., JR., AND SAWYER, W. D. 1973 Role of Pili in the Virulence of *Neisseria gonorrhoeae*. Infect Immun, **8,** 255.

RODAS, C. U., AND RONALD, A. R. 1974 Comparison of Three Serological Tests in Gonococcal Infection. Appl Microbiol, **27,** 695.

RUDOLPH, A. H. 1972 Control of Gonorrhea. JAMA, **220,** 1587.

SAYEED, Z. A., BHADURI, U., HOWELL, E., AND MEYERS, H. L., JR. 1972 Gonococcal Meningitis. JAMA, **219,** 1730.

SCHMIDT, H., HJØRTING-HANSEN, E., AND PHILIPSEN, H. P. 1961 Gonococcal Stomatitis. Acta Derm Venereol, **41,** 324.

SCHROETER, A. L., AND LUCAS, J. B. 1972 Gonorrhea—Diagnosis and Treatment. Obstet Gynecol, **39,** 274.

STOLZ, E., AND SCHULLER, J. 1974 Gonococcal Oro- and Nasopharyngeal Infection. Br J Vener Dis, **50,** 104.

THOMPSON, T. R., SWANSON, R. E., AND WIESNER, P. J. 1974 Gonococcal Ophthalmia Neonatorum. JAMA, **228,** 186.

TOEWS, W. H., AND BASS, J. W. 1974 Skin Manifestations of Meningococcal Infection. Am J Dis Child, **127,** 173.

VOLK, J., AND KRAUS, S. J. 1973 Asymptomatic Meningococcal Urethritis. Br J Vener Dis, **49,** 511.

WATKO, L., AND BROWNLOW, W. J. 1975 Antibiotic Susceptibility of *Neisseria gonorrhoeae* Isolated in the Western Pacific in 1971. Br J Vener Dis, **51,** 34.

WIESNER, P. J., TRONCA, E., BONIN, P., PEDERSEN, A. H. B., AND HOLMES, K. K. 1973 Clinical Spectrum of Pharyngeal Gonococcal Infection. N Engl J Med, **288,** 181.

YOW, M. D., BAKER, C. J., BARRETT, F. F., AND ORTIGOZA, C. O. 1973 Initial Antibiotic Management of Bacterial Meningitis (Selection in Relationship to Age). Medicine, **52,** 305.

chapter 22

Corynebacterium and Diphtheria

George S. Schuster

CORYNEBACTERIUM DIPHTHERIAE

General Characteristics. *C. diphtheriae* are gram positive, nonmotile, nonsporing, nonencapsulated, somewhat pleomorphic bacteria. They occur as straight, slightly curved, crooked, or seemingly branched rods frequently swollen at one or both ends. The cells contain bands or beads which stain with methylene or toluidine blue. These are called metachromatic granules or Babès-Ernst granules and are composed of highly polymerized polyphosphates.

C. diphtheriae can be divided into three distinct morphological and cultural types that are called gravis (rough), mitis (smooth), and intermedius (rough or smooth). There is no relationship between these morphological types and virulence.

Growth and Nutrition. The diphtheria bacillus, an aerobe and facultative anaerobe will grow on a simple medium but a medium enriched with animal protein is more suitable. Media commonly used are Loeffler's serum medium, or selective media such as blood or chocolate agar containing potassium tellurite.

Antigenic Composition. *C. diphtheriae* contains thermolabile, alkali-soluble surface protein (K) antigens that are responsible for agglutination reactions. Less specific thermostable carbohydrate (O) antigens have been found in the interior of the bacterial cell. Various combinations of O and K antigens constitute the antigenic structure of the serotypes of *C. diphtheriae*. Lipid antigens are also present but are less specific than the agglutinogens.

Diphtheria Toxin. Pathogenic diphtheria bacilli produce a lethal exotoxin. Toxigenicity is characteristic only of diphtheria bacilli lysogenized by β-prophage or a closely related phage which carries the *tox*$^+$ gene for formation of diphtheria toxin. Loss of prophage by a toxigenic strain converts it to a nontoxigenic strain, which, in turn, can be made toxigenic by reinfection. While the *tox*$^+$ gene controls the synthesis of toxin, expression also relates to the physiology and metabolism of the diphtheria bacillus: toxin is synthesized in high amounts when exogenous Fe^{2+} is depleted.

In man and rabbits, diphtheria toxin is lethal in doses less than 0.1 μg/kg. When exposed to formalin, the toxin is converted to a toxoid that has no toxicity but is antigenically undistinguishable from the toxin. Vaccines prepared from toxoid elicit protective antibodies against all diphtheria toxins.

Diphtheria toxin completely blocks amino acid incorporation in cells. In cell-free extracts and in living animals, the toxin interferes with the incorporation of amino acids in polypeptide chains by inactivation of the translocation factor.

DIPHTHERITIC INFECTIONS

Clinical Course. Diphtheria is the principal disease caused by *C. diphtheriae*. Initially there is a localized infection of the nasal or pharyngeal mucous membranes. The symptoms arise from diphtheria toxin acting either locally or systemically. Diphtheria bacilli on the mucosal surface initially form exotoxin, which causes the local degeneration of epithelial cells and profuse exudation. The initial lesions are grayish white spots which spread laterally to coalesce and deepen but never ulcerate. The inflammatory response is relatively severe, and fibrinous exudation, erythrocytes, and tissue debris form a "pseudomembrane" which covers the affected area.

In a severe case, the diphtheritic membrane spreads rapidly to occlude the airway. The patient is very ill and the symptoms are quite severe. The profound toxemia seriously affects the heart and nervous system and less often and less severely affects kidneys, adrenals, spleen, and liver. Severe edema may develop in the neck (bull neck), and bronchopneumonia is not infrequent.

Complications involving the oral cavity directly are rare. Cases have been described in which the entire mucous membrane of the oral cavity was covered with a thick, firmly attached, yellowish membrane. A case has been reported in which a lesion, covered with a whitish membrane, developed in the lower lip of a child. The site of erupting deciduous teeth and the corners of the mouth also have been the sites for diphtheritic involvement.

Localized diphtheritic infections may occur on lips, nares, and, less often, conjunctivae. Membrane formation is rare, and the systemic symptoms are usually mild but occasionally they are severe. The middle and external ears may be affected by a very chronic otitis media of diphtherial origin.

Diphtheria bacilli are also involved in ulcerative, indolent, chronic cutaneous infections in warm or tropical climates (figs. 22/1 and 22/2). This infection, often called desert sore or tropical ulcer according to the circumstances of its occurrence, arises at the site of a minor injury. It develops into a persistent ulcer, often lasting for months.

Immunological Aspects. Immunity to infection by diphtheria bacilli is essentially antitoxic. The human infant is naturally immune to diphtheria only by passive transfer of antitoxin from an immune mother. Where immunization is not practiced, immunity in older children and in adults is dependent on natural contact with diphtheria toxin. Recovery from an untreated initial infection with a highly virulent strain is possible only if the individual can survive until antibodies develop. Immunity develops with less danger when the diphtheritic infection is caused by a moderately virulent strain. The degree of immunity achieved by natural immunization is variable and transient and diminishes with time, unless boosted by repeated antigenic stimuli.

Mass artificial immunization is effective in substantially reducing the prevalence of diphtheria. In an artificially immunized population, however, most mothers are not sufficiently immune to provide significant passive protection to their offspring. Thus, artificial immunization should be done at an early age. Mass artificial immunization is effective in controlling diphtheria only when about 70% of a population is effectively immunized.

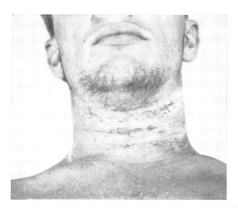

Figure 22/1. Cutaneous diphtheria of the neck. (AFIP A44723-1.)

The Schick Test. The degree of immunity to diphtheria can be measured by the Schick test. The technique of the test is to inject diphtheria toxin and controls intracutaneously into the flexor surface of the arms. A positive, negative, pseudoreaction, or combined reaction occurs at the test sites. In a positive reaction, erythema, superficial necrosis, and a brownish pigmentation develops in 24 hours and lasts for more than a week at the test site. There is no reaction at the control site. In the negative reaction, there is a brief transient response at either the test or control site. In the pseudoreaction, an erythema develops at both control and test sites within 18 hours, increases for not more than 48 hours, and disappears within 3 or 4 days. This reaction indicates immunity plus an allergy. In the combined reaction, the control and test sites both go through the successive stages of an allergic reaction but the control reaction subsides within 3 or 4 days, whereas the test reaction persists, indicating an absence of immunity.

Immunization. Active immunization for diphtheria is accomplished by various preparations of toxoid. These consist essentially of a purified toxoid administered as fluid or an alum-precipitated compound. The toxoid is given in three successive doses for the immunization of children. It is not so suitable for immunization of adults because of their systemic reaction to the bacillary proteins, which is not likely to occur in children. Severe local and systemic reactions may result from the use of toxoids, even when a preliminary skin test indicates no sensitivity to them. A combined tetanus, pertussis and diphtheria toxoid is available for primary immunization in young children and a highly purified toxoid preparation is now available for administration to older children and adults.

Passive immunity to diphtheria can be established by the injection of antitoxin. It is only of short duration but has the somewhat restricted usefulness of protecting highly susceptible individuals exposed directly to the disease.

Laboratory Diagnosis. Specimens are obtained from the primary lesion. Initial growth and isolation is accomplished on Loeffler's medium, tellurite medium, and blood agar. Growth on blood agar and no growth on tellurite agar indicates no diphtheria bacilli. Growth of typical diphtheria bacilli on tellurite agar indicates their presence. Diagnosis should be made also by injecting the suspected bacteria subcutaneously or intracutaneously into protected and unprotected guinea pigs or rabbits. If the bacteria are toxigenic, a local lesion with superficial necrosis develops in unprotected animals, which die in one to four days. The gel diffusion test is also used to determine toxigenicity. In this test a paper impregnated with diphtheria antitoxin is incorporated in agar containing serum.

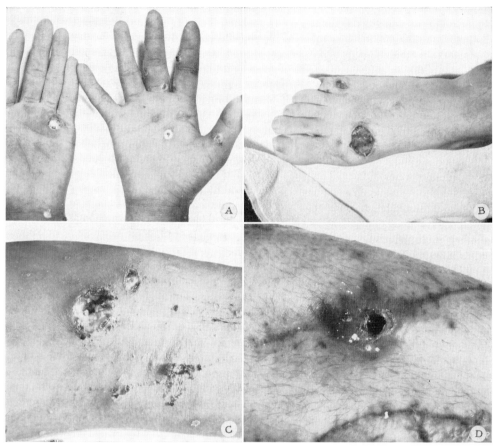

Figure 22/2. Cutaneous lesions caused by *Corynebacterium diphtheriae.* (*A,* AFIP 44847-1; *B,* AFIP L-4360-1; *C,* AFIP 44847-2; *D,* AFIP A-45659-1.)

Suspected bacilli are streaked on the agar surface. If diphtheria bacilli are present a line of antigen-antibody precipitate forms.

Treatment. Immediate therapy is imperative. Suspected diphtheria should be treated immediately with from 100 to 500 units/lb of antitoxic serum, depending upon the severity of the symptoms. Bacteriological diagnosis should be accomplished as quickly as possible for confirmation of the clinical diagnosis. Penicillin, erythromycin, or the tetracyclines are useful adjuncts in the treatment of diphtheria.

Control. The control of diphtheria requires the active immunization of children. Immunization should be done universally by the time the child is 3 months old, at 1 year of age, and again at school age. Such a regimen furnishes adequate protection until adolescence. Further immunization or boosting of immunity in adults is complicated by their reaction to some component of diphtheria vaccine and is dependent on their immunity status as determined by Schick testing. While untoward reactions are seldom fatal, they are prevalent enough to preclude mass immunization of adults.

ADDITIONAL READING

BARKSDALE, W. L. 1971 *Corynebacterium diphtheriae* and Its Relatives. Bacteriol Rev, **34,** 378.

BEZJAK, V., AND FARSEY, S. J. 1970 *Corynebacterium diphtheriae* in Skin Lesions in Ugandan Children. Bull WHO, **43,** 643.

BRAY, J. P., BURT, E. G., POTTER, E. V., POON-KING, T., AND EARLE, D. P. 1972 Epidemic Diphtheria and Skin Infections in Trinidad. J Infect Dis, **126,** 34.

BROOKS, G. F., BENNETT, J. V., AND FELDMAN, R. A. 1974 Diphtheria in the United States, 1959–1970. J Infect Dis, **129,** 172.

CASTELLANI, A. 1957 Tropicaloid Ulcer; a General Account. Parasitology, **8,** 38.

COLLIER, R. J. 1975 Diphtheria Toxin: Mode of Action and Structure. Bacteriol Rev, **39,** 54.

COX, J. C. 1975 New Method for the Large-scale Preparation of Diphtheria Toxoid: Purification of Toxin. Appl Microbiol, **29,** 464.

CROMBACH, W. H. J. 1974 Morphology and Physiology of Coryneform Bacteria. Antonie Van Leeuwenhoek, **40,** 361.

DOBIE, R. A., AND TOBEY, D. N. 1979 Clinical Features of Diphtheria in the Respiratory Tract. JAMA, **242,** 2197.

FELDMAN, R. A. 1973 Epidemic Diphtheria and Skin Infection in Trinidad. J Infect Dis, **127,** 207.

GIBSON, L. F. 1973 Variation among Strains of *Corynebacterium diphtheriae* During an Outbreak in a Restricted Environment. J Hyg, **71,** 691.

GILL, D. M., PAPPENHEIMER, A. M., JR., AND UCHIDA, T. 1973 Diphtheria Toxin, Protein Synthesis, and the Cell. Fed Proc, **32,** 1508.

HATANO, M. 1956 Effect of Iron Concentration in the Medium on Phage and Toxin Production in a Lysogenic, Virulent *Corynebacterium diphtheriae.* J Bacteriol, **71,** 121.

JOHNSON, W. D., AND KAYE, D. 1970 Serious Infection Caused by Diphtheroids. Ann NY Acad Sci, **174,** 568.

LAIRD, W., AND GROMAN, N. 1973 Rapid, Direct Tissue Cultures Test for Toxigenicity of *Corynebacterium diphtheriae.* Appl Microbiol, **25,** 709.

MANGE, R. 1956 Sinus Diphtheria, Diphtherial Sinusitis and Carriers of Bacteria. Pract Oto-Rhino-Laryngol, **17,** 351.

MAXIMESCU, P., OPRISAN, A., POP, A., AND POTORAC, E. 1974 Further Studies on *Corynebacterium* Species Capable of Producing Diphtheria Toxin (*C. diphtheriae, C. ulcerans, C. ovis*). J Gen Microbiol, **82,** 49.

MAXIMESCU, P., POP, A., OPRISAN, A., AND POTORAC, E. 1974 Diphtheria Tox⁺ Gene Expressed in *Corynebacterium* Species Other than *C. diphtheriae.* J Hyg Epidemiol Microbiol Immunol, **18,** 324.

MAXUMDER, D. N. G. 1969 Observations in Diphtheritic Myocarditis. J Indian Med Assoc, **52,** 315.

MILLER, L. W., OLDER, J., DRAKE, J., AND ZIMMERMAN, S. 1972 Diphtheria Immunization. Am J Dis Child, **123,** 197.

PAPPENHEIMER, A. M., JR. 1977 Diphtheria Toxin. Annu Rev Biochem, **44,** 69.

PAPPENHEIMER, A. M., JR., AND GILL, D. M. 1973 Diphtheria. Science, **182,** 353.

PODLEVSKIY, A. F. 1954 Diphtheria of Mucosa of Tongue, Mouth, and Lips. Pediatriya, **4,** 81.

RYAN, W. J. 1972 Throat Infection and Rash Associated with an Unusual Corynebacterium. Lancet, **2,** 1345.

SINCLAIR, M. C., OVERTON, R., AND DONALD, W. J. 1971 Alabama Diphtheria Outbreak. Health Serv Rep, **86,** 107.

SOMERVILLE, D. A. 1972 The Microbiology of the Cutaneous Diphtheroids. Br J Dermatol, **86** (Suppl 8), 16.

TRINCA, J. C. 1975 Combined Diphtheria-Tetanus Immunization of Adults. Med J Aust, **2,** 543.

UCHIDA, T., AND PAPPENHEIMER, A. M., JR. 1974 Diphtheria Toxin and Mutant Proteins. Jpn J Med Sci Biol, **27,** 93.

chapter 23

Mycobacteria

George S. Schuster

The mycobacteria include *Mycobacterium tuberculosis* (the human tubercle bacillus) and *Mycobacterium bovis* (the bovine tubercle bacillus). *Mycobacterium avium* primarily infects birds, occasionally swine, and seldom humans. *Mycobacterium ulcerans* causes cutaneous tuberculosis. *Mycobacterium paratuberculosis* (Johne's bacillus) causes an enteric infection in cattle. In addition, there are four groups of acid-fast bacilli that are not very pathogenic for guinea pigs (or rabbits), but sometimes do cause a mild form of human pulmonary tuberculosis. They are called atypical mycobacteria. Group I includes the photochromogens that form a bright yellow pigment when exposed to light. Group II includes the scotochromogens that produce a reddish-orange pigment, whether exposed to light or not. There is a group (III) of nonchromogens; still another group (IV) are referred to as rapid growers.

Mycobacterium leprae causes leprosy or Hansen's disease in humans.

MYCOBACTERIUM TUBERCULOSIS

Morphological Characteristics. *M. tuberculosis* appears as primarily slender, curved rods that are nonmotile, nonsporing, form no demonstrable capsule, but contain characteristic glycogen and polymetaphosphate granules and large mesosomes. *M. avium* is occasionally filamentous, with true branching. The cell walls of tubercle bacilli contain up to 60% lipid, as compared to as much as 20% in gram negative cell walls and 1 to 4% in gram positive cell walls. They are somewhat hydrophobic and relatively impermeable to basic dyes. However, at the boiling point of water, appropriate dyes penetrate the cell wall and stain the interior. Tubercle bacilli retain such dyes even when exposed to acidified solvents (see Ziehl-Neelsen method of staining). Hence, they are called acid-fast microorganisms. Tubercle bacilli appear to be gram positive.

Cultivation and Nutrition. The human tubercle bacillus can be cultured on three general types of media. The first type is an enriched solid medium that is used for initial isolation of tubercle bacilli from an infection. A second type of medium contains a nonionic detergent or wetting agent and provides dispersed growth of tubercle bacilli that have been adapted to artificial cultivation. The third type of medium for tubercle bacilli is chemically defined. Growth is slow, but maximal growth is eventually achieved with this medium.

Chemical Composition. The pathogenicity of tubercle bacilli has been studied with regard to proteins, polysaccharides, and lipids. Proteins comprise up to half of the dry weight of the cell. When administered to nontuberculous animals in very large amounts, they cause fever, hemorrhage, and a slight anemia. In very small amounts they are extremely toxic for tuberculous humans or animals. Such protein is an essential component of the hypersensitive reaction that occurs in tuberculosis. When linked to a waxy factor of the tubercle bacillus and injected into animals, proteins cause a typical tuberculin hypersensitivity.

The polysaccharide fraction of tubercle bacilli comprises only a small portion of their total substance. Tuberculocarbohydrates are not primarily toxic for the normal human or animal body, do not cause the formation of tubercles, and do not produce the tuberculin type of hypersensitivity. Anaphylactic hypersensitivity may develop to the carbohydrates when they are linked to proteins.

The cells of tubercle bacilli and other mycobacteria contain from 20 to 40% lipid that is composed of neutral fats, phospholipids, and waxes: as much as 60% of the cell wall is composed of lipid. Mycosides are glycolipids composed of covalently linked carbohydrates and lipids. The lipids include an interesting group of large saturated fatty acids known as mycolic acids. Virulence of the tubercle bacillus is associated with a mycoside (6, 6'-dimycolyltrehalose). This has the ability to inhibit polymorphonuclear (PMN) leukocyte migration *in vitro* and is lethal to mice. Wax D, another mycoside of high molecular weight, has the capacity to enhance the immunogenicity of many antigens. It is commonly used in a water-in-oil emulsion known as Freund's adjuvant. When wax D is mixed with the proteins of the tubercle bacillus or even saprophytic mycobacteria, it readily induces a delayed-type hypersensitivity. Another lipid fraction, which is quite firmly bound in the cell wall, is related to acid fastness.

TUBERCULOSIS

Introduction. Tuberculosis is an infection with tubercle bacilli which affects principally the lungs, but may involve lymph nodes (scrofula), meninges (meningeal tuberculosis), kidneys (renal tuberculosis), bone or spine (Pott's disease), skin (lupus) (fig. 23/1), and oral cavity. It may take the form of a general infection (miliary tuberculosis), involving one or more of the organs. On the other hand, it may appear to be nothing more than a mild bronchitis. In the individual with little resistance, it is sometimes a fulminating disease, with much destruction of the affected organs.

Clinical Appearance and Pathogenesis. *Primary Infection.* When tubercle bacilli enter the tissues of a nonimmune individual, usually by inhalation, they establish a localized primary infection in which the local reaction is at first negligible. The lower lobes and anterior segments of the upper lobes of the lungs are usually the sites of primary infection. Infection is followed by regional multiplication of organisms, some of which are carried by the lymphatics and bloodstream to numerous sites throughout the body. The patient at this time is asymptomatic or only has mild symptoms of fatigue and irritability. After 2 to 8 weeks, seroconversion

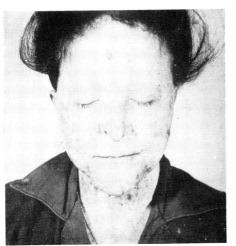

Figure 23/1. Recurrent lupus vulgaris. (AFIP 58-15052-15.)

occurs and the patient demonstrates a positive reaction to the tuberculin skin test. This corresponds to activation of the macrophage response. Although primary infection is accompanied by active multiplication within the foci, the activated macrophages become capable of containing the primary infection. Thus, the activated macrophage response limits the infection. When delayed hypersensitivity develops and granulomatous inflammation occurs, characteristic lesions known as tubercles are formed. The pulmonary focus and granulomatous lesion in the hilar lymph nodes together are called the primary complex. The next stage in the response consists of caseation necrosis wherein the necrotic centers of the lesions become semisolid, and remain as such, rather than softening to form pus. Primary tubercles, particularly in young people, may heal by fibrosis and calcification, producing characteristic radiographic findings. These are called the Ghon complex. In most cases, infection is contained and due to lymphocyte memory the patients retain tuberculin reactivity and immunity from primary reinfection for life.

In approximately 10% of primary infections immunity is inadequate to contain the infection and regional parenchymal multiplication is followed by progressive tissue destruction and liquefaction, followed by discharge of lesions, producing cavitation. This may result in extension of the disease via the bronchi.

Reactivation Disease. Much adult tuberculosis is due to reactivation of dormant foci remaining following primary infection. These frequently are in the lung and persist due to a favorable environment, especially good oxygenation. Reactivation may or may not be associated with identifiable factors such as diabetes, silicosis or corticosteroid therapy.

Once reactivation has occurred the lesion undergoes liquefaction and cavitation and the organisms proliferate. They may enter the bronchi and spread to other parts of the lung and be transmitted to other individuals by aerosol. Extrapulmonary lesions usually develop as a result of reactivation of dormant lesions seeded during primary infection. Indeed, almost 15% of tuberculosis cases involve extrapulmonary sites. Almost any organ may be the site of lesions but especially the lymph nodes, pleura, bones and joints, genitourinary system and peritoneum. The oral cavity is not infrequently involved. If a lesion ruptures into a pulmonary vein miliary or disseminated tuberculosis may result.

Two general types of tissue reactions are evident histologically during infection with tubercle bacilli. The exudative lesion, seen during initial infection, is characterized by inflammation, fluid exudation and accumulation of PMN leukocytes around the bacteria. The productive or granulomatous lesions form when hypersensitivity develops. The macrophages become concentrically arranged in the form of epithelial cells to form the characteristic tubercles (fig. 23/2). In the center, some cells may fuse to form multinucleate giant cells. Outside the concentric layer of cells is a layer of lymphocytes and proliferating fibroblasts, resulting in fibrosis.

ORAL TUBERCULOSIS

Tuberculous lesions, usually circumscribed and walled-off, may occur in any oral tissue or organ. Oral tuberculosis lesions have been reported in the tongue, mandible, maxilla, lip, alveolar process, alveolar sockets, gingivae, cheeks, pharynx, tonsils, salivary glands, and nasal cavity (fig. 23/3). The

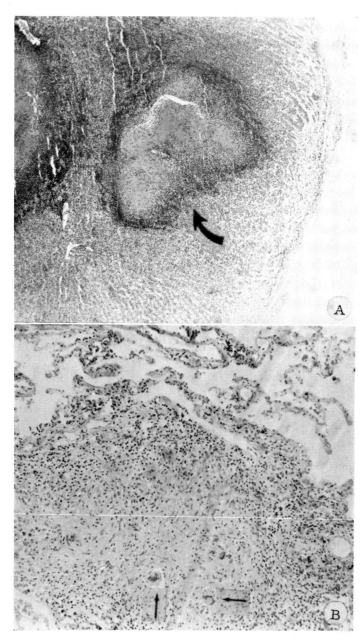

Figure 23/2. Generalized tuberculosis. (*A*) Tubercles, with central caseation about which there is extensive cellular infiltration with erythrocytes and mononuclear cells. Alveoli filled with hemorrhagic exudate. (*B*) Higher magnification of tubercle showing fibrosis and numerous giant cells. (AFIP 162451.)

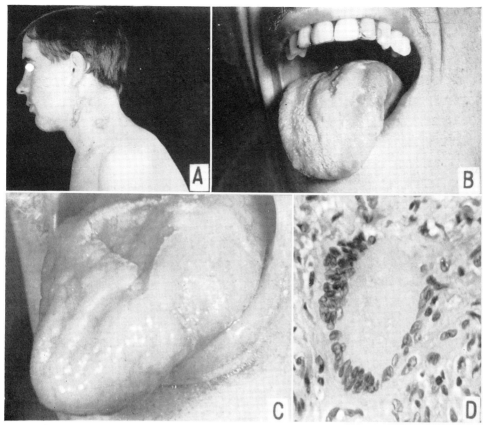

Figure 23/3. Tuberculosis about the oral cavity. (*A*) Tuberculosis of lymph nodes, and scrofula. (*B*) and (*C*) Tuberculosis of the tongue. (*D*) Tubercle. (*A*, AFIP 13926; *B*, AFIP AMH8680; *C*, AFIP 218869; *D*, AMH8680.)

types of lesions encountered have been described as ulcers, gummata, fissures, lupus, hypertrophic gingivitis, tuberculoma, "mouse-eaten" furrowed ulcerations, and granulomas.

Tubercular infection of oral tissues may arise under proper conditions from either an exogenous (from disseminated tubercle bacilli in the oral cavity) or endogenous (via the circulatory system) source of microorganisms. Usually, oral infection is dependent upon a generalized pulmonary involvement, influenced by a concurrent lowering of resistance to infection and possible increase in virulence of the involved microorganisms. Oral tuberculosis has been reported to occur in 3.5% of patients with systemic lesions, and rarely in those who have no systemic infection. Primary infection of the oral tissues does occur without systemic infection, but it is rare. The amount of lymphoid tissue in the area influences tuberculous infection, for the incidence is much less in the anterior than it is in the posterior part of the oral cavity, coinciding with the distribution of lymphoid tissue in these areas. Much protection is afforded against tubercular infection by the flushing and antibacterial action of saliva,

and undoubtedly by the antagonistic action of other oral microorganisms. Trauma from tooth extraction or constant low-grade infection predisposes to oral tuberculous infection if other conditions are favorable.

Tuberculous infection is found in periapical areas or in tooth sockets after extraction in patients with long-standing pulmonary infection. The incidence of this type of infection is about 8%. In tuberculous patients, after extraction, healing is delayed and the socket is filled with a mass of granulation tissue which is sometimes called "tuberculous granulations." This tissue is characterized by numerous small pink or dark red elevations which bleed easily if disturbed. If the granulation tissue is removed by curettage, a healthy blood clot forms, usually followed by normal healing.

Tuberculosis of oral mucous membranes results from advanced pulmonary infection, where it has been found to occur in approximately 20% of consecutive autopsies of tuberculous patients. The incidence of clinically discernible oral lesions in patients with pulmonary tuberculosis has been reported as up to 1.44%. The more common pathological lesions of the oral mucosa are ulcerative, miliary, and infiltrative, and the less common are the granuloma, tuberculous fissure, and cold abscess. The ulcerative type is the most common. The mucous membranes of the soft and hard palate are most often affected. The surface of the tongue is occasionally affected, with the lesions occurring near the base where they are not likely to be discovered by the usual clinical examination. Lesions are found less often upon the buccal mucosa. The oral tuberculous lesion of soft tissue is initiated in lymphoid tissue, where it produces chronic inflammation, loss of stratified squamous epithelium, and ulceration. Hyperplasia, degeneration, and leukocytic infiltration of the deeper tissues occur, together with granulation and tubercle formation.

Tuberculous lesions also occur, though rarely, in the maxilla and mandible, where they usually cause an osteomyelitis. The development of swelling is characteristic of the disease, and there may or may not be pain. When fully developed, the swelling ruptures spontaneously and sinuses are established through which small sequestra are discharged. The mandible seems to be affected more often than the maxilla, but there are few valid data to indicate how often infection of either area occurs. Infection of the mandible or maxilla is regarded as primary if the mucous membrane is not initially affected, and secondary if the mucous membrane is attacked first with subsequent involvement of the underlying bone.

Several cases of tuberculosis of the salivary glands have been reported in the literature, affecting mostly people in the second and third decades of life. The parotid gland is affected most often and the sublingual gland is seldom affected. In more than three-fourths of the cases there was no family or personal history of tuberculosis. There appear to be two types of salivary tubercular lesions. One is chronic and encapsulated, requiring many years to develop, the other is acutely inflammatory, requiring only a few days or weeks to develop. Clinically, they first appear as small swellings or tumors which are usually freely movable.

Immunity. Initial infection with tubercle bacilli results in an allergy to tuberculoprotein that modifes the reaction to reinfection. The effect of tuberculin allergy on reinfection by tubercle bacilli was originally demonstrated by Robert Koch (Koch phenomenon) in guinea pigs. When virulent tubercle bacilli are inoculated into a normal guinea pig, a persistent ulcer develops after several weeks at the site of the inoculation and tubercles are found in the regional lymph nodes. In a tuberculous guinea pig, injection of tubercle bacilli produces a transient, superficial ulcer which appears faster, is more acute but is well circumscribed and heals quickly, and the regional lymph nodes are unaffected. Thus, initial infection or exposure to tubercle bacilli in either guinea pigs or man results in sensitization or altered tissue reactivity that modifies any reinfection. Modifying factors are the inability of tubercle bacilli to multiply as rapidly in the sensitized animal as in the normal animal and the slowness with which the tubercle bacilli spread in lymphatics of the sensitized animal. Immunity or altered reactivity in tuberculosis relates to the state of the macrophages. Tubercle bacilli survive quite well in the macrophages of a normal animal. On the other hand, following exposure to tubercle bacilli macrophages become activated and then have an increased bactericidal activity, thus disposing of the organisms. The development of tuberculin sensitivity is both partially protective and potentially harmful. The exposure of a sensitive individual to tubercle bacilli may result in severe reactions in the lung and may cause the spread of the disease.

Epidemiology. The incidence of tuberculosis has gradually decreased in the United States over the last 100 years. At the beginning of the decline, the incidence of tuberculosis and the mortality rate was highest in children, but active disease and mortality rate of tuberculosis was lowest in old age. Since that time, the risk of exposure has decreased in children, and the mortality rate has shifted from a peak in childhood to the current group of elderly individuals. This group had a high rate of exposure to tuberculosis in childhood and most acquired a primary infection that established henceforth a dormant focus of viable tubercle bacilli. The relatively high incidence of infection in the present elderly group is caused principally by reactivation of their dormant tuberculosis foci.

Active Immunization. Most current attempts at active immunization of man use a vaccine composed of living, attenuated tubercle bacilli. An attenuated bovine strain developed by Calmette and Guérin (BCG) is used almost universally, but a live vaccine is also made of strains of the vole bacillus (*Mycobacterium microti*). The efficacy of such vaccines has ranged from 0 to 80% in several studies and the reasons for such variation are not clear. Even with a vaccine, a question remains as to the necessity of vaccination, especially in western populations. Furthermore, BCG has been associated with a variety of adverse reactions. Such reactions, coupled with tuberculin conversion, making the tuberculin skin test virtually useless as a screening measure, makes the recommendation that vaccination against tuberculosis be used only under limited circumstances seem prudent.

Tuberculin and the Tuberculin Reaction. An experimental animal or human sensitized to tubercle bacilli through infection or by vaccination reacts characteristically to several soluble components of the cells, termed tuberculins. The active constituents are the proteins of the bacilli. There are several types of tuberculin, the more important of which are:

1. Original or old tuberculin (OT), which is prepared by evaporating a 6-week broth culture to approximately ¹⁄₁₀ its original volume, after which any remaining intact cells are removed by filtration.

2. Purified protein derivative (PPD), which is a protein fraction precipitated by trichloroacetic acid or ammonium sulfate from the autoclaved supernatants of cultures of tubercle bacilli grown in synthetic media.

A method of testing for tuberculin sensitivity (Mantoux test) is to inject PPD intracutaneously on the flexor surface of the forearm. The test is positive if within 24 to 48 hours an indurated area of inflammation, 10 mm or more in diameter, develops at the site.

A less sensitive method of tuberculin testing is the patch test, in which a small piece of filter paper, impregnated with tuberculin, is taped to the skin. The test is positive if an inflammatory, often vesiculated, reaction develops after several days.

A single positive tuberculin reaction indicates present or previous infection with tubercle bacilli but tells nothing of the current activity of the process. A positive test within several months of previously negative tests indicates that the individual is undergoing or recovering from an initial infection. A negative test is particularly useful in excluding tuberculosis during diagnosis and in epidemiological studies.

Bacteriological Diagnosis. Tubercle bacilli may be found in the sputum or urine, in the intestinal tract from swallowed sputum, or in infected tissue. They may be detected in sputum, intestinal contents, or urine by examining a direct smear for acid-fast bacilli. The tubercle bacilli may be cultured on appropriate media, with visible growth occurring after incubation for two to five weeks, or they may be inoculated into the groin or thigh muscle of a guinea pig.

Treatment. After 1940 several chemicals came into use which radically changed the treatment of tuberculosis. Streptomycin and *para*-aminosalicylic acid (PAS), either singly or in combination, were put into common use in the United States. PAS requires relatively large oral doses to be effective in the treatment of tuberculosis and produces gastrointestinal side effects. Thus, it is not generally used as a primary drug. Streptomycin, which is rapidly active against tubercle bacilli, was considered most effective against tuberculosis in the exudative phase. However, the organisms may become resistant to it, for the treatment of tuberculosis is necessarily prolonged. Consequently, there is also serious danger of permanent damage by the streptomycin to the eighth cranial nerve. Isonicotinic

acid hydrazide (isoniazid or INH) then came into use as the single most effective drug for treatment of tuberculosis. It is relatively inexpensive, has low toxicity, and is effective when given orally, even in small doses. Rifampin has also come into use as a very effective drug for treating tuberculosis, particularly when used in combination with isoniazid. Rifampin is absorbed well when given orally, and is relatively nontoxic. Similarly, ethambutol hydrochloride is effective when used in combination with isoniazid. There are other chemotherapeutics that can be used in the treatment of tuberculosis, although they are usually used when the primary drugs cannot be used because of allergy or development of microbial resistance. These drugs include pyrazinamide, ethionamide, cycloserine, viomycin, capreomycin, and kanamycin.

Isoniazid can be used successfully for prophylactic chemotherapy of tuberculosis. It has brought about a decrease of 50% in active cases of tuberculosis when applied to persons that have recently become tuberculin positive. Its use has been particularly effective when used to treat household contacts.

MYCOBACTERIUM LEPRAE

The cells of *M. leprae* are acid-fast, gram positive, nonspore-forming, nonmotile rods. They stain more easily and are less acid-fast than *M. tuberculosis*. *M. leprae* is an obligate parasite of man, in whom they grow profusely in tissues and organs, causing leprosy. *M. leprae* has not been cultured *in vitro* and is not readily transmitted to laboratory animals or higher primates. By serial passage in certain strains of mice, transmissible mutants arise which eventually establish a progressive infection. *M. leprae* also infects the foot pad of mice, but even after serial passage, remains confined to the foot pad. Recent evidence indicates that the armadillo is susceptible to infection with leprosy bacilli.

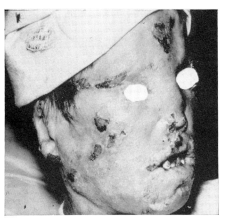

Figure 23/4. Advanced leprosy. (AFIP 43.)

Leprosy

Course and Appearance. At the present time leprosy is prevalent in Central and South America, Southeast Asia, China, Africa, and India; the incidence is highest in Central Africa. It is estimated that there are as many as 5,000,000 lepers in the world today.

Transmission of leprosy usually requires long and close contact between a person with the disease and a susceptible person, children being the most susceptible. The incubation period ranges between 2 and 3 years, but may be as long as 30 years.

Essentially two types of disease develop, the cutaneous and the neural. The cutaneous disease is more acute and progresses more rapidly. It is characterized by the development of large masses of granulation tissue, called lepromas, which occur superficially, causing distortion and mutilation (figs. 23/4 and 23/5). The neural type is longer in development and duration. It affects principally the nerves, causing localized areas of anesthesia or paralysis. This can result in deformities of the feet and hands (fig. 23/6), loss of facial expression, inability to close the eyes, and an increased incidence of minor trauma leading to secondary infection.

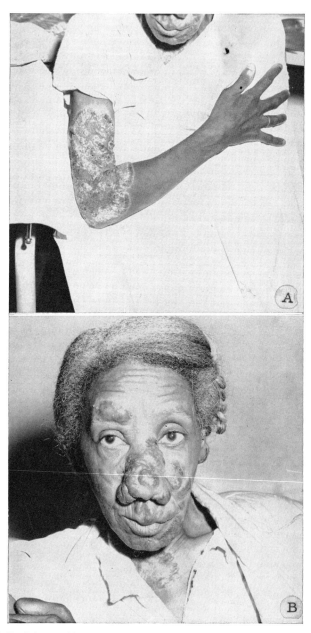

Figure 23/5. Advanced lepromatous leprosy. (*A*, AFIP 54-18444; *B*, AFIP 54-18443.)

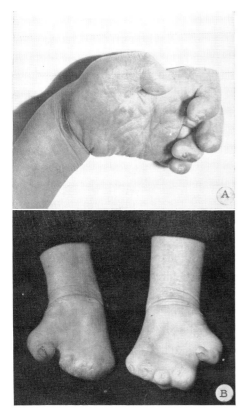

Figure 23/6. Lepromatous leprosy showing "claw" hand (A) and extensive destruction of the fingers (B). (AFIP 45-14075.)

While numerous leprosy bacilli are found in both types of the disease, the most organisms are found in the nodular type. Most lesions of leprosy are found in the cooler portions of the body. In addition to the typical lesions which appear about the nose and face, leprosy also affects the mucous membranes of the lips, mouth, and nasopharynx. Initial lesions are usually flat nodules which develop first as mere swellings in the lips (lepromas). In later stages of leprosy, the tongue may be affected by lesions ranging from a mild glossitis to nodules along the anterior third, and less commonly the whole tongue. In the late stages, nodular lesions may appear in the hard and soft palate and the uvula, sometimes causing perforation of the palate.

Pathology. Pathologically, there are two principal phases of leprosy, lepromatous and tuberculoid.

Lesions of the lepromatous type develop in infected persons who have little or no resistance or when the disease is in a progressive phase. The leprosy bacilli multiply in macrophages with a characteristically foamy cytoplasm that are termed lepra cells; in these cells the organisms are abundant. In advanced disease, the membranes of the lepra cells are destroyed and the freed leprosy bacilli

form globular masses which are also sometimes found in the foreign body type of giant cells.

Skin lesions of the tuberculoid type develop in infected persons with considerable resistance or in a healing phase of disease. The lesions contain few bacilli and fibrosis is prominent.

Diagnosis. The diagnosis of leprosy is by clinical examination and by the microscopic demonstration of leprosy bacilli in tissue from suspected lesions or in scrapings from the nasal mucosa. Leprosy may be confused with syphilis, yaws, tuberculosis of the skin, ringworm, and neuritis.

Lepromin, analogous to tuberculin, is used in a skin test for leprosy. It is more useful in determining prognosis or phase of the disease than in actual diagnosis because of possible false positive reactions.

Control of Leprosy. The control of leprosy by segregation is still in current use, even though the disease is not very communicable. The modern forms of segregation are institutional or in the home. It might seem that compulsory segregation would eliminate leprosy in one generation but it does not. The detection of early leprosy is difficult, and it is during this stage that the disease is most easily transmitted to children. Since compulsory segregation is akin to corporal punishment, lepers often attempt to escape detection and will resist segregation as long as possible, thereby defeating the attempt at prevention.

Since 1921 a modified form of compulsory segregation has been practiced in the United States, with lepers being confined to the National Leprosarium at Carville, Louisiana. The National Leprosarium receives and cares for lepers who are referred to it by local or state health authorities or go voluntarily in order to receive treatment. Home segregation of lepers is very difficult and not very satisfactory.

Treatment. Diaminodiphenysulfone, or related sulfone compounds are drugs of choice in the treatment of leprosy. They produce a gradual improvement over several years, although resistance may occur after prolonged treatment. There is some indication that rifampin may be useful in the treatment of leprosy.

ADDITIONAL READING

ADDINGTON, W. W. 1979 The Treatment of Pulmonary Tuberculosis. Arch Int Med, **139**, 1391.

ANITA, N. H. 1974 The Significance of Nerve Involvement in Leprosy. Plast Reconstr Surg, **54**, 55.

ARANGO, L., BREWIN, A. W., AND MURRAY, J. F. 1973 The Spectrum of Tuberculosis as Currently Seen in a Metropolitan Hospital. Am Rev Respir Dis, **108**, 805.

ARBOUR, M., AND L'ARCHEVEQUE, A. 1973 Tuberculosis of Atypical Mycobacterium. Union Med, **102**, 2122.

BANNER, A. S. 1979 Tuberculosis Clinical Aspects and Diagnosis. Arch Intern Med, **139**, 1387.

BALENTINE, J. D., CHANG, S. C., AND ISSAR, S. L. 1976 Infection of Armadillos with *Mycobacterium leprae*. Arch Pathol Lab Med, **100,** 175.

BLUMBERG, B. S., MELARTIN, L., GUINTO, R., AND LE-CHAT, M. 1970 Lepromatous Leprosy. J Chronic Dis, **23,** 507.

BROWNE, S. G. 1975 The Drug Treatment of Leprosy. Practitioner, **215,** 493.

BURRELL, R., AND LEWIS, D. M. 1975 Further Studies on the Effect of Lung Antibodies on the Pathogenesis of Tuberculosis. J Lab Clin Med, **86,** 741.

BUSYGINA, M. V. 1965 Conditions of the Oral Cavity of Children of Lepromatous Patients. Stomatologiia (Mosk), **44,** 38.

BYRD, C. B., NELSON, R., AND ELLIOTT, R. C. 1972 Isoniazid Toxicity. JAMA, **220,** 1471.

CALDERARI, G. 1965 Considerations on a Case of Tubercular Osteitis of the Mandible. Intern Stomatol Pract, **16,** 287.

CHEN, T. S. N., DRUTZ, D. J., AND WHELAN, G. E. 1976 Hepatic Granulomas in Leprosy. Arch Pathol Lab Med, **100,** 182.

CHRISTENSEN, W. I. 1974 Genitourinary Tuberculosis: Review of 102 Cases. Medicine, **53,** 377.

CHUN, Y. E., CHANG, C. H. J., AND NYKA, W. 1972 New Observations Concerning the Development of Resistant Bacilli in Pulmonary Tuberculosis. Clin Med, **79,** 15.

COCHRANE, R. G., AND DAVEY, T. F. (EDS.) 1964 *Leprosy in Theory and Practice,* Ed. 2. Wright, Bristol, England.

COLOMBO, E. 1964 Tuberculosis of the Mucosa of the Hard Palate. Arch Ital Otolaryngol, **75,** 667.

COMSTOCK, G. W. 1975 False Tuberculin Test Results. Chest, **68S,** 465S.

DANNENBERG, A. M., JR., ANDO, M., AND SHIMA, K. 1972 Macrophage Accumulation, Division, Maturation, and Digestive and Microbicidal Capacities in Tuberculous Lesions; III. The Turnover of Macrophages and Its Relation to Their Activation and Antimicrobial Immunity in Primary BCG Lesions and Those of Reinfection. J Immunol, **109,** 1109.

DARLINGTON, C. C., AND SOLMAN, I. 1935 Oral Tuberculous Lesions. Am Rev Tuberc, **35,** 147.

DAVIS, R. K., BAER, P. N., ARCHARD, H. O., AND PALMER, J. H. 1964 Tuberculous Sclerosis with Oral Manifestations. Report of Two Cases. Oral Surg, **17,** 395.

DEL RIO, A. L. 1936 Clinical Contribution to the Study of Leprosy of the Ear, Nose, and Throat. Ann Laringol, **36,** 80.

DONOHUE, W. B., AND BOLDEN, T. E. 1961 Tuberculosis of the Salivary Glands. Oral Surg, **14,** 576.

EHRENKRANZ, N. J., AND KICKLIGHTER, J. L. 1972 Tuberculosis Outbreak in a General Hospital: Evidence for Airborne Spread of Infection. Ann Intern Med, **77,** 377.

FEIN, S. 1974 Tuberculous Cervical Lymphadenitis (Scrofula). J Oral Surg, **32,** 31.

FELTON, C. P., AND JONES, J. M. 1973 Acute Forms of Tuberculosis. Med Clin North Am, **57,** 1395.

FITCH, H. B., AND ALLING, C. C. 1963 Leprosy, Oral Manifestations. J Periodontol, **33,** 40.

GARDNER, J. A., AND HANFT, R. J. 1961 A Tuberculosis Granuloma of the Oral Mucosa and Cervical Lymph Glands. Oral Surg, **14,** 406.

GEPPERT, E. F., AND LEFF, A. 1979 The Pathogenesis of Pulmonary and Miliary Tuberculosis. Arch Int Med, **139,** 1381.

GLASSROTH, J., ROBINS, A. G., AND SNIDER, D. E. 1980 Tuberculosis in the 1980's. N Engl J Med, **302,** 1441.

GODAL, T., AND NEGASSI, K. 1973 Subclinical Infection in Leprosy. Br Med J, **3,** 557.

GOLDEN, G. S., McCORMICK, J. B., AND FRASER, D. W. 1977 Leprosy in the United States, 1971–73. J Infect Dis, **135,** 120.

GONDZIK, W., AND JARZYNKA, W. 1964 Histopathological Studies on the Dental Pulp in Normal Subjects and in Pulmonary Tuberculosis Patients. Rocz Pomorskiej Akad Med Szczecin, **10,** 319.

GUNNELS, J. J., BATES, J. H., AND SWINDOLL, H. 1974 Infectivity of Sputum-Positive Tuberculous Patients on Chemotherapy. Am Rev Respir Dis, **109,** 323.

HARADA, K. 1976 The Nature of Mycobacterial Acid-Fastness. Stain Technol, **51,** 255.

HARRIS, B. C., TAYLOR, C. G., AND WADE, W. W., JR. 1973 Miliary Tuberculosis with Oral Manifestations. J Oral Surg, **31,** 305.

HIRSH, F. S., AND SAFFOLD, O. E. 1976 *Mycobacterium kansasii* Infection with Dermatologic Manifestations. Arch Dermatol, **112,** 706.

HJORTING-HANSEN, E. 1965 Leprotic Granuloma in the Maxilla. Int J Lepr, **33,** 83.

HUTT, M. S. R. 1974 *Mycobacterium ulcerans* Infection. Br J Dermatol, **91,** 34.

JOHNSTON, R. F., AND WILDRICK, K. H. 1974 The Impact of Chemotherapy on the Care of Patients with Tuberculosis. Am Rev Respir Dis, **109,** 636.

JOLLY, H. W., JR. 1975 Atypical Mycobacterial Infections of the Skin: Treatment. Dermatol Dig, **14,** 16.

KIRCHHEIMER, W. F., AND SANCHEZ, R. M. 1973 Leprosy-Susceptibility of Armadillos. Microbios, **1,** 31.

KENNEDY, C., AND KNOWLES, G. K. 1975 Miliary Tuberculosis Presenting with Skin Lesions. Br Med J, **3,** 356.

KÖDEL, G. 1964 Tubercular Infection in Maxillar-Dental Cysts. Rev Fr Odonto-stomatol, **11,** 1477.

KÖDEL, G. 1964 Tuberculosis of the Jaws and Adjacent Regions. Stoma, **17,** 22.

KRONVALL, G., STANFORD, J. L., AND WALSH, G. P. Studies of Mycobacterial Antigens, with Special Reference to *Mycobacterium leprae*. Infect Immun, **3,** 1132.

KWAPINSKI, J. B. G., BECHELLI, L. M., HADDAD, N., AND SIMAO, E. T. 1975 Impairment of Reactivity to Lepromin by Mycobacterial Antigens Related to, or Identical with, *Mycobacterium leprae*. Can J Microbiol, **21,** 896.

LAGERLÖF, B. 1964 Tuberculous Lesions of the Oral Mucosa. Oral Surg, **17,** 1735.

LEFF, A., AND GEPPERT, E. F. 1979 Public Health and Preventive Aspects of Pulmonary Tuberculosis. Arch Int Med, **139,** 1405.

LEIKER, D. L. 1966 Classification of Leprosy. Lepr Rev, **37,** 7.

LIGHTERMAN, I. 1962 Leprosy of the Oral Cavity and Adnexa. Oral Surg, **15,** 1178.

LYE, R. H. 1974 Primary Pulmonary Tuberculosis: A Retrospective Study in Rochdale Children. Practitioner, **212,** 715.

MANSFIELD, R. E., AND BINFORD, C. H. 1976 The Histopathologic Diagnosis of Leprosy. South Med J, **69,** 986.

MARILL, F. G. 1965 Tuberculosis Macrocheilitis. Bull Soc Fr Dermatol Syph, **72,** 362.

MAZUNDER, J. K. 1953 A Survey on Oral Manifestations of Tropical Diseases. Int Dent J, **4,** 209.

McCLATCHY, J. K. 1971 Mechanism of Action of Isoniazid on *Mycobacterium bovis* Strain BCG. Infect Immun, **3,** 530.

McDONALD, P. J., MURRAY, C. J., AND McDONALD, H. M. 1974 Antibiotics, Antiseptics, and Tubercle Bacilli. Med J Aust, **2,** 41.

MEISELS, A., AND FORTIN, R. 1975 Genital Tuberculosis: Cytologic Detection. Acta Cytol, **19,** 79.

MILLER, R. L., KRUTCHKOFF, D. J., AND GRAMMARA, B. S. 1978 Human Lingual Tuberculosis. Arch Pathol Lab Med, **102**, 360.

NAVALKAR, R. G., PATEL, P. J., AND DALVI, R. R. 1974 Immunological Studies on Leprosy: Separation and Evaluation of the Antigens of *Mycobacterium leprae.* J Med Microbiol, **8**, 319.

NOORDEEN, S. K. 1969 Chemoprophylaxis in Leprosy. Lepr India, **41**, 247.

ORD, R. J., AND MATZ, G. J. 1974 Tuberculous Cervical Lymphadenitis. Arch Otolaryngol, **99**, 327.

OWENS, D. W. 1974 General Medical Aspects of Atypical Mycobacteria. South Med J, **67**, 39.

PODLESKI, W. K., AND PODLESKI, U. G. 1973 Circulating Cytotoxic Lymphocytes in Human Tuberculosis. Am Rev Respir Dis, **108**, 791.

PORRES, J. M. 1973 Isolation of *Mycobacterium rhodochrous* from a Cutaneous Lesion. Arch Dermatol, **108**, 411.

RADFORD, A. J. 1973 The Nomenclature of *Mycobacterium ulcerans* Infections. Trans R Soc Trop Med Hyg, **67**, 885.

RAMOS, A. D., HIBBARD, L. T., AND CRAIG, J. R. 1974 Congenital Tuberculosis. Obstet Gynecol, **43**, 61.

REA, T. H., AND LEVAN, N. E. 1975 Erythema Nodosum Leprosum in a General Hospital. Arch Dermatol, **111**, 1575.

READ, J. K., HEGGIE, C. M., MEYERS, W. M., AND CONNOR, D. H. 1974 Cytotoxic Activity of *Mycobacterium ulcerans.* Infect Immun, **9**, 114.

REICHART, P., ANANATASAN, T., AND REZNIK, G. 1976 Gingiva and Periodontium in Lepromatous Leprosy. J Periodontol, **47**, 455.

REICHMAN, L. B. 1973 Routine Follow-up of Inactive Tuberculosis—A Practice That Has Been Abandoned. Am Rev Respir Dis, **108**, 1442.

REICHMANN, J. 1965 Tuberculosis of the Parotid Gland. Zentralbl Chir, **90**, 689.

Ridley, D. S. 1974 Histological Classification and the Immunological Spectrum of Leprosy. Bull WHO, **51**, 451.

RUBIN, E. H. 1927 Tuberculosis of the Buccal Mucous Membrane. Am Rev Tuberc, **16**, 39.

SAHN, S. A., AND NEFF, T. A. 1974 Miliary Tuberculosis. Am J Med, **56**, 495.

SBARBARO, J. A. 1975 Tuberculosis: The New Challenge to the Practicing Clinician. Chest, **68S**, 436S.

SCHWARTZ, S. H. 1972 Tuberculosis: Surveillance or Control. Am Rev Respir Dis, **106**, 897.

SHAPIRO, C. D. K., HARDING, G. E., AND SMITH, D. W. 1974 Relationship of Delayed-type Hypersensitivity and Acquired Cellular Resistance in Experimental Airborne Tuberculosis. J Infect Dis, **130**, 8.

SHENGOLD, M. A., AND SHEINGOLD, H. 1951 Oral Tuberculosis. Oral Surg, **20**, 29.

SOLOMON, D. A., AND GRACEY, D. R. 1974 Modern Concepts in Treating Tuberculosis. Geriatrics, **29**, 110.

STEAD, W. W. 1975 Goals and Productivity of Tuberculosis Screening. Chest, **68S**, 446S.

STEVENSON, D. K. 1974 Pulmonary Tuberculosis. Practitioner, **212**, 320.

TAYLOR, R. G., AND BOOTH, D. F. 1964 Tuberculosis Osteomyelitis of the Mandible. Oral Surg, **18**, 7.

TIZES, R., AND ZUCKERMAN, S. 1972 Tuberculosis in Suburbia—New Indices for an Old Disease. Am J Public Health, **62**, 1586.

TORTORELLI, A. F. 1964 Tuberculosis of the Mouth. J Clin Stomatol Conf, **5**, 13.

TRAUTMAN, J. R. 1965 The Management of Leprosy and Its Complications. N Engl J Med, **273**, 756.

TSUKAMURA, M., MIZUNO, S., MURATA, H., NEMOTO, H., AND YUGI, H. 1974 A Comparative Study of Mycobacteria from Patients' Room Dusts and from Sputa of Tuberculous Patients. Source of Pathogenic Mycobacteria Occurring in the Sputa of Tuberculous Patients as Casual Isolates. Jpn J Microbiol, **18**, 271.

VIOLANTE, E. 1964 On Tuberculosis of the Salivary Glands. Gior Ital Chir; **20**, 709.

WEAVER, R. A. 1976 Tuberculosis of the Tongue. JAMA, **235**, 2418.

WERELDS, R. J. 1965 The Possible Role of the Tooth in Oral Tuberculosis. Acta Stomatol Belg, **62**, 361.

WINBLAD, B. 1975 Male Genital Tuberculosis—The Possibility of Lymphatic Spread. Acta Pathol Microbiol Scand, Sect A, **83**, 425.

WINBLAD, B., BUCHEK, M., AND HOLM, S. 1975 Experimental Male Genital Tuberculosis—Appraisal of Protective Value of BCG Vaccination. Acta Pathol Microbiol Scand, Sect A, **83**, 415.

WOLSTENHOLME, G. E. W., AND O'CONNOR, M. (EDS.) 1963 *Pathogenesis of Leprosy.* Little, Brown, Boston.

ZANOLLI, P. 1964 Tuberculosis of the Parotid Gland. Chir Patol Sper, *12*, 148.

chapter 24

Yersinia, Francisella, and Pasteurella

George S. Schuster

The organisms described in this chapter are all gram negative, facultative or aerobic rods. They cause zoonoses, infections that are naturally transmitted between lower vertebrates and man. Included are the *Yersinia*, that causes plague and other infections; *Francisella*, that causes tularemia; and the pasteurellae.

YERSINIA PESTIS

Morphology and Cultivation. *Y. pestis* is a gram negative, nonmotile rod, usually 1 to 2 μm in length, that shows bipolar staining. Under less than optimal growth conditions plague bacilli are pleomorphic. Virulent strains produce a large capsule.

The plague bacillus is facultative, growing either aerobically or anaerobically at an optimum temperature of 28 C. A large inoculum is required to initiate growth in ordinary nutrient media, so complex media have been devised for obtaining growth from small inocula and for primary isolation. Repeated subculturing of the plague bacillus anaerobically reduces its virulence.

Virulence. *Y. pestis* is highly virulent. When freshly isolated from human or rodent infections, only a few plague bacilli are fatal in a guinea pig. Virulence can be maintained by repeated passage in susceptible animals, storage of cultures at 4 C or by drying from the frozen state. Diminution of virulence is effected by rapid, repeated subculture, culturing in the presence of ethanol, passage through immune animals, or by bacteriophage action.

Plague bacilli contain a toxin which resembles an exotoxin in that it can be easily converted into a toxoid. It also produces a lipopolysaccharide endotoxin that behaves pharmacologically similar to those of enteric bacilli but has a greater LD_{50} for animals.

Antigenic Structure. Virulent plague bacilli possess at least ten different antigens. Immunological methods have defined an "envelope" or capsular (F1) antigen, a somatic antigen, and the toxin. Virulent strains produce more of the envelope antigens than do avirulent strains. The envelope antigen, composed of a heat-labile protein, is antiphagocytic, highly soluble in water, difficult to demonstrate as a definite capsule, and is thermolabile. It seems to be an essential immunizing antigen. The somatic antigen is of unproved immunological significance.

Bacteriophages. Numerous bacteriophages specific for the plague bacillus have been isolated. Attempts to use bacteriophage in the treatment of experimental plague have not been successful, at least in part because the phage may lyse the infecting plague bacilli enough to release lethal amounts of the toxin.

PLAGUE

Plague in the United States. Plague has existed in Hawaii since 1899 and since 1900 it has occurred in several cities in the continental United States. Wild rodent or sylvatic plague is now prevalent in the western United States. The three groups of rodents constituting the primary reservoirs are ground squirrels, wood rats, prairie dogs, and occasionally sage brush voles and meadow mice. Human plague has been contracted from wild rodents directly or through their fleas throughout the western states.

Human Plague. Plague is transmitted to man from infected rats or other rodents by the bite of infected fleas. Except in pneumonic plague, direct transfer of *Y. pestis* from person to person rarely, if ever, occurs. Following the flea bite type of infection the organisms enter the lymphatics and reach the lymph nodes, usually in the groin where they cause them to become enlarged and tender, forming buboes (literally a swelling in the groin). An initial bacteremia may distribute the bacilli to the spleen, liver, and bone marrow. If the action of the reticuloendothelial system is sufficient to remove the circulating bacilli, the initial bacteremia or septicemia develops.

Bubonic plague has an average incubation period of 3 or 4 days, sudden onset, high fever, unusually rapid pulse, disturbed sensorium, prostration, and average mortality from 60 to 90% within 3 to 5 days. As plague bacilli die they release toxin, which causes widespread hemorrhagic and degenerative changes.

A less common but very dangerous type of human plague is the primary pneumonic variety. Originating in the pneumonia secondary to bubonic plague, this highly contagious form of the disease is transmitted from man to man by droplets of infected sputum. The plague bacilli multiply uninhibited in the lungs, release large quantities of toxin, and cause death within two days.

Immunity. In humans, recovery from an attack of plague produces solid immunity and reinfection is rare. Acquired immunity is essentially antiinfectious and to a lesser extent antitoxic.

Several types of vaccines, consisting of formalin- or heat-killed virulent bacilli or living avirulent bacilli, have been used to immunize against plague infection. The degree of vaccine efficacy under field conditions is not certain.

Antisera for passive immunization are commonly obtained from rabbits and horses. A variety of antigens have been used: killed plague cultures, filtrates of broth cultures, live virulent bacilli, live avirulent bacilli, toxoids, "envelope" antigens, and F1 antigen.

Laboratory Diagnosis. Culture of organisms for the laboratory diagnosis of plague is dangerous and maximal care must be exercised. The methods of diagnosis used must produce rapid results. Bacteriological diagnosis consists of the identification of *Y. pestis* in gram stained smears of sputum or tissue exudate from a bubo. *Y. pestis* can be isolated by culturing on blood agar. Plague bacilli can be rapidly identified by fluorescent antibody staining or lysis with appropriate bacteriophage. Animal inoculation, particularly guinea pigs, is sometimes used if the specimen is grossly contaminated with other bacteria.

Treatment. The early use of streptomycin, chloramphenicol, or tetracyclines reduces the mortality rate of plague below 5%. A few strains of *Y. pestis* become resistant to streptomycin, which may be overcome by the concurrent administration of either chloramphenicol or tetracycline.

Control and Prevention. The best method for the control of plague is the eradication of commensal rats, other rodents, and fleas. The rodent-flea-rodent cycle can be broken at least temporarily by insecticides and rodenticides.

YERSINIA PSEUDOTUBERCULOSIS AND YERSINIA ENTEROCOLITICA

Y. pseudotuberculosis and *Y. enterocolitica*, both are relatively large pleomorphic, gram negative, sometimes motile rods that exhibit bipolar staining. They are distinguished from each other by differences in biochemical characteristics, susceptibility to bacteriophages, the pathogenicity by antigenic differences, and by differences in susceptibility to antibiotics.

The most common manifestation of *Y. enterocolitica* is an acute gastroenteritis or enterocolitis, especially in children. It also may cause terminal ileitis or mesenteric lymphadenitis. The organisms are usually transmitted in food or water but person-to-person transmission may occur as well.

Y. pseudotuberculosis infection usually manifests as terminal ileitis or mesenteric lymphadenitis. The probable route of transmission to man is through food contaminated with animal excreta.

FRANCISELLA AND TULAREMIA

Francisella tularensis. *F. tularensis* is a gram negative, pleomorphic microorganism that is primarily rod-shaped, although coccoid forms predominate in young cultures and rods in older cultures. It is a facultative anaerobe but grows best aerobically. *F. tularensis* stains satisfactorily with crystal violet and carbol fuchsin but not with methylene blue.

F. tularensis is cytotropic and accordingly difficult to cultivate. It reproduces by budding rather than by binary fission. It will grow on initial isolation on cystine-glucose-blood agar or in enriched broth media. After initial isolation, simpler media can be used for growth. *F. tularensis* can be cultured also in chick embryo tissue, in embryonated eggs, where it grows mostly in the yolk sac, and in albino mice.

Smooth and rough colonial variants of *F. tularensis* occur, most nonsmooth strains being avirulent and most smooth forms being virulent.

Antigens. Several kinds of antigens have been extracted from *F. tularensis*, but only a single antigenic type has been identified. The cell wall antigens demonstrated include a soluble, specific polysaccharide antigen that gives a wheal-type reaction in the skin of convalescent human patients; a protein antigen which elicits agglutinins; and an endotoxin whose role in pathogenesis is similar to that of *Salmonella typhi*.

Tularemia. Tularemia occurs most frequently in the United States and Russia, although it has been reported from European countries, Canada, Mexico, Venezuela, and Japan. It has occurred in virtually every one of the United States. Tularemia occurs seasonally, in the summer in the western United States and in the winter months in the eastern United States.

In the United States, tularemia is primarily an infection of wild mammals, but the principal sources of human infection are the cottontail rabbit and, in the western states, the jack rabbit. Tularemia is usually transmitted from animal to animal (and occasionally to man) by bloodsucking insects.

F. tularensis survives in the environment, in water and soil, and in animal products, which serve as alternative media for its transmission to man. It is unusually hazardous to work with in the laboratory and pneumonic form may result from inhalation of infected droplets.

The clinical manifestations of tularemia generally resemble those of bubonic plague. Tularemia may simulate several other diseases such as influenza or pneumonia. In man the clinical diseases are ulceroglandular; typhoidal, oculoglandular, glandular, pulmonary, or ingestive types. The mortality rate varies with the type of disease.

The incubation period of tularemia is from 2 to 5 days but may extend to 10 days. Prodromal symptoms are rare and the onset is sudden. The disease has a febrile, influenza-like nature, with headaches, fever, chills, profuse sweats, body pain, nausea, vomiting, and prostration. Fever from 102 to 104 F (39 to 40C) is constantly present during the first 2 to 4 weeks of the disease, although it may persist for months, with an initial rise, a remission, and a secondary rise.

In the ulceroglandular type of tularemia, a primary lesion in the form of a small red papule usually but not always develops at the site of infection, which is commonly the upper extremities, face, or conjunctivae. This papule enlarges and ulcerates, forming an indolent ulcer with raised edges and a ragged floor (fig. 24/1). From the site of the initial infection, *F. tularensis* invades along superficial and deep lymphatics, producing dermal lymphangitic nodules, regional lymphadenitis, and buboes.

In most cases with a favorable prognosis, the antibody titer begins to rise about 1 week after the onset of the disease, coinciding with the disappearance of the initial bacteremia and the beginning of the abatement of lesions and symptoms. In unfavorable cases, a septicemia develops from foci of necrosis or is continually present, producing miliary foci of necrosis in many organs and glands.

Eighty percent of primary lesions of tularemia occur about the fingers, but initial lesions may occur at any site about the body, including the oral cavity and face. Primary infection of the oral cavity usually results from eating flesh infected with *F. tularensis*, or it may be carried by contaminated hands to the face or oral cavity. The initial oral lesion of tularemia closely resembles the chancre of syphilis, which often leads to delayed diagnosis of the disease. In addition to primary lesions of the oral cavity, secondary lesions associated with tularemic infection may occur. Such secondary infection of the oral cavity usually produces small grayish white areas on the tongue, gums, and buccal mucosa which eventually become ulcerated. These ulcers are coated superficially with thin layers of

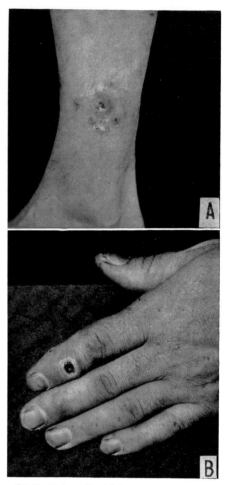

Figure 24/1. Tularemia: (*A*) leg lesion; (*B*) lesion on the index finger. (*A*, AFIP 218885-1; *B*, AFIP 85387-2.)

fibrin and only a few contaminating microorganisms. If tularemic infection is continued, the oral lesions may simulate Vincent's infection, or Vincent's infection may be superimposed on the tularemic infection. If the pharyngotonsillar region is involved, the lesions may resemble those of diphtheria. The continuation of the oral lesions is dependent upon the systemic disease, for the ulcers regress upon the abatement of the systemic disease, following adequate treatment. Facial lesions heal with scarring but oral lesions heal without residual tissue changes.

Diagnosis. The diagnosis of tularemia is based on a history indicative of exposure to the infection, clinical findings, culture of *F. tularensis*, particularly from blood, and serological tests. Definite diagnosis of tularemia requires identification of organisms from exudates or special culture media, such as cystine-glucose-blood agar, by specific fluorescent antibodies or by an agglutination test. Also allergic tests have been used. During the first week of tularemia intracutaneous injection of homologous antiserum produces a wheal and erythema response. After antibodies appear, a similar response is elicited by the polysaccharide. A delayed-type hypersensitivity also is demonstrable by intracutaneous injection of protein antigen. An attack of tularemia results in immunity sufficient to either prevent or greatly mitigate a second infection.

Treatment. Streptomycin effectively cures tularemia. The tetracyclines and chloramphenicol also are effective, but since they are bacteriostatic, relapse may result if treatment is halted prematurely. Immunization with attenuated types of vaccine provides some resistance in man, especially against respiratory infections.

PASTEURELLA MULTOCIDA AND PASTEURELLOSIS

Bacteriology of Pasteurella multocida. *P. multocida*, the species name implying the killing of many kinds of animals, is a common cause of fowl cholera in birds and mammalian hemorrhagic septicemia, syndromes generically termed pasteurellosis. This species is composed of short, ellipsoidal, gram negative, nonmotile, nonsporing rods that exhibit bipolar staining and possess polysaccharide capsules with chemical composition varying among serogroups.

Pasteurellosis. *P. multocida* normally parasitizes the upper respiratory tract and less often the intestinal tract of mammals and fowl. It is considered a true commensal in cats, dogs, and some rodents. These ordinarily innocuous strains produce disease when they acquire virulence from repeated animal passage or because of lowered resistance of the host, usually owing to debilitation, or both. Low resistance and high virulence result in fowl cholera, or acute hemorrhagic septicemia in a variety of animals. Evidently an endotoxin causes many of the symptoms seen in pasteurellosis. It is now recognized that *P. multocida* can infect man, although the number of proved human infections is quite small. The most common known source of human infection has been an animal bite, usually a cat, dog, or rabbit. The clinical manifestations of the human infection are quite variable, ranging from localized swelling and abscess formation to bronchiectasis, pneumonia, meningitis, and septicemia. Diagnosis of human pasteurellosis rests on clinical findings, cultivation and identification of the causative organism, and by infection of animals, by agglutination with specific antisera, and penicillin-sensitivity tests. At present, penicillin seems to be the most effective therapeutic agent.

ADDITIONAL READING

ALFROD, R. H., JOHN, J. T., AND BRYANT, R. E. 1972 Tularemia Treated Successfully with Gentamicin. Am Rev Respir Dis, **106,** 265.

ALLUISI, E. A., BEISEL, W. R., BARTELLONI, P. J., AND COATES, G. D. 1973 Behavioral Effects of Tularemia and Sandfly Fever in Man. J Infect Dis, **128,** 710.

ASAKAWA, Y., AKAHANE, S., KAGATA, N., NOGUCHI, M., SAZAZAKI, R., AND TAMURA, K. 1973 Two Community Outbreaks of Human Infection with *Yersinia enterocolitica.* J Hyg (Camb), **71,** 715.

BENNETT, L. G., AND TORNABENE, T. G. 1974 Characterization of the Antigenic Subunits of the Envelope Protein of *Yersinia pestis.* J Bacteriol, **117,** 48.

BIBEL, D. J., AND CHEN, T. H. 1976 Diagnosis of Plague: An Analysis of the Yersin-Kitasato Controversy. Bacteriol Rev, **40,** 633.

BRADFORD, W. D., NOCE, P. S., AND GUTMAN, L. T. 1974 Pathologic Features of Enteric Infection with *Yersinia enterocolitica.* Arch Pathol, **98,** 17.

BUTLER, T., LEVIN, J., LINH, N. N., CHAU, D. M., ADICKMAN, M., AND ARNOLD, K. 1976 *Yersinia pestis* Infection in Vietnam; II. Quantitative Blood Cultures and Detection of Endotoxin in the Cerebrospinal Fluid of Patients with Meningitis. J Infect Dis, **133,** 493.

CAVANAUGH, D. C., ELISBERG, B. L., LLEWELLYN, C. H., MARSHALL, J. D., JR., RUST, J. H., WILLIAMS, J. E., AND MEYER, K. F. 1974 Plague Immunization; V. Indirect Evidence for the Efficacy of Plague Vaccine. J Infect Dis, **129** (Suppl), S37.

CHEN, T. H., AND MEYER, K. F. 1974 Susceptibility and Antibody Response of *Rattus* Species to Experimental Plague. J Infect Dis, **129** (Suppl), S62.

COOPER, A., MARTIN, R., AND TIBBLES, J. A. R. 1973 Pasteurella Meningitis. Neurology, **23,** 1097.

FOSHAY, L. 1950 Tularemia. Ann Rev Microbiol, **4,** 313.

FRANCIS, D. P., HOLMES, M. A., AND BRANDON, G. 1975 *Pasteurella multocida*: Infection after Domestic Animal Bites and Scratches. JAMA, **233,** 42.

HAWES, S. C. 1973 Bubonic Plague. NZ Med J, **77,** 389.

HANNUKSELA, M., AND AHVONEN, P. 1975 Skin Manifestation in Human Yersiniosis. Ann Clin Res, **7,** 368.

JOHNSON, R. H., AND RUMANS, L. W. 1977 Unusual Infections Caused by *Pasteurella multocida.* JAMA, **237,** 146.

KOHL, S. 1979 *Yersinia enterocolitica* Infections in Children. Pediatr Clin North Am, **26,** 433.

MARSHALL, J. D., JR., BARTELLONI, P. J., CAVANAUGH, D. C., KADULL, P. J., AND MEYER, K. F. 1974 Plague Immunization; II. Relation of Adverse Clinical Reactions to Multiple Immunizations with Killed Vaccine. J Infect Dis, **129** (Suppl), S19.

MASSEY, E. D., AND MANGIAFICO, J. A. 1974 Microagglutination Test for Detecting and Measuring Serum Agglutinins of *Francisella tularensis.* Appl Microbiol, **27,** 25.

MEYER, K. F., CAVANAUGH, D. C., BARTELLONI, P. J., AND MARSHALL, J. D., JR. 1974 Plague Immunization; I. Past and Present Trends. J Infect Dis, **129** (Suppl), S13.

MEYER, K. F., SMITH, G., FOSTER, L. E., MARSHALL, J. D., JR., AND CAVANAUGH, D. C. 1974 Plague Immunization; IV. Clinical Reactions and Serologic Response to Inoculations of Haffkine and Freeze-Dried Plague Vaccine. J Infect Dis, **129** (Suppl), S30.

KLOCK, L. E., OLSEN, P. F., AND FUKUSHIMA, T. 1973 Tularemia Epidemic Associated with the Deerfly. JAMA, **226,** 149.

OHARA, S., SATO, T., AND HOMMA, M. 1974 Serological Studies on *Francisella tularensis, Francisella novicida, Yersinia philomiragia,* and *Brucella abortus.* Int J Syst Bacteriol, **24,** 191.

QUAN, T. J., MEEK, J. L., TSUCHIYA, K. R., HUDSON, B. W., AND BARNES, A. M. 1974 Experimental Pathogenicity of Recent North American Isolates of *Yersinia enterocolitica*. J Infect Dis, **139,** 341.

SUZUKI, E., AND SHIMOJO, H. 1973 Isolation of *Yersinia pseudotuberculosis* from an Appendix in Man. Jpn J Microbiol, **17,** 429.

TOIVANEN, P., TOIVANEN, A., OLKKONEN, L., AND ANATAA, S. 1974 Is the Incidence of *Yersinia enterocolitica*

Infection Increasing? Acta Pathol Microbiol Scand, **82,** 303.

VELIMIROVIC, B. 1972 Plague in South-East Asia; a Brief Historical Summary and Present Geographical Distribution. Trans R Soc Trop Med Hyg, **66,** 479.

VISELTEAR, A. J. 1974 The Pneumonic Plague Epidemic of 1924 in Los Angeles. Yale J Biol Med, **47,** 40.

chapter 25

Brucella and Brucellosis

George S. Schuster

BRUCELLA

The genus *Brucella* comprises six recognized species with *Brucella melitensis*, *Brucella abortus*, and *Brucella suis* being the most common. The other species described include *Brucella neotomae*, found in desert wood rats; *Brucella ovis*, causing epididymitis and abortion in sheep; and *Brucella canis*, causing epididymitis and abortion in dogs.

Morphology and Metabolism. All species of the brucellae are gram negative, not acid-fast, nonsporing, usually nonmotile, sometimes encapsulated, and occur singly, in pairs, or in short chains. Although the cells are typically short rods, cocci or coccobacilli may predominate. Brucellae form smooth (S), intermediate (I), rough (R), mucoid (M), and G type colonies. The virulent and strongly antigenic brucella is the S type which undergoes spontaneous smooth to rough variation. Loss of virulence and changed antigenicity are correlated with changes in colonial morphology in the R type. The transition from S to R type may be sudden and complete but there may arise a transient or intermediate (I) type. The colonies of the mucoid (M) type mutate to the R type either in liquid or on solid media. G type colonies appear infrequently among S type during initial isolation of brucellae from infected uteri. Brucellae are difficult to grow on initial isolation except on enriched media. All species are aerobic and *B. abortus* requires 5 to 10% CO_2 for initial isolation. Several components of media inhibit the growth of brucellae.

Antigenic Composition. S strains have distinctive antigenic compositions, which progressively lose specificity during the usually gradual transformation from S to R phases in culture. S forms of the three *Brucella* species contain two characteristic heat-stable antigens, termed A and M. These antigens are toxic polysaccharide-lipid-protein complexes. A and M antigens of the three species are closely related but not identical. Furthermore, their amounts and distribution on the cell surfaces would allow for antigenic variations among species.

ANIMAL BRUCELLOSIS

Animal brucellosis is primarily an infection of goats, sheep, swine, and cattle. It causes great economic loss in livestock because of decreased milk supply, failure to produce offspring because of loss of fertility or abortion, and overall decrease in market value. Although it is a secondary disease of man, and is seldom if ever transmitted from person to person it can pose a threat to human health.

HUMAN BRUCELLOSIS

Human brucellosis (commonly, undulant fever) is usually acquired through contact with infected animals or materials. The route of infection with brucellae is through the alimentary tract (ingestion), conjunctiva and skin (contact), and lungs (inhalation). Organisms entering a host can gain access to lymphatics. There often is local lymphadenopathy and subsequent bacteremia following bacterial multiplication and dissemination from the primarily involved nodes. Subsequent localization of the organisms occurs particularly in the reticuloendothelial system. Brucellae have been observed inside phagocytes where they are protected from antibodies and antibiotics. There is a granulomatous response in infected tissues that may, in some cases, lead to abscess formation. After an extremely variable incubation period, ranging from 3 to 60 days, the disease begins either insidiously or abruptly. Symptoms of disease that develop are weakness, evening rise in temperature, chills, sweats, anorexia, headaches, loss of weight, backache, splenomegaly, abdominal tenderness, rheumatism, arthritis, and anemia. The nonspecific symptoms may be accompanied by nervousness and mental depression. In human beings, brucellosis may assume many forms, ranging from an acute or undulant form to a recurrent type of disease which may persist for years. The human disease generally has been divided into two main types, acute or undulant and chronic. The acute type relates to the occur-

313

rence of focal lesions in the vascular or central nervous system. The chronic granulomatous type occurs when the organisms exist intracytoplasmically. Patients recovering from brucellosis may develop complications related to chronic granulomatous lesions in bones, joints, bursea, meninges, endocardium, lungs, liver, spleen, epididymis, testes, and kidneys. In many instances these lesions cannot be differentiated histologically from those of tuberculosis. A chronic localized pulmonary brucellosis occurs in humans. The symptoms are fever, productive coughing, chest pains, choking sensations, hoarseness, and chills, together with many of the other usual symptoms of generalized brucellosis. Joints are often involved as a complication of brucellosis with the most common manifestations generalized being polyarthritis. Spondylitis is an infrequent complication of brucellosis, resembling tuberculosis of the spine.

Brucellae are sometimes a cause of ocular lesions. The central nervous system is involved not infrequently, with brucellae invading cerebrospinal fluid or cerebral tissue. Other complications of brucellosis are granulomatous panarteritis, miliary peritonitis, urinary infections, salpingitis, epididymitis, and orchitis.

Immunity. While serum antibodies, as measured by agglutinin, precipitin, opsonin, or bactericidal tests occur early in the disease, they do not prevent reinfection by brucellosis.

Hypersensitivity. Hypersensitivity plays a significant role in human brucellosis. In nonsensitized individuals the organisms are phagocytized but some almost always survive to pass to the regional lymph nodes. Some take up an intracellular existence within liver, spleen, lymph nodes, and bone marrow. Subsequently, the organisms are killed, releasing endotoxin, which elicits the characteristic clinical symptoms of the disease. Hypersensitivity also seems to be an important factor mediating chronic brucellosis, for affected individuals are quite sensitive dermally and systemically to brucella antigens.

Laboratory Diagnosis of Brucellosis. Laboratory diagnosis of human brucellosis depends on isolation and identification of the causal organisms and the performance of agglutination tests. Diagnosis by culture is difficult because the organisms are present in the blood, urine, and feces only intermittently and in small numbers. Usually blood or other tissue is cultured for as long as a month in tryptose or trypticase soy broth. It is useful to inoculate the cultures into guinea pigs. The injection of suspected material into the yolk sacs of embryonated eggs is sometimes superior to either of the above procedures.

Perhaps the most commonly used laboratory diagnostic procedure is the agglutination test. A titer of 1:160 in an individual with appropriate symptoms is usually considered significant. A fluctuating or rising titer is particularly suggestive of infection. Antigenic cross reactions may occur between brucellae and *Francisella tularensis* or *Vibrio cholerae*.

The brucella skin test is mostly for detection of hypersensitivity. Antigen is injected intradermally into the forearm and observed in 24 to 48 hours. In a hypersensitive individual, usually not in the early stages of the disease, an edematous area develops, usually not larger than 2.5 cm in diameter.

Treatment and Control. The antibiotics which have been used in the treatment of brucellosis are the tetracyclines and streptomycin. Several regimens have been followed in order to overcome the high relapse rate and to treat brucellosis more effectively. One such procedure is the administration of a tetracycline and streptomycin. Such combinations of antibiotics have produced a significantly lower relapse rate.

Prevention of human brucellosis is mainly dependent upon control of the animal sources of infection. Available vaccines are suitable mainly for animals. Control of dairy product processing as well as animal surveillance and immunization have greatly reduced the dangers of brucellosis in the United States.

ADDITIONAL READING

ALTON, G. G., MAW, J., ROGERSON, B. A., AND MCPHERSON, G. G. 1974 The Serological Diagnosis of Bovine Brucellosis; an Evaluation of the Complement Fixation Serum Agglutination and Rose Bengal Tests. Aust Vet J, **51,** 57.

BERTRAND, J. L., AND GUEYFFIER, C. 1974 *Brucella endocarditis*; a General Review with Reference to 46 Observations from Medical Literature and One Personal Observation. Lyon Med, **231,** 123.

BRUCELLOSIS: A SYMPOSIUM. 1950 American Association of the Advancement of Science, Washington, D.C.

BUCHANAN, T. M., BAHER, L. C., AND FELDMAN, R. A. 1974 Brucellosis in the United States, 1960–72; an Abattoir-associated Disease. Part I, Clinical Features and Therapy. Medicine, **53,** 403.

BUSCH, L. A., AND PARKER, R. L. 1972 Brucellosis in the United States. J Infect Dis, **125,** 289.

COGHLAN, J. D., AND LONGMORE, H. J. A. 1973 The Significance of Brucella Antibodies in Patients in a Rural Area. Practitioner, **211,** 645.

ELBERG, S. S. 1973 Immunity to Brucella Infection. Medicine, **52,** 339.

FARRELL, I. D., HINCHLIFFE, P. M., AND ROBERTSON, L. 1975 The Use of the Conglutinating Complement Fixation Test in the Diagnosis of Human Brucellosis. J Hyg (Camb), **74,** 29.

FARRELL, I. D., ROBERTSON, L., AND HINCHLIFFE, P. M. 1975 Serum Antibody Response in Acute Brucellosis. J Hyg (Camb), **74,** 23.

FOLEY, B. V., CLAY, M. M., AND O'SULLIVAN, D. J. 1970 A Study of a Brucellosis Epidemic. Ir. J Med Sc, **3,** 457.

KULSHRESHTHA, R. C., ATAL, P. R., AND WAHI, P. N. 1973 A Study on Serological Tests for the Diagnosis of

Human and Bovine Brucellosis. Indian J Med Res, **61,** 1471.

MANN, P. G., AND RICHENS, E. R. 1973 Aspects of Human Brucellosis. Postgrad Med J, **49,** 523.

McCULLOUGH, N. B. 1970 Microbial and Host Factors in the Pathogenesis of Brucellosis. In *Infectious Agents and Host Reactions*, edited by S. Mudd. W. B. Saunders, Philadelphia.

McDIARMID, A. 1973 Some Veterinary Aspects of the Eradication of Brucellosis. Postgrad Med J, **49,** 526.

ROBERTSON, L., FARRELL, I. D., AND HINCHLIFFE, P. M. 1973 The Sensitivity of *Brucella abortus* to Chemotherapeutic Agents. J Med Microbiol, **6,** 549.

YOUNG, E. J., AND SUVANNOPARRAT, U. 1975 Brucellosis Outbreak Attributed to Ingestion of Unpasteurized Goat Cheese. Arch Intern Med, **135,** 240.

chapter 26

Haemophilus and Bordetella

George S. Schuster

HAEMOPHILUS SPECIES

The genus *Haemophilus* is a group of facultatively anaerobic, gram negative coccoid bacilli, which cannot synthesize essential components of their enzyme systems that are furnished by blood. These include the "X" (heat-stable) factor that acts like hematin and supplies porphyrins and the "V" (heat-labile) factor that is NAD or NADP. Of the 14 recognized species *Haemophilus influenzae*, *Haemophilus aegyptius* (Koch-Weeks bacillus), *Haemophilus suis*, and *Haemophilus haemolyticus* require both X and V factors. *Haemophilus ducreyi* requires only X factor, whereas *Haemophilus parainfluenzae* and *Haemophilus parahaemolyticus* require only V factor. *H. influenzae* is associated with acute respiratory infections, and causes purulent meningitis. *H. ducreyi* produces soft chancre or chancroid. *H. aegyptius* is a biotype which causes a highly contagious conjunctivitis, termed pinkeye.

HAEMOPHILUS INFLUENZAE

Morphology and Metabolism. Fully virulent *H. influenzae* are small encapsulated coccobacilli but it is not unusual to see cocci, bacilli, and long filaments in a single culture. Primary isolation of *H. influenzae* is best accomplished on chocolate blood agar in which both the X and V factors have been released from the red blood cells. On chocolate agar, fully virulent, encapsulated strains form relatively small, mucoid, transparent colonies showing a characteristic iridescence when viewed by oblique light during the first 6 to 8 hours of incubation.

Antigenic Structure. The encapsulated strains have been divided into six immunological types designated as a, b, c, d, e, and f, based on capsular swelling and agglutination and precipitation reactions. Antigenically, *H. influenzae* resembles the pneumococcus, for all of their type-specific capsules are carbohydrates. Nonspecific somatic, protein antigens are also present in *H. influenzae*. Virulence of *H. influenzae* is at least partially related to the polysaccharide capsule which interferes with phagocytosis.

Genetic Variations. *H. influenzae* undergoes smooth to rough variations at a relatively rapid rate. The species undergo transformations mediated by DNA with regard to drug resistance and to formation of specific capsular antigens.

Diseases Caused by *H. influenzae*. *H. influenzae* and its close relatives, *H. haemolyticus*, *H. parainfluenzae*, and *H. parahaemolyticus*, are indigenous to the human pharynx. *H. haemolyticus* and *H. parainfluenzae* are essentially nonpathogenic, except for rare cases of subacute endocarditis. *H. parahaemolyticus* is frequently associated with acute pharyngitis and occasionally with subacute endocarditis. *H. influenzae* is associated with pharyngitis, sinusitis, and otitis media, and less frequently it is involved in primary pneumonia, empyema, endocarditis, pyoarthrosis, and obstructive laryngotracheal infection with bacteremia in young children. A less frequent but very serious disease mediated by *H. influenzae* is primary pyogenic meningitis in children under 3 years of age. Another disease is a secondary complication of infections of the respiratory tract, notably in pandemic influenza.

It has been reported that children between the ages of 6 months and 2 years may develop a buccal cellulitis as a result of infection by *H. influenzae* b. This begins as a swelling of the cheek with central erythema that rapidly progresses to a lesion without a distinct border but having a reddish discoloration surrounded by a purplish area. Occasionally, the entire lesion is purple-red in color. There may be regions of erythematous buccal mucosa accompanying the buccal lesion. These must be differentiated from trauma, erysipelas and streptococcal cellulitis, usually by blood cultures.

Diagnosis. Prompt bacteriological diagnosis of infections with *H. influenzae* is essential to therapy. *H. influenzae* may be identified rapidly in spinal fluid, exudate from middle ear or joints, empyema fluid, nasopharyngeal mucus, or sputum by staining, capsular swelling, and a precipitin test for type-specific polysaccharide. Cultures should be made from such specimens and from the blood, and the diagnosis verified by demonstration of capsular swelling by type-specific antiserum.

Treatment. Prior to 1938, nearly all patients with *H. influenzae* meningitis died. Ampicillin and chloramphenicol together are now recommended in treating meningitis and other infections caused by *H. influenzae*.

Immunity. Immunity develops with increasing age from inapparent exposure to *H. influenzae* during the normal course of life. During the first 3 years, when there is relatively little immunological resistance, the individual is most susceptible. Resistance to *H. influenzae* parallels development of other immunologic protection suggesting its importance.

HAEMOPHILUS AEGYPTIUS

A bacterial species was observed by Koch in 1883 and isolated by Weeks in 1887 from a human conjunctivitis known as pinkeye. It was named the Koch-Weeks bacillus and was indistinguishable from nonencapsulated *H. influenzae*. However, it is immunologically distinct and also differs in rather subtle cultural characteristics. It is now recognized as *H. aegyptius*, a biotype of *H. influenzae*.

HAEMOPHILUS DUCREYI

H. ducreyi, commonly called Ducrey's bacillus, is a small gram negative rod with the common characteristics of the genus *Haemophilus*. *H. ducreyi* is the cause of about 10% of all venereal infections, producing soft chancre or chancroid on the genitalia and lymphatic swellings (buboes), and abscesses in the groin (figs. 26/1 and 26/2). This disease is often confused clinically with syphilis. Hypersensitivity to the bacillus is used as the basis for a diagnostic

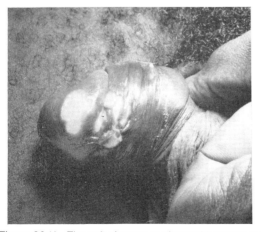

Figure 26/1. The soft chancre or chancroid caused by *Haemophilus ducreyi*. (AFIP.)

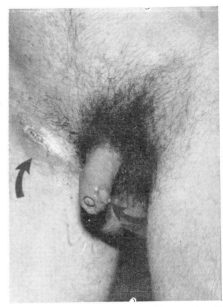

Figure 26/2. New, acute chancroid, showing the involvement of adjacent lymph node. (AFIP.)

cutaneous test. Immunity to chancroid does not develop, and untreated infections may persist for years. Chloramphenicol is useful in prophylaxis and treatment.

BORDETELLA

The genus *Bordetella* is made up of three species of strictly aerobic gram negative coccobacilli (*Bordetella pertussis*, *Bordetella bronchiseptica*, and *Bordetella parapertussis*).

Morphology and Metabolism. *B. pertussis*, the cause of whooping cough, is a short, ovoid, gram negative, nonmotile, and nonsporing bacillus that does not require either X or V factors. Cell morphology is also more constant than that of *H. influenzae*. Encapsulated and noncapsulated types occur, with the former having smooth colonial characteristics. Complex media (*e.g.*, Bordet-Gengou agar media) are required for the growth of virulent *B. pertussis*. It has little or no action on most carbohydrates and develops a marked alkalinity in broth.

Antigenic Structure and Variation. Freshly isolated *B. pertussis* are antigenically homogeneous. When initially isolated, the encapsulated coccobacillus is termed a phase 1 type. It is fully virulent, has pili-type appendages and requires enriched media. Subsequent culturing brings about variations, analogous to smooth to rough variation, that results in a stepwise change through phase 2 and 3 types to type 4 cells that are pleomorphic and will grow on unenriched media. Phase 4 cells are not virulent and have no filaments or capsules. Several types of toxin have been identified including a heat labile toxin, a lipopolysaccharide endotoxin, a histamine sensitizing factor, a lymphocytosis promoting factor, hemagglutinins and possibly an islet activating protein. These are intimately involved in infection, disease and immunity.

Whooping Cough. B. pertussis is transmitted in droplets from one human respiratory tract to another; no intermediate vectors or fomites of importance have been demonstrated. Human infection has three clinical phases, each lasting about 2 weeks: the catarrhal, the paroxysmal or spasmodic, and the convalescent. From 7 to 14 days after exposure, the catarrhal stage begins with coryza, sneezing, and mild but progressive cough. The bacilli multiply on the epithelium of the trachea and bronchi and their toxic components cause irritation and coughing. The paroxysmal stage is characterized by violent repetitive coughing, which forcefully empties the lungs and is followed by sudden forceful croaking or whooping inspiration. The infection may spread even to the alveoli and often results in interstitial pneumonia or secondary infection. Thick, ropy, mucinous bronchial secretions may obstruct the lower airways and produce atelectasis. Allergy to protein fractions of B. pertussis may contribute to the clinical manifestations of whooping cough.

Immunity. The immunity that develops from an attack of whooping cough prevents a second attack except in rare instances. During convalescence, antibodies to B. pertussis appear in the serum, persist for several months, and gradually decrease or even disappear. The relationship of humoral antibodies to immunity to whooping cough is uncertain. Clinical immunity may be partially cellular. There is no satisfactory way to measure individual immunity to whooping cough. Nevertheless, immunization with killed phase I B. pertussis is an effective protective measure.

Laboratory Diagnosis. The bacteriological diagnosis of whooping cough entails the obtaining of a culture of the causal organisms on a Bordet-Gengou agar plate containing penicillin to inhibit gram positive bacteria. Identification is made by microscopic examination of gram stained smears and by agglutination with specific antiserum. Since agglutinin for B. pertussis does not appear in the serum of a patient until the third week of infection or later, it has no practical diagnostic value.

Treatment. B. pertussis is sensitive *in vitro* to erythromycin, with chloramphenicol and tetracyclines as alternative agents. If administered early enough erythromycin may shorten the paroxysmal manifestations. Supportive treatment is very important.

Prevention and Control. Whooping cough affects 90% of the nonimmunized population, usually in childhood. The disease is controlled by active immunization of infants (age 2 months) in a primary course of three injections at monthly intervals and with booster shots given at 1 year of age, and 5 years later. The immunizing agent consists of killed phase I organisms or extracts of these organisms. These preparations are combined with diphtheria and tetanus toxoids to form a vaccine. The use of such vaccines has greatly reduced morbidity due to whooping cough caused by B. pertussis. It does not protect against whooping cough caused by B. parapertussis.

ADDITIONAL READING

AFTANDELIANS, R., AND CONNOR, J. D. 1973 Bactericidal Antibody in Serum During Infection with *Bordetella pertussis*. J Infect Dis, **128,** 55.

AFTANDELIANS, R. V., AND CONNOR, J. D. 1974 *Bordetella pertussis* Serotypes in a Whooping Cough Outbreak. Am J Epidemiol, **99,** 343.

BENNETT, N. 1973 Whooping Cough in Melbourne. Med J Aust, **2,** 481.

BORSKA, K., AND SIMKOVICOVA, M. 1972 Studies on the Circulation of *Bordetella pertussis* and *Bordetella parapertussis* in Populations of Children. J Hyg Epidemiol Microbiol Immunol, **16,** 159.

DAVIES, J. L., LAUGHTON, C. R., AND MAY, J. R. 1974 An Improved Test for *Haemophilus influenzae* Precipitins in the Serum of Patients with Chronic Respiratory Disease. J Clin Pathol, **27,** 265.

FAROOKI, Z. O., HENRY, J. G., AND GREEN, E. W. 1974 *Haemophilus influenzae* Pericarditis Associated with Meningitis; a Treatable Fatal Disease. Clin Pediatr, **13,** 609.

INTERNATIONAL SYMPOSIUM ON PERTUSSIS. 1978 National Institutes of Health, Bethesda, Md.

KHAN, W., ROSS, S., RODRIQUEZ, W., CONTRONI, G., AND SAZ, A. K. 1974 *Haemophilus influenzae* Type B Resistant to Ampicillin. JAMA, **229,** 298.

KULENKAMPFF, M., SCHWARTZMAN, J. S., AND WILSON, J. 1974 Neurological Complications of Pertussis Inoculation. Arch Dis Child, **49,** 46.

NORDEN, C. W., AND MICHAELS, R. 1973 Immunologic Response in Patients with Epiglottitis Caused by *Haemophilus influenzae* Type B. J Infect Dis, **128,** 777.

MORSE, S. I., AND MORSE, J. H. 1976 Isolation and Properties of Leukocytosis and Leukocytosis Promoting Factor of *Bordetella pertussis*. J Exp Med, **143,** 1483.

PARTON, R., AND WARDLAW, A. C. 1974 Cell-Envelope Proteins of *Bordetella pertussis*. J Med Microbiol, **8,** 47.

PITTMAN, M. 1970 *Bordetella pertussis*: Bacterial and Host Factors in the Pathogenesis and Prevention of Whooping Cough. In *Infectious Agents and Host Reactions*, edited by S. Mudd. W. B. Saunders, Philadelphia.

RAPKIN, R. H., AND BAUTISTA, G. 1972 *Haemophilus influenzae* Cellulitis. Am J Dis Child, **124,** 540.

ROSS, R., MUNOZ, J., AND CAMERON, C. 1969 Histamine Sensitizing Factor, Mouse Protective Antigens and Other Antigens of Some Members of the Genus *Bordetella*. J Bacteriol, **99,** 57.

SIMS, W. 1972 Pathogenicity of Human Oral Strains of Haemophili: Enzymes, Anaerobiosis and Effects on Mice and Rabbits. Arch Oral Biol, **17,** 745.

TURK, D. C., AND MAY, J. R. 1967 *Haemophilus influenzae; Its Clinical Importance*. English Universities Press, London.

WARDLAW, A. C., PARTON, R., AND HOOKER, M. J. 1976 Loss of Protective Antigen, Histamine-Sensitizing Factor and Envelope Polypeptides in Cultural Variants of *Bordetella pertussis*. J Med Microbiol, **9,** 89.

chapter 27

Enterobacteriaceae and the Enteric Gram Negative Microbial Flora

George S. Schuster

ENTEROBACTERIACEAE

The family Enterobacteriaceae contains several groups of saprophytic and pathogenic bacteria inhabiting the intestinal tract of man and animals. Others are plant parasites or soil inhabitants and decomposers of organic material. Although they are enteric inhabitants, *Bacteroides* species, *Pseudomonas* species, *Clostridium* species, and enterococci are usually not included in the Enterobacteriaceae. The typical members are the enteric bacilli, gram negative rods that may vary considerably in size and shape. They are glycolytic, producing acid or acid and gas. Nearly all species reduce nitrate to nitrite. These common characteristics cannot be used to differentiate individual members from each other.

Even when all the differential characteristics available are applied, individual species cannot be clearly differentiated and the groups blend into one another, with many intergrading types. Table 27/1 follows closely but not completely the classification of *Bergey's Manual of Determinative Bacteriology*, 8th edition, in listing the most important enteric bacteria. Based upon DNA analyses, several changes have been proposed in the taxonomy of the Enterobacteriaceae, mostly in *Klebsiella* and *Proteus*. These are being incorporated into the current literature and may provide a basis for later reclassification.

Morphology of the Enterobacteriaceae. The Enterobacteriaceae are small, gram negative, nonsporeforming rods. They may be motile by petrichous flagella, or nonmotile. Enteric bacteria may possess a well defined capsule, a loose capsule or slime layer, or no capsule. Many species have pili (fimbriae) for attachment to surfaces or transfer of genetic information.

Physiological and Cultural Characteristics. Enterobacteriaceae are facultative organisms that have diverse biochemical properties. Under anaerobic conditions, they ferment carbohydrates but aerobically they utilize the trichloroacetic acid (TCA) cycle. The different organism vary in the carbohydrates they ferment, although all ferment glucose. The pathway used in metabolism and the end products produced, such as gas formation, are useful in specifically identifying these organisms. Gram negative enteric bacilli are resistant to some bacteriostatic dyes and surface-active compounds such as bile salts. Selective media containing such compounds facilitates the isolation of the enteric bacilli from fecal specimens. Four biochemical characteristics have been applied to differentiate the coliform-dysentery-typhoid groups. These characteristics, collectively known as the IMViC reactions are indole production, methyl red acid determination, acetylmethylcarbinol production (Voges-Proskauer reaction), and the utilization of citrate. Antigenic analysis, especially that based on the schema of Kauffmann and White, has been used to differentiate coliform-dysentery-typhoid groups.

Antigenic Structure of the Enterobacteriaceae. The antigenic characteristics of enterobacteria are important in their classification and epidemiology. Enterobacteriaceae contain three types of antigens: H, O, and K. Those that are motile contain the protein H antigen in their flagella. The variations in flagella antigen are likely due to differing amino acid sequences.

The polysaccharide O antigen is a somatic antigen present in the cell wall. Within some genera the O antigens are diverse structurally, such that they can be used for serologic subgrouping.

The K or capsular antigens are polysaccharides. They may exist as a true capsule or as an overlying layer that blocks O antigen from reacting with homologous antibodies. Vi antigen is a type of K antigen found in only certain species, such as *Salmonella typhi*. It plays a role in the pathogenesis of typhoid fever.

In addition to differential antigens, all Enterobacteriaceae possess a common antigen (EAC), that appears to be present on the outer surface of the

Table 27/I
Enteric bacteria

1. **Coliform Bacilli:** *Escherichia coli, Enterobacter aerogenes, Klebsiella pneumoniae, Klebsiella ozaenae, Klebsiella rhinoscleromatis, Serratia marcescans, Edwardsiella tarda, Citrobacter freundii*
2. **Proteus-Providence Group:** *Proteus vulgaris, Proteus mirabilis, Proteus morganii, Proteus rettgeri,* genus *Providencia*
3. **Salmonella:**
   a. Causing human diseases: *Salmonella typhi; Salmonella paratyphi* A; *Salmonella schottmulleri; Salmonella hirschfeldii*
   b. Causing diseases of animals and birds—also humans: *Salmonella typhimurium, Salmonella cholerasuis, Salmonella enteritidis, Salmonella gallinarum, Salmonella arizonae, Salmonella salamae, Salmonella boutenae*
      NOTE: Attempts have been made to reduce the salmonellae to three species; *Salmonella cholerae-suis, Salmonella typhi,* and *Salmonella enteritidis,* with more than 1000 serotypes.
   c. Diseases of animals and birds only: *Salmonella anatum, Salmonella gallinarum, Salmonella pullorum*
4. **Shigella:** *Shigella dysenteriae, Shigella boydii, Shigella flexneri, Shigella sonnei.*
5. **Vibrio:** *Vibrio cholerae*
6. **Aeromonas group:** *Aeromonas hydrophila, Aeromonas punctata, Aeromonas salmonicida*
7. ***Pseudomonas aeruginosa***, and 28 other recognized species
8. **Flavobacterium:** 12 species widely distributed in the environment

---

bacteria and may play a role in host-bacteria interactions. They can be detected by hemagglutination or hemolysis of antigen covered erythrocytes.

Colicins. Enteric bacilli produce colicins which are able to attach themselves to specific receptors on other susceptible enteric bacilli. They then kill them by blocking phosphorylation, protein synthesis, or by degradation of nucleic acids. They are selective in their activity, attacking only susceptible strains. This helps to stabilize the enteric microbiota.

COLIFORM BACILLI

Escherichia coli. *E. coli* universally inhabits human and animal intestinal tracts. These organisms are gram negative, nonsporing, occasionally encapsulated, variably motile bacilli. *E. coli* is aerobic or facultatively anaerobic and is easily grown on common laboratory media.

E. coli is not very pathogenic for either man or animals, ordinarily serving a useful purpose in the intestinal tract, where it is a major source of vitamin K and in some persons a secondary source of B vitamins. It is an opportunist, however, and produces disease when the resistance of the intestinal tract or adjacent areas is lowered sufficiently for it to invade the tissues. Within the immediate confines of the intestinal tract, infantile diarrhea and adult gastroenteritis are common infections caused by several O groups of *E. coli.* At least two mechanisms are involved. Invasive strains penetrate the intestinal wall and cause infections resembling bacillary dysentery. Others produce an enterotoxin that causes a cholera-like disease.

E. coli is often the cause of urinary tract infections. It gains entrance to the urinary tract via the urethra, bladder, and ureters to the kidney. There it commonly causes a cystitis (infection of the bladder), but its suppurative infections of the kidney are persistent and difficult to control. *E. coli* often relates to infections of the gall bladder, peritonitis, appendicitis, and other infections along the intestinal tract, including wounds. *E. coli* is frequently encountered in gram negative bacteremias and septicemias.

While *E. coli* is generally sensitive to most antibiotics used to treat gram negative infections single or multiple resistance to such agents is often present or soon develops in treatment. As a lifesaving measure, more toxic agents are used such as gentamycin, kanamycin, streptomycin, polymyxin, or colistin. Maintenance of fluid balance is critical in management of diarrhea.

Enterobacter. The genus *Enterobacter* has been well characterized only relatively recently. Previously it was not distinguished, especially in clinical isolates. *Enterobacter* species are short, frequently encapsulated, gram negative rods that are usually motile.

The two main species are *Enterobacter aerogenes* and *Enterobacter cloacae.* They can cause similar infections, often of the urinary tract. *E. aerogenes* is often found as a secondary pathogen in that it superinfects a primary infection. *E. aerogenes* may be found in wound infections, blood, and sputum, as a primary agent or a commensal.

Klebsiella pneumoniae. *K. pneumoniae,* at one time called Friedlander's bacillus, is a gram negative, nonsporing, nonmotile, facultatively anaerobic rod. *Klebsiella* species are classified serologically into at least 80 antigenic types.

K. pneumoniae is present in less than 5% of all normal human respiratory tracts. It is also present in the feces of about 5% of normal individuals. It is the cause of less than 3% of all cases of pneumonia and is associated with a few inflammatory suppurative infections. Pneumonia caused by *K. pneumoniae* is highly fatal if untreated and may be attended by such profound changes in the lung as necrosis, abscess formation, and cavitation. The residual lung damage may be so great as to require surgical intervention.

K. pneumoniae is susceptible to most antibiotics that act on gram negative bacteria, except ampicillin and carbenicillin. Cephalosporin is usually effective. Nalidixic acid and nitrofurantoin are effective in treating infections of the urinary tract.

Serratia. The genus *Serratia*, of which *Serratia marcescens* is best known, is composed of gram negative motile rods that form a red pigment, prodigiosin. They have long been considered to be nonpathogenic but it now seems more likely that they are opportunistic pathogens. They are susceptible to aminoglycoside antibiotics, chloramphenicol, and trimethoprim-sulfamethoxazole.

Edwardsiella. A relatively new genus, *Edwardsiella*, was created in 1965 to include a group of motile, gram negative, lactose-negative bacilli that resemble but are considered distinct from the salmonellae. They are found in humans and other mammals and reptiles. They cause acute gastroenteritis and serious septic infections. *Edwardsiella tarda* is the type species.

Citrobacter. The genus *Citrobacter* contains three species, *Citrobacter freundii*, *Citrobacter diversus*, and *Citrobacter amalonaticus*. At one time, these bacteria were called paracolon bacilli. The citrobacteria resemble but are distinct from salmonellae. While these bacilli are not considered to be true enteric pathogens since they are found in normal feces, they also are associated with human diarrhea, urinary tract infections, and assorted septic infections. They are sensitive to chloramphenicol, and aminoglycoside antibiotics.

Proteus-Providencia Group. The Proteus-Providencia group of the Enterobacteriaceae consists of gram negative, lactose-negative, motile bacilli that deaminate phenylalanine. *Proteus* species produce abundant urease, and grow at an alkaline pH, the latter property helping distinguish them from other enteric bacilli.

The genus *Proteus* contains two clinically important species, *Proteus vulgaris* and *Proteus mirabilis*. It has been suggested that *Proteus morganii* be called *Morganella* and *Proteus rettgeri* be called *Providencia rettgeri*. The most important pathogens are *Proteus vulgaris* and *Proteus morganii*. *Proteus vulgaris* and *Proteus mirabilis* have the peculiar characteristic of "swarming" or intermittent spreading while growing on a moist agar surface. Swarming complicates isolation of other bacterial species mixed with *Proteus* species.

The *Proteus* species are antigenically heterogeneous and have been subdivided on the basis of O, H and K antigens but thus far this is not a useful epidemiologic tool. Certain strains designated by the letter X contain three O antigenic components by which they are divided into OX2, OX19, and OXK groups. These react with antibodies of individuals with rickettsial infections. The cross-reaction (Weil-Felix test) is utilized in the diagnosis of such infections as typhus.

Proteus strains are widely distributed and are involved in the decay of protein. *Proteus* strains are rarely found in large numbers in the intestinal tract except when there is some disturbance, as in diarrhea. They are involved in urinary tract and wound infections. *Proteus* species are sensitive to aminoglycosides and trimethoprim-sulfamethoxazole. Only *P. mirabilis* is sensitive to ampicillin and cephalothin.

The genus *Providencia* now contains the enteric bacteria that were formerly assigned to *Proteus inconstans*. These bacilli occur in the feces of normal individuals, as well as those with diarrhea.

SALMONELLA

Taxonomy of Salmonella. The genus *Salmonella* is composed of a biochemically and serologically diverse group of organisms that infects humans and many animal species. Most are motile, produce H_2S from thiosulfate and gas from glucose fermentation; they rarely ferment lactose. The antigenic structure of the genus *Salmonella* has been used to classify them according to the schema of Kauffman and White. By the use of H, O, and Vi antigens and their respective antibodies, about 1500 serotypes of salmonella have been identified by cross-absorption and cross-reaction tests. The salmonella are divided into groups A-I based on common O antigens. Minor O determinants which are also found and H antigens allow for additional divisions of the groups into serotypes or species. The proposed alternative classification scheme to that of Kauffman-White differs in that there are only three species of *Salmonella*, *Salmonella typhi*, *Salmonella cholerae-suis*, and *Salmonella enteritidis*. The Kauffman-White scheme designates each antigenic type as a species whereas the alternate scheme designates the antigenic types as serotypes of *S. enteritidis*.

Poultry products are the largest source of nontyphoid salmonellosis. Improperly cooked or stored meat may permit growth of the organisms, resulting in infection. Dried eggs may also act as a source, either directly or as a contaminant when used in other food products. Household pets including turtles, may harbor salmonella and act as a source of infection.

The clinically distinct diseases resulting from salmonella infections depend on the species involved, the number of microorganisms ingested, and the resistance of the susceptible individual. These diseases are gastroenteritis ("food poisoning"), typhoid and other enteric fevers, and septicemia. The latter condition usually arises from a localized focus of infection in some organ.

Salmonella gastroenteritis is usually caused by *S. enteritidis*, serotype *typhimurium*, although any species can cause it. It has an incubation period of about 24 hours, and is characterized by sudden onset, abdominal pain, nausea, vomiting, diarrhea, and fever. It usually lasts 2 to 5 days and is self-limiting.

Typhoid fever is exclusively a human disease caused by *S. typhi*. Milder enteric fevers are caused by *Salmonella paratyphi*, *Salmonella schottmuelleri*, and *Salmonella hirschfeldii*. Typhoid fever has an incubation period of less than 14 days, during which the bacteria multiply intracellularly in lymphoid tissue. Onset is insidious with headache, malaise, anorexia, and a febrile period in which body temperature increases stepwise to an average of 104 F (40 C). The disease continues for about 3 weeks, with the temperature returning to normal after a period of gradual remission during the third week.

The incubation period of the milder enteric fevers is usually less than 10 days and the duration is similar to or less than that of typhoid fever. Although less severe, the symptoms are similar to those of typhoid fever.

Salmonellae may localize in joints, heart, lungs, or other organs and produce local abscesses. From such foci, salmonellae enter the bloodstream causing a septicemia, with a high, rheumatic-type fever.

Immunity in Salmonella. A lasting immunity develops during an attack of typhoid fever. Immunity to salmonellosis relates to anti-O and anti-Vi antibodies. Anti-H antibodies have no apparent protection. However, a high antibody titer may be present during relapses or fatal, terminal stages of the disease due to the bacilli multiplying intracellularly.

Pathogenicity of Salmonella. In man, *Salmonella* species are transmitted from sick human beings, animals, or healthy carriers to susceptible individuals. Temporary and permanent carriers are common. Salmonellae leave the infected or carrier individual in feces or urine which contaminates milk, food, or water and gain entrance into the body through the intestinal tract. The organisms pass through the epithelium into the subepithelial tissue. After penetration, the organisms are ingested by macrophages where they multiply and may be carried to other sites. The ability of the organisms to survive intracellularly may be due to surface O antigens or the Vi antigen, since those organisms containing the latter antigen are more virulent than those lacking it.

The exact role of endotoxin in salmonella infections is not clear but it may be responsible for fever and possibly shock during bacteremia. It also may cause localization of leukocytes in the tissue due to activation and resulting chemotactic properties of complement. Several species of *Salmonella* contain enterotoxin, although its role in salmonellosis is not understood.

Major epidemics of typhoid fever are caused by contaminated drinking water or food. Wherever adequate sanitary measures have been applied, typhoid fever has nearly disappeared. Small outbreaks are sometimes traced to typhoid carriers among institutional or restaurant food handlers. Vaccines prepared from *S. typhi* cells have long been used prophylactically. The vaccines have proven to be somewhat successful in children but none has proven to be entirely effective in preventing disease.

Laboratory Diagnosis of Salmonella. The laboratory diagnosis of salmonella infection consists principally of the isolation and identification of the causative microorganisms or the demonstration of a rise in specific agglutinins within one or two weeks after the onset of the disease. Stool specimens are the best source of organisms during acute gastroenteritis. Blood cultures are best for detection of enteric fevers and septicemia. In typhoid bone marrow cultures may be positive, even after blood becomes negative. Urine also may be positive.

Treatment of Salmonella Infections. The treatment of typhoid fever and other salmonella infections centers around generalized supportive care of the patient and antibiotics. Ampicillin or chloramphenicol are the drugs of choice, although resistance to these has occurred. In such cases trimethoprim-sulfamethoxazole has proved effective. Ampicillin, possibly with cholecystectomy may be used in chronic carriers.

Prevention and Control of Salmonella Infections. Considerable success has been achieved in salmonella control by modern methods of livestock slaughter, better control and supervision of meat, eggs, and other animal products consumed by man, proper sewage disposal, and a carefully controlled water supply. The detection and control of human salmonella carriers have greatly helped to control typhoid fever and other human salmonelloses. Active immunization is not as effective as are sanitary procedures and the elimination of carriers.

THE SHIGELLAE

Shigella are primarily human pathogens that cause infections of the intestinal tract characterized primarily by diarrhea. Although fermentation reactions are useful for separation and differentiation, final identification of the various species is dependent upon their antigenic structure. The recognized species are *Shigella dysenteriae*, *Shigella boydii*, *Shigella flexneri*, and *Shigella sonnei*. *S. flexneri* and *S. dysenteriae* are the most common causes of dysentery.

Bacteriological Characteristics of the Shigellae. The morphology of the shigellae closely resembles that of the other enteric bacteria. They are gram negative, nonmotile, nonsporing rods. The shigellae are not very resistant to either physical or chemical agents and do not survive for long in the environment. They are particularly sensitive to acids; hence, if they are to be isolated from feces they must be cultured promptly or they will die from the acid produced by other fecal bacteria.

Pathogenicity of Shigella. The causal organisms are usually transmitted to the digestive tract of the susceptible individual in contaminated food or water. They penetrate the epithelial cells of the terminal ileum and colon, multiply and cause cell death and sloughing of the lining. The incubation period may be as short as 24 hours, and the onset of the disease is characterized by abdominal pain and cramps caused by an acute inflammatory reaction of the mucous membranes of the large bowel and occasionally the terminal ileum. Ulceration may occur, with hemorrhage and the production of mucin. Septicemia does not occur and the infection is self-limited. During the severe diarrhea, dehydration and disturbance of the electrolyte balance are frequent concomitants. Shigellae produce a heat-labile enterotoxin that can cause fluid accumulation in ileal loops of rabbits. The role of the toxin in disease is not clear since invasive but nontoxigenic strains of *S. dysenteriae* can cause disease. It may be responsible for the watery diarrhea that occurs in *Shigella*-induced dysentery.

Immunity in Shigella. Abundant humoral antibodies are formed during a dysenteric infection. However, recovery from the disease is not correlated to the appearance of specific antibodies. Individuals living in regions where the dysentery bacilli are indigenous become resistant if not immune to recurrent attacks of bacillary dysentery. Local tissue immunity may be the most important protective factor. Although shigella vaccines have been prepared which induce a high antibody titer, they are not effective.

Laboratory Diagnosis of Shigella. The laboratory diagnosis of dysentery consists principally of the isolation and identification of the causal microorganisms.

Diagnosis of dysentery retrospectively by the demonstration of specific agglutinin formation is not very practical. The demonstration of a rise in antibody titer during the course of the disease is the only significant demonstration of specific antibody formation. Serological typing and biochemical studies are necessary for complete diagnosis and identification.

Treatment of Shigella. Although many do not seek treatment and the disease may be self-limiting, antimicrobial therapy decreases severity and mortality of the disease. Especially in the debilitated and young children and in older individuals, antibiotic therapy is indicated. While ampicillin is the drug of choice, most shigella are sensitive to tetracyclines, streptomycin, sulfonamides, kanamycin, chloramphenicol, nalidixic acid, and colistin. However, trimethoprim-sulfamethoxazole also is effective. Shigella are notorious for their ability to quickly develop drug resistance.

Prevention and Control of Shigella. The control of bacillary dysentery requires careful disposition of excreta. Careful consideration must also be given to the detection of subclinical or symptomless cases which may become carriers. No convalescent case should be released while still discharging dysentery bacilli. Food and water must be protected and flies must be controlled.

THE VIBRIOS

The genus *Vibrio* is composed of five recognized species and a number of biotypes which are variously parasitic, pathogenic, and widely distributed as saprophytes in water and soil. *Vibrio cholerae* causes cholera, a water-borne gastrointestinal disease of areas with inadequate sanitation, which normally affects only human beings. *Vibrio* strains not capable of producing true cholera have been isolated in tropical areas. El Tor and Celebes vibrios differ from *V. cholerae* by being hemolytic and less virulent. El Tor vibrios are antigenically similar to the cholera vibrio, but they produce only a mild diarrheal disease. The Celebes vibrios are similar to the El Tor vibrios but are more pathogenic. Other *Vibrio* species that are not pathogenic for man produce disease in birds, animals, or fish.

Vibrio cholerae. *V. cholerae* is a gram negative, nonsporing, slightly curved rod that is markedly pleomorphic under adverse conditions. The cells are actively motile by a single polar flagellum. It is considered a facultative anaerobe. A biotype of *V. cholerae* was first isolated at the El Tor quarantine station on the Sinai Peninsula. Other similar types were isolated and for a time these bacteria were considered to be distinct species. The classic and El Tor types are similar and both are now considered as biotypes of the same species.

Pathogenesis of Cholera. Cholera is primarily acquired by the ingestion of the cholera vibrio in contaminated water or food. The incubation period ranges from 1 to 5 days but is commonly no longer than 3 days. At the end of the incubation period cholera begins suddenly with the development of abdominal cramps, nausea, vomiting, and diarrhea. In the more severe form there is a voluminous liquid feces (rice water stools) discharged that is composed of mucous, epithelial cells, and 10^6 or more vibrios per milliliter, but it contains practically no protein. Patients with cholera may discharge as much as 10 to 15 liters of fluid per day, resulting in an extracellular fluid deficit, metabolic acidosis, and hypokalemia of sufficient severity to quickly produce shock and death. In either mild or severe cholera, the vibrios do not invade or disrupt the intestinal mucosa. They are able to maintain themselves in large numbers on the surface of the intestinal mucosa where they produce the cholera enterotoxin, which at submicrogram levels is able to stimulate a net flow of fluids and electrolytes from cells into the lumen of the gut, producing the symptoms characteristic of the disease.

Laboratory Diagnosis of Vibrio. Laboratory procedures essential to the exact diagnosis of cholera are the detection and identification of the organisms. Essential to diagnosis is the cultivation of *V. cholerae* from stools, but not from vomitus, in which they are inconstant. Many types of media have been used for cultivation, but the usual enteric media are suboptimal for growth and isolation. Specialized media are available for growth of *V. cholerae*. Once isolated they can be identified by staining with fluorescein-labeled specific antisera and by biochemical and agglutination tests.

Treatment of Vibrio. The current treatment of cholera consists of the restoration of lost liquids and electrolytes, usually resulting in dramatic recovery. This is accomplished by the intravenous administration of isotonic sodium chloride containing appropriate amounts of sodium bicarbonate or sodium acetate and potassium chloride. The administration of tetracycline will also assist in preventing intestinal fluid loss by decreasing the number of organisms. While antibiotics are useful in the treatment of cholera, they are not a complete substitute for fluid and ion restoration.

Prevention and Control of Cholera. The prevention and control of cholera are problems of public and private hygiene, mostly concerned with removing factors that favor the spread of the disease. Certainly, decontamination of drinking water is an important measure, as is the improvement of environmental sanitation. Safeguarding food and drinks by control of manufacturing processes or conditions under which they are sold, particularly during epidemics, is important in checking the spread of the disease. The early detection and isolation of cholera victims, particularly those without severe signs, are important life-saving and control measures. Various methods have been used to treat convalescent and contact carriers. Many of those concerned with prevention and control of cholera

believe that the parenteral administration of killed vaccines is useful.

OROFACIAL INFECTIONS

Gram negative enteric bacteria may inhabit the oropharynx and, as a result, produce infections of this region. These are a particular problem in elderly and chronically ill patients and those in whom antibiotic therapy has depressed the gram positive bacterial population. In the chronically ill patient, such infections become more common as the level of illness increases and the level of self-care decreases. The organisms found include *Escherichia coli*, *Enterobacter* species, *Pseudomonas aeruginosa*, *Proteus* species, *Klebsiella* species, and other members of the Enterobacteriaceae. These have been isolated from soft tissue infections and osteomyelitis, most often as a component of a mixed infection. The pattern of infections suggests that many are secondary infections or exacerbations of subacute infections. Many patients have had antibiotics for several days or weeks in association with some oral surgical procedure or infection. Acute infections with the enteric bacteria appear usually as a low grade fever and an obvious swelling filled with thick, possibly foul smelling purulent material. Treatment usually involves drainage and adjunctive antibiotic therapy. However, since these organisms are resistant to many antibiotics, they must be selected with particular care.

ADDITIONAL READING

BEECHAM, H. J., COHEN, M. L., AND PARKIN, W. E. 1979 *Salmonella typhimurium*; Transmission by Fiberoptic Upper Gastrointestinal Endoscopy. JAMA, **241**, 1013.

BLAKE, P. A., ALLEGRA, D. T., SNYDER, J. D., et al. 1980 Cholera—A Possible Endemic Focus in the United States. N Engl J Med, **302**, 305.

BLISSETT, M. L., ABBOTT, S. L., AND WOOD, R. M. 1974 Antimicrobial Resistance and R Factors in Salmonella Isolated in California (1971–1972). Antimicrob Agents Chemother, **5**, 161.

BORLAND, E. D. 1975 Salmonella Infection in Dogs, Cats. Tortoises and Terrapins. Vet Rec, **96**, 401.

BRAN, J. L. 1973 Skin Infection Due to *Salmonella enteritidis*. NY State J Med, **73**, 1118.

BRENNER, D. J., AND FALKOW, S. 1971 Molecular Relationships among Members of the Enterobacteriaceae. Adv Genet, **16**, 81.

BRENT, P., AND VOSTI, K. L. 1973 Methods for Serogrouping *Escherichia coli*. Appl Microbiol, **25**, 208.

CARPENTER, C. C. J. 1971 Cholera; Diagnosis and Treatment. Bull NY Acad Med, **47**, 1192.

CARPENTER, C. C. J. 1972 Cholera and Other Enterotoxin-related Diarrheal Diseases. J Infect Dis, **126**, 551.

CLEMENTI, K. J. 1975 Treatment of *Salmonella* Carriers with Trimethoprim-Sulfamethoxazole. Can Med Assoc J, **112**, 28S.

COLLINS, C. M. 1973 Importation of Cholera into New Zealand, 1972. NZ Med J, **78**, 105.

COSTERTON, J. W., INGRAM, J. M., AND CHENG, K. J. 1974

Structure and Function of the Cell Envelope of Gram-Negative Bacteria. Bacteriol Rev, **38**, 87.

DATTA, N., AND OLARTE, J. 1974 R Factors in Strains of *Salmonella typhi* and *Shigella dysenteriae* I Isolated During Epidemics in Mexico; Classification by Compatibility. Antimicrob Agents Chemother, **5**, 310.

DAVIES, J. W., COX, K. G., SIMON, W. R., AND BOWMER, E. J. 1972 Typhoid at Sea; Epidemic Aboard an Ocean Liner. Can Med Assoc J, **106**, 877.

DIEM, L. V., AND ARNOLD, K. 1974 Typhoid Fever with Myocarditis. Am J Trop Med Hyg, **23**, 218.

DONTA, S. T. 1975 Changing Concepts of Infectious Diarrheas. Geriatrics, **30**, 123.

DUPONT, H. L. 1978 Enteropathogenic Organisms. Med Clin North Am, **62**, 945.

DUPONT, H. L., FORMAL, S. B., HORNICK, R. B., SNYDER, M. J., LIBONATI, J. P., SHEAHAN, D. G., LABREE, E. R., AND KALAS, J. P. 1971 Pathogenesis of *E. coli* diarrhea. N Engl J Med, **285**, 1.

DUPONT, H. L., HORNICK, R. B., SNYDER, M. J., LIBONATI, J. P., FORMAL, S. B., AND GANGAROSA, E. J. 1972 Immunity in Shigellosis; I, II. J Infect Dis, **125**, 12.

ETKIN, S., AND GORBACH, L. S. 1971 Studies on Enterotoxin from *Escherichia coli* Associated with Acute Diarrhea in Man. J Lab Clin Med, **78**, 81.

FIELD, M. 1971 Intestinal Secretion; Effect of Cyclic AMP and Its Role in Cholera. N Engl J Med, **284**, 1137.

FINEGOLD, D. C. 1970 Hospital-Acquired Infections. N Engl J Med, **283**, 1384.

FORMAL, S. B., SEMSKI, P., JR., GIANNELLA, R. A., AND AUSTIN, S. 1972 Mechanisms of *Shigella* Pathogenesis. Am J Clin Nutr, **25**, 1427.

GANGAROSA, E. J. 1971 The Epidemiology of Cholera; Past and Present. Bull NY Acad Med, **47**, 1140.

GANGAROSA, E. J., BEISEL, W. R., CHANYS, B., SPRINZ, H., AND PRAPONT, P. 1960 The Nature of the Gastrointestinal Lesion in Asiatic Cholera and Its Relation to Pathogenesis; A Biopsy Study. Am J Trop Med Hyg, **9**, 125.

GANGAROSA, E. J., AND FAICH, G. A. 1971 Cholera; the Risk to American Travelers. Ann Intern Med, **74**, 412.

GARROWAY, R. Y., AND ORDWAY, C. B. 1980 *Serratia marcescens* Osteomyelitis: Report of Two Cases. J Trauma, **20**, 1007.

GORBACH, S. L. 1971 Intestinal Microflora. Gastroenterology, **60**, 1110.

GOULD, K. L., GOOCH, J. M., AND CHING, G. Q. L. 1972 Epidemiologic Salmonellosis in Hawaii. Amer J Public Health, **62**, 1216.

GRADY, G. F., AND KEUSCH, G. T. 1971 Pathogenesis of Bacterial Diarrheas; I, II. N Engl J Med, **285**, 831.

GRAHNEIS, H. 1974 Effectiveness of Oral Inactivated Typhoid Vaccine. Acta Microbiol Acad Sci Hung, **21**, 129.

GREGORY, J. E., STARR, S. P., AND OMDAL, C. 1974 Wound Infection with *Shigella flexneri*. J Infect Dis, **129**, 602.

GYLES, C. L. 1972 Plasmids in Intestinal Bacteria. Am J Clin Nutr, **25**, 1455.

HARDING, J. W., BRADDOCK, G. T. T., AND CROYDON, E. A. P. 1970 Successful Treatment of Osteomyelitis Caused by *Pseudomonas aeruginosa*. J Clin Pathol, **23**, 653.

HENDRIX, T. R. 1971 The Pathophysiology of Cholera. Bull NY Acad Med, **47**, 1169.

HOFFMAN, T. A., RUIZ, C. J., COUNTS, G. W., SACHS, J. M., AND NITZKIN, J. L. 1975 Waterborne Typhoid Fever in Dade County, Florida; Clinical and Therapeutic Evaluation of 105 Bacteremic Patients. Am J Med, **59**, 481.

HOLMGREN, J., AND LONNROTH, I. 1976 Cholera Toxin and the Adenylate Cyclase-activating Signal. J Infect Dis, **133**, S64.

HONE, R., FITZPATRICK, S., KEANE, C., GROSS, R. J., AND ROWE, B. 1973 Infantile Enteritis in Dublin Caused by *Escherichia coli* 0142. J Med Microbiol, **6**, 505.

HORNICK, R. B., GREISMAN, S. E., WOODWARD, T. E., DUPONT, H. L., DAWKINS, A. T., AND SNYDER, M. J. 1970 Typhoid Fever; Pathogenesis and Immunologic Control. N Engl J Med, **283**, 686.

JAMES, T. 1973 History of Medicine; the Story of the Enteropathic *Escherichia coli*. S Afr Med J, **47**, 1476.

KÉTYI, I., RAUSS, K., AND VERTENYI, A. 1974 Oral Immunization against dysentery. Acta Microbiol Acad Sci Hung, **21**, 81.

KEUSCH, G. T., AND GRADY, G. F. 1972 The Pathogenesis of *Shigella* diarrhea; I. Enterotoxin Production by *Shigella dysenteriae*. J Clin Invest, **51**, 1212.

KUBINYI, L., KISS, I., AND LENDVAI, G. 1974 Epidemiological-Statistical Evaluation of Oral Vaccination against Infantile *Escherichia coli* Enteritis. Acta Microbiol Acad Sci Hung, **21**, 187.

KUROSKY, A., MARKEL, D. E., TOUCHSTONE, B., AND PETERSON, J. W. 1976 Chemical Characterization of the Structure of Cholera Toxin and Its Natural Toxoid. J Infect Dis, **133** (Suppl), S14.

LAFORCE, F. M., HOPKINS, J., TROW, R., AND WANG, W. L. L. 1976 Human Oral Defenses against Gram-Negative Rods. Am Rev Respir Dis, **114**, 929.

LAMM, S. H., TAYLOR, A., JR., GANGAROSA, E. J., ANDERSON, H. W., YOUNG, W., CLARK, M. H., AND BRUCE, A. R. 1972 Turtle-associated Salmonellosis; I. An Estimation of the Magnitude of the Problem in the United States, 1970–1971. Am J Epidemiol, **95**, 511.

LERNER, A. M. 1974 Persistent Carrier of *Escherichia coli* in Sputum. JAMA, **227**, 315.

LEVIN, M. M., DUPONT, H. L., KHODABANDELOU, M., AND HORNICK, R. B. 1973 Long-Term Shigella-Carrier State. N Engl J Med, **288**, 1169.

LEWIS, J. N., LOEWENSTEIN, M. S., GUTHRIE, L. C., AND SUGI, M. 1972 *Shigella sonnei* Outbreak on the Island of Maui. Am J Epidemiol, **96**, 50.

LOVE, W. C., GROSS, R. J., GORDON, A. M., AND ROWE, B. 1972 Infantile Gastroenteritis Due to *Escherichia coli* 0142. Lancet, **2**, 355.

MACKENJEE, M. K. R., COOVADIA, H. M., AND NAIDOO, L. S. 1974 Salmonella Osteomyelitis. S Afr Med J, **48**, 591.

McCOY, J. H. 1974 Trends in Salmonella Food Poisoning in England and Wales, 1941–1972. J Hyg (Camb), **74**, 271.

MEITERT, T., SULEA, I. T., GOGULESCU, L., BARON, E., TEMPEA, C., AND ISTRATI, G. 1974 Immunogenic Value of Live, Inactivated and Cell-free Dysentery Vaccines. Acta Microbiol Acad Sci Hung, **21**, 103.

MEL, D. M., ARSIC, B. L., RADOVANOVIC, M. L., KALJALOVIC, R., AND LITVINJENKO, S. 1974 Safety Tests in Adults and Children with Live Oral Typhoid Vaccine. Acta Microbiol Acad Sci Hung, **21**, 161.

OBERDOERSTER, F., AND THILO, W. 1974 A New Inactivated Oral Cholera Vaccine. Acta Microbiol Acad Sci Hung, **21**, 213.

PIERCE, N. F., GREENOUGH, W. B., AND CARPENTER, C. C. J., JR. 1971 *Vibrio cholerae* Enterotoxin and Its Mode of Action. Bacteriol Rev, **35**, 1.

RAUSS, K., KÉTYI, I., SZENDREI, L., AND VERTENYI, A. 1974 Immunization of Infants against *Escherichia coli* Enteritis. Acta Microbiol Acad Sci Hung, **21**, 181.

RICHARDSON, A. 1975 Salmonellosis in Cattle. Vet Rec, **96**, 329.

ROBERTS, D., BOAG, K., HALL, M. L. M., AND SHIPP, C. R. 1975 The Isolation of Salmonellas from British Pork Sausages and Sausage Meat. J Hyg (Camb), **75**, 173.

ROSE, H. D., HECKMAN, M. G., AND UNGER, J. D. 1973

Pseudomonas aeruginosa Pneumonia in Adults. Am Rev Respir Dis, **107**, 416.

ROSENBAUM, B. J. 1972 Modern Concepts in the Treatment of Cholera. Milit Med, **137**, 26.

ROWE, B., TAYLOR, J., AND BITTELHEIM, K. A. 1970 An Investigation of Traveller's Diarrhoea. Lancet, **1**, 1.

SACK, D. A., WELLS, J. G., MERSON, M. H., SACK, R. B., AND MORRIS, G. K. 1975 Diarrhoea Associated with Heat-Stable Enterotoxin-producing Strains of *Escherichia coli*. Lancet, **2**, 239.

SALETTI, M., AND RICCI, A. 1974 Experiments with Cholera Toxin Detoxified with Glutaraldehyde. Bull WHO, **51**, 633.

SALMONELLOSIS IN THE UNITED STATES, 1968–1974. 1976 From the Center for Disease Control. J Infect Dis, **133**, 483.

SASLAW, M. S., NITZKIN, J. L., FELDMAN, R., BAINE, W., PFEIFFER, K., AND PEARSON, M. 1975 Typhoid Fever; Public Health Aspects. Am J Public Health, **65**, 1184.

SHIGETA, S., AND ISHIDA, N. 1974 Studies of *Pseudomonas aeruginosa* Infections among Hospitalized Patients; I. Isolation and Identification of Nonfermentative Gram-Negative Rods. Jpn J Microbiol, **18**, 9.

SIEBELING, R. J., NEAL, P. M., AND GRANBERRY, W. D. 1975 Evaluation of Methods for the Isolation of *Salmonella* and *Arizona* Organisms from Pet Turtles Treated with Antimicrobial Agents. Appl Microbiol, **29**, 240.

SMITH, D. G. 1973 The *Proteus* Swarming Phenomenon. Sci Prog, **60**, 487.

SMYSER, C. F., AND SNOEYENBOS, G. H. 1973 Fluorescent-Antibody Methods for Detecting Salmonellae in Animal By-products. Avian Dis, **17**, 99.

SOJKA, W. J., WRAY, C., HUDSON, E. B., AND BENSON, J.

A. 1975 Incidence of Salmonella Infection in Animals in England and Wales, 1968–73. Vet Rec, **96**, 280.

SVENNERHOLM, A. M., HOLMGREN, J., AND OUCHTERLONY, O. 1975 Experimental Studies on Cholera Immunization. Acta Path Microbiol Scand, Sect C, **83**, 221.

TAYLOR, H. M. 1974 Cholera in Volunteers and in Naturally Infected Patients. J Infect Dis, **129**, 478.

TOPPING, J. W., POPKES, D. L., AND DISANTO, D. A. 1974 Salivary *Pseudomonas aeruginosa*. Oral Surg, **38**, 42.

VALENTI, W. M., TRUDELL, R. G., AND BENTLEY, D. W. 1978 Factors Predisposing to Oropharyngeal Colonization with Gram-Negative Bacilli in the Aged. N Engl J Med, **298**, 1108.

WALKER, J. H. 1971 Typhoid and Paratyphoid Immunization. Practitioner, **206**, 478.

WASHINGTON, J. A., II 1976 Laboratory Approaches to the Identification of Enterobacteriaceae. Hum Pathol, **7**, 151.

WATSON, W. A. 1975 Salmonella Infection and Meat Hygiene; Poultry Meat. Vet Rec, **96**, 351.

WERNER, S. B., ROBERTO, R. R., AND CHIN, J. 1972 Importation of Shiga Bacillus Dysentery into California. Calif Med, **116**, 20.

WHIPP, S. C., MOON, H. W., AND LYON, N. C. 1975 Heat-stable *Escherichia coli* Enterotoxin Production *in Vivo*. Infect Immun, **12**, 240.

WILLIAMS, B. M. 1975 Environmental Considerations in Salmonellosis. Vet Rec, **96**, 318.

WRIGHT, C., KOMINOS, S. D., AND YEE, R. B. 1976 *Enterobacteriaceae* and *Pseudomonas aeruginosa* Recovered from Vegetable Salads. Appl Environ Microbiol, **31**, 453.

chapter 28

Clostridium

George S. Schuster

CLOSTRIDIA

The genus *Clostridium*, composed of gram positive, obligately anaerobic, sporulating rods, is divided into more than 60 species. Some are frankly pathogenic but many of the saprophytic species inhabit the soil where they decompose organic matter and fix nitrogen. A few species are important in industrial fermentations. Pathogenic species inhabit soils and the intestinal tracts of man and domesticated animals. They cause tetanus, gas gangrene, enterocolitis, and botulism. Tetanus and botulism are each caused by single species, *Clostridium tetani* and *Clostridium botulinum*, respectively. Enterocolitis may be caused by several different species and at least five or six species are primarily involved in gas gangrene.

The identification of the clostridia associated with human or animal disease is by means of (1) cultural characteristics, (2) biochemical activities, (3) spore formation and the morphology of the spore, (4) production of specific toxins and their identification by neutralization with homologous antitoxins, and (5) requirements for special media and conditions.

The pathogenicity of the clostridia for the most part depends upon their production of powerful exotoxins either outside the body in foodstuffs or in local infections in the tissues. Disease production by the gas gangrene group is partially attributable to the production *in vivo* of lytic enzymes, which assist in the spread of infection and the dissemination of the breakdown products of tissue.

CLOSTRIDIUM TETANI

Morphology of *C. tetani*. *C. tetani* is a gram positive, obligately anaerobic, sporulating rod with a spherical, terminal spore. It is flagellated and therefore motile. The bacteria and its spores are normal inhabitants of the soil and the intestinal tract of man and animals. The spores of *C. tetani* are very resistant to physical and chemical agents.

Growth and Metabolism of *C. tetani*. The tetanus bacillus grows optimally at 37 C if the oxidation-reduction potential is reduced suffi-

ciently. Carbohydrates are not fermented by the tetanus bacillus but the complex nutritional requirements can be met by blood agar or cooked meat medium. Swarming occurs on blood agar, with growth spreading over the surface of the agar, making colony isolation difficult.

Antigenic Structure of *C. tetani*. *C. tetani* has been divided into at least 10 serotypes, based upon their flagellar (H) antigen. Other antigens include a somatic (O) and a spore antigen. Tetanus toxins are antigenically identical, regardless of the serotype from which they are derived.

Tetanus. Tetanus (or commonly lockjaw) is essentially a tonic spasm of striated muscle caused by the neurotoxin of *C. tetani*.

The chief reservoir of tetanus cells or spores is the soil, from which they find their way into wounds, burns, or other injuries. If conditions are suitable, as in traumatized tissue or puncture wounds with a sufficiently low oxidation-reduction potential, the spores germinate in 2 to 50 days and the bacilli multiply locally, producing a toxin which usually is disseminated to nearby peripheral nerves and eventually to the central nervous system. The toxin probably travels within the nerve trunk in the tissue spaces between individual nerve fibers: it is not clear how it enters the central nervous system. Tetanus can, on occasion, occur in a localized form, adjacent to the site of inoculation, but more frequently it is generalized in nature.

The earliest manifestation of tetanus is muscle stiffness, followed by spasm of the masseter muscles, trismus or lockjaw, the classic symptoms of tetanus. As the disease progresses tetanic spasms cause clenching of the jaws, flexing of the arms, extension of the legs and arching of the back. These spasms are brief but may be frequent. Occasionally, the spasms may be severe enough to produce bone fracture. Respiratory complications such as aspiration pneumonia are common. The disease may persist over several weeks and death may occur during one of the spasms due to contractions in the muscles of respiration. Injuries close to the head have a poor prognosis. Patients who recover usually have no permanent sequelae.

327

Tetanus toxin is released mostly after cessation of cellular growth. Tetanus toxin, a simple protein with a molecular weight of about 68,000, is among the most poisonous produced by bacteria. When crystallized it contains more than 30 million lethal doses for mice per milligram of protein. It is readily converted by formaldehyde into a stable toxoid, which is useful for active immunization. Tetanus toxin acts at the synaptosome. It binds to the gangliosides in the synaptic membranes and is dependent upon the number and position of sialic acid residues. Toxin produces excitation of the central nervous system by blocking synaptic inhibition in the spinal cord, presumably at inhibitory terminals. Such elimination of inhibitory responses of the nerve fibers permits the uncontrolled spread of impulses initiated in the central nervous system, resulting in an exaggerated reflex response of the skeletal muscles. The pattern of response is determined by the strongest muscles at a given joint.

Laboratory Diagnosis of C. tetani. The initial diagnosis and treatment of tetanus depends on the presence of certain clinical symptoms. Time is of the essence in treatment and it should not wait on the few days required to isolate and identify C. tetani. Nevertheless, the causative bacteria should be cultured and isolated. Identification of C. tetani relates to morphological, serological and cultural characteristics, especially sporulation and type of terminal spore produced, hemolysis of blood, swarming, staining with fluorescent antibodies, toxin production, and its neutralization in a mouse protection test.

Treatment of C. tetani. Initial treatment consists of immediate excision of the lesion to allow its exposure to the air. Excision is followed by the administration of antitoxin to neutralize as much as possible of the toxin before it becomes fixed to the tissues. Large doses of penicillin, or a suitable alternate, should be administered. Supportive care to maintain respiratory functions and control spasms is also important.

Prevention and Control of Tetanus. Some time after World War I, toxoid came into use for active immunization against tetanus. The usual practice is to immunize during the first year of life with a multiple vaccine containing tetanus toxoid, diphtheria toxoid, and pertussis vaccine in a course of three injections about a month apart. A booster dose is given a year later and when entering elementary school. Booster vaccinations at 10-year intervals are given to those who are regularly exposed to a risk of infection. Previously immunized individuals who are wounded should have an immediate booster dose of toxoid. Wounded individuals not previously immunized should be given human tetanus immune globulin as well as toxoid injections for future protection.

HISTOTOXIC CLOSTRIDIAL INFECTIONS

Gas Gangrene. Gas gangrene is essentially a rapidly spreading edematous myonecrosis accompanied by profound toxemia and prostration, which results from the infection of severe wounds and the invasion of muscle by species of Clostridium, especially Clostridium perfringens, Clostridium novyi, Clostridium bifermentans, Clostridium histolyticum, and Clostridium septicum.

The cells of the principal species of Clostridium involved in gas gangrene are all relatively large gram positive rods that form oval, subterminal spores greater in diameter than the vegetative cell.

Wound Infection and the Pathogenesis of Gas Gangrene. The development of gas gangrene is intimately related to the general problem of wound infection. The organisms most commonly found in wounds are the Clostridium species, nonsporulating bacteria of fecal origin (enterococci and enterobacteriaceae), and pyogenic cocci (staphylococci and streptococci). Factors which influence the course of a wound infection are the nature of the contaminating bacteria; the location, nature, and severity of the wound; the presence of extraneous material in the wound; the condition of the patient, including immunity response; and perhaps most important of all, the promptness and adequacy of treatment. Infected wounds that do not develop into gas gangrene exhibit approximately three phases. In the primary stage, which lasts about a week, clostridia and streptococci predominate. During the secondary stage, which lasts from 2 to 3 weeks, there is a gradual transition from the primary anaerobic infection to one dominated by the pyogenic cocci, accompanied by the enterococci and enterobacteriaceae. Finally, the latter gradually disappear, leaving a simple pyogenic infection by staphylococci and streptococci.

Cytotoxic clostridial infections usually result from the introduction of the causal clostridia or their spores by contamination of wounds with soil. The intensity of the infection can vary from a simple contamination of the wound of short duration without frank disease, to anaerobic cellulitis, to the most serious condition of all, known as clostridial myonecrosis or gas gangrene, which can develop within several hours. In simple wound contamination the clostridia may be present without obvious pathology. Anaerobic cellulitis occurs when the clostridia infect tissue damaged by direct trauma or ischemia. Organisms spread through subcutaneous tissue and along fascial plans, but do not invade healthy tissue. There is extensive clostridial growth and gas is a prominent feature. There is not an extreme toxemia present, as occurs in clostridial myonecrosis.

In myonecrosis during the first few hours follow-

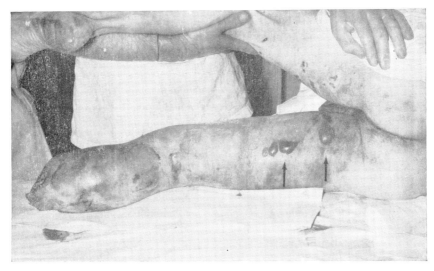

Figure 28/1. Gas gangrene. Note gas bubbles which have formed beneath the skin. (AFIP.)

ing the initiation of the infection, there is at first connective tissue destruction adjacent to healthy muscle. Characteristic of the onset of the infection is a rapidly spreading edema, which first involves subcutaneous connective tissue and then connective tissue of muscles. Accompanying the edema, gas may develop and distend the tissue (fig. 28/1). The resulting pressure tends to spread the infection. As the disease progresses, more and more tissue is involved and muscle tissue adjacent to the wound is discolored. The infection is rapidly destructive and more foul smelling if the proteolytic species are present. Gas gangrene results in a severe toxemia and prostration caused by the absorption of the products of tissue injury and dissolution. Although the patient usually remains mentally alert, coma and delirium sometimes precede death. Characteristically there is a reduced blood pressure and death results from circulatory failure.

Streptococcal myositis may appear similar to gas gangrene except that it is caused by anaerobic streptococci, there is only focal muscle involvement, the discharge from the wound is purulent, and toxemia is inconstant.

C. perfringens is also a cause of food poisoning. It is induced some 12 hours after eating foods, particularly meat, that are contaminated with *C. perfringens*. It occurs in the form of a self-limited gastroenteritis. A more serious enteric infection, enteritis necroticans, has been described. It is an acute inflammatory infection of the small intestines that causes a high mortality.

Laboratory Diagnosis of Cytotoxic Clostridial Infections. The demonstration of typical gram positive bacilli in exudate from infected wounds is indicative of cytotoxic clostridial infections. It is also useful to culture specimens both aerobically and anaerobically. Growth of typical gram positive bacilli anaerobically but not aerobically indicates a positive clostridial infection. Positive identification of clostridia requires the determination of their biochemical characteristics.

Treatment of Cytotoxic Clostridial Infections. The treatment of clostridial wound infections requires surgical debridement, and, in the case of gas gangrene, the complete removal of infected muscle. Polyvalent antitoxin is useful, as is hyperbaric oxygen in the treatment of clostridial myonecrosis. Penicillin prevents spread of the infection and prevents a bacteremia.

ANTIBIOTIC-ASSOCIATED COLITIS

Certain antibiotics, including clindamycin, ampicillin, and neomycin, have been associated with development of diarrhea and pseudomembranous enterocolitis. This appears to be due to enterotoxin-producing strains of *Clostridium difficile. C. difficile* is usually present in low numbers in the normal intestinal flora of some individuals and may be resistant to various antibiotics. Administration of these drugs selects for the resistant strains that overgrow in the gastrointestinal tract. Production of the enterotoxin results in the symptomatology, but the toxin's mode of action is not known. Cessation of the use of the antibiotic will result in resolution of most cases. Vancomycin has been used successfully to treat *C. difficile* enterocolitis, although there have been reports of deaths after the vancomycin was stopped.

BOTULISM

Bacteriological Characteristics of *Clostridium botulinum*. *C. botulinum*, widely distributed in soils, is a gram positive, sporeforming, motile, anaerobic rod. The organisms under strictly anaerobic conditions produce a characteristic and very potent lethal exotoxin.

Botulinum Toxin. Botulism normally is an intoxication resulting from the consumption of food in which *C. boutulinum* has grown and produced exotoxin. There are eight serologically distinct types of the organism based on the type of toxin produced. Botulinum toxin is the most potent toxin known. One microgram of purified toxin contains about 2,000,000 minimum lethal doses for a mouse. The toxins are relatively heat-labile, being inactivated at 100 C for 10 min. They are resistant to the gastric acids and intestinal proteolytic enzymes.

Toxin is absorbed largely from the small intestine, appearing in the lymphatics, then the bloodstream. The toxin acts at the myoneural junction to produce paralysis of the cholinergic nerve fibers at the point of release of acetylcholine. It suppresses release of acetylcholine. Death occurs following paralysis of respiratory organs.

Clinical Manifestations. Typically symptoms of botulism begin 12 to 36 hours after ingestion of contaminated food. The onset of the disease is relatively gradual.

The following symptoms are characteristic of the disease in man:

1. Either an arrest of secretion or the hypersecretion of salivary glands and the glands in the buccopharyngeal mucosa.
2. More or less complete inability to hold the eyelids open, dilatation of pupils, paralysis in accommodation, diplopia and internal strabismus.
3. Dysphagia, aphonia, constipation, and retention of urine.
4. General weakness of all voluntary muscles.
5. An absence of fever and sensory and mental disturbances.
6. Depression of respiration and circulation.

Death is caused by asphyxia resulting from respiratory paralysis or heart failure.

Until recently it was assumed that botulism could be caused only by ingestion of preformed toxin. However, it has been recognized that in infants botulism may occur following elaboration of toxin from organisms in the gastrointestinal tract. In many instances, the cases followed ingestion of honey contaminated with botulinum spores, suggesting this food as a possible source of the illness in these children.

Laboratory Diagnosis of *C. botulinum*. The demonstration of *C. botulinum* as a cause of food poisoning depends upon the detection of the toxin or the bacilli either in the contents of the intestinal tract of the victim or in the food eaten by him.

Prevention and Control of *C. botulinum*. On the whole, the prevention of botulism is simple. All preserved foods which are obviously spoiled should be avoided, but *C. botulinum* often toxifies food without obvious signs of spoilage. Exposure to 100 C for 15 min or its equivalent can be relied on for detoxification. The botulinal toxins can be converted into effective toxoids by formaldehyde but no clear-cut indications have been defined for their general use. Polyvalent type A, B, and E antitoxin should be administered intramuscularly as a prophylactic to all who have consumed a known toxified food but have not yet exhibited symptoms of botulism. Therapeutic value of the antitoxins has not been convincingly demonstrated.

ADDITIONAL READING

AFONJA, A. O., JAIYEOLA, B. O., AND TUNWASHE, O. L. 1973 Tetanus in Lagos: A Review of 228 Adult Nigerian Patients. J Trop Med Hyg, **76,** 171.

BARTLETT, J. G., CHANG, T., TAYLOR, N. S., AND ONDERDONK, A. B. 1979 Colitis Induced by *Clostridium difficile*. Rev Infect Dis, **1,** 370.

BARTLETT, J. G., WILLEY, S. H., CHANG, T., AND LOWE, B. 1979 Cephalosporin-associated Pseudomenbranous Colitis Due to *Clostridium difficile*. JAMA, **242,** 2683.

BARTLETT, J. G., TEDESCO, F. J., SHULL, S., LOWE, B., AND CHANG, T. 1980 Symptomatic Relapse after Oral Vancomycin Therapy of Antibiotic Associated Pseudomembranous Colitis. Gastroenterology, **78,** 431.

BLAKE, P. A., FELDMAN, R. A., BUCHANAN, T. M., BROOKS, G. F., AND BENNETT, J. V. 1976 Serologic Therapy of Tetanus in the United States, 1965–1971. JAMA, **235,** 42.

BOROFF, D. A., AND GUPTA, D. 1971 Botulinum Toxin. In *Microbial Toxins*, Vol. IIA, p. 1, edited by S. Kadis, T. C. Montie, and S. J. Ajl. Academic Press, New York.

COCKEY, R. R., AND TATRO, M. C. 1974 Survival Studies with Spores of *Clostridium botulinum* Type E in Pasteurized Meat of the Blue Crab *Callinectes sapidus*. Appl Microbiol, **27,** 629.

FINEGOLD, S. M. 1980 Anaerobic Infections. Surg Clin North Am, **60,** 49.

GEORGE, W. L., ROLFE, R. D., SUTTER, V. L., AND FINEGOLD, S. M. 1979 Diarrhea and Colitis Associated with Antimicrobial Therapy in Man and Animals. Am J Clin Nutr, **32,** 251.

GORBACH, S. L., AND THADEPALLI, H. 1975 Isolation of *Clostridium* in Human Infections; Evaluation of 114 Cases. J Infect Dis, **131,** S81.

GUNN, R. A. 1979 Epidemiologic Characteristics of Infant Botulism in the United States. Rev Infect Dis, **1,** 642.

HOBBS, B. C. 1974 *Clostridium welchii* and *Bacillus cereus* Infection and Intoxication. Postgrad Med J, **50,** 597.

ITO, K. A., CHEN, J. K., LERKE, P. A., SEEGER, M. L., AND UNVERFERTH, J. A. 1976 Effect of Acid and Salt Concentration in Fresh-Pack Pickles on the Growth of *Clostridium botulinum* Spores. Appl Environ Microbiol, **32,** 121.

KELLETT, C. E. 1939 The Early History of Gas Gangrene. Ann Med Hist, **1,** 452.

KWAN, P. L., AND LEE, J. S. 1974 Compound Inhibitory to *Clostridium botulinum* Type E Produced by a *Mor-*

axella Species. Appl Microbiol, **27,** 329.

LENNER, S. 1943 Experience with Gas Gangrene in Field Hospitals on the Western Front. War Med, **3,** 660.

LERNER, P. I. 1974 Antimicrobial Considerations in Anaerobic Infections. Med Clin North Am, **58,** 533.

MacLENNAN, J. D. 1962 The Histotoxic Clostridial Infections of Man. Bacteriol Rev, **26,** 177.

McCLUNG, L. S. 1956 The Anaerobic Bacteria with Special Reference to the Genus *Clostridium*. Ann Rev Microbiol, **10,** 173.

MERSON, M. H., AND DOWELL, V. R., JR. 1973 Epidemiologic, Clinical and Laboratory Aspects of Wound Botulism. N Engl J Med, **289,** 1005.

MILLER, L. G. 1975 Observations on the Distribution and Ecology of *Clostridium botulinum* Type E in Alaska. Can J Microbiol, **21,** 920.

NAKAMURA, M., AND SCHULZE, J. A. 1970 *Clostridium perfringens* Food Poisoning. Annu Rev Microbiol, **24,** 359.

NIILO, L. 1975 Measurement of Biological Activities of Purified and Crude Enterotoxin of *Clostridium perfringens*. Infect Immun, **12,** 440.

PETERSON, D. R., EKLUND, M. W., AND CHINN, N. M. 1979 The Sudden Infant Death Syndrome and Infant Botulism. Rev Infect Dis, **1,** 630.

POLEN, R. A., AND BROWN, L. W. 1979 Infant Botulism. Pediatr Clin North Am, **26,** 345.

PRINCE, A. S., AND NEU, H. C. 1979 Antibiotic-associated Pseudomembranous Colitis in Children. Pediatr Clin North Am, **26,** 261.

RAIBAUD, P., DUCLUZEAU, R., DUBOS, F., AND SACQUET, E. 1972 Spore Formation and Germination of *Clostridium perfringens* in the Digestive Tract of Holoxenic and Axenic Mice. J Appl Bacteriol, **35,** 177.

ROBERTS, T. A., KEYMER, I. F., BORLAND, E. D., AND SMITH, G. R. 1972 Botulism in Birds and Mammals in Great Britain. Vet Rec, **91,** 11.

SAKAGUCHI, G., OHISHI, I., KOZAKI, S., SAKAGUCHI, S., AND KITAMURA, M. 1974 Molecular Structures and Biological Activities of *Clostridium botulinum* Toxins. Jpn J Med Sci Biol, **27,** 95.

SEBALD, M., JOUGLARD, J., AND GILLES, G. 1974 Type B Botulism in Man Due to Cheese. Ann Microbiol (Paris), **125,** 349.

SELLIN, L. C. 1981 The Action of Botulinum Toxin at the Neuromuscular Junction. Med Biol, **59,** 11.

SHIMIZU, T., KONDO, H., AND SAKAGUCHI, G. 1974 Immunological Heterogeneity of *Clostridium botulinum* Type B Toxins. Jpn J Med Sci Biol, **27,** 99.

SILVA, J., JR., AND FEKETY, R. 1981 Clostridia and Antimicrobial Enterocolitis. Annu Rev Med, **32,** 327.

SMITH, L. D. S. 1979 Virulence Factors of *Clostridium perfringens*. Rev Infect Dis, **1,** 254.

SMITH, M. J. A., AND MYALL, R. W. T. 1976 Tetanus; Review of the Literature and Report of a Case. Oral Surg, **41,** 451.

UEMURA, T., GENIGEORGIS, C., RIEMANN, H. P., AND FRANTI, C. E. 1974 Antibody against *Clostridium perfringens* Type A Enterotoxin in Human Sera. Infect Immun, **9,** 470.

VAN BEEK, A., ZOOK, E., YAW, P., GARDNER, R., SMITH, R., AND GLOVER, J. L. 1974 Nonclostridial Gas-forming Infections; a Collective Review and Report of Seven Cases. Arch Surg, **108,** 552.

VAN HEYNINGEN, W. E., AND MELLANBY, J. 1971 Tetanus Toxin. In *Microbial Toxins*, Vol. IIA, p. 69, edited by S. Kadis, T. C. Montie, and S. J. Ajl. Academic Press, New York.

chapter 29

The Aerobic Spore-forming Bacilli

George S. Schuster

Bacillus anthracis. *B. anthracis* is the only member of the aerobic genus *Bacillus* that is commonly considered to be a significant pathogen. However, *Bacillus cereus, Bacillus subtilis,* and *Bacillus sphaericus* have been reported capable of causing meningitis, endocarditis, and osteomyelitis. *B. anthracis* is a large aerobic, gram positive, encapsulated sporeforming rod (fig. 29/1). It is non-hemolytic, which differentiates it from most other members of the genus *Bacillus.* Sporulation occurs readily under almost all conditions except in the living body where encapsulation is most prominent. Spores are very resistant, contaminating soils, the chief source of animal infection, for many years. They withstand boiling water for 10 min and dry heat (140 C) for 3 hours.

Anthrax bacilli possess capsular and somatic antigens and antigens that make up a complex exotoxin. The capsule is unusual in that it is a high molecular weight polypeptide consisting of D-glutamic acid. The somatic antigen is a polysaccharide component of the cell wall. The immunogenic toxin has been divided into three distinct antigenically active components; protective antigen, lethal factor, and edema factor.

B. anthracis undergoes genetic variation with regard to spore formation, virulence, sensitivity to chemotherapeutic agents, nutritional requirements, bacteriophages, and lysozyme. Virulence relates essentially to two factors, capsule formation and exotoxin production, and only strains that produce both are fully virulent. The capsule interferes with phagocytosis and is important in pathogenesis, especially in the early stages and infection. Anticapsular antibodies, however, are not protective. The signs and symptoms of anthrax are due to the cumulative effects of the toxin acting on the central nervous system. Toxemia can result in respiratory failure, anoxia and death.

Anthrax. In animals, the spores of *B. anthracis* enter the body through some break in the oral or intestinal mucosa. The incubation period is only a day or two, followed by an acute, fulminating disease that may terminate fatally within a few hours and usually in less than 1 day. In man, the organisms enter the body through breaks or wounds of the skin and the oral and intestinal mucosa or by inhalation. In the skin, a vesicle called a malignant pustule develops 2 to 5 days after infection (fig. 29/2). It begins as a papule that becomes filled with bluish-black fluid. This ruptures revealing a black eschar surrounded by an inflammatory ring. The infection may remain localized or disseminate. In the pulmonary infection, the primary manifestation is an acute pneumonia that leads to respiratory distress and cyanosis. In the intestinal tract it causes an acute enteritis.

Anthrax infection of the oral cavity has been caused by unsterilized tooth brushes made from bristles contaminated with anthrax spores. In a typical case, the hard palate was initially infected, causing considerable swelling and eventually discharging a straw-colored fluid. The patient was quite ill with a temperature which ranged from 100 to 102 F (38 to 39 C). The bone of the area became involved and as the infection continued, most of the palatal and alveolar bone was progressively destroyed. As the lesion developed, more and more of the area was involved, with extensive edema. The teeth were overly erupted and were apparently without bony support. Pustules with bright red bases appeared on the mucosal surface, many of which developed into vesicles that broke and scabbed, with eventual resolution. Treatment of the patient with antianthrax serum abated the symptoms, and there was gradual recovery. Either animals or humans that survive an attack of anthrax are usually resistant to reinfection, and vaccines have proved useful to control outbreaks in animals and humans.

Laboratory Diagnosis of Anthrax. The laboratory procedures useful for the diagnosis of anthrax are demonstration of characteristically large bacilli in tissue specimens stained with gram stain, culturing, and inoculation of samples into guinea pigs or mice.

Treatment of Anthrax. The anthrax bacillus is sensitive to penicillin, tetracycline, erythromycin,

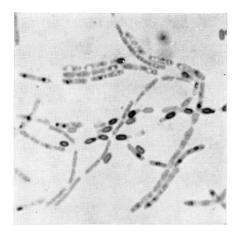

Figure 29/1. Antrax bacilli undergoing sporulation (×1850). (From Max Poser, Bausch and Lomb Optical Company.)

and chloramphenicol, with penicillin being the drug of choice and tetracycline being the best alternate. Cutaneous anthrax responds favorably to chemotherapy. Pulmonary anthrax is quite resistant to chemotherapy and its mortality rate is very high.

Prevention and Control of Anthrax. Anthrax is epidemic in Asia, Africa, and the Middle East, where it causes a heavy loss. It has occurred in Texas, Louisiana, South Dakota, Nebraska, and California. Worldwide, the human cases are estimated to range up to 100,000 annually. The few cases of anthrax that occur in the United States are in those who contact infected livestock, or who process imported hair, wool, or hides. The most successful control of animal anthrax relates to the use of attenuated vaccines. A vaccine made of protective antigens is also useful in protecting workers and veterinarians.

ADDITIONAL READING

BRACHMAN, P. S. 1970 Anthrax. Ann NY Acad Sci, **174,** 577.

CHRISTIE, A. B. 1973 The Clinical Aspects of Anthrax. Postgrad Med J, **49,** 565.

HEYWORTH, B., ROPP, M. E., VOOS, U. G., MEINEL, H. I., AND DARLOW, H. M. 1975 Anthrax in the Gambia; an Epidemiological Study. Br Med J, **4,** 79.

HUGH-JONES, M. E., AND HUSSAINI, S. N. 1974 An Anthrax Outbreak in Berkshire, Vet Rec, **94,** 228.

KAUFMAN, A. F., FOX, M. D., AND KOLB, R. C. 1973 Anthrax in Louisiana, 1971; an Evaluation of the Sterne Strain Anthrax Vaccine. J Am Vet Med Assoc, **163,** 442.

MORBIDITY AND MORTALITY WEEKLY REPORTS. 1968 Animal Anthrax in California, **17,** 279.

MORBIDITY AND MORTALITY WEEKLY REPORTS. 1969 Anthrax in New Jersey, **18,** 212.

MORBIDITY AND MORTALITY WEEKLY REPORTS. 1969 Cutaneous Anthrax in North Carolina, **18,** 40.

PLOTKIN, S. A., BRACHMAN, M., UTELL, M., BUMFORD, F. H., AND ATCHISON, M. M. 1960 An Epidemic of Inhalation Anthrax: The First in the Twentieth Century; I. Clinical Features. Am J Med, **29,** 992.

RONAGHY, H. A., AZADEH, B., KOHOUT, E., AND DUTZ, W. 1972 Penicillin Therapy of Human Anthrax. Curr Ther Res, **14,** 721.

SMITH, I. M. 1973 A Brief Review of Anthrax in Domestic Animals. Postgrad Med J, **49,** 571.

TUAZON, C. U., MURRAY, H. W., LEVY, C., SOLNY, M. N., CURTIN, J. A., AND SHEAGREN, J. N. 1979 Serious Infections from *Bacillus* sp. JAMA, **241,** 1137.

VANNESS, G. B. 1971 Ecology of Anthrax. Science, **172,** 1303.

WEBSTER, A. 1973 Inhibiting Effect of Antibiotics on Anthrax Vaccination. Aust Vet J, **49,** 545.

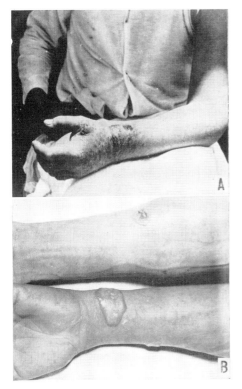

Figure 29/2. The cutaneous lesions of anthrax. (*A*, AFIP 218885-7; *B*, AFIP D45409-10.)

chapter 30

Spirochetes and Spirochetal Diseases

George S. Schuster

SPIROCHAETALES

The spirochetes are classified in the order Spirochaetales. Nonpathogenic spirochetes are generally large, free-living forms in water or sewage, or parasites of marine life. The species which are pathogenic for man, include only members of the three genera, *Treponema*, *Leptospira*, and *Borrelia*. They are differentiated primarily by their morphology.

TREPONEMA PALLIDUM AND RELATED SPIROCHETES

Morphology of *T. pallidum*. The causative agents of venereal and endemic syphilis (*T. pallidum*), yaws (*Treponema pertenue*), pinta (*Treponema carateum*), rabbit syphilis (*Treponema cuniculi*), and some of the oral spirochetes (*Treponema microdentium* and *Treponema mucosum*) cannot be definitely differentiated morphologically. They do differ in the diseases or lack of diseases they produce. *T. pallidum* (as well as the other related spirochetes) is a thin, spiral microorganism (fig. 30/1). Since the breadth of the cells ranges from 0.09 to 0.5 μm, their observation in films with an ordinary light microscope is difficult. Staining is not particularly helpful for observing the spirochetes unless the dye or some component is deposited to increase their volume and breadth. Spirochetes can be seen by dark-field or phase-contrast microscopy. Electron microscopy has revealed much of the internal morphology of spirochetes.

T. pallidum is similar structurally to other spirochetes (fig. 30/2). It consists of a multilayered cytoplasmic membrane, six thin fibrils which are located between the cytoplasmic membrane and the cell wall, a muramic acid containing cell wall, and a thin outer envelope. Pathogenic strains also appear to have a capsule-like layer not present in nonpathogens. *Treponema* species also contain intracytoplasmic tubules.

The cells of *T. pallidum* are flexible and elastic and have distinctive movement and motility, undergoing a sustained type of movement that involves rapid rotation. Their flexibility allows them to move among intercellular spaces.

Metabolism and Cultivation of *T. pallidum*. All attempts to culture fully pathogenic *T. pallidum* have been unsuccessful. Tissue cultures have not been successful because they are inherently aerobic, whereas *T. pallidum* is strictly anaerobic. The human and some other mammalian bodies may offer a nutritional factor that is not supplied *in vitro*.

Serial infection of the testicles of living rabbits has been the most successful method of propagating and maintaining virulent strains of *T. pallidum*. The Syrian hamster is also useful, but the infection is not so characteristic as it is with the rabbits.

Cultural procedures and animal inoculation have resulted in the isolation of several treponemal strains, some of which have maintained their pathogenicity in susceptible animals for considerable time. Cultured strains are antigenically heterogeneous, whereas the pathogenic Nichols and Noguchi strains resemble *T. pallidum*. Cultured strains are considered not to be identical with *T. pallidum*.

The fully virulent *T. pallidum* can be kept viable for about a week in an anaerobic maintenance medium but it does not reproduce. The organisms apparently do metabolize in it, for penicillin, even at very low concentrations will kill them after being exposed to it for 5 hours or so.

The cultured strains of spirochetes that resemble *T. pallidum* metabolize glucose and require exogenous fatty acids, coenzymes, bicarbonate, a variety of amino acids, and purines and pyrimidines.

T. pallidum is sensitive to temperature, for their survival time decreases as the temperature increases between 20 C and 40 C. Sensitivity of *T. pallidum* to increased temperature was used as the basis for fever therapy of syphilis. In blood or blood products at refrigerator temperature, the spirochetes do not survive for more than 48 hours. Contaminated whole blood used in transfusions is

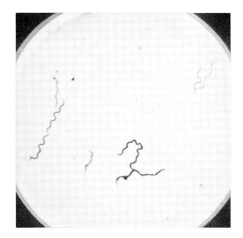

Figure 30/1. *Treponema pallidum* (×1000). (From Max Poser, Bausch and Lomb Optical Company.)

not a source of infections after being maintained for 4 days at refrigerator temperature.

SYPHILIS

Venereal Syphilis. Syphilis, caused by *T. pallidum*, is a venereal disease with a long clinical course and protean manifestations. It occurs naturally only in man and is usually propagated by sexual contacts between adults, except when it is transmitted congenitally from mother to fetus. In the Middle East and Balkans endemic syphilis occurs which is propagated by nonvenereal contact between children or children and adults.

In the primary and secondary stages of syphilis, *T. pallidum* grows and survives well in the oral cavity and the genitalia. Transmission of *T. pallidum* by the genital organs accounts for from 90 to 95% of syphilitic infections. The overwhelming proportion of extragenital infections occurs about the mouth as a result of transmission of the organisms from the oral cavity when kissing or by oral sex. Syphilis is seldom but occasionally transmitted indirectly by fomites. In the secondary stage of syphilis, there are many organisms in the skin. In the latter stages of syphilis, an individual may disseminate few or no spirochetes. The treponemes may be transmitted through the placental barrier of an infected, pregnant woman to a fetus. However, *T. pallidum* does not always infect the fetus.

After inoculation the organisms undergo rapid multiplication and are widely disseminated via the perivascular lymphatics and the systemic circulation. This takes place before development of the primary lesion. In man the incubation time required to produce an initial lesion averages about 3 weeks. The shortest incubation periods have resulted from the accidental inoculation of individuals with contaminated instruments. At the end of the primary incubation period a chancre develops, although a generalized systemic syphilitic infection may occur without its appearance. The chancre is usually single and painless (fig. 30/3). It appears at first as an erythematous macule, then as a papule which enlarges, becomes infiltrated, and eventually erodes. The base of the chancre is reddish brown. When fully developed it has a narrow, copper-colored, beveled border and is well demarcated from the surrounding skin or mucous membrane. It is indurated, hence it is called a hard chancre. The floor of the chancre produces a serosanguineous discharge and is covered by an adherent fibrinous membrane.

In the oral regions, the most frequent sites for the development of a chancre are the lips and tongue, the gingiva seldom being involved (fig. 30/6). When chancres occur on tonsils, they are often mistaken for diphtheria. Extraorally, initial infection and chancre formation may occur in or about

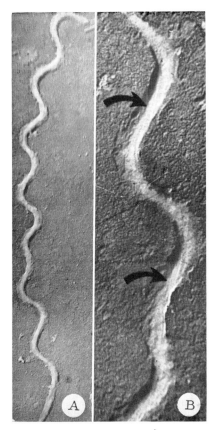

Figure 30/2. (*A*) *Treponema pallidum* from exudate of primary chancre. (*B*) The same spirochete at higher magnification showing an axial band (*arrows*) around which the main body of the spirochete is wound. (Reproduced with permission from R. H. A. Swain: Electron Microscopic Studies of the Morphology of Pathogenic Spirochetes. *Journal of Pathology and Bacteriology,* **69,** 117, 1955.)

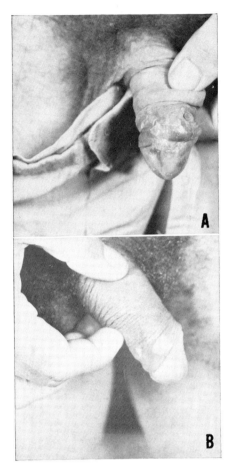

Figure 30/3. Chancre of the penis. (*A*, AFIP 59-12783; *B*, AFIP 59-12654.)

the eyes of dentists or health personnel. The chancre, if not secondarily infected, usually heals within 2 weeks but occasionally it may persist for as long as 6 weeks after initial onset. As the lesion subsides healing occurs with or without scarring.

After the chancre heals, the infection enters a secondary stage, with an average duration of about 2 years. This stage is characterized by a generalized spirochetal infection and by systemic manifestations. The integument teems with spirochetes. The symptoms are fever, headache, malaise, and fatigue.

Cutaneous eruptions manifest themselves as macules or papules (figs. 30/4 and 30/5). The lesion of the mucous membranes of the mouth and throat is the recurrent mucous patch and is due to local vasculitis (figs. 30/7 and 30/8). These lesions are small, grayish, slightly raised areas. Mucous patches disseminate numerous spirochetes into the oral cavity. The mucous and cutaneous eruptions of the secondary stage of syphilis persist or recur for 2 or 3 years. Recurrent outbreaks of secondary syphilitic lesions gradually become less extensive and further apart, finally subsiding as the infection

becomes latent. Secondary disease also may be characterized by generalized immunologic phenomena such as immune-complex nephritis (due to deposition of antigen-antibody complexes in the glomerular basement membrane), arthritis, and arthralgia.

In the latent stage, the infection shifts from a generalized type to a focal type, in which there are no specific subjective symptoms. Onset depends on some altered reactivity of the host cells and tissues to the spirochetes. As immunity develops, the many spirochetes of the secondary stage are reduced and they survive in restricted areas. Latency may continue for only a few months or for a lifetime.

The subsequent course of the syphilitic infection varies. About one-half of untreated patients remain asymptomatic. During a quite long period of time (up to 10 years) the remainder of untreated patients develop symptoms indicating a late or tertiary form of syphilis. The slow but persistent reactions occurring during this period may be hyperergic, chronic, proliferative, inflammatory, and destructive; they involve the viscera, and the skeletal, cardiovascular and central nervous systems. A very characteristic lesion of late syphilis is the gumma, probably arising from an immunological reaction. This lesion is quite destructive and may affect any tissue or organ of the body (fig. 30/9). Very few spirochetes are present in a gumma, certainly insufficient to produce the extensive damage found, unless an allergic reaction of the tissues to spirochetes is involved.

The principal lesions of late syphilis are gummas and nodular or noduloulcerative syphilids of the skin. These lesions are similar histologically but differ in gross appearance. The lungs, bronchi, and trachea are seldom affected in late syphilis. Gummas occur frequently in the oral cavity and in the larynx and vocal cords, however, resulting in a painless but persistent hoarseness. Next to the skin, the skeleton is most commonly involved in late syphilis. The changes in bone are usually a destructive osteitis or hypertrophic periosteitis, from which no bone is immune. The joints may be involved, commonly with hydroarthrosis.

Central Nervous System Syphilis. The central nervous system may be invaded by *T. pallidum* at any time from 10 days or more before the chancre appears until 4 or 5 years after latency develops, but not thereafter, apparently due to the development of an immunity. About 30% of those initially involved develop asymptomatic neurosyphilis but only about half develop late symptomatic neurosyphilis, if untreated.

Asymptomatic neurosyphilis is characterized by any of the following changes in the cerebrospinal fluid: an increase in the number of lymphocytes; an increase in the protein content, principally globulin

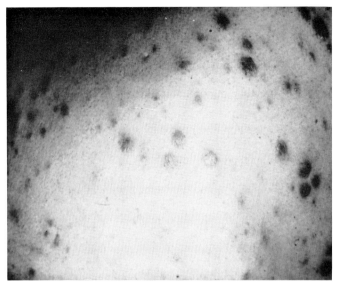

Figure 30/4. Cutaneous eruptions of the secondary syphillis. (AFIP 58-13966-45.)

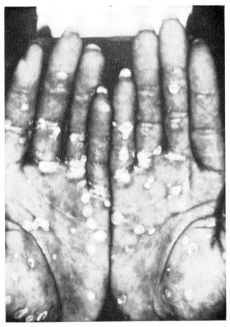

Figure 30/5. Palmar cutaneous manifestations of secondary syphilis. (AFIP 56-7603-9.)

which can be detected by the colloidal gold reaction; and the appearance of a positive complement-fixation test.

The reactions occurring in symptomatic neurosyphilis are acute or subacute meningitis, meningovascular syphilis, tabes dorsalis, general paresis, and optic atrophy. Acute meningitis is rare, develops more often in early than late syphilis, and resembles bacterial meningitis. Subacute meningitis may extend for weeks or months. Meningovascular syphilis is usually chronic and mild with prominent vascular changes consisting of narrowing, occlusion, or rupture of blood vessels. Tabes dorsalis, sometimes called locomotor ataxia, results from degeneration of the posterior roots and columns of the spinal cord and malfunction of certain cranial nerves. General paresis is produced by a chronic meningoencephalitis, resulting in progressive atrophy of the brain and loss of motor and mental function. If untreated the disease is usually fatal within 3 to 4 years.

Congenital Syphilis. Another form of syphilis arises from prenatal infection. A syphilitic mother may infect her child at any time before birth through the placental circulation. Syphilitic infection of the unborn child interferes with its normal growth and development. A syphilitic child at birth may present with a variety of manifestations, of varying degrees of severity. These include hepatosplenomegaly, jaundice, hemolytic anemia, skin lesions, and damage to the long bones. The child may have no lesions or be dead at birth.

Congenital syphilis may be manifest in the oral cavity as delayed dentition and abnormal development of two groups of teeth, the upper central incisors and the first permanent molars. These abnormal teeth have been termed Hutchinsonian teeth and mulberry molars, respectively. Hutchinsonian incisors are characterized by being widely separated, with crowns that converge toward the incisal edge, giving rise to the term, pegged teeth (figs. 30/10 and 30/11). The incisal edge of Hutchinsonian teeth is usually notched, often singly. The mulberry molar does not develop correctly, resulting in defective cusps which are not properly oriented and which are covered by defective enamel. The incidence of dental defects in prenatal syphilis

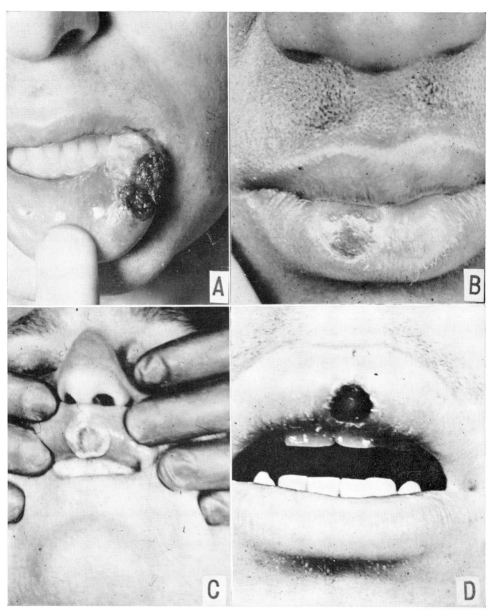

Figure 30/6. Primary syphilitic chancres of the lip. (*A*, AFIP B251B; *B*, AFIP 358; *C*, AFIP LS360.)

indicates that they occur in about 38% of all affected children.

IMMUNOLOGICAL ASPECTS OF SYPHILIS

Immune Response. During the initial infection with *T. pallidum*, humoral antibodies are detectable by the time the chancre appears. IgG and IgM antibodies persist for a long time in untreated patients. In treated patients IgM declines but IgG persists for many years. Syphilis proceeds through its clinical stages despite the presence of humoral antibodies.

In early syphilis, cell-mediated immunity is inhibited. Lymphocytes demonstrate reduced response specifically to treponemal antigens. However, individuals with late secondary and tertiary syphilis do exhibit cell-mediated immunity to treponemal antigens. These antigens can inhibit migration of leukocytes from syphilitic individuals.

Thus, neither humoral nor cell-mediated immunity is sufficient to provide protection against syphilis. However, persons with untreated syphilis have a relative resistance to syphilis, and chancre development following a second infection is unusual.

Serologic Reactions. *Wassermann Antigen.* The fixing of complement by syphilitic sera is due to an antibody termed Wassermann antibody. The original complement-fixation tests used as antigen

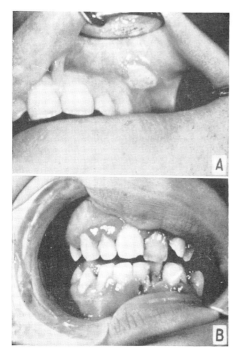

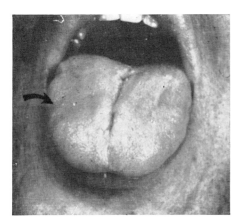

Figure 30/7. Secondary syphilitic manifestations. (*A*) Mucous patch adjacent to the mucobuccal fold. (*B*) Mucous patch in the upper right maxillary gingiva. (*A*, AFIP 363; *B*, AFIP.)

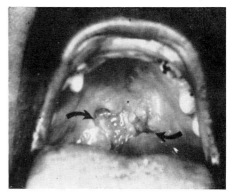

Figure 30/9. Palatal perforation resulting from syphilitic gumma. (AFIP 218663.)

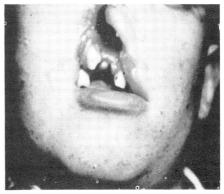

Figure 30/10. Congenital syphilitic manifestations in an adult. (AFIP 356.)

Figure 30/8. Mucous patch of the tongue. (AFIP 218663.)

One is that it is a true antibody to a lipoidal component of *T. pallidum*. A different explanation is that treponemes and other bacteria cause the disintegration of human tissue during an infection, releasing cardiolipin as a hapten. According to this concept, the appearance of the Wassermann antibody is an autoimmune response.

Over the years two common types of serological tests have been devised using cardiolipin-lecithin antigen, the Wassermann and Kolmer complement-fixation tests and the flocculation test, of which an alcoholic extract of the livers of stillborn syphilitic infants. Subsequently, it was found that the alcoholic extracts of a wide variety of tissues were equally effective as antigen. The specific principal is a phospholipid, termed cardiolipin (diphosphatidyl glycerol) which is, however, fully reactive only when supplemented with lecithin and cholesterol. Mostly a highly purified preparation is used, termed VDRL antigen after the Venereal Disease Research Laboratory.

Two theories have been put forth to explain the occurrence of the Wassermann antibody in man.

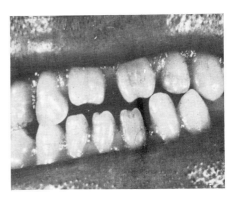

Figure 30/11. Hutchinsonian teeth. (AFIP 218547-4.)

there are numerous modifications. Commonly both complement-fixation and flocculation tests are called a serological test for syphilis (STS). It has become evident that the Wasserman antibody occurs in high titer during a more or less definite period in individuals with a variety of infectious and noninfectious diseases. Thus, these tests may demonstrate a high proportion of false positive reactions and some false negative reactions in late untreated syphilis. In some individuals with no treponemal infection, the Wassermann antibody titer may remain high for months or years. However, the tests are inexpensive and demonstrate the changing antibody titers in the individual.

Immobilization Phenomenon of T. pallidum. Syphilitic serum contains an antibody specific for an antigenic component of T. pallidum, which immobilizes it in the presence of complement. T. pallidum immobilization (TPI) test was devised for its detection in syphilitic infections. This test is particularly useful in detecting biologically false positive cases, as determined by STS, but otherwise is not used very much clinically. The TPI test is specific for syphilis and yaws, but it does not differentiate between them or other treponemal infections.

Immunofluorescence Tests. Fluorescent antibody tests are being utilized to a greater extent now in the diagnosis of syphilis and are available in several forms. Fluorescent treponemal antibody (FTA) tests use lyophilized organisms of the Nichols strain of T. pallidum as an antigen. This is fixed to a slide, followed by test serum. After any reaction has occurred fluorescein-labeled antihuman immunoglobulin is applied and the presence of reacting antibody in the patient's serum determined by fluorescent microscopy. A currently used variation of this test is the FTA-ABS (fluorescent treponemal antibody absorption) test. In this test the patient's serum is absorbed with another species of Treponema to remove antibodies to shared, nonspecific group antigens. The absorbed serum is reacted with nonviable Nichols strains of T. pallidum followed by labeled antihuman globulin, and if serum contains specific antibody, which is usually against T. pallidum, it reacts in this indirect immunofluorescence test, as in the FTA test. Another variation is the IgM-FTA-ABS test that is specific for IgM antibodies and is useful for differentiating between passively transferred antibodies and actively formed antibodies in possible cases of congenital syphilis.

Hemagglutination Tests. A hemagglutination method for serodiagnosis of syphilis is available and is particularly useful for screening. This test, the TPHA test, involves sensitizing tanned erythrocytes with treponemal antigens. When these react with specific antispirochetal antibodies, the eryth-

rocytes are agglutinated. This test may be performed by microtitration.

Thus, there are a variety of immune reactions associated with syphilis. Both humoral and cell-mediated immune reactions have protective functions and some may participate in the pathogenesis of the disease. However, the immune responses are also very useful in diagnosis of these infections.

Laboratory Diagnosis of T. pallidum. The inability to culture T. pallidum on laboratory media hampers the laboratory diagnosis of syphilis. An early method of laboratory diagnosis was the dark-field examination of an exudate from a suspected lesion for spirochetes and this still may be useful in instances where the individual has not turned seroreactive. It is not useful for oral lesions due to the presence of indigenous treponemes that are morphologically indistinguishable from T. pallidum. Positive identification has been made of T. pallidum in smears of exudate from a suspected lesion on slides by the fluorescent antibody technique (FTA test). This technique differentiates T. pallidum from other spirochetes, especially nonpathogenic contaminants.

The wide variety of serological tests described above are useful for the laboratory diagnosis of syphilis. The immunofluorescence and hemagglutination tests are coming into more widespread use but those using the Wassermann antigens are still widely used, especially for screening since they are inexpensive and demonstrate changes in antibody titers. The TPI test is useful in detecting biologically false positive reactions.

Treatment of T. pallidum Infection. Penicillin is now the drug of choice in the treatment of syphilis. Slowly absorbed or repository types of penicillin are most widely used. Intramuscular injection of penicillin G-benzathine, 2.4 million units per week, for 2 weeks, is quite effective. Patients allergic to penicillin may be given 500 mg tetracycline 4 times a day for 12 days. About the only drawback to the use of penicillin is the Jarisch-Herxheimer reaction which is caused by the release of spirochetal endotoxin following lysis of the spirochetes. This toxic reaction is usually seen following treatment of primary or secondary syphilis and is uncommon in late syphilis. It usually manifests as headache, fever, and malaise. It resolves in a day although reactions in late syphilis may result in cardiovascular or nervous system damage.

Epidemiology and Control of T. pallidum. A syphilitic is highly contagious during both the primary and secondary stages. The disease is acquired principally during sexual contact, but dental and medical personnel may acquire it accidentally during their treatment of syphilitic patients. Occasionally, the disease may be acquired by nonsexual contact in barber shops and beauty parlors. Another factor complicating the control of syphilis is that many syphilitics, particularly women, are often unaware that they have the disease. If such an individual is sexually promiscuous, they may transmit the disease to many of their contacts. Control relates to early identification and treatment of all syphilitics and their contacts. The several prophylactic procedures such as the use of a condom, cleansing of the genitalia with soap and water, application of calomel ointment and vaccines, have not controlled syphilis. While the use of penicillin is quite successful in treating syphilis, it has not been useful as a prophylactic.

TREPONEMA PERTENUE AND YAWS

Treponema pertenue. The causative agent of yaws is morphologically indistinguishable from *T. pallidum*. *T. pertenue* has not been satisfactorily cultivated in artificial media. In rabbits, it does not reproduce as rapidly as *T. pallidum* and few cells can be obtained for study. Our knowledge of this organism is limited. No significant immunological difference has been demonstrated between *T. pertenue* and *T. pallidum*.

Yaws. Yaws is an endemic disease of worldwide distribution in hot and wet climates; it seldom occurs in the temperate zone. It is found in the tropics of Central and South America, the West Indies, Africa, India, Southeast Asia, Indonesia, Northern Australia, and the islands of the South Pacific. Worldwide, an estimated 50 million people have yaws.

There are several modes of yaws infection. Usually it is acquired by contact, the organisms entering the body through abrasions in the integument. The incubation period of yaws is about 2 weeks to a month. The initial lesion, known colloquially as "mother yaw," appears as single or multiple papules or granulomas which ulcerate, crust over, and heal with scarring over the next 1 to 2 months, while evidence of a generalized infection develops.

Usually after 1 to 3 months, secondary flat-topped granulomas as large as 3 cm in diameter diffusely involve the skin. The secondary lesions, which may persist for years, teem with spirochetes and are known as "daughter yaw" or papillomatous frambeside which gives to yaws the synonym frambesia. These lesions may heal without scarring but recurrences may continue for several years. The palms of the hand and the plantar surfaces of the feet may be affected with painful and incapacitating frambesides, known as "crab yaws" from the crab-like gait of such individuals. Bones and joints may be involved with arthritis and hydrarthrosis, respectively. As the disease progresses, the lesions in the skin, bone, and joints tend to become very destructive. Yaws persists throughout the lifetime of about 25% of cases, without *per se* causing death.

The symptoms of yaws are quite diagnostic. Laboratory diagnosis is similar to that of syphilis. Penicillin is the choice treatment for either control or eradication.

ENDEMIC SYPHILIS OR BEJEL

The causal spirochete of endemic syphilis or bejel is morphologically identical with *T. pallidum* and *T. pertenue*. The disease it produces in human beings differs slightly from those of venereal syphilis and yaws.

Endemic syphilis occurs throughout the Middle East and in the Balkans. It is acquired primarily in childhood but occasionally is transmitted congenitally.

The initial lesion of endemic syphilis seldom occurs on the genital organs, but is most often oral or cutaneous. The course of the disease is somewhat similar to that of venereal syphilis, except that the stages are likely to be more prolonged and late lesions have a predilection for bone and mucous membranes. The best treatment is penicillin, administered as in venereal syphilis.

TREPONEMA CARATEUM AND PINTA

Treponema carateum. *T. carateum* the cause of pinta is morphologically and serologically similar to *T. pallidum* and *T. pertenue*. It has not been cultured, but has been successfully transferred to chimpanzees and experimentally from man to man to establish its causal relationship to pinta.

Pinta. Pinta, which has been described by many synonyms such as mal del pinto, carate, and azul, was for years thought to be a cutaneous mycosis. In 1938, a spirochete was discovered in active lesions and subsequently shown to be the causal organism. Pinta is prevalent in tropical and subtropical areas of the western hemisphere where there are an estimated 1,400,000 cases, but it also occurs in Africa, the Middle East, India, and the Philippines. Pinta is not venereal but is transferred from person to person by contact. It affects all age groups and if not treated it may persist for a lifetime.

Pinta progresses through three distinct stages. The incubation period is from 7 to 20 days and the primary stage extends to a year or more. The primary lesion is a papule which slowly develops into an erythematosquamous patch that spreads slowly around the affected area. Adjoining patches develop and coalesce with the original one. The secondary stage begins 6 to 12 months or more after onset with skin rashes and papules for which the name "pintid" has been proposed. Primary and secondary stages are not sharply delineated, for secondary lesions may occur simultaneously with the primary lesions. After several years or more, the tertiary stage begins, usually to continue for life if untreated. The lesions of this stage are characterized by achromic or pigmented spots, erythema, follicular keratosis, and keratoderma.

The treatment of pinta is similar to that of syphilis and yaws. The drug of choice is penicillin.

THE LEPTOSPIRAE AND LEPTOSPIROSIS

Morphology. *Leptospira* species range from pathogenic types causing human fevers and infections of a wide variety of animals (collectively termed leptospiroses) to harmless parasites. They are distinguished from other spirochetes by their very fine spirals and by their tapered and curved or hooked ends.

Growth and Cultivation of Leptospira. The leptospirae are the least difficult of the pathogenic spirochetes to cultivate, growing aerobically on a simple medium. They grow best in liquid or on semisolid media. They do not grow satisfactorily on most solid media. Cultivation in simple media decreases virulence, which can be maintained or even revived by the addition of emulsions of fresh tissue such as liver. The leptospirae utilize long chain unsaturated fatty acids as a source of carbon and energy and can use inorganic ammonium salts as a nitrogen source.

Species and Classification of Leptospira. The genus *Leptospira*, first established by Noguchi in 1917, was divided into saprophytic and parasitic species. The saprophytic types have been referred to as *Leptospira biflexa*, but in the 8th Edition of *Bergey's Manual of Determinative Bacteriology* only *Leptospira interrogans* was recognized. The parasitic leptospirae are divided into several serological groups and these are, in turn, separated into serotypes. The etiologic agents of the various leptospiroses are considered to be the various serogroups of *L. interrogans*. For example, Weil's disease is due to the serogroup *icterohaemorrhagiae*.

Antigenic Structure. The genus *Leptospira* includes a large number of serologically distinct groups. These serogroups are differentiated and characterized by agglutination reaction. The serogroups are not recognized taxons but have been given names that imply that they are different species. The serogroups serve primarily for diagnostic purposes and no formal classification has been established. Eighteen serogroups have been proposed: each serogroup is made up of one or more serotypes and there are more than 150 serotypes. The immunological forms appear to be quite stable, and are widely distributed as to host affected and geographic occurrence.

Epidemiology of Leptospira. The leptospirae are widely distributed in rodents and wildlife mammals, which are their natural hosts, but their geographic distribution is variable. They can survive for several weeks in surface waters under optimal conditions.

Human leptospiral infections are usually acquired directly or indirectly from infected rodents or other mammals. The spirochetes persist in the renal tubules of small rodents and larger wild mammals, and are shed in the urine. The organisms gain entrance through the mucosa of eyes, nose, mouth, throat, or abraded skin. Infection is related to occupation (agricultural workers, slaughterhouse workers, sewer workers, and miners). Leptospiral infection that occurs when swimming is common. It may also occur in soldiers who must live in close contact with their environment.

Clinical Types of Human Leptospirosis. Human leptospiroses range from extremely severe to moderate and relatively mild infections. The classical severe form of leptospirosis is spirochetal fever, spirochetal jaundice, or more commonly Weil's disease. A more moderate form of leptospirosis is canicola fever. In addition, a large number of diseases are produced in particular geographical locations; they are given such local names as canefield fever, seven-day fever, autumnal fever, Fort Bragg fever, mud fever, and ricefield fever. They correspond to either Weil's disease or canicola fever.

Weil's Disease. Weil's disease, the most virulent leptospirosis, is caused by several leptospira serotypes, especially of the serogroup *icterohaemorrhagiae*. The organisms gain entrance into the body through the skin or mucous membranes. The incubation period is usually from 7 to 13 days. Onset, marked by fever and rigor, is usually sudden and dramatic. The disease occurs in three stages. The first stage, in which a leptospiremia occurs, lasts about a week. It is characterized by a high temperature (104 F; 40 C), malaise, debility, headache, muscular pain, intestinal disturbances and abdominal pain, and sore throat, and sometimes pneumonia occurs near the end of the first stage.

The second stage of Weil's disease, which occupies a few days, is the most critical period of the infection and is characterized by the initiation of the immunological response. Death is most frequent during the second stage, though it may occur earlier. Acute renal failure is not unusual and is the cause of death in most cases. Jaundice is pronounced, the temperature is lower and a rash occurs in 10% of patients.

In the third stage, beginning in the 3rd week, fever may persist or recur but signs and symptoms abate, jaundice decreases, kidney function increases, the antibody titer increases, cardiac action improves, and convalescence begins, lasting from 6 to 12 weeks, or even as long as 6 months. Mortality ranges from 5 to 30%, perhaps averaging about 10%.

Canicola Fever. Canicola fever is an example of

a milder type of leptospirosis than Weil's disease. It is transmitted by direct contact, by contact with excreta, or by bathing in contaminated water. The course of the disease and the symptoms are similar to those of Weil's disease but less severe.

Laboratory Diagnosis. The bacteriological diagnosis of the leptospiral fevers consists of the demonstration of the causal organisms and the detection of specific antibodies for the involved serotype. The organisms can be demonstrated by culture of body fluids or tissues in fluid or semisolid suitable media. *Leptospira* may be isolated from contaminated specimens by intraperitoneal inoculation of hamsters and guinea pigs. Direct demonstration by microscopic techniques may be a useful adjunct.

Antibodies can be detected by agglutination tests. The number of antigens used in the test depends in part upon the number of serotypes in a given geographic area. The microscopic agglutination test is the most useful strain-specific serologic test. Negative immunological tests throughout the course of an illness indicate the absence of leptospirosis. The presence of leptospiral antibodies indicates a leptospiral infection or residual antibodies from past leptospiral infection.

Treatment. Leptospiral infections may be treated with penicillin, tetracycline, the macrolide antibiotics and streptomycin. Recovery is enhanced if treatment is started during the first 2 days after onset. If delayed past the 4th or 5th day, the course of the illness may not be altered.

BORRELIA RECURRENTIS AND OTHER SPIROCHETES ASSOCIATED WITH RELAPSING FEVER

***Borrelia recurrentis* and Closely Related Spirochetes.** The borreliae that cause relapsing fever are widely distributed and may infect many varieties of animals such as mice, chipmunks, foxes, dogs, and particularly rats. It is suspected that rodents may be the principal reservoir of pathogenic borreliae, for many are infected in endemic areas. In man the disease is seldom transferred by direct contact with rodents but usually by ticks or lice. Tick-borne infections are considered to represent the transmission of the disease from animals to man, while the louse-borne disease is considered to represent transfer of the infection from man to man.

Relapsing Fever. The borreliae responsible for relapsing fever are usually transferred to man by the bit of an infected tick or louse or by crushing such insect vectors on the skin with the fingers. The incubation period is approximately 7 days. Prodromal symptoms are slight or absent and the onset is sudden with fever of 104 to 106 F (40 to 41 C), chills, sweats, generalized aches and pains, ma-

laise, nausea, vomiting, and diarrhea. A febrile period of 3 or 4 days is succeeded by an afebrile period of more than a week, only to be followed by another febrile period of approximately the same duration as the first but of less severity. Thus, there are successive febrile and afebrile periods, with the febrile periods gradually decreasing in severity until the disease terminates, usually after about 3 months if untreated. The bacteriological diagnosis of relapsing fever consists of the demonstration of the spirochetes in blood by dark-field microscopy, by the use of stained blood films, or by inoculation into young white rats.

Antibiotics have been used in the therapy of relapsing fever. Tetracyclines and chloramphenicol are the most effective antimicrobial agents. Streptomycin may modify the course of the disease.

ADDITIONAL READING

ACKERMAN, A. B., GOLDFADEN, G., AND COSMIDES, J. C. 1972 Acquired Syphilis in Early Childhood. Arch Dermatol **106**, 92.

BABUDIERI, B., CASTELLI, M., AND PISONI, F. 1973 Comparative Tests with Formolized and Irradiated Vaccines Against Leptospirosis. Bull WHO, **48**, 587.

BARKIN, R. M., GUCKIAN, J. C., AND GLOSSER, J. W. 1974 Infection by *Leptospira ballum*; a Laboratory-Associated Case. South Med J, **67**, 155.

BERNFELD, W. K. 1971 Hutchinson's Teeth and Early Treatment of Congenital Syphilis. Br J Vener Dis, **47**, 54.

BHATTACHARJEE, S. P. 1955 Congenital Syphilis. J Indian Med Assoc, **25**, 439.

BLOUNT, J. H., DARROW, W. W., AND JOHNSON, R. E. 1973 Venereal Disease in Adolescents. Pediatr Clin North Am, **20**, 1021.

BRADLAW, R. V. 1953 Dental Stigma of Prenatal Syphilis. Oral Surg, **6**, 147.

BROWN, W. J. 1973 Epidemiological Treatment of Veneral Disease Contacts. Br J Vener Dis, **49**, 139.

CATTERALL, R. D. 1972 Systemic Disease and the Biological False Positive Reaction. Br J Vener Dis, **48**, 1.

CAVE, V. G., AND NIKITAS, M. A. 1976 Venereal Disease—Clinical and Laboratory Diagnosis. Mt Sinai J Med, **43**, 795.

CHAPEL, T. A. 1980 The Signs and Symptoms of Secondary Syphilis. Sex Transm Dis **7**, 161.

CHRISTMAS, B. W., TENNENT, R. B., PHILIP, N. A., AND LINDSAY, P. G. 1974 Dairy Farm Fever in New Zealand; a Local Outbreak of Human Leptospirosis. NZ Med J, **79**, 901.

CSONKA, G. W., 1953 Clinical Aspects of Bejel. Br J Vener Dis, **29**, 95.

CUTTER, J. C. 1972 Prophylaxis in the Venereal Diseases. Med Clin North Am, **56**, 1211.

DANS, P. E. 1975 Treatment of Gonorrhea and Syphilis; II. Syphilis. South Med J, **68**, 1295.

DODGE, R. W. 1973 Human Serological Response to Louse-borne Relapsing Fever. Infect Immun, **8**, 891.

ELLINGHAUSEN, H. C., JR. 1973 Growth Temperatures, Virulence, Survival, and Nutrition of Leptospires. J Med Microbiol, **6**, 487.

ELSAHY, N. I. 1976 Syphilitic Elephantiasis of the Penis and Scrotum. Plast Reconstr Surg, **57**, 601.

FAIER, A. D. 1952 Primary Gingival Syphilitic Lesions—Report of a Case. J Oral Surg, **10**, 159.

FARKAS, P. S., KNAPP, A. B., LIEBERMAN, H., GUTTMAN, I., MAYAN, S., AND BLOOM, A. A. 1981 Markedly Elevated Creatinine Phosphokinase, Cotton Wool Spots and Pericarditis in a Patient with Leptospirosis. Gastroenterology, **80**, 587.

FISCHMAN, A., AND MUNDT, H. 1971 Test Pattern of Yaws Antibodies in New Zealand. Br J Vener Dis, **47**, 91.

FIUMARA, N. J. 1974 Acquired Syphilis in Three Patients with Congenital Syphilis. N Engl J Med, **290**, 119.

FIUMARA, N. J. 1980 Treatment of Primary and Secondary Syphilis. JAMA, **243**, 2500.

FIUMARA, N. J., GRANDE, D. J., AND GIUNTA, J. L. 1978 Papular Secondary Syphilis of the Tongue. Oral Surg, **45**, 540.

FRANK, A. S. T. 1964 Temporomandibular Dysfunction Associated with Cerebral Syphilis. Oral Surg, **18**, 327.

GARNER, M. F. 1972 The Serological Diagnosis of Treponemal Infection. NZ Med J, **75**, 353.

GRIN, E. I. 1956 Endemic Syphilis and Yaws. Bull WHO, **15**, 959.

GUTHE, T., AND WILLCOX, R. R. 1954 *Treponematoses, a World Problem.* World Health Organization, Columbia University Press.

HARMUKSELA, M., AND KARAHARJU, E. O. 1972 Syphilis of the Spine. Br J Vener Dis, **48**, 397.

HARRISON, L. W. 1956 The Oslo Study of Untreated Syphilis, Review and Commentary. Br J Vener Dis, **32**, 70.

HOLT, S. C. 1978 Anatomy and Chemistry of Spirochetes. Microbiol Rev, **42**, 114.

HOLZEL, A. 1956 Jarisch-Herxheimer Reaction following Penicillin Treatment of Early Congenital Syphilis. Br J Vener Dis, **32**, 175.

HORNE, G. 1952 Oral Manifestations of Syphilis. Practitioner, **168**, 140.

HUDSON, E. H. 1958 *Non-venereal Syphilis: A Sociological and Medical Study of Bejel.* Livingstone, Ltd., Edinburgh and London.

HUNTER, E. F. 1975 The Fluorescent Treponemal Antibody-Absorption (FTA-ABS) Test for Syphilis. CRC Crit Rev Clin Lab Sci, **5**, 315.

IDSOE, O., KIRALY, K., AND CAUSSE, G. 1973 Venereal Disease and Treponematoses—The Epidemiological Situation and WHO's Control Programme. WHO Chron, **27**, 410.

IZZAT, N. N., DACRES, W. G., KNOX, J. M., AND WENDE, R. 1970 Attempts at Immunization against Syphilis with Avirulent *Treponema pallidum.* Br J Vener Dis, **46**, 451.

KAMPMEIER, R. H. 1973 Venereal Disease Control. Am J Hosp Pharm, **30**, 774.

KEOGH, C., AND KING, A. 1956 Syphilis of the Mouth and Upper Respiratory Tract. Practitioner, **177**, 691.

LAWSON, J. H. 1971 Leptospirosis. Br J Hosp Med, **5**, 357.

LAWSON, J. H. 1972 Leptospirosis in the West of Scotland. Scott Med J, **17**, 220.

LUCAS, J. B. 1972 The National Venereal Disease Problem. Med Clin North Am, **56**, 1073.

MARQUEZ, F., REIN, C. R., AND ARIAS, O. 1955 Mal del Pinto in Mexico. Bull WHO, **13**, 299.

MAZUNDER, J. K. 1953 A Survey on Oral Manifestations of Tropical Diseases. Int Dent J, **4**, 209.

METZGER, M. 1979 Role of Humoral versus Cellular Mechanisms of Resistance in the Pathogenesis of Syphilis. Br J Vener Dis, **55**, 94.

MILLER, J. N. 1971 Development of an Experimental Syphilis Vaccine. Med Clin North Am, **56**, 1217.

MILLER, R. L. 1973 Pustular Secondary Syphilis. Arch Dermatol, **108**, 727.

MORTON, R. S. 1973 Social Indicators and Venereal Diseases. Br J Vener Dis, **49**, 155.

NATHAN, A. S., AND LAWSON, W. 1964 Syphilitic Osteomyelitis of the Mandible. Oral Surg, **17**, 284.

NELSON, K. E., AGER, E. A., GALTON, M. M., GILLESPIE, R. W. H., AND SULZER, C. R. 1973 An Outbreak of Leptospirosis in Washington State. Am J Epidemiol, **98**, 336.

NICOL, C. S. 1971 Venereal Disease in Women—I. Br Med J, **2**, 328, 383.

NOTOWICZ, A., AND MENKE, H. E. 1973 Atypical Primary Syphilitic Lesions on the Penis. Dermatologica, **147**, 328.

NOTOWICZ, A., MENKE, H. E., STOLZ, E., AND VUZEVSKI, V. D. 1975 Solitary Papular Lesions on the Penis in Insufficiently Treated Early Syphilis. Dermatologica, **150**, 26.

OLANSKY, S. 1972 Serodiagnosis of Syphilis. Med Clin North Am, **56**, 1145.

PARKER, J. D. J. 1972 Uncommon Complications of Early Syphilis. Br J Vener Dis, **48**, 32.

PETROZZI, J. W., LOCKSHIN, N. A., AND BERGER, B. J. 1974 Malignant Syphilis. Arch Dermatol, **109**, 387.

PREBBLE, E. E. 1957 Infection and Re-infection in Early Syphilis. Br J Vener Dis, **33**, 112.

RATHLEV, T. 1975 Investigations on *in Vitro* Survival and Virulence of *T. pallidum* under Aerobiosis. Br J Vener Dis, **51**, 196.

REIF, J. S., AND MARSHAK, R. R. 1973 Leptospirosis; a Contemporary Zoonosis. Ann Intern Med, **79**, 893.

SCHROETER, A. L., LUCAS, J. B., PRICE, E. V., AND FALCONE, V. H. 1972 Treatment for Early Syphilis and Reactivity of Serologic Tests. JAMA, **221**, 471.

SHENBERG, E., AND TORTEN, M. 1973 A New Leptospiral Vaccine for Use in Man; I. Development of a Vaccine from Leptospira Grown on a Chemically Defined Medium. J Infect Dis, **128**, 642.

SHOTTS, E. B., JR., ANDREWS, C. L., AND HARVEY, T. W. 1975 Leptospirosis in Selected Wild Mammals of the Florida Panhandle and Southwestern Georgia. J Am Vet Med Assoc, **167**, 587.

SMITH, J. L. 1971 Neuro-Ophthalmological Study of Late Yaws. Br J Vener Dis, **47**, 223.

SMITH, J. L. 1973 Acute Blindness in Early Syphilis. Arch Ophthalmol, **90**, 256.

SMITH, R. M. 1965 Gumma of the Palate. Oral Surg, **20**, 29.

SULZER, C. R., GLOSSER, J. W., ROGERS, F., JONES, W. L., AND FRIX, M. 1975 Evaluation of an Indirect Hemagglutination Test for the Diagnosis of Human Leptospirosis. J Clin Microbiol, **2**, 218.

TABER, L. H., AND FEIGIN, R. D. 1979 Spirochetal Infections. Pediatr Clin North Am, **26**, 377.

TITCHE, L. L. 1972 Tertiary Syphilis of the Mouth. Arch Otolaryngol, **96**, 460.

WEBSTER, B. 1970 Venereal Disease Control in the United States of America. Br J Vener Dis, **46**, 406.

WIDEMANN, A. 1948 Syphilis of the Mucous Membrane of the Mouth. Z Stomatologie, **45**, 143.

WILLCOX, R. R. 1972 Some Aspects of the Epidemiology of the Venereal Diseases as a World Problem. Public Health, **86**, 225.

WILLCOX, R. R. 1974 Changing Patterns of Treponemal Disease. Br J Vener Dis, **50**, 169.

WILSON, J. 1973 Syphilis and Yaws; Diagnostic Difficulties and Case Report. NZ Med J, **78**, 494.

WILSON, J., AND MAUGER, D. G. 1973 Syphilis in Pregnancy Supervening on Yaws; Case Report. NZ Med J, **77**, 384.

WRIGHT, D. J. M., AND GRIMBLE, A. S. 1974 Why Is the Infectious Stage of Syphilis Prolonged? Br J Vener Dis, **50**, 45.

chapter 31

Transitional Groups of Bacteria

George S. Schuster

THE MYCOPLASMAS

In 1898 Nocard and Roux found the etiological agent of a type of bovine pleuropneumonia to be a small, highly pleomorphic, very fragile microorganism cultivable in a cell-free medium. Twenty-five years later a similar microorganism was found to cause agalactia, an inflammatory disease of the udder in sheep and goats. Similar microorganisms have been isolated from animals, the genitourinary tracts of humans, and from nearly all healthy human mouths and throats. Similar saprophytic organisms have been isolated from sewage, manure, humus, and soil. Based on their resemblance to the etiological agent of bovine pleuropneumonia, these microorganisms were named pleuropneumonia-like organisms, and commonly have been called PPLO.

PPLO are currently placed in the class Mollicutes. Those that require sterols are placed in the genus *Mycoplasma*, and those not requiring sterols are placed in the genus *Acholeplasma*.

Relationship of PPLO to L Organisms. Related to the PPLO by colonial and morphological similarities but not related taxonomically, are the "L" forms of bacteria. L forms are bacterial cells that have lost their rigid cell walls. The L_1 organism was first recognized as a pleuropneumonia-like variant of *Streptobacillus moniliformis*. Subsequently L-phase organisms were found to arise either spontaneously or by induction from many bacterial species. The L nomenclature was applied specifically to only seven strains, termed L_1 through L_7. Similarities between L types and PPLO are found in regard to internal structure, lack of conventional cell wall, pleomorphism, colonial appearance, resistance to antibiotics, particularly penicillin, and susceptibility to antibodies in the absence of complement. However, the L type is a laboratory-induced variant of conventional bacterial cells and has not been isolated directly *in vivo*. Under suitable conditions L types often revert to the familiar vegetative form but mycoplasmas do not.

Morphology. Mycoplasmas range in size from 200 to 300 nm in diameter. They are bounded by a trilaminar membrane but lack a rigid cell wall. Due to the latter characteristic they may assume a number of morphologic forms such as cocci, cocci with tubules, filaments, branching filaments and pear-shaped cells (figs. 31/1 and 31/2).

On solid media mycoplasma form colonies that are 20 to 600 μm in diameter and have the appearance of a fried egg.

The cells have a typical genome consisting of a single circular double-stranded DNA molecule that is quite small; its molecular weight is approximately 5×10^8.

Physiology and Metabolism. Most species of mycoplasma are facultative anaerobes, although they grow better under aerobic conditions. The organisms can be divided into two broad groups, the fermentative and the nonfermentative. In the former, adenosine triphosphate (ATP) is derived from glycolysis while other pathways provide ATP in the latter group.

The mycoplasmas can be cultured in or on infusion or digest media. Essential growth factors for mycoplasmas are present in ascitic fluid and animal sera. Except for *Acholeplasma* species, the mycoplasmas require fatty acids and cholesterol. Saprophytic species of the mycoplasmas grow in media containing no sera or similar growth factors.

Penicillin, crystal violet, and potassium tellurite may facilitate the isolation of mycoplasmas from mixed cultures.

Mycoplasmal Disease in Man. The principal human disease definitely related to mycoplasma is an atypical pneumonia, caused by *Mycoplasma pneumoniae*. *M. pneumoniae* is immunologically distinct from other human mycoplasmas. After an incubation period of 2 to 3 weeks, there is a gradual onset of fever, headache, and a nonproductive cough. In the early stages physical findings may be minimal. As the disease progresses, loud rales become prominent. Untreated disease may last up to 3 weeks. Initial diagnosis is made on clinical grounds. Laboratory diagnosis is by direct culturing of sputum or pharyngeal swabbings and the bacteria are identified by hemadsorption, β-hemolysis of

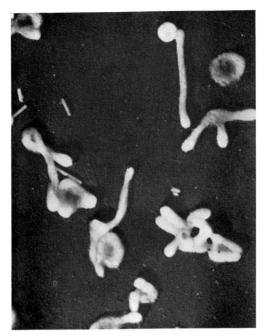

Figure 31/1. Various cellular forms of the mycoplasma of goat pleuropneumonia seen in a 24-hour serum broth culture (×10,080). (Reproduced with permission from E. Klieneberger-Nobel and F. W. Cuckow: A Study of the Organisms of Pleuropneumonia Group by Electron Microscopy. *Journal of General Microbiology*, **12**, 95, 1955.)

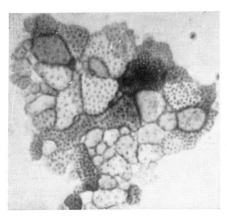

Figure 31/2. Pleuropneumonia-like organisms from a lung of a bronchiectatic rat, showing intracellular granules. (Reproduced with permission from E. Kleineberger-Nobel: Methods for the Study of the Cytology of Bacterial and Pleuropneumonia-like Organisms. *Quarterly Journal of Microscopic Science*, **91**, 340, 1950.)

guinea pig erythrocytes, by staining with homologous fluorescein-labeled antibody, or by inhibition of growth by specific antibody. Tetrazolium also inhibits the organism's growth. Treatment of primary atypical pneumonia is uncertain, although tetracyclines do affect the course of the disease. Erythromycin is also used for treatment.

STREPTOBACILLUS MONILIFORMIS

It is now generally agreed that a group of gram negative bacilli isolated from humans that develop a fever after animal bites and to which a multitude of names have been applied belong to a single species, *Streptobacillus moniliformis*.

Bacteriological Characteristics of Streptobacillus. *S. moniliformis* is a CO_2 requiring, facultatively anaerobic, gram negative, pleomorphic, nonencapsulated, nonmotile, sometimes pathogenic microorganism. It occurs *in vivo* and under optimal culture conditions as a bacillus. Under less satisfactory culture conditions it occurs as long chains of relatively large irregular vegetative bacilli interspersed with cocci and coccoid swellings. It also occurs as the small filterable L type first described by Klieneberger-Nobel in 1935 specifically as L_1.

The L_1 colony of *S. moniliformis*, composed of coccoid or coccobacillary units, is seldom more than 0.2 mm in diameter. It contains a central dark brown center embedded in agar and surrounded by a delicate, translucent peripheral zone composed of large, swollen bodies, amorphous material, and extracellular fatty droplets.

Streptobacillus Infections. The human diseases produced by *S. moniliformis* include a milk-borne disease termed Haverhill fever and rat-bite fever. Rat-bite fever also is caused by *Spirillum minor*. The source of *S. moniliformis* is usually the bite of a rodent, the initial wound healing without inflammation. The incubation period is usually from 1 to 3 days but in some instances is as long as 3 weeks. The local wound becomes inflamed and indurated and there is lymphangitis and regional lymphadenitis. The onset of symptoms is sudden, with chills and fever, the subsequent course of which may be either relapsing or septic. A rash always develops, either at the first or later exacerbations of fever. In contrast to spirillar rat-bite fever, arthritis is a common complication in the bacillary disease; severe sore throat and congestion of the pharyngeal mucous membrane are also frequent complications. Mortality is about 15%. Penicillin or tetracycline are both effective in the treatment of streptobacillary infections. Treatment is complicated by persistence in the body of the L_1 form, which is resistant to penicillin.

ACTINOBACILLUS

Members of the genus *Actinobacillus* cause septicemia or granulomatous lesions in animals. One human pathogen associated with this genus is *Actinobacillus actinomycetemcomitans*, a small, nonmotile, nonencapsulated, gram negative coccobacillus. It grows best at 37 C on serum or blood agar in an atmosphere of 10% CO_2.

This organism is found in the human oral cavity. Most clinical isolates have been found in blood and bone although some have been found in lesions also infected with *Actinomyces* species. A number of cases of subacute bacterial endocarditis due to this organism have been described.

Strains of *A. actinomycetemcomitans* have been isolated from plaque of cases of juvenile periodontitis. The organisms produced a heat-labile toxin that was capable of destroying isolated human polymorphonuclear leukocytes and had toxic effects on human monocytes. This organism may play a role in the pathogenesis of juvenile periodontitis by compromising antibacterial host defenses in the periodontal region. Also, the consequent release of lysosomal contents from such cells may damage surrounding connective tissue, further contributing to the disease process.

THE BARTONELLA GROUP

The family Bartonellaceae, a group of blood parasites, contains two genera, *Bartonella* and *Grahamella*. *Bartonella* contains a single species, *Bartonella bacilliformis*, infecting man but not naturally infecting animals. *Grahamella* species do not affect man. *B. bacilliformis* causes Oroya fever, a febrile hemolytic anemia, and verruga peruana, a benign skin eruption which is a continuing or secondary phase of Oroya fever. Collectively, this syndrome is known as bartonellosis or Carrion's disease.

Characteristics of *B. bacilliformis*. *B. bacilliformis* is a gram negative, nonacid-fast, pleomorphic, flagellated, predominantly rod-shaped microorganism.

In size, morphology, staining characteristics, intracellular parasitism, and employment of an arthropod vector, *B. bacilliformis* resembles the rickettsiae. In cultivability, flagellation, and possession of a cell wall, *B. bacilliformis* resembles bacteria. *Bartonella* species exhibit stages closely resembling the bizarre forms of the mycoplasma.

Bartonellosis. *B. bacilliformis* is indigenous to certain mountainous regions of Peru, Ecuador, and Colombia. Man is the reservoir host and the organism is transmitted from man to man by the bite of sand flies (*Plebotomus* species).

The incubation period averages about 20 days but may range from 10 days to several months. Onset is abrupt with fever as high as 104 F (40C), intermittent chills, intense pain, and abundant sweating. Subsequent symptoms of Oroya fever are intense pain in bones, joints, and muscles, fever, sweating, petechiae, and dull red papules, extreme pallor of skin and mucosa and a rapidly progressive hemolysis resulting in anemia in which erythrocyte and hemoglobin values fall to 25% of normal. The duration of the disease is usually 4 to 5 weeks. Fatal, fulminating cases may terminate in 10 days but usually linger for a month. About 1 month following recovery from Oroya fever, a benign skin eruption (verruga peruana) develops, which was originally thought to be unrelated to Oroya fever. During this phase, the microorganisms do not invade erythrocytes but are to be found in the cytoplasm of endothelial cells. The wart-like lesions persist for from one month to several years. The most prominent symptoms are intermittent pain and fever, usually most severe during the eruption of the lesions.

Bartonellosis responds dramatically to treatment with penicillin, chloramphenicol, or tetracycline. Secondary infections with salmonellae are common and require a broad-spectrum antibiotic for effective treatment.

ADDITIONAL READING

BRANDE, A. I., AND SIEMIENSKI, J. 1968 Production of Bladder Stones by L-Forms. Trans Assoc Am Physicians, **81**, 323.

CHANOCK, R. M. 1965 Mycoplasma Infections of Man. N Engl J Med. **273**, 1199, 1257.

CHARACHE, P. 1970 Cell Wall-defective Bacterial Variants in Human Disease. Ann NY Acad Sci, **174**, 903.

CLYDE, W. A., JR. 1971 *Mycoplasma pneumoniae* Pneumonia. Milit Med, **136**, 20.

COLE, B. C., OVERALL, J. C., JR., LOMBARDI, P. S., AND GLASGOW, L. A. 1976 Induction of Interferon in Ovine and Human Lymphocyte Cultures by Mycoplasmas. Infect Immun, **14**, 88.

DIENES, L., AND WEINBERGER, H. J. 1951 The L Form of Bacteria. Bacteriol Rev, **15**, 245.

ENGEL, L. D., AND KENNY, G. E. 1970 *Mycoplasma salivarium* in Human Gingival Sulci. J Periodontol Res, **5**, 163.

EVANS, C. A., KENNY, G. E., WANG, S. P., AND LANGER, E. E. 1976 A Search for Mycoplasmas and Chlamydiae in Acne Lesions. J Invest Dermatol, **67**, 283.

FAUR, Y. C., WEISBURD, M. H., WILSON, M. E., AND MAY, P. S. 1974 Mycoplasmas, and T-Mycoplasmas. Appl Microbiol, **27**, 1041.

FOY, H. M., KINNEY, G. E., McMAHAN, R., KAISER, G., AND GRAYSTON, J. R. 1970 *Mycoplasma pneumoniae* in the Community. Am J Epidemiol, **93**, 55.

FOY, H. M., NUGENT, C. G., KENNY, G. E., McMAHAN, R., AND GRAYSTON, J. R. 1971 Repeated *Mycoplasma pneumoniae* Pneumonia after 4½ Years. JAMA, **216**, 671.

FURNESS, G. 1973 T-Mycoplasmas; Some Factors Affecting Their Growth, Colonial Morphology, and Assay on Agar. J Infect Dis, **128**, 703.

GUPTA, U., OUMACHIGUI, A., AND HINGORANI, V. 1973 Microbial Flora of the Vagina with Special Reference to Anaerobic Bacteria and Mycoplasma. Indian J Med Res, **61**, 1600.

HAYFLICK, L. (ed.) 1967 Biology of the *Mycoplasma*. Ann NY Acad Sci, **143**, 1.

KLIENEBERGER-NOBEL, E. 1962 *Pleuropneumonia-like Organisms (PPLO) Mycoplasmataceae.* Academic Press, New York.

LERER, R. J., AND KALAVSKY, S. M. 1973 Central Nervous

System Disease Associated with *Mycoplasma pneumoniae* Infection; Report of Five Cases and Review of the Literature. Pediatrics, **52,** 658.

MARDH, P. A., AND TAYLOR-ROBINSON, D. 1973 New Approaches to the Isolation of Mycoplasmas. Med Microbiol Immunol, **158,** 259.

McCORMACK, W. M., ROSNER, B., AND LEE, Y. 1973 Colonization with Genital Mycoplasmas in Women. Am J Epidemiol, **97,** 240.

MOGABGAB, W. J. 1973 Protective Efficacy of Killed *Mycoplasma pneumoniae* Vaccine Measured in Large-Scale Studies in a Military Population. Am Rev Respir Dis, **108,** 899.

MUFSON, M. A. 1970 *Mycoplasma hominis* I in Respiratory Tract Infections. Ann NY Acad Sci, **174,** 798.

NAFTALIN, J. M., WELLISCH, G., ZAHANA, Z., AND DIENGOTT, D. 1974 *Mycoplasma pneumoniae* Septicemia. JAMA, **228,** 565.

NIVAYAMA, G., AND GRACE, J. T., JR. 1971 Mycoplasmas (PPLO) and Human Neoplasms. Tohoku J Exp Med, **105,** 257.

NOAH, N. D. 1974 *Mycoplasma pneumoniae* Infection in the United Kingdom—1967-1973. Br Med J, **2,** 544.

PACHAS, W. N. 1970 The Role of Mycoplasma in Some Unusual Conditions of the Kidney and the Urinary Tract. Ann NY Acad Sci, **174,** 786.

PETERS, D., AND WIGAND, R. 1955 Bartonellaceae. Bacteriol Rev, **19,** 150.

RAZIN, S. 1978 The Mycoplasmas. Microbiol Rev, **42,** 414.

SLOTS, J., REYNOLDS, H. S., AND GENCO, R. J. 1980 *Actinobacillus actinomycetemcomitans* in Human Periodontal Disease; a Cross-Sectional Microbiological Investigation. Infect Immun, **29,** 1013.

TAICHMAN, N. S., DEAN, R. T., AND SANDERSON, C. J. 1980 Biochemical and Morphological Characterization of the Killing of Human Monocytes by a Leukotoxin Derived from *Actinobacillus actinomycetemcomitans.* Infect Immun, **28,** 258.

TARR, P. I., LEE, Y. H., ALPERT, S., SCHUMACHER, J. R., ZINNER, S. H., AND McCORMACK, W. M. 1976 Comparison of Methods for the Isolation of Genital Mycoplasmas from Men. J Infect Dis, **133,** 419.

THOMAS, L. 1973 Experimental Mycoplasma Infections as a Model of Rheumatoid Arthritis. Fed Proc, **32,** 143.

THOMSEN, A. C. 1975 The Occurrence of Mycoplasmas in the Urinary Tract of Patients with Chronic Pyelonephritis. Acta Pathol Microbiol Scand, Sect B, **83,** 10.

TSAI, C. C., McARTHUR, W. P., BAEHNI, P. C., HAMMOND, B. F., AND TAICHMAN, N. S. 1979 Extraction and Partial Characterization of Leukotoxin from a Plaque-derived Gram-Negative Microorganism. Infect Immun, **25,** 427.

WATANABE, T. 1975 Proteolytic Activity of *Mycoplasma salivarium* and *Mycoplasma orale*; I. Med Microbiol Immunol, **161,** 127.

WATANABE, T., MISHIMA, K., FUJITA, O., HORIKAWA, T., NOGUCHI, T., ISHIZU, T., AND KINOSHITA, S. 1972 Possible Role of Mycoplasmas in Periodontal Disease. Bull Tokyo Med Dent Univ, **19,** 93.

chapter 32

Actinomycetes and Actinomycosis

George S. Schuster

There are a number of pathogenic microorganisms that resemble both bacteria and fungi. Some of these microorganisms are included in the order Actinomycetales. This order contains the genera *Actinomyces, Arachnia, Bifidobacterium, Bacterionema,* and *Rothia.* They resemble in many ways both the pathogenic fungi and the corynebacteria and diphtheroids. The *Nocardia,* members of a different family in this order, more closely resemble the mycobacteria (some are acid-fast) and have less resemblance to fungi. Another related family, the *Streptomyces,* more closely resembles the fungi than do the others.

Actinomycosis is a disease of human beings and some species of animals that is caused by species of *Actinomyces,* although there have been reports of cases due to *Arachnia* and *Bifidobacterium.* It is generally recognized that *Actinomyces bovis,* which is the type species, is the cause of actinomycosis or lumpy jaw in cattle. The human oral species are generally considered to be *Actinomyces israelii,* the principal cause of human actinomycosis; *Actinomyces naeslundii,* that is essentially nonpathogenic, although human infections have been reported; *Actinomyces viscosus* that has been implicated in periodontal disease and may play a role in some cases of human actinomycosis; and *Actinomyces odontolyticus,* an isolate from deep dentinal caries.

Certain of the characteristics of the actinomyces strains resemble both bacteria and fungi, and they have often been considered to be transitional between the two groups of microorganisms. Most of the more fundamental characteristics of the actinomycetes indicate that they are, in fact, bacteria. They are anaerobic or facultative, in contrast to the pathogenic fungi that are uniformly aerobic. Because their cell membranes contain no sterols they are not sensitive to the polyenes that can act on pathogenic fungi. They are sensitive to antibacterial chemotherapeutic agents that have no effect on pathogenic fungi. The cell walls of the actinomycetes are similar to those of bacteria in that they contain muramic acid and do not contain chitin or glucans that are typical of the cell walls of fungi. They are procaryotic, for they lack a nuclear membrane. The actinomycetes form mycelia in tissue or in culture and they can form branching filaments. However, the diameter of these filaments is similar to that of the cells of bacilli and are not as wide as those of fungi. Thus, they more correctly are considered to be bacteria rather than fungi.

Clinical Course and Manifestations. Human actinomycosis may involve almost any area of the body. Primary lesions occur most frequently in the oral cavity, face, or neck (figs. 32/1 and 32/2). The abdominal cavity and the lungs are other frequent sites of infection. Clinically, four types of actinomycosis have been distinguished according to the area of initial infection. These four types are: (1) cervicofacial, (2) abdominal, (3) cutaneous, and (4) thoracic.

The initial lesion of the more prevalent cervicofacial infection is usually found in the oral cavity. The onset of the disease is insidious and, if it does not follow some surgical procedure or injury, is first noticed as a persistent swelling, usually in the parotid or mandibular regions. The swelling is not painful, although it may be if secondarily infected. If the disease develops following surgical procedures, healing of the wound is slow, and swelling persists or even increases. With such symptoms diagnosis of actinomycosis is difficult, for the symptoms are those of cellulitis or residual osteitis with a different or more common etiology. A dark red or purplish skin overlaying a very hard and board-like swelling is characteristic of actinomycosis. As the infection progresses, points of fluctuation develop extraorally, abscesses form, and multiple sinuses appear. Bone involvement is rare in the early stages of the disease, but later a true osteomyelitis may develop, with considerable bone destruction. When this occurs the infection may burrow upward toward the spine or cranial region, often causing death.

Primary thoracic actinomycosis is not uncommon, and it may be caused either by *A. israelii* or by aerobic *Nocardia* species. The pulmonary infec-

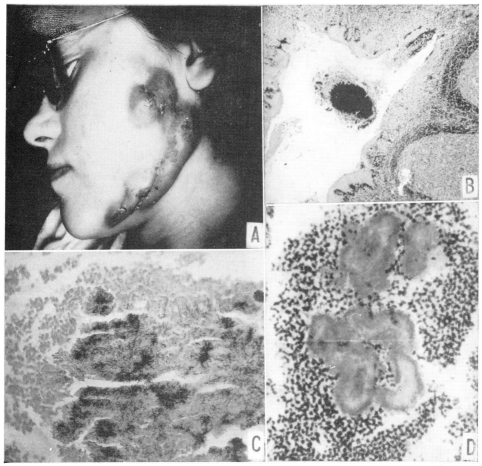

Figure 32/1. (*A*) Facial actinomycosis. (*B*) "Sulfur" granule in tissue (×35). (*C*) *Actinomyces* in the skin (×160). (*D*) "Sulfur" granule in tissue (×340). (*A*, AFIP 88; *B*, AFIP 137912; *C*, from Max Poser, Bausch and Lomb Optical Company; *D*, AFIP 89.)

tion occurs with low-grade fever, coughing, and expectoration of bloody sputum. As the disease progresses, draining sinuses extending to external chest wall or to the heart are established by direct invasion. The patient gradually loses weight, becomes anemic, and has a severe pulmonary infection.

Cutaneous infections are usually the result of traumatic implantation of organisms. They are first seen as small subcutaneous swellings that slowly enlarge and soften. The lesions rupture to the surface and sinus tracts form. They also can burrow deeper into the tissues, invading and destroying bone.

Abdominal actinomycosis may be caused by the invasion of the intestinal mucosa by actinomycetes from the oral cavity, or by the extension of a pulmonary infection. It initially appears as a palpabal abdominal mass that simulates appendicitis. Infection may spread to the liver, spleen, or spinal column.

Actinomycosis is a persistent disease which may show signs of regression, only to recur with renewed vigor. The actinomycetes elicit an immunological reaction which is not very consistent. Opsonins, agglutinins, precipitins, and complement-fixing antibodies occur, but they are not useful in diagnosis, and their role in resistance is unknown.

Pathogenesis of Actinomycosis. Since *A. israelii* normally inhabits tonsils, carious teeth, and calculus deposits, any open wound in the mouth such as those caused by the extraction of teeth, accidents, or pulp exposure provides a pathway for the introduction of the organisms into susceptible tissue. However, the simple introduction of potentially pathogenic actinomycetes into oral tissues does not necessarily lead to infection. Several factors seem to be involved in actinomycosis. A single inoculation of susceptible animals with actinomycetes from a proven case seldom causes infection, whereas repeated inoculation frequently does, indicating that some form of tissue sensitization may

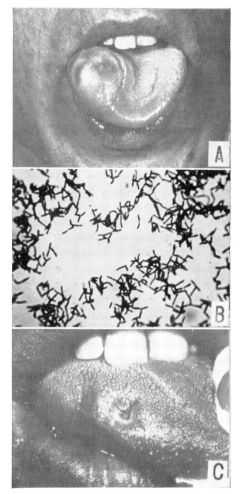

Figure 32/2. Actinomycosis. (*A*) Lesion involving the tongue. (*B*) Causal Actinomycetes. (*C*) Lesion after treatment. (Reproduced with permission from L. Dorph-Petersen and J. J. Pindborg: Actinomycosis of the Tongue. *Oral Surgery, Oral Medicine, and Oral Pathology,* **7,** 1178, 1954.)

play a role in the process of infection. Trauma associated with surgery, injury, or less often such chronic irritation as calculus beneath the gingival margin predisposes to infection.

During an infection, the pathogenic actinomyces form characteristic but not necessarily specific granules that are commonly visible by ordinary observation. These granules, often called "sulfur" granules because of their resemblance to precipitated sulfur, are present in the tissues of the lesion, but are most easily found in the exudate and pus of the lesion. Sulfur granules may vary considerably in size and composition, but their central portion consists of delicate intertwining filaments. The peripheral filaments are surrounded by gelatinous sheaths, giving them a club-like appearance. Granules are found, however, without peripheral clubs. The tiny branching filaments in granules stain positive with gram stain or they may appear as gram positive beads. When stained with hematoxylin and eosin, the central portion is basophilic, while the periphery is eosinophilic.

Laboratory Diagnosis of Actinomycosis. A laboratory method for diagnosis of actinomycosis consists of detecting sulfur granules in pus or exudate from a suspected lesion by ordinary visual observation. Pus for observation of the granules can be collected directly into a sterile test tube or obtained indirectly from deeper lesions by aspiration with needle and syringe and then placed in a tube. Rotation of the tube will distribute the pus thinly over its surface so that the larger granules can be more easily observed directly. Or the pus can be crushed between a cover glass and slide and stained with gram stain for observation of granules too small to see by direct vision.

Cultivation is also useful for diagnosis. Specimens of exudate or tissue should be cultured in enriched media and incubated both aerobically and anaerobically at 37 C. Thioglycollate broth is especially useful for distinguishing *A. israelii* from other species by the hard colonies it produces vs. the more easily disrupted colonies of the others. Except for *A. viscosus* the catalase test can be used to distinguish the catalase-negative *Actinomyces* from *Corynebacterium* and *Propionibacterium.*

Treatment of Actinomycosis. Treatment of actinomycosis is complicated by the large tissue areas involved and the hard swelling, but exploration and drainage of sinus tracts, and excision of damaged tissue greatly facilitates chemotherapy. Combined treatment consisting of surgical intervention and chemotherapy has effected an 80 to 90% cure rate. Antibiotic therapy should be intensive and prolonged, perhaps weeks to months. Treatments with penicillin, erythromycin, tetracycline, cephalosporin, clindamycin, and lincomycin have been reported as successful.

ADDITIONAL READING

BACH, M. C., MONACO, A. P., AND FINLAND, M. 1973 Pulmonary Nocardiosis. JAMA, **224,** 1378.

BOSSUYT, M. 1964 Cervico-facial Actinomycosis. Acta Stomatol Belg, **61,** 25.

BROCK, D. W., GEORG, L. K., BROWN, J. M., AND HICKLIN, M. D. 1978 Actinomycosis Caused by *Arachnia propionica*; Report of 11 Cases. Am J Clin Pathol, **59,** 66.

BUJAK, J. S., OTTESEN, E. A., DINARELLO, C. A., AND BREMER, V. J. 1973 Nocardiosis in a Child with Chronic Granulomatous Disease. J Pediatr, **83,** 98.

COLEMAN, R. M., GEORG, L. K., AND ROZZELL, A. R. 1967 *Actinomyces naeslundii* as an Agent of Human Actinomycosis. Appl Microbiol, **18,** 420.

CRAN, J. A., AND HAUNAM, A. G. 1963 Cervico-facial Actinomycosis. Aust Dent J, **8,** 106.

CURIONI, C., AND VIANELLO BOTE, D. 1964 Clinical Contribution to the Knowledge of Facial Actinomycosis. Mondo Odontostomatol, **6**, 275.

DEGNAN, E. J. 1963 Cervico-facial Actinomycosis Treated with Prolonged Penicillin and Tetracycline Therapy. Oral Surg, **16**, 757.

EASTRIDGE, C. E., PRATHER, J. R., HUGHES, F. A., JR., YOUNG, J. M., AND McCAUGHAN, J. J., JR. 1972 Actinomycosis; a 24-Year Experience. South Med J, **65**, 839.

ELLEN, R. P., AND BALCERZAK-RACZKOWSKI, I. B. 1975 Differential Medium for Detecting Dental Plaque Bacteria Resembling *Actinomyces viscosus* and *Actinomyces naeslundii*. J Clin Microbiol, **2**, 305.

ENG, R. H. K., CORRADO, M. L., CLERI, D., CHERUBIN, C., AND GOLDSTEIN, E. J. C. 1981 Infection Caused by *Actinomyces viscosus*. Am J Clin Pathol, **75**, 113.

ENGEL, D., VAN EPPS, D., AND CLAGETT, J. 1976 *In Vitro* and *in Vivo* Studies on Possible Pathogenic Mechanisms of *Actinomyces viscosus*. Infect Immun, **14**, 548.

FILLERY, E. D., BOWDEN, G. H., AND HARDIE, J. M. 1978 A Comparison of Strains Designated *Actinomyces viscosus* and *Actinomyces naeslundii*. Caries Res, **12**, 299.

GERGELY, L., AND HERPAY, Z. 1964 Demonstration of *Actinomyces israelii* in Carious Cavities. Fogorvosi Szemle, **57**, 298.

GUTSHIK, E. 1976 Case Report; Endocarditis Caused by *Actinomyces viscosus*. Scand J Infect Dis, **8**, 271.

HAMNER, J. E. 1965 Anterior Maxillary Actinomycosis; Report of Case. J Oral Surg, **23**, 60.

HANRATTY, W. J., AND NAEVE, H. F. 1964 Actinomycosis with Pathologic Fracture of Mandible. Oral Surg, **18**, 303.

HERTZ, J. 1957 Actinomycosis; Oral, Facial and Maxillary Manifestations. J Int Coll Surg, **28**, Part I, 539.

JOHNSON, H., PULASKI, E. J., AND THOMPSON, C. W. 1957 Actinomycosis of Mandible. US Armed Forces Med J, **8**, 1214.

LACA, E. 1964 Primary Actinomycosis of the Parotid Gland. Torax, **13**, 234.

LANGENEGGER, J. J. 1965 Actinomyces and Their Effects on Oral Tissues. J Dent Assoc S Afr, **20**, 1.

LARSEN, J., BOTTONE, E. J., DIRKMAN, S., AND SAPHIR, R. 1978 Cervicofacial *Actinomyces viscosus* Infection. J Pediatr, **93**, 797.

LEAFSTEDT, S. W., AND GLEESON, R. M. 1977 Cervicofacial Actinomycosis. Am J Surg, **130**, 496.

MONTOLEONE, L. 1963 Actinomycosis. J Oral Surg, **21**, 313.

PEABODY, J. W., JR., AND SEABURY, J. H. 1957 Actinomycosis and Nocardiosis. J Chronic Dis, **5**, 374.

PINE, L., HOWELL, A., JR., AND WATSON, S. J. 1960 Studies of the Morphological, Physiological and Biochemical Characteristics of *Actinomyces bovis*. J Gen Microbiol, **23**, 403.

SAUNDERS, J. M., AND MILLER, C. H. 1980 Attachment of *Actinomyces naeslundii* to Human Buccal Epithelial Cells. Infect. Immun, **29**, 98.

SLACK, J. M., LANDFRIED, S., AND GERENCSER, M. A. 1971 Identification of Actinomyces and Related Bacteria in Dental Calculus by Fluorescent Antibody Technique. J Dent Res, **50**, 78.

SPRAGUE, W. G., AND SHAFER, W. G. 1963 Presence of Actinomyces in Dentigerous Cyst; Report of Two Cases. J Oral Surg, **21**, 243.

THADEPALLI, H., AND RAO, B. 1979 *Actinomyces viscosus* Infection of the Chest in Humans. Am Rev Respir Dis, **120**, 203.

VASARINSH, P. 1968 Primary Cutaneous Nocardiosis. Arch Dermatol, **98**, 489.

chapter 33

Rickettsial and Chlamydial Infections

George S. Schuster

RICKETTSIAE

Physiochemical Characteristics. The genus *Rickettsia*, family Rickettsiaceae, contains 10 species, divided into spotted fever, typhus, and scrub typhus groups. Also included in the Rickettsiaceae are *Coxiella burnetii*, the cause of Q fever and *Rochalimaea quintana*, the agent that causes trench fever. *C. burnetii* resembles the typical rickettsiae in many of its physiological aspects, while *R. quintana*, previously classified as a species of *Rickettsia*, resembles them in its route of transmission and some features of its disease. Members of the genus *Rickettsia* are small coccobacilli, 0.3 to 0.5 μm $\times$ 0.8 to 2.0 μm, that are similar to gram negative bacteria in their fine structure and chemical composition. The cell walls of rickettsiae seem to have endotoxic activity. The cells have a cytoplasmic membrane, contain both DNA and RNA, and members of the genera *Rickettsia* and *Coxiella* mulitply by transverse fission. All members of the genus *Rickettsia* are obligate intracellular parasites. Special stains are needed to demonstrate rickettsiae in cell preparations. While most strains of the rickettsiae are rather unstable and fragile, *C. burnetii* is one of the more resistant nonspore-forming microorganisms.

Growth of Rickettsia. Rickettsiae are commonly cultured in embryonated eggs or in tissue cultures derived from laboratory animals. Laboratory animals are useful for primary isolation and virulence studies. *Rochalimaea quintana* differs from rickettsiae in that it can be cultivated on relatively simple bacteriological media. The natural hosts of rickettsiae include a variety of mammals and arthropods. Mammals, including man, are infected by inoculation of the organisms into the skin during feeding of an infected arthropod and, conversely, new arthropods can become infected by feeding on infected mammals. Arthropods often serve as both a vector and a reservoir, because the rickettsiae can be transferred from arthropod to arthropod transovarially.

Pathogenesis. Rickettsiae have an affinity for the endothelial cells of small blood vessels, causing their hyperplasia. Perivascular infiltration and local thrombosis permit blood to leak into the surrounding tissues. Inflammation of the blood vessels, particularly in the skin and brain, causes the rash and terminal shock that are common clinical signs of a rickettsial infection. Although it has not been characterized, there appears to be a toxin that participates in the pathogenesis of rickettsial diseases.

Treatment. *Rickettsia* and *Rochalimaea* species are resistant to sulfonamides but they are inhibited by *p*-aminobenzoic acid. Penicillin and streptomycin only slightly inhibit rickettsiae and are of no therapeutic value. Broad spectrum antibiotics (*e.g.*, oxytetracycline, chlortetracycline, deoxycycline, and chloramphenicol) are quite useful for rickettsial infections.

Diagnosis. Rickettsial infections can be diagnosed by identification of the causative organism, either by infection of laboratory animals or serologically. At best, however, isolation of rickettsiae is a hazardous procedure that is technically difficult. If rickettsiae are isolated they can be identified by neutralization with specific antisera.

Serological procedures are most useful for diagnosis of rickettsial infections. One of the most useful of such tests is the Weil-Felix test. Rickettsiae and strains of *Proteus*, referred to as OX strains, share common heat-stable antigens. The Weil-Felix test is based on the agglutination of the *Proteus* strains by antibodies formed against these common antigens during some of the rickettsial infections. Antibodies to group-specific and type-specific antigens may be detected by complement-fixation tests. Immunofluroescence and agglutination reactions are also useful in diagnosis of rickettsial infections, particularly those in which the Weil-Felix test is negative.

353

TABLE 33/1

Rickettsial diseases, causal agents, and insect vectors

Disease	Causal Agent	Insect Vector	Weil-Felix Reaction
1. European epidemic louse borne typhus	*Rickettsia prowazekii*	Human body louse (*Pediculus corporis*); human head louse (*Pediculus capitis*)	Positive OX-19
2. Brill's disease (recrudescent epidemic typhus)	*R. prowazeki*	(Recrudescence of previous infection)	Usually negative
3. Endemic murine flea-borne typhus	*Rickettsia typhi*	Rat louse (*Polydax spinulosus*); rat flea (*Ceratophyllus fasciatus* and *anisus*); rat mite (*Liponyssus bacoti*); flea (*Xenopsylla cheopis*)	Positive OX-19
4. South African tick-bite fever	*Rickettsia conorii*	Common dog tick (*Haemaphysalis leachi*); hare tick (*Amblyomma hebraeum*)	Positive OX-19, OX-2
5. North Queensland tick typhus.	*Rickettsia australis*	Tick (*Ixodes holocyclus*)	Positive OX-19, OX-2
6. North Asian tick-borne rickettsiosis	*Rickettsia sibiricus*	Ticks (*Dermacentor nuttalli; Dermacentor silvarium; Haemaphysalis concina*)	Positive OX-19, OX-2
7. Scrub typhus (Tsutsugamushi disease)	*Rickettsia tsutsugamushi*	Chigger mites (*Trombicula akamushi* and *Trombicula deliensis*)	Positive OX-K
8. Trench fever	*Rochalimaea quintana*	Human louse (*P. corporis*)	Negative
9. Rocky Mountain spotted fever	*Rickettsia rickettsii*	American dog tick (*Dermacentor variabilis*); Rocky Mountain wood tick (*Dermacentor andersoni*); Lone Star tick (*Amblyomma americanum*); South American tick (*Amblyomma cajennense*); brown dog tick (*Rhipicephalus sanguineus*); rabbit tick (*Haemaphysalis leporis palustris*)	Positive OX-19, OX-2
10. Fièvre boutonneuse	*R. conorii*	Dog ticks (*Rhipicephalus sanguineus*)	Positive OX-19, OX-2
11. Q fever (Query fever)	*Coxiella burnetii*	Cattle ticks (*Boophilus annulatus microplus* and *Haemaphysalis bispinosa*); Lone Star tick (*A. americanum*); Rocky Mountain wood tick (*Dermacentor andersoni*); North African ticks (*Hyalomma savignyi* and *Hyalomma dromedarii*)	Negative
12. Rickettsialpox	*Rickettsia akari*	House mouse mite (*Allodermanyssus sanguineus*)	Negative

The principal human rickettsial infections, their causal agents, the arthropod vector, and their principal serological reactions are listed in table 33/1.

RICKETTSIAL DISEASES

European Epidemic Louse-Borne Typhus. European epidemic louse-borne typhus is caused by *Rickettsia prowazeki*, which is transmitted from man to man by body or head lice. The incubation period of typhus averages about 12 days. The disease, usually lasting for less than 20 days, is divided into four phases, each characterized by definite symptoms, but there is fever in all stages. The first, or invasion stage, lasts 3 days. The second stage, which lasts for 4 days, is characterized by a rash that begins on the trunk and spreads to the extremities (figs. 33/1 and 33/2). The third stage, characterized by prostration, delirium, and collapse, lasts

until the 12th day after onset and terminates in a crisis in which the patient is desparately ill. If the patient survives the crisis, and if there are no complications, he enters the fourth stage in which there is usually a satisfactory recovery. However, there are often a variety of complications, many of which are quite severe. Mortality of the disease is related to age, for death seldom occurs in children less than 5 years old, and the mortality rate increases with age so that after age 50 it may be as high as 60%. Treatment is principally symptomatic, but chloramphenicol and tetracyclines have been used successfully to treat the disease. Recovery from an initial typhus infection confers resistance to a second attack. Several types of typhus vaccines have been used for active immunization. Their application has reduced the severity of the disease and perhaps reduces its incidence also.

Brill's Disease. Brill's disease, also known as

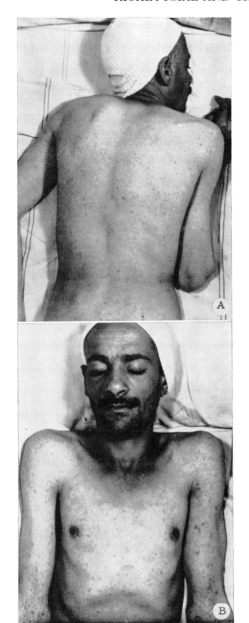

Figure 33/1. Typhus rash, 10th day: (*A*) back view; (*B*) front view. (AFIP 60-1001.)

Endemic Murine Flea-Borne Typhus. This form of typhus is caused by *Rickettsia typhi*, which naturally infects several species of rats. *R. typhi* is transferred between rats by rat lice or rat fleas and from rats to human beings by the fleas. The disease is characterized by abrupt onset of fever, headache, malaise and a maculopapular rash that begins on the trunk and spreads to the extremities. Involvement of the face, palms, and soles is rare. Murine typhus is not as severe as epidemic typhus having a mortality rate of less than 5%.

Scrub Typhus (Tsutsugamushi Disease). Scrub typhus, which occurs in India, Southeast Asia, the East Indies, Northern Australia, and many islands of the Southwest Pacific is caused by *Rickettsia tsutsugamushi* (fig. 33/3). It is transmitted to man by trombiculid mites. It is a very severe febrile illness, with the usual symptoms of typhus. The disease lasts about 3 weeks and has a fatality rate of up to 50%. Broad spectrum antibiotics are highly effective in suppressing the growth of *R. tsutsugamushi* but recrudescences are common and recovery ultimately depends on antibody formation.

Trench Fever. More than one million cases of trench fever occurred during World War I and World War II. The causal organism is *Rochalimaea quintana*, which is transmitted to man by the human body louse, *Pediculus corporis*. The incubation period of the disease, which in man is from 2 weeks to 2 months, is followed by a febrile disease which normally lasts for no longer than a month. It has the characteristics of typhus. The mortality rate is low.

Rocky Mountain Spotted Fever. Rocky Mountain spotted fever, occurring in 43 states of

recrudescent epidemic typhus, is a rickettsial infection with symptoms similar, if not identical to European epidemic louse-borne typhus. It was first described as occurring in New York among recent immigrants, particularly those from Eastern Europe, where epidemic typhus was common. The disease represents a recrudescence of a latent typhus infection acquired previously, for it is not acquired from lice in the usual way. Such asymptomatic carriers may harbor the rickettsiae for many years and are probably the reservoir of classic typhus.

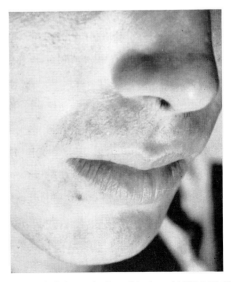

Figure 33/2. Primary lesion of typhus. (AFIP A44-256.)

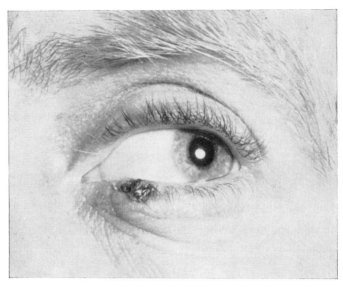

Figure 33/3. Scrub typhus showing eschar of eyelid. (AFIP 1st MFL 86-1.)

the United States and in Canada, Mexico, and South America, is caused by *Rickettsia rickettsii*. A reservoir of the rickettsia is maintained in rabbits and small rodents and it is transmitted among animals by ticks. In the western United States the organism is transmitted to man by the wood tick *Dermacentor andersoni*, in the eastern United States and Mexico by the dog tick *Dermacentor variabilis*, and in South America by other ticks. The incubation period of Rocky Mountain spotted fever is no longer than 2 weeks. The onset is sudden with headache, fever and chills. Rash appears from the 3rd to 7th day, and a temperature as high as 107 F (41 C) occurs which may continue for 2 or 3 weeks. Convalescence is slow and complications are frequent. No lasting immunity results from a primary infection. Mortality has ranged from 40% in children to 80% in adults, although the mortality rate is much lower at the present time because of vaccination and antibiotic therapy. Initial diagnosis and treatment should be done on the basis of clinical findings. Laboratory diagnosis is useful for confirmation of infection. Chloramphenicol and tetracycline are used for treatment with success. At present in the United States, nearly two-thirds of all cases occur east of the Mississippi. The disease is not uncommon, for over 1100 cases were reported in the United States during 1977, many occurring in the Mid Atlantic region. Foci of the disease also have been reported in the Cape Cod area and in Virginia.

Q Fever (Query Fever). Q fever clinically resembles influenza and primary atypical pneumonia, and is unique among rickettsioses in three ways: transmission to man is usually not arthropod-borne; no skin rash develops; and patients do not develop agglutinins for *Proteus* strains. The causal rickettsia, *Coxiella burneti*, is probably maintained in various rodents, among which it is spread by a number of species of ticks. They transmit it to domesticated animals, in which it produces mild disease and from which it is excreted in milk and feces. *C. burneti* is unusually resistant to heat and drying, and may survive pasteurization in milk. It also persists for long periods in the dried effluvia of infected animals, whence it is acquired directly or indirectly by susceptible cattle and man. Transfer from infected to susceptible persons is possible but rare. Very likely, Q fever is or will be globally distributed.

The incubation period of Q fever is about 3 weeks. Infection may be unapparent or produce a very mild illness. Clinically recognized Q fever has a sudden onset and is influenza-like. A severe febrile illness lasts about 2 weeks on the average, but fever may continue for several months. Pneumonitis is a common accompaniment. Mortality is very low. Differential diagnosis is quite difficult and is most readily established retrospectively when specific antibodies develop. Recovery is usually uncomplicated, although rather slow.

Rickettsialpox. Since rickettsialpox was first recognized in New York City in 1946, it has been reported in many major cities, as well as some foreign countries. It is caused by *Rickettsia akari*, which is transmitted by the common house mouse mite vector *Allodermanyssus sanguineus*. Because of the mild nature of rickettsialpox, it may often go unrecognized and actually be more common and widespread than is currently reported.

The general pathology of rickettsialpox is unknown. The most distinctive of the lesions is the initial skin lesion, which develops about the bite of the infected mite after about a week. The lesion is a firm red papule, 1 to 2.5 cm in diameter, which vesiculates, then forms a black eschar which scabs and heals after 2 or 3 weeks, with some scarring. The systemic reactions which occur in rickettsialpox are fever, chills, sweating, backache, sore throat, and muscular pain. Concurrent with or within a week after the onset of fever, a rash of wide distribution appears which has been described as maculopapular, discrete, and erythematous. Vesicles develop after a few days and heal without scarring. Oral lesions of a transient nature have been reported in rickettsialpox. Although they have not been found consistently, vesicles do occur on the tongue and palate.

The diagnosis of rickettsialpox is based on clinical symptoms and on the complement-fixation test. In many ways the disease resembles varicella (chickenpox), variola (smallpox), tick typhus, Rocky Mountain spotted fever, scrub typhus, and to a lesser extent, tularemia and plague.

Control of Rickettsial Diseases. Rickettsial infections may be controlled by antibiotics, immunization, or by disrupting the transmission cycles of the causative rickettsia. Epidemic typhus may be prevented by delousing humans with DDT. Elimination of rodents and their parasites helps control murine typhus, scrub typhus, and rickettsialpox. Clearing of infested land and use of protective clothing will help prevent spotted fever. Avoiding infected animals and proper pasteurization of milk will help control Q fever. Proper disposal of garbage and control of mice will control rickettsialpox.

CHLAMYDIAE

The genus *Chlamydia* contains two species, *Chlamydia trachomatis* and *Chlamydia psittaci*, which can be further divided into many different strains on the basis of their antigenic composition, host range, virulence, and pathogenic effects. The chlamydia are obligate intracellular parasites, and do not synthesize adenosine triphosphate (ATP), but in many ways resemble bacteria. The chlamydia have cell walls similar to those of gram negative bacteria, they contain both DNA and RNA, they divide by binary fission, and they are susceptible to antibiotics. Chlamydiae have a life cycle that involves two alternate forms, the elementary body and the reticulate body (fig. 33/4). The elementary

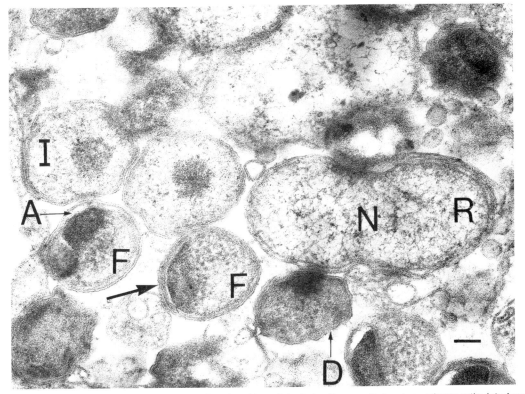

Figure 33/4. Electron micrograph of *Chlamydia psittaci* in an infected yolk sac cell showing various particulate forms of the organism: the early stage of the division (*N*) of a reticulate body (*R*); intermediate body (*I*); less condensed elementary bodies (*F*) whose membranes are closely apposed (*arrow*) except for a distention adjacent to the nucleoid (*A*) and irregularly shaped highly condensed elementary bodies (*D*). (Courtesy of Dr. J. W. Costerton and reproduced with the permission of the National Research Council of Canada from the *Canadian Journal of Microbiology*, **21**, 1433–1447, 1975.)

body is taken into a host cell by phagocytosis, and while remaining within the cytoplasmic vacuole reorganizes into a noninfectious reticulate body. This form multiplies by binary fission within the cytoplasmic vacuole. As the number of reticulate bodies increases, their size decreases and small elementary bodies appear. The developmental cycle is completed within about 48 hours by reorganization of the reticulate bodies into hundreds of infectious elementary bodies which are released by rupture of the host cell to infect other cells.

All chlamydia share a common genus-specific antigen. C. trachomatis strains also share species- and type-specific antigens to varying degrees. Antibodies can be detected in sera by complement-fixation, immunofluroescence, or neutralization tests.

Chlamydia infect a wide range of animal hosts, including birds, mice, cats, dogs, and humans. The mechanism by which they cause disease is not known, but in general, the chlamydiae are not very pathogenic. However, many of these diseases may have a latent stage which permits the disease to recur following treatment. Chlamydial infections are usually easily controlled or cured by chemotherapy. C. trachomatis is susceptible to sulfonamides and both C. trachomatis and C. psittaci are susceptible to broad spectrum antibiotics.

CHLAMYDIAL INFECTIONS

Trachoma. Trachoma, a disease of the eye caused by C. trachomatis, is found naturally only in man and is the greatest single cause of blindness. It is found in nearly every country and fluorishes in areas with poor public sanitation and personal hygiene. It is transmitted primarily by hand to eye contact or by fomites. Flies may transmit the disease. Onset is sudden, with inflamed conjunctivae. Within a few weeks characteristic follicles form beneath the conjunctival surface, followed later by vascularization of the cornea and pannus. This may result in partial or complete blindness. The conjunctivae may become scarred and the normal flow of tears is disturbed, resulting in bacterial infections of the eyes.

Trachoma may be diagnosed by its clinical symptoms or by isolation of the causative organism from conjunctival scrapings in embryonated eggs or tissue cultures; location of cytoplasmic inclusions in conjunctival cells by staining or fluorescent antibodies; or by detection of trachoma-specific antibodies in eye secretions.

Inclusion Conjunctivitis. Inclusion conjunctivitis is a prevalent inflammatory eye infection that is sometimes termed inclusion blenorrhea or swimming pool conjunctivitis. The causal organism is a strain of C. trachomatis. At present, disease in the adult likely results from contamination of the eyes by genitourinary exudates on the hands or fomites. The conjunctivitis resembles the early stages of trachoma, but usually it does not progress to a chronic disease. Inclusion conjunctivitis is usually a disease of the newborn, acquired during birth from an infected maternal genital tract. The disease is difficult to diagnose clinically and final diagnosis depends upon the demonstration of characteristic basophilic granular inclusions (Thygeson bodies) in the cytoplasm of epithelial cells from the affected area or by isolating the agent in cell cultures. Immunofluorescence studies have allowed differentiation of the causative organism of inclusion conjunctivitis from that of trachoma. Inclusion conjunctivitis is benign and self-limited, and leaves no residual damage. It can be cured readily with sulfonamides, tetracyclines, or chloramphenicol.

Neonatal Pneumonia. Chlamydia trachomatis may cause infant pneumonitis: the children usually become ill at 1 to 4 months of age. They have prominent respiratory symptoms of cough and wheezing but lack fever. Chlamydial conjunctivitis may precede the onset of pneumonia.

Nongonococcal Urethritis (NGU). Chlamydiae are the leading identified cause of nongonococcal urethritis in males; perhaps 25 to 50% of cases are due to C. trachomatis. Many men with gonorrhea will have NGU that will manifest itself after treatment of gonorrhea, especially if the gonorrhea is treated with penicillin since the Chlamydia are not sensitive to these agents. The infection may be transmitted to females producing symptomatic or asymptomatic infections, especially of the cervix.

Lymphogranuloma Venereum. Lymphogranuloma venereum (also known by a variety of other names) is a protean venereal disease of world-wide distribution, although it occurs most often in the tropics. The causative agent of lymphogranuloma venereum usually is a strain of C. trachomatis.

Lymphogranuloma venereum is usually transmitted by sexual contact either with those who have frank disease or with asymptomatic carriers. Incubation periods are variable, but they appear to be generally between 10 and 30 days. Primary lesions appear most often in the genital or anorectal regions and the oral cavity, according to the site of contact (fig. 33/5). Nonvenereal infection often involves the hands, particularly the fingers of dentists and other medical personnel. The primary lesion usually appears first as a distinct vesicle which later ruptures, leaving a shallow, grayish ulcer or chancre. It is not painful and heals without scarring. The initial stages of the infection are not accompanied by systemic reactions.

In an initial oral infection, the tongue is most often affected with a painless, blister-like lesion. As the disease progresses, the tongue is enlarged, with

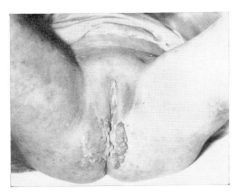

Figure 33/5. Perianal lesions of lymphogranuloma venereum. (AFIP D-45421.)

zones of scarring and retraction. Such symptoms are sometimes mild, at other times severe. Deep grooves are often found on the dorsum of the tongue, with zones of intense red coloration and loss of superficial epithelium, or, alternatively, grayish opaque papules may develop. The dorsum of the tongue may be painful to salts or sour foods. When only the margins of the tongue are involved, the subjective symptoms are few. The lesions on the tongue are generally of long duration; sometimes the lesions subside spontaneously only to recover their original aspects.

Within 7 days to as long as 2 months after appearance of the initial lesion, a painful regional lymphadenitis occurs, with varying degrees of enlargement. In the majority of cases the affected lymph nodes suppurate, forming abscesses and fistulas. Adenopathy may subside after several months but the fistulous tracts usually persist for years. During the intermediate stage of the disease the constitutional symptoms are variable but consist of headache, fever, vomiting, lassitude, and skin eruptions, indicating a generalized infection.

In the later stages of the disease, which may not be manifest in all those infected, the manifestations are esthiomene, the urethro-genital-perineal syndrome, penoscrotal elephantiasis, rectal stenosis, and/or plastic induration of the penis. During this stage the skin and sense organs and the cardiovascular, respiratory, digestive, genitourinary, and nervous systems may be affected. In general, the latter-day manifestations are accompanied by weakness, loss of weight, mental changes, and anemia.

Laboratory procedures useful in the diagnosis of lymphogranuloma venereum include examination of stained films of pus or tissue sections, including affected lymph nodes, for intracellular organisms. Perhaps the most common diagnostic aid, although not necessarily the most used, is the Frei test in which antigen and control material are injected intradermally. The test is positive if the papule raised by the antigen is larger than the control

papule. The Frei test becomes positive within 6 months after infection and remains so for many years. A false-positive reaction sometimes may be obtained, particularly in syphilis.

Treatment with tetracyclines cures the acute signs and decreases complications.

Ornithosis and Psittacosis. Caused by *C. psittaci*, psittacosis is the term applied to infections of psittacine birds such as parrots and parakeets, while ornithosis refers to infection of nonpsittacine birds. Birds may have latent infections which become active with increased stress. The organisms may be transmitted to other birds by contact, droplets, or infected droppings. Once infected, the birds lose weight and have diarrhea and discharge from the eyes. The infection is usually fatal to the birds. Humans usually acquire the disease from birds by inhalation of infected material in which the organisms may persist for a prolonged period; direct human spread has been observed.

In man, the infection may be asymptomatic or appear as a mild to moderately severe respiratory infection. The incubation period ranges from 6 to 15 days. The more severe forms have a sudden onset with signs and symptoms of bronchitis and bronchopneumonia. High fever may occur and a cough is common. Prior to treatment the patient is severely ill.

The clinical signs of these infections are not sufficiently characteristic to establish a diagnosis. Laboratory diagnosis of human infection is based on isolation of the organism from blood or sputum, or from infected material and identification by neutralization of infectivity, a complement-fixation test, or immunofluorescence.

Broad spectrum antibiotics are useful for treating ornithosis and psittacosis.

ADDITIONAL READING

DAWSON, C. 1973 Therapy of Diseases Caused by Chlamydia Organisms. Int Ophthalmol Clin **13,** 93.

DUPONT, H. C., HORNECK, R. B., DAWKINS, A. T., HEINER, G. G., FABRIKANT, I. B., WISSEMAN, C. L., AND WOODWARD, T. E. 1974 Rocky Mountain Spotted Fever; A Comparative Study of the Active Immunity Induced by Inactivated and Viable Pathogenic *Rickettsia rickettsii*. J Infect Dis, **128,** 340.

HAND, W. L., MILLER, V. B., AND REINARZ, J. A. 1970 Rocky Mountain Spotted Fever; a Vascular Disease. Arch Intern Med, **125,** 879.

HATTWICK, M. A., PETERS, A. H., O'BRIEN, R. J., AND HANSON, B. 1976 Rocky Mountain Spotted Fever; Epidemiology of an Increasing Problem. Ann Intern Med, **84,** 732.

KELSEY, D. S. 1979 Rocky Mountain Spotted Fever. Pediat Clin North Am, **26,** 367.

LENNETTE, E. H., AND SCHMIDT, N. F. (eds). 1969 *Diagnostic Procedures for Viral and Rickettsial Diseases,* Ed. 4. American Public Health Association, New York.

LUMICAO, G. G., AND HEGGIE, A. D. 1979 Chlamydial Infections. Pediatr Clin North Am, **26,** 269.

MAULITZ, R. M., AND IMPERATO, P. J. 1974 Rocky Mountain Spotted Fever in an Urban Setting. NY State J Med, **74,** 1403.

ORIEL, J. D., POWIS, P. A., REEVE, P., MILLER, A., AND NICOL, C. S. 1974 Chlamydial Infections of the Cervix. Br J Vener Dis, **50,** 11.

PAOVONEN, J. 1979 Chlamydial Infections; Microbiological, Clinical and Diagnostic Aspects. Med Biol, **57,** 135.

REEVE, P. 1970 Trachoma and Inclusion Conjunctivitis Agents in The British Isles. Mod Trends Med Virol, **2,** 186.

ROSE, H. M. 1949 The Clinical Manifestations and Laboratory Diagnosis of Rickettsialpox. Ann Intern Med, **31,** 871.

SCHACHTER, J. 1978 Chlamydial Infections. N Engl J Med, **298,** 428.

SCHACHTER, J., AND GROSSMAN, M. 1981 Chlamydial Infections. Annu Rev Med, **32,** 45.

VIANNA, N., AND HINMAN, A. R. 1971 Rocky Mountain Spotted Fever on Long Island; Epidemiologic and Clinical Aspects. Am J Med, **51,** 725.

WEISS, E. 1973 Growth and Physiology of Rickettsiae. Bacteriol Rev, **37,** 259.

chapter 34

Mycotic Infections

George S. Schuster

The fungi are plant-like organisms that are widely distributed in water and soil and on living and dead and decaying plants. Of the 200,000 or so species very few are human parasites or pathogens. Pathogenic fungi are restricted to yeasts and molds. They are generally immotile and have no leaves, stems or roots. Since they are not photosynthetic, they must exist as parasites or saprophytes. While the fungi are much less differentiated than the usual plants, they are more differentiated and complex than bacteria. The yeasts exist as a single cells (*i.e.*, they are monomorphic), while the molds exist either as single cells or as multicellular filamentous colonies (*i.e.*, they are dimorphic). However, the uninucleated individual cells of fungi can differentiate into sexually distinct cells, single yeast cells, multinucleated filamentous strands, or bodies that produce spores.

In addition to being pathogenic for humans, fungi are also pathogenic for other mammals, birds, and plants, often with serious consequences. However, they perform many useful functions as soil scavengers, as producers of antibiotics, organic acids, hormones, and in the production of such foods as cheese, bread, and ethanol for beverages.

MORPHOLOGY

The cells of fungi resemble those of higher plants in that they have a distinct nucleus, with a limiting membrane, nucleoli, an endoplasmic reticulum, mitochondria, and other organelles. Some have an external coating like a slime layer or a capsule. Yeasts usually exist as spherical or oval cells that are from 2 to 15 μm in diameter. Occasionally, yeast cells form chains of individual cells that adhere together. Molds may exist in a yeast form but their principal vegetative form is the hypha. Hyphae are tubules that range from 2 to 10 μm in diameter and grow by producing side branches or by elongation. As they grow, they form an intertwining mass which is termed a mycelium. As the mass increases in size it forms a colony or thallus. As the thallus forms, hyphae that penetrate the culture media to absorb the nutrients are known collectively as the vegetative mycelium. On the other hand, the hyphae that project above the surface of the thallus form the aerial mycelium. If the aerial mycelia bear reproductive cells or spores such aerial hyphae are collectively known as the reproductive mycelium.

Hyphae may be either septate or nonseptate. The nonseptate hyphae are usually multinucleate (coenocytic) while the septate hyphae usually contain only one nucleus in each compartment.

CANDIDIASIS

Candidiasis, caused by species of the genus *Candida*, may vary from a benign localized infection of skin or mucous membranes to an acute, disseminated infection of lung or intestine which often terminates fatally within a relatively short period of time, particularly when there is septicemia, endocarditis, or meningitis. Onset is generally related to factors that lower resistance either locally or generally. Candidiasis is worldwide in distribution and occurs in all races and at all ages.

Eight species of *Candida* are commonly isolated

from man: *C. albicans, C. tropicalis, C. pseudo-tropicalis, C. krusei, C. rugosa, C. guilliermondi, C. parapsilosis,* and *C. stellatoidea.* Of these, *C. albicans* is most frequently pathogenic.

C. albicans. *C. albicans* is an oval, thin-walled, budding, yeastlike cell 2 to 5 μm in diameter when it is first obtained from a lesion. Positive identification can be made best from the growth on corn-meal agar, which contains characteristic budding cells and chlamydospores (figs. 34/1 and 34/2). *C. albicans* can also be differentiated from nonpathogenic species by the formation of germ tubes growing out from the cell after about 90 min in serum at 37 C.

Candidal Infection. It is generally recognized that there are a number of clinical and pathological entities attributable to *C. albicans* and collectively referred to as candidiasis. They involve many structures. Some infections remain localized and benign; others are disseminated and acute. Candidiasis generally falls into three broad categories, cutaneous, systemic, and chronic mucocutaneous. Cutaneous candidiasis involves infection of the skin, mucous membranes, and nails by endogenous *Candida* and may result from chronic maceration of these areas, physiological changes in the host or a compromised immune status. From the localized lesions, the organisms may disseminate directly or hematoge-

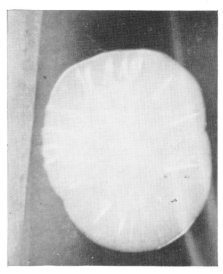

Figure 34/2. Colonial form of *Candida albicans.* (AFIP 218663-1-53.)

nously. The initial infection is more likely to involve the skin, or mucosa of the mouth or other portions of the gastrointestinal tract, the vagina, and the lungs. Systemic candidiasis follows dissemination directly in tissues, resulting in infection of the urinary and gastrointestinal tracts, the middle ear and mastoids, vagina, pleura, or diaphragm, depending on the location of the initial infection. Also, from the initial infection, the yeast cells can invade blood vessels and disseminate to almost any area of the body.

Candidiasis in Infants. An acute and definitive infection of *C. albicans* is oral candidiasis of infants, commonly called thrush. The original lesions develop in otherwise healthy infants often within eight or nine days after contact with an infected birth canal. The disease is then usually transmitted to other infants in a ward or nursery by nipples, pacifiers, and contaminated utensils until it becomes epidemic. The lesions are characterized by whitish, flaky, loosely adherent membranes covering part or all of the tongue, lips, gingivae, or buccal mucous membrane. Less frequently the uvula, fauces, and soft palate are involved. Beneath the membrane, the mucosa is bright red and moist. The incidence of oral candidiasis in the newborn has been reported as ranging from less than one percent to more than 18%, but a more realistic incidence is less than 5%.

The gastrointestinal tract of infants also may be infected with *C. albicans.* The esophagus is the most frequent site, with lesions of the stomach and intestine being less common. Esophageal infections are characterized by the development of a whitish pseudomembrane sometimes of sufficient size to occlude the esophagus. Ulcerations may develop

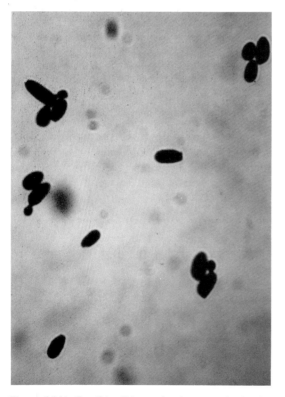

Figure 34/1. *Candida albicans* showing reproduction by budding.

and sometimes cause fatal bleeding. As evidenced from autopsies, membrane formation may occur in gastric and intestinal infections, sometimes with ulceration and perforation.

Candidal infection of the respiratory tract occurs in infants but not so often as in the intestinal tract. When the tonsils and larynx are involved, the disease resembles diphtheria. The pharynx may be involved, with the infection sometimes extending through the eustachian tube to involve the ear or mastoids.

Next to oral candidiasis, superficial cutaneous candidiasis of infants is most common. It usually begins in the perianal region and spreads to thigh or abdomen, but rarely the back. Weeping lesions occur about the neck or axillary region, and almost the entire cutaneous surface may be involved.

Systemic candidiasis in infancy results from dissemination of the yeast in the blood usually preceded by extensive cutaneous candidiasis. Clinical features are suggestive: anorexia, severe vomiting, progressive wasting, severe diarrhea, and sudden collapse.

Candidiasis in Adults. In the adult, oral candidiasis may be either subacute or chronic, or occasionally may take an acute course. The subacute adult type is characterized by white, cream-colored, or grayish plaques, surrounded by erythema, scattered over all or part of the oral mucous membranes. When a patch is removed, usually with difficulty, the remaining base appears brightly inflamed. In the chronic adult form of candidiasis, which may relate to the development of hypersensitivity, there is a dry, red buccal mucosa, with little or no covering membrane, sometimes in the form of patches. The tongue has a "raw-beef," shiny appearance and is dry, fissured, cracked, and swollen. Since the entire mucous membrane is dry and burning, the mastication of anything but bland foods is difficult, and nutritional deficiencies may complicate the situation if the disease continues for a long time.

Candidal infection of the lips, often called perlèche, is a symmetrical erosion of the labial commissures. The upper layers of the epidermis are lost, while those beneath are red in appearance. Deep cracks, sometimes covered with a gray or white membrane, develop in the folds at the corner of the mouth. A somewhat similar lesion develops in riboflavin deficiency, from which this type of candidiasis is difficult to differentiate. It is probable that nutritional deficiency predisposes to candidal infection of the lips, and that perlèche is the infection of vitamin deficiency lesions by C. albicans.

Candidal vulvovaginitis is often associated with diabetes, pregnancy, or seen in women taking hormones, including birth control pills. Lesions appear as gray-white pseudomembranous patches on the vaginal mucosa. A yellowish discharge may also be present.

Cutaneous candidal lesions may be localized, generalized, and allergic (candidiids). Wetting of the skin and other factors which lower resistance predispose to this type of infection. The region about the fingernails is the most common site of cutaneous candidal infection (onychia and paronychia). Intertrigo, commonly involving the axillae, gluteal folds, and groin, and occasionally the webs of the toes and the perianal region, is an example of a generalized cutaneous candidal infection. Generalized infection of the smooth skin may occur, usually related to oral or other localized grouped vesicular candidal lesions occurring over the hands, arms, or body surface.

Chronic Mucocutaneous Candidiasis. Chronic mucocutaneous candidiasis is a syndrome resulting from proliferation of C. albicans in which the cutaneous structures become chronically infected (fig. 34/3). It is not a single entity but represents the final common pathway resulting when one or more of the defense mechanisms that normally restrict C. albicans proliferation is defective. Organisms apparently penetrate the membrane of viable epithelial cells and exist as intracellular parasites. The degree of involvement varies from patient to patient and in a patient at different times. The classic lesions are verrucous, with tissue projections growing out from the skin. The lesions appear early and become chronic, with development of extensive epithelial hyperplasia. Most patients have deficiencies in their cell-mediated immunity. Apparently, any of the T-dependent immunodeficiencies may permit this condition to develop. Other abnormalities such as endocrinopathies, leukemias and thymomas may contribute to the pathogenesis. Chronic mucocutaneous candidiasis also is seen in patients with no apparent immunological defects.

Laboratory Diagnosis of Candidiasis. Laboratory methods useful in the diagnosis of candidiasis are microscopic examination of stained tissue sections, microscopic examination of a gram stained film of hydroxide-cleared pus, sputum, or scrapings of suspected lesions, and direct culture. Sabouraud's glucose agar (with chloramphenicol or without antibiotic) is most useful for initial isolation of Candida species.

A method for determining the presence of candidal infection is by examining under a microscope a portion of the membrane from a suspected lesion treated with potassium hydroxide until it has been cleared. C. albicans appears in tissue as a fine, branching, nonsegmented mycelial net, sometimes with small, oval, budding, thin-walled cells, and clusters of microspores scattered about the microscopic field.

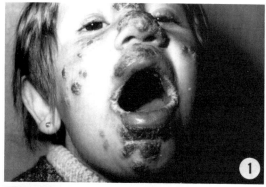
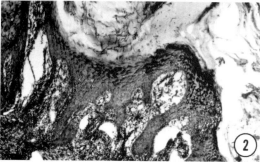
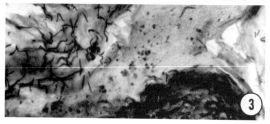

Figure 34/3. Chronic mucocutaneous candidiasis and disseminated histoplasmosis in a 14-year-old girl. The oral lesions show thick white scales alternating with eroded red areas. Histologically, there was hyperkeratosis and parakeratosis. Pseudohyphae were associated with leukocytes. (Courtesy of Dr. Leopoldo F. Montes and reproduced with permission from J. Kriner *et al.*: Chronic Mucocutaneous Candidiasis and Disseminated Histoplasmosis. *Journal of Cutaneous Pathology, 7*, 58, 1980; Munksgaard International Publishers Ltd., Copenhagen, Denmark.)

Treatment of Candidiasis. It is useful in the treatment of candidiasis to institute all measures that will improve the general health of the patient. The antibiotics available for the treatment of candidiasis are amphotericin B and nystatin.

GEOTRICHOSIS

Geotrichosis is thought to be an uncommon chronic disease caused by one or more species of *Geotrichum*, a common fungal inhabitant of the upper respiratory and gastrointestinal tracts. As with candidiasis, infection with *Geotrichum* species is most often associated with situations which lower resistance of the host.

***Geotrichum* Species.** The various infective species of *Geotrichum*, particularly *G. candidum*, can be demonstrated from the lesions by direct examination or they can be isolated by appropriate cultural techniques. In tissue, the organisms appear as oblong or rectangular cells. Microscopic examination of the growth in culture reveals hyphae which segment into rectangular arthrospores; spherical cells up to 10 to 12 μm in diameter can be seen which are also segmented from the hyphae.

Infection. Four clinical forms of geotrichosis occur: oral, intestinal, bronchial, and pulmonary. In geotrichosis of the oral cavity, white membranous patches are found which are difficult to distinguish from the lesions of candidiasis. Intestinal geotrichosis presents a more confusing picture since the clinical picture is variable and species of the fungus are often present in the intestine of normal individuals. Bronchial geotrichosis, a more common form, is characterized by bronchitis, coughing, and gelatinous sputum, streaked with blood. Clinically, it resembles acute tuberculosis, with extensive involvement of the lungs (pulmonary).

Diagnosis. Clinical symptoms, direct microscopic examination and culture are appropriate methods for the diagnosis of geotrichosis. In specimens fungal cells appear oblong, rectangular, or spherical. In culture rectangular arthrospores and spherical cells up to 12 μm in diameter are characteristically produced.

Treatment of Geotrichosis. The prognosis of geotrichosis is good, especially if adequate treatment is instituted. Treatment of the pulmonary form is similar to that of tuberculosis. The polyene antibiotics are effective in treating oral and intestinal geotrichosis.

HISTOPLASMOSIS

Histoplasmosis is caused by *Histoplasma capsulatum*. Before 1935, histoplasmosis was considered to be uniformly fatal. However, later surveys indicate that a self-limited clinically undetected chronic pulmonary infection with *H. capsulatum* is widespread, affecting an estimated 30 million people in at least 22 countries, whereas progressive histoplasmosis of either the acute pulmonary or disseminated type is relatively rare.

***H. capsulatum*.** In the yeast form in tissues, *H. capsulatum* appears as small oval bodies. On Sabouraud's glucose agar, this fungus grows slowly, producing white, cottony aerial mycelia, which microscopically show branching, septate hyphae bearing chlamydospores.

Clinical Course. Histoplasmosis is primarily a benign disease of man. Patients with a subclinical disease are asymptomatic, although the illness may be evident on radiographic examination.

The acute pulmonary form of the disease is characterized by sudden onset of fever, malaise, cough, chest pains and dyspnea. There is a focal granuloma and lymphadenitis that heals, often with calcification, resembling tuberculosis radiographically. The illness may range from a subclinical form to a severe flu-like illness. Recovery is usually rapid, with development of strong immunity although progressive disease occurs in a fraction of a percentage of the cases.

The chronic progressive pulmonary form may appear like acute pulmonary disease, but with exaggerated symptoms. However, there is slow progression of the disease with necrosis, caseation and cavitation, resembling tuberculosis.

The disseminated type can occur at any age but usually is seen in severely debilitated older individuals, middle-aged men, or infants. It has a rapid, fatal course. Mucocutaneous lesions are characteristic of disseminated histoplasmosis. The oral lesions of histoplasmosis occur on the lips, buccal mucosa, palate and tongue. They are granulomatous and may persist as nodules or they may ulcerate. These lesions may simulate carcinoma or tuberculosis.

Epidemiology. *Histoplasma* has been isolated from animals, soil and bird feces. It is usually acquired exogenously from contaminated dust and is not apparently transmitted from animal to animal. Pulmonary disease results when the individual inhales the organisms. Progressive disseminated disease may occur with spread of the fungus throughout the body after varying periods of time.

Diagnosis. The diagnosis of histoplasmosis depends to a great extent on the clinical manifestation although it may be confused with tuberculosis, carcinoma, leukemia and Hodgkin's disease. Also required for diagnosis are detection of the organisms by microscopy, culture and isolation.

H. capsulatum appears in tissues as small, oval, yeast-like cells that appear to have a capsule, although they do not possess such a structure. The organism is usually intracellular in mononuclear leukocytes in the peripheral blood, and in macrophages elsewhere, particularly in the spleen and bone marrow. It may be cultivated from blood, biopsy material, or sputum.

Several immunological tests are also available including a skin test similar to the tuberculin test for detection of hypersensitivity to *Mycobacterium tuberculosis*. This test uses a culture filtrate called histoplasmin for detecting hypersensitivity to the organism.

Treatment. Amphotericin B is most effective for treatment. This may be combined with surgical removal of localized lesions for management of chronic pulmonary histoplasmosis.

SPOROTRICHOSIS

Sporotrichosis, caused by *Sporothrix schenckii*, is a chronic, granulomatous mycotic disease and has been reported from every continent, with the areas of greatest prevalence being the North Central United States and Mexico.

S. schenckii. *S. schenckii* seldom can be found by direct microscopic examination of unstained human pus or tissue. The tissue phase in human beings, which is difficult to differentiate from normal cellular constituents, is polymorphic, assuming such shapes as rings and hollow spheres. In biopsy specimens, an asteroid body has been described which is somewhat analogous to the sulfur granule seen in actinomycosis (fig. 34/4). In culture, *S. schenckii* is dimorphic, occurring in either a mycelial or a yeast phase.

Clinical Course and Appearance. There are five local types of sporotrichosis which relate to the area of tissue involved, including the lymphatics, skin, mucous membranes, skeleton, and viscera. The upper extremities are most often involved.

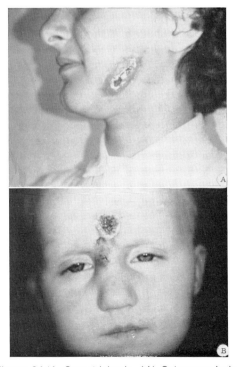

Figure 34/4. Sporotrichosis. (*A*) Cutaneous lesion of sporotrichosis resembling actinomycosis. (*B*) An uncommon localized lymphangitic type of cutaneous sporotrichosis. (Reproduced with permission from W. M. Mikkelsen, R. L. Brandt, and E. R. Harrell: Sporotrichosis. *Annals of Internal Medicine,* **47,** 435, 1957.)

Sporotrichosis begins as an ulcer at the site at which the causative fungus enters the body, frequently at a site of trauma. The injury fails to heal, then ulcerates. This is followed by an infection which progresses along lymphatics to regional lymph nodes, where ulceration occurs. Infection seldom extends beyond regional lymph nodes, although sometimes a disseminated form occurs which involves no characteristic area or tissue. The lesions of cutaneous sporotrichosis occur as plaques, follicles, nodules, and papules and may represent a previous sensitization to the organism. Mucosal sporotrichosis more commonly involves the nose, mouth or pharynx with erythematous, ulcerative, suppurative, or vegetative lesions. When the oral cavity is the site of the initial infection, the mucosal lymphatics may be involved locally. Oral lesions also may be derived from a hematogenous dissemination and resemble those occurring on the skin.

Laboratory Diagnosis of Sporotrichosis. The microscopic examination of tissue fluid specimens, although sometimes useful, cannot be depended on for a positive diagnosis. More dependable is direct culture, which is easily accomplished on blood agar or Sabouraud's agar. Animal inoculation (mice, rats) is also useful in diagnosis but direct culture is preferred.

Treatment. Potassium iodide is specifically curative and thus is the treatment of choice for sporotrichosis. It is administered for up to 4 to 6 weeks after apparent recovery. Amphotericin B, stilbamidine, and dihydroxystilbamidine also have been reported successful.

NORTH AMERICAN BLASTOMYCOSIS

North American blastomycosis is a chronic, infectious, granulomatous disease caused by *Blastomyces dermatitidis*. It often resembles tuberculosis, from which it may be difficult to distinguish. Blastomycosis is mostly restricted to midwestern and southeastern United States but sporadic cases have been described from all the states.

B. dermatitidis. In tissues, *B. dermatitidis* appears as spherical or oval, thick-walled, yeast-like cells that reporduce by budding. When cultured at 37 C, *B. dermatitidis* retains its yeast-like characteristics but at 25 C, this organism grows in a mycelial form.

Clinical Course. Human infection with *B. dermatitidis* is apparently from exogenous sources and occurs by a pulmonary route. There is no man-to-man spread. Once lesions appear the regional lymphatics become involved, with resulting lymphadenopathy. Blastomycosis appears in a pulmonary, cutaneous, or systemic form. Although infection is by the pulmonary route, it may be asymptomatic and the first manifestations are cutaneous. Skin

lesions begin as small, firm papules, with satellite lesions that coalesce (fig. 34/5). The lesions break down and discharge pus that contains numbers of the organisms. There is a granulatomatous inflammatory reaction and a mononuclear cell infiltration. As the disease progress a mass of tissue forms that ulcerates and drains pus from multiple openings, simulating actinomycosis. The disease spreads slowly through subcutaneous tissues while healing and scar formation occur in the center of the lesion. Such lesions may be seen on any body surface or in the oral cavity. Pulmonary blastomycosis resembles histoplasmosis or tuberculosis. The systemic form results from dissemination from a pulmonary lesion and may appear in any organ system. Initial infection by *B. dermititidis* is not easily established, but once present, progresses steadily. Spontaneous resolution is rare.

Diagnosis. Laboratory diagnostic procedures are direct microscopic examination of tissue or exudates and cultural procedures and biopsy. Immu-

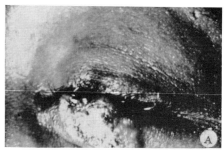

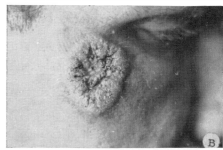

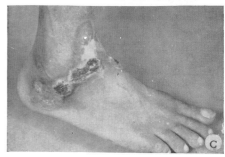

Figure 34/5. The cutaneous lesions of North American blastomycosis. (*A*) Eyelid, (*B*) face, and (*C*) ankle. (*A*, AFIP 57-10448; *B*, AFIP 53-2219; *C*, AFIP 55-15884.)

nological procedures are skin and complement-fixation tests. Cutaneous hypersensitivity is determined by the use of a culture filtrate, termed blastomycin, which is analogous to tuberculin. Consequently, the blastomycin skin test is quite similar to the tuberculin test.

Treatment of North American Blastomycosis. Success in treatment has been reported with the aromatic diamidines (stilbamidine, 2-hydroxystilbamidine) but the course of treatment is long and relapses are frequent. Amphotericin B is the most useful treatment.

COCCIDIOIDOMYCOSIS

Coccidioidomycosis occurs in North America, especially the southwestern United States, and Central South America. It is caused by *Coccidioides immitis*, a fungus that is widely distributed in soils and in dust. In some areas of the southwestern United States as much as 80% of the population reacts to coccidioidin skin tests suggesting that a great number of cases are asymptomatic or not distinguished from other respiratory infections. It also may present with various clinical manifestations including a nondisseminated and a disseminated form.

C. immitis. *C. immitis* occurs in distinct phases in tissue and in culture. From an arthrospore, it develops in tissue and body fluids and exudates into a nonbudding spherule packed with endospores. In reproduction the spherules rupture, the endospores are set free and develop into full-sized spherules. In culture, mycelial growth occurs which can develop from either spherules or arthrospores. Spherules do not form during cultivation *in vitro*, but can be produced in the yolk sac of embryonated eggs.

Clinical Appearance. Coccidioidomycosis is primarily a respiratory infection. The organisms usually enter the human body by inhalation of spores in contaminated dust, initiating the respiratory infection. There is no known man-to-man or animal-to-animal transmission of the disease.

Nondisseminated coccidioidomycosis is characterized by upper respiratory involvement with nasopharyngitis. It is self-limiting. Pleural pain, chills, and a nonproductive cough are common. A pulmonary form may develop with symptoms of acute pneumonia. Complications are not common although dissemination sometimes occurs. Less commonly, patients develop erythematous skin lesions within 2 to 20 days after onset of the disease (fig. 34/6). Primary skin lesions are rare.

In disseminated coccidioidomycosis that develops from severe cases of primary disease, there is also a respiratory infection and progressive debilitation that usually takes a rapid course. It is characterized by fever, production of mucopurulent spu-

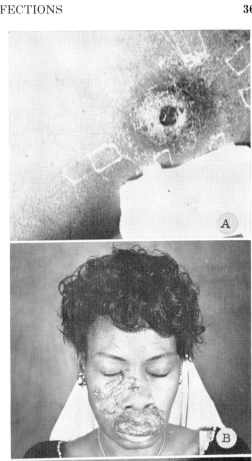
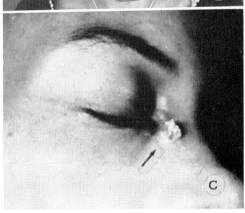

Figure 34/6. Cutaneous lesions of coccidioidomycosis. (*A*, AFIP 57-11831; *B*, AFIP; *C*, AFIP 56-7603-32.)

tum, and weight loss. Lesions appear in subcutaneous tissues, bones and internal organs. This form usually progresses to a fatal outcome within a year. The oral manifestations appear as purple nodules, which are of several weeks duration. Other oral manifestations are erythema exudativum multiforme and erythema nodosum.

Diagnosis. Diagnosis of coccidioidomycosis relates to the clinical symptoms and laboratory procedures. The symptoms are likely to be confused with tuberculosis, North American blastomycosis, histoplasmosis, influenza, upper respiratory infections, and neoplastic diseases. Laboratory procedures include animal inoculation (mice or guinea pigs), microscopic detection of the causative organisms in sputum or body fluids, skin testing and serological tests.

A culture filtrate of medium in which the organisms have been grown, known as coccidioidin, comparable to tuberculin or histoplasmin, may be used as a skin test material for detection of hypersensitivity.

Treatment. The treatment of coccidioidomycosis is mostly symptomatic but amphotericin B is useful.

PARACOCCIDIOIDOMYCOSIS

Paracoccidioidomycosis is a mycotic disease limited to Central and South America. It is caused by *Paracoccidioides brasiliensis*, a fungus somewhat similar to *Blastomyces dermatitidis*.

P. brasiliensis. *P. brasiliensis* appears as two types of thickwalled, yeast-like cells. One type is a single-budding cell, the other a multiple-budding cell. The single-budding cells resemble *B. dermatitidis*, but the multiple-budding cells are differential and diagnostic for *P. brasiliensis*.

Clinical Apppearance. South American blastomycosis has varying clinical manifestations which to a certain extent are mediated by the site of inoculation and the organ or tissue infected.

Primary infection often is pulmonary and inapparent. The organisms are then transported to the oral mucosa by macrophages. Occasionally initial infection occurs in the skin, producing ulceration and invasion of subcutaneous tissues. The infection then spreads locally producing secondary lesions. Lymphatic spread may further disseminate the infection, and hematogenous dissemination may result in invasion of the lungs and brain.

Paracoccidioidomycosis is usually classified into mucocutaneous, visceral, lymphatic, and mixed forms. The lesion common to the various clinical forms is an ulcerative granuloma. Almost any oral tissue may be involved in paracoccidioidomycosis, including the tongue, lips, gingiva, palate, tonsils, and buccal mucosa. Lesions in the throat or oral cavity are so painful during swallowing that they interfere with the intake of food. Ulcerative stomatitis and gingivitis are common to paracoccidoidomycosis. Lymphatic spread results in hard, painful nodes that adhere to the skin, soften, then ulcerate. Visceral involvement results in lesions in the spleen, liver, pancreas, intestines and kidneys.

Treatment. Paracoccidioidomycosis is chronic and eventually almost always fatal unless some form of treatment is instituted. Sulfonamide therapy has been effective in some cases. Amphotericin B is the only drug that is very useful for treatment of the disseminated disease.

CRYPTOCOCCOSIS

Cryptococcosis is caused by inhalation of dust and bird droppings contaminated by a yeast-like organism, *Cryptococcus neoformans*. The disease may be chronic, wasting, and highly fatal, although there are many subclinical cases, especially in the United States. It involves the respiratory tract and has a predilection for the central nervous system, being the most common cause of mycotic meningitis.

C. neoformans. *C. neoformans* occurs as a thickwalled, heavily encapsulated oval yeast. The cells reproduce only by budding, usually by a single bud. *C. neoformans* can be grown on all the usual media.

Pathogenesis of C. neoformans. Most commonly cryptococcosis occurs in the respiratory tract, where it has the characteristics of a chronic lung infection, with few evident or distinctive symptoms. The pulmonary disease *per se* seldom progresses sufficiently to cause death, but in a considerable fraction of cases it disseminates to the central nervous system or other organs. Following dissemination it may produce ulcers or granulomas, particularly in the spleen, kidneys, liver and mesenteric lymph nodes. Bone abscesses also may occur. Clinical disease has a high fatality rate.

C. neoformans is only weakly antigenic and the immunological response plays little or no part in the course of the disease. Some degree of hypersensitivity to *C. neoformans* develops but this has not been useful in diagnosis. Laboratory diagnostic procedures entail direct examination of tissue fluid or exudates, culturing, and animal inoculation.

Treatment of Cryptococcosis. Treatment of cryptococcosis is by amphotericin B.

MUCORMYCOSIS

The organisms involved in mucormycosis (*phycomycosis*) are in the order Mucocales, particularly *Absidia*, *Mucor*, and *Rhizopus* species. These are ordinarily nonpathogenic saprophytes found in soil and starchy foods (the common bread molds are phycomycetes) which can under proper conditions produce disease. Mucormycosis is an opportunistic fungous disease that occurs in the presence of severe depression of resistance. The patients may have debilitating conditions such as diabetes with acidosis, renal failure, leukemia, cirrhosis, severe burns, or even infections such as tuberculosis, syphilis, or amebic colitis. They are often being treated with therapeutic agents such as antibiotics, antineoplastic drugs, steroids, or other immunosuppressive regimens.

Clinical Course and Appearance. The classic picture of mucormycosis is orbital cellulitis and meningoencephalitis in an acidotic diabetic. In acidotic patients primary infection often occurs in the nose due to *Rhizopus oryzae* or *Rhizopus arrezus*. These species are the most common causes of this type of infection because they possess the enzyme ketoreductase, and acidotic patients generally have ketone bodies in their serum.

In pulmonary disease seen in patients with malignancies such as leukemia or lymphoma, primary lung infection occurs. Growth on the bronchial mucosa penetrates the wall. The causative organisms have an affinity for blood vessels and lymphatics and may be found in the vessel walls. They can penetrate into the lumen to produce thrombosis. Ulceration due to ischemia and local invasion may be present and the lungs show necrosis and cavitation. Organisms are regularly found in the margins of the ulcer craters and there is a polymorphonuclear leukocyte infiltrate around the margin. Gastrointestinal mucormycosis may occur in which the intestinal or gastric mucosa is invaded, and there have been reports of disseminated disease.

In cervicofacial disease the organisms enter by way of the nose or mouth, then by direct extension reach the paranasal sinuses, orbit, and cranial cavity. Discrete ulcerations of varying size may occur. The organisms invade the walls of blood vessels and proliferate, causing thrombosis and subsequent necrosis. Symptoms may include unilateral headache, facial pain, periorbital numbness, swelling of the eyelid, eye irritation, lacrimation and blurring of the vision (fig. 34/7).

Involvement of the nasal cavity results in rhinorrhea, epistaxis, nasal stuffiness, a dark, blood-stained discharge and a reddish-black necrotic appearance of the septum and turbinates. A dull steady pain over the sinus is a common finding. Necrotic lesions of the hard and soft palate may be present as sharply demarcated areas of black-grey eschar covering the surface mucosa.

Diagnosis. Although the majority of cases have been diagnosed at necropsy, phycomycosis may be diagnosed by clinical manifestations, usually coupled with a history of debilitating disease. Detection of the fungi in tissue and exudates by microscopic observation is useful. In tissues the fungi appear as broad, nonseptate hyphae. Culturing may be helpful in diagnosis but since these organisms are common laboratory contaminants, it is not definitive.

Treatment. Treatment involves control of the underlying debilitating condition to the extent possible coupled with chemotherapy and possible surgical excision of localized septic areas. Desensitization with autogenous vaccines and administration of iodides are used in the treatment, but amphotericin B also is beneficial.

MADUROMYCOSIS

Maduromycosis is a distinct clinical entity caused by 13 or more fungal species. Mycetoma is a term applied to localized granulomatous and suppurative lesions that affect the skin, subcutaneous tissues, bone, fascia of feet and hands. The causative agents are either actinomyces or several species of fungi. The fungi commonly involved are *Aspergillus jeanselmi*, *Allescheria boydii*, *Madurella grisea*, and *Madurella mycetomi*. The initial lesions are papules, nodules, or vesicles, which are at first characterized by remission and recurrence. As the disease progresses, abscesses and fistulas develop and the infection spreads to bone and other deep tissues, until the foot or leg becomes club-shaped and enlarged to several times its normal size. The primary mycosis usually is not systemic, but secondary bacterial infections occur with systemic manifestations.

Laboratory Diagnosis of Maduromycosis. Laboratory diagnosis may be made by direct microscopic examination of pus or fluid from lesions or fistulas. Isolation of the causal organism by culturing is useful in diagnosis, but animal inoculation is not.

Treatment of Maduromycosis. Although the disease is chronic, it is slowly and surely progressive and the prognosis is poor unless the affected limb is amputated. Death usually results from secondary bacterial infection, rather than by direct action of the causal fungus. Polyene antibiotics may be useful in some cases.

RHINOSPORIDIOSIS

Rhinosporidiosis, caused by *Rhinosporidium seeberi*, is a chronic disease affecting principally the mucous membranes of the nasopharynx, but also sometimes affecting the upper respiratory tract. It is rare in humans, but the causal organism is apparently widespread in nature and infects both man and such domestic animals as horses, mules, and cattle.

R. seeberi. *R. seeberi* has not as yet been definitely cultured. Its life cycle in tissues begins as a thin-walled, round corpuscle. As it enlarges the corpuscle becomes double-walled. The nucleus but not the cytoplasm of the corpuscle then divides repeatedly until some 2,000 to 4,000 nuclei are produced; the cytoplasm then divides, enveloping each nucleus to form numerous individual mature spores.

Pathogenesis of Rhinosporidiosis. The regions most often affected by rhinosporidiosis are the nostrils and nasopharynx and the soft palate. Except for the upper respiratory tract, rarely are other areas of the body involved. The principal lesions of the disease are sessile but sometimes pedunculated polyps, which are red, bleed easily,

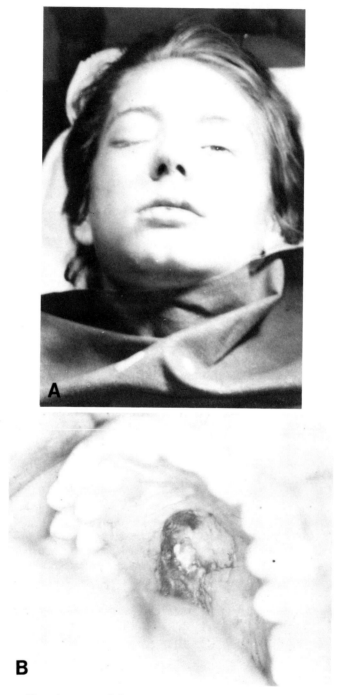

Figure 34/7. Rhinomaxillary phycomycosis in 16-year-old male diabetic. (*A*) Appearance at time of admission to hospital. There is edema in the right perinasal and periorbital areas, anesthesis of the right infraorbital region, loss of corneal reflex, and ptosis of the upper right eyelid. (*B*) Palatal ulcer. Note black necrotic tissue at margin. (Courtesy of Dr. Thomas D. Moye, Jr., and reproduced with permission from T. D. Moye and R. J. Caudill: Rhinomaxillary Phycomycosis; Report of a Case. *Journal of Oral Surgery,* **38,** 132, 1980.)

and sometimes enlarge sufficiently to obscure the passageway, interfering with breathing.

Treatment of Rhinosporidiosis. Though many drugs have been tested none has proved definitely effective. Surgical intervention seems to be the most useful measure, but recurrence is likely unless extensive amounts of unaffected tissue are removed.

CHROMOBLASTOMYCOSIS

Chromoblastomycosis is an uncommon, noncontagious disease of mixed fungal origin that results in chronic cutaneous granulomatous nodular growths on the head, neck, and trunk. The fungal species most often involved are *Fonsecaea pedrosoi*, *Fonsecaea compacta*, *Phialophora verrucosa*, and other *Fonsecaea* species.

Mycotic Agents of Chromoblastomycosis. *F. pedrosoi* is somewhat variable as to the type and color of its colonies. Usually it is slow-growing and forms dark brown to black colonies. *F. compacta* also grows slowly, producing a characteristic heaped, brittle colony, black in color. *P. verrucosa* is slow-growing and forms greenish brown colonies. It produces conidia from cup-like structures that are situated either laterally or terminally on aerial hyphae. In either unstained or stained sections of infected tissue, the organisms are seen as spherical or oval, thick-walled, sometimes septate bodies.

Pathogenesis of Chromoblastomycosis. The various causative agents of chromoblastomycosis exist saprophytically in the environment, in some instances in soils, and accidentally gain entrance into the body through some abrasion or wound. Most cases have occurred in tropical and subtropical areas but are by no means restricted to them.

Chromoblastomycosis is slow in developing, chronic, and usually involves the skin of the face or trunk with a granulomatous, inflammatory reaction. Occasionally an extremity will be affected. The initial lesion resembles that of ringworm. After some time, new lesions develop peripherally along superficial lymph channels. The affected areas have a raised cauliflower appearance. Such lesions are ordinarily painless unless secondarily infected. In diagnosis, clinical observations should be supplemented by microscopy of the exudates, histological examination of tissue, cultural studies, and animal inoculation.

Treatment of Chromoblastomycosis. There is no specific therapy for chromoblastomycosis. The treatment of choice has been surgical excision of the cutaneous lesion, unless it is extensive, supplemented by iodide or polyene antibiotic therapy.

ASPERGILLOSIS

Many species of *Aspergillus* are widespread in the environment. Certain of these species, particularly *Aspergillus fumigatus*, are occasional pathogens for man, causing a disease known as aspergillosis.

***Aspergillus* Species.** Species of *Aspergillus* appear as fragmented mycelia and characteristic spore heads and spores.

Pathogenesis of Aspergillosis. Human aspergillosis is largely an occupational disease affecting agricultural or industrial workers who must handle or come into close contact with material contaminated with aspergillus spores, although not infrequently severe burns become infected with these organisms.

Aspergillosis is essentially an inflammatory granulomatous reaction involving most commonly the ear, bronchi and lungs, bones, nasal and maxillary sinuses, genitalia, and the integument, either primarily or secondarily. Pulmonary infection may simulate tuberculosis, bronchopneumonia, tracheitis, or bronchitis. So closely does it simulate these diseases that differential diagnosis is difficult.

Treatment of Aspergillosis. Antibiotic treatment has not only been generally useless but in some instances seems to favor the development and spread of the aspergilli and contributes to a fatal outcome. However, amphotericin B is sometimes useful for treatment.

THE DERMATOMYCOSES

A number of fungi infect the superficial skin, rarely invade the deeper tissues, and never cause systemic infections. These superficial skin infections are known as the dermatomycoses. Species of the three genera, *Microsporum*, *Trichophyton*, and *Epidermophyton* are the most common etiological agents, although yeasts or other fungi causing systemic infections, such as *Candida albicans*, may be involved. Since several species can cause identical lesions in the same area of the body and since a single species can cause different lesions in different areas of the skin, considerable confusion has arisen over the classification and naming of the various manifestations. The dermatomycoses are usually classified according to the area of body affected, regardless of the responsible fungus, using a binomial system. The generic name for such a disease is tinea (literally, a gnawing worm; colloquially, ringworm), followed by a term describing its location, such as pedis (foot) (fig. 34/8), capitis (head), barbae (beard), unguium (nail), corporis (body), favosa (scalp), cruris (groin), and imbricata (scaly skin). Other names sometimes used are tinea versicolor (changeable in color), tinea nigra (dark or black), and tinea albigena (white or without color). Sometimes all mycoses of smooth skin are classified as tinea glabrosa.

The clinical features of mycotic infections are quite variable and may resemble those of neoplastic or bacterial diseases. In most instances, therefore, identification of the causal organism is essential to the specific diagnosis of the disease. The morphological and cultural characteristics of the dermatophytes are the principal basis for their identification, and in some instances, their physiological properties. Certain properties are generally com-

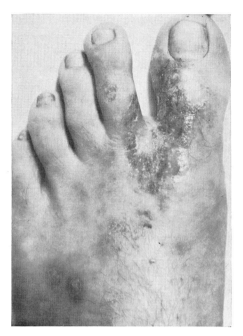

Figure 34/8. Tinea pedis. (AFIP A-44904).

mon to the dermatophytes: asexual spore formation, simple nutritional requirements, growth at
room temperature, and growth in media either sufficiently acid or alkaline to suppress bacterial
growth. Other characteristics serve for differentiation.

ADDITIONAL READING

ABERNATHY, R. S. 1973 Treatment of Systemic Mycoses.
Medicine, **52,** 385.

ALLEN, A. M., AND TAPLIN, D. 1973 Epidemic *Trichophyton mentagrophytes* Infections in Servicemen.
JAMA, **226,** 864.

AUFDEMORTE, T. B., AND McPHERSON, M. A. 1978 Refractory Oral Candidiasis. Oral Surg, **46,** 776.

BAKER, R. D. 1970 The Phycomycoses. Ann NY Acad
Sci, **174,** 592.

BARDANA, E. J., JR., GERBER, J. D., CRAIG, S., AND
CIANCIULLI, F. D. 1975 The General and Specific Hu-
moral Immune Response to Pulmonary Aspergillosis.
Am Rev Respir Dis, **112,** 799.

BAUM, C. L., AND SCHWARZ, J. 1955 Coccidioidomycosis;
a Review. Am J Med Sci, **230,** 82.

BAYER, A. S., YOSHIKAWA, T. T., GALPIN, J. E., AND
GUZE, L. B. 1976 Unusual Syndromes of Coccidioidomycosis: Diagnostic and Therapeutic Considerations. A
Report of 10 Cases and Review of the English Literature. Medicine, **55,** 131.

BHAGWANDEEN, S. B. 1974 North American Blastomycosis in Zambia. Am J Trop Med Hyg, **23,** 231.

BODENHOFF, J. 1965 Some Important Mycotic Infections
with Oral Manifestations. Tandlaegebladet, **69,** 77.

BRADFORD, L. G., AND MONTES, L. F. 1972 Perioral Dermatitis and *Candida albicans*. Arch Dermatol, **105,**
892.

BUDTZ-JÖRGENSEN, E. 1973 Cellular Immunity in Acquired Candidiasis of the Palate. Scand J Dent Res, **81,**
360.

BUDTZ-JÖRGENSEN, E., AND BERTRAM, U. 1970 Denture
Stomatitis; II. The Effect of Antifungal and Prosthetic
Treatment. Acta Odontol Scand, **28,** 282.

CAWSON, R. A. 1965 Thrush in Adult Out-Patients. Dent
Pract (Bristol), **15,** 361.

CHICK, E. W. 1973 Opportunistic Are the Fungi. Chest,
63, 3.

CHMEL, H., GRIECO, M. H., AND ZICKEL, R. 1973 Candida
Osteomyelitis—Report of a Case. Am J Med Sci, **266,**
299.

CIEGLER, A. 1975 Mycotoxins; Occurrence, Chemistry,
Biological Activity. Lloydia, **38,** 21.

COHEN, S. G., AND GREENBERG, M. S. 1980 Rhinomaxillary Mucormycosis in a Kidney Transplant Patient.
Oral Surg, **50,** 33.

CRAIG, E. L., AND SUIE, T. 1974 *Histoplasma capsulatum*
in Human Ocular Tissue. Arch Ophthalmol, **91,** 285.

CRUICKSHANK, G., VINCENT, R. D., CHERRICK, H. M.,
AND DERBY, K. 1977 Rhinocerebral Mucormycosis. J
Am Dent Assoc, **95,** 164.

CUSH, R., LIGHT, R. W., AND GEORGE, R. B. 1976 Clinical
and Roentgenographic Manifestations of Acute and
Chronic Blastomycosis. Chest, **69,** 345.

DAVENPORT, J. C., AND WILTON, J. M. A. 1971 Incidence
of Immediate and Delayed Hypersensitivity to *Candida albicans* in Denture Stomatitis. J Dent Res, **50,**
892.

DAVIES, R. R., AND DENNING, T. J. V. 1972 Growth and
Form in *Candida albicans*. Sabouraudia, **10,** 180.

DAVIS, C. M., GARCIA, R. L., AND RIORDON, J. P. 1972
Dermatophytes in Military Recruits. Arch Dermatol,
105, 558.

DIAMOND, R. D., ROOT, R. K., AND BENNETT, J. E. 1972
Factors Influencing Killing of *Cryptococcus neoformans* by Human Leukocytes *in Vitro*. J Infect Dis, **125,**
367.

DOTO, I. L., TOSH, F. E., FARNWORTH, S. F., AND FUR-
COLOW, M. L. 1972 Coccidioidin, Histoplasmin, and
Tuberculin Sensitivity among School Children in Mar-
icopa County, Arizona. Am J Epidemiol, **95,** 464.

DRAKE, T. E., AND MAIBACK, H. I. 1973 Candida and
Candidiasis. Postgrad Med, **83,** 120.

DWYER, J. M. 1981 Chronic Mucocutaneous Candidiasis.
Annu Rev Med, **32,** 491.

ECHOLS, R. M., SELINGER, D. S., HALLOWELL, C., GOOD-
WIN, J. S., DUNCAN, M. H., AND CUSHING, A. H. 1979
Rhizopus Osteomyelitis. Am J Med, **66,** 141.

EDWARDS, J. E., JR., FOOS, R. Y., MONTGOMERIE, J. Z.,
AND GUZE, L. B. 1974 Ocular Manifestations of Candida
Septicemia; Review of Seventy-Six Cases of Hematog-
enous Candida Endophthalmitis. Medicine, **53,** 47.

EDWARDS, L. B., ACQUAVIVA, F. A., AND LIVESAY, V. T.
1973 Further Observations on Histoplasmin Sensitivity
in the United States. Am J Epidemiol, **98,** 315.

ERDOS, M. S., BUTT, K., AND WEINSTEIN, L. 1972 Mucor-
mycotic Endocarditis of the Pulmonary Valve. JAMA,
222, 951.

EVERS, R. H., AND WHEREATT, R. R. 1974 Pulmonary
Sporotrichosis. Chest, **66,** 91.

FEIGIN, R. D., SHACKELFORD, P. G., EISEN, S., SPITLER,
L. E., PICKERING, L. K., AND ANDERSON, D. C. 1974
Treatment of Mucocutaneous Candidiasis with Trans-
fer Factor. Pediatrics, **53,** 63.

FELTON, F. G., MUCHMORE, H. G., AND McCARTHY, M.
A. 1974 Epidemiology of Cryptococcosis; I. Environ-
mental Distribution of Cryptococci in Oklahoma.
Health Lab Sci, **11,** 201.

FELTON, F. G., MUCHMORE, H. G., McCARTHY, M. A.,
MONROE, P. W., AND RHOADES, E. R. 1974 Epidemiology of Cryptococcosis; II. Evaluation of Patient's Environment. Health Lab Sci, **11,** 205.

FISCHER, J. B., AND KANE, J. 1974 The Laboratory Diagnosis of Dermatophytosis Complicated with *Candida albicans*. Can J Microbiol, **20**, 167.

FISHBACH, R. S., WHITE, M. L., AND FINEGOLD, S. M. 1973 Bronchopulmonary Geotrichosis. Am Rev Respir Dis. **108**, 1388.

FITZGERALD, E., LLOYD-STILL, J., AND GORDON, S. L. 1975 Candida Arthritis; a Case Report and Review of the Literature. Clin Orthop, **106**, 143.

FORREST, J. V. 1973 Common Fungal Diseases of the Lungs; II. Histoplasmosis. Radiol Clin North Am, **11**, 163.

GAINES, J. D. 1973 Diagnosis of Deep Infection with *Candida*. Arch Intern Med, **132**, 699.

GARTENBERG, G., BOTTONE, E. J., KEUSCH, G. T., AND WERTZMAN, I. 1978 Hospital-acquired Mucormycosis (*Rhizopus rhizopodiformis*) of Skin and Subcutaneous Tissue. N Engl J Med, **299**, 1115.

GELLER, R. D., MAYNARD, J. E., AND JONES, V. 1973 Coccidioidin Sensitivity among Southwestern American Indians. Am Rev Respir Dis, **107**, 301.

GISSLEN, H., HERSLE, K., AND MOBACKEN, H. 1974 Topical Treatment of Cutaneous Candidiasis with 5-Fluorocytosine Compared with Nystatin. Dermatologica, **148**, 362.

GRAPPEL, S. F., BISHOP, C. T., AND BLANK, F. 1974 Immunology of Dermatophytes and Dermatophytosis. Bacteriol Rev, **38**, 222.

GREEN, R. 1976 Blastomycosis of the Lung and Parotid Gland; Case Report. Milit Med, **141**, 100.

HABTE-GSBR, E., AND SMITH, I. M. 1973 North American Blastomycosis in Iowa; Review of 34 Cases. J Chronic Dis, **26**, 585.

HARDIN, H. F., AND SCOTT, D. I. 1974 Blastomycosis; Occurrence of Filamentous Forms *in Vivo*. Am J Clin Pathol, **62**, 104.

HOFFORTH, G. A., JOSEPH, D. L., AND SHUMRICK, D. A. 1973 Deep Mycoses. Arch Otolaryngol, **97**, 475.

HOLBROOK, W. P., AND KEPPAX, R. 1979 Sensitivity of *Candida albicans* from Patients with Chronic Oral Candidiasis. Postgrad Med J, **55**, 692.

JACOBS, P. H. 1978 Fungal Infection in Childhood. Pediatr Clin North Am, **25**, 357.

JENKINS, W. M. M., THOMAS, H. C., AND MASON, D. K. 1973 Oral Infections with *Candida albicans*. Scott Med J, **18**, 192.

JOHNSON, J. E., III, RADIMER, G., DiSALVO, A. F., AJELLO, L., AND BIGLER, W. 1970 Histoplasmosis in Florida. Am Rev Respir Dis, **101**, 299.

KAMMER, R. B., AND UTZ, J. P. 1974 Aspergillus Species Endocarditis; the New Face of a Not So Rare Disease. Am J Med, **56**, 506.

KANNAN-KUTTY, M., AND TEH, E. C. 1974 *Rhinosporidium seeberi*; an Electron Microscopic Study of Its Life Cycle. Pathology, **6**, 63.

KAPLAN, W. 1973 Epidemiology of the Principal Systemic Mycoses of Man and Lower Animals and the Ecology of Their Etiologic Agents. J Am Vet Med Assoc, **163**, 1043.

KEPRON, M. W., SCHOEMPERLEN, C. B., HERSHFIELD, E. S., ZYLAK, C. J., AND CHERNIACK, R. M. 1972 North American Blastomycosis in Central Canada. Can Med Assoc J, **106**, 243.

KIRKPATRICK, C. H., AND ALLING, D. W. 1978 Treatment of Chronic Oral Candidiasis with Clotrimazole Troches. N Engl J Med, **299**, 1201.

KIRKPATRICK, C. H., AND SMITH, T. K. 1974 Chronic Mucocutaneous Candidiasis; Immunologic and Antibiotic Therapy. Ann Intern Med, **80**, 310.

KROLL, J. J., EINBINDER, J. M., AND MERZ, W. G. 1973 Mucocutaneous Candidiasis in a Mother and Son. Arch Dermatol, **108**, 259.

LEWIS, J. L., AND RABINOVICH, S. 1972 The Wide Spectrum of Cryptococcal Infections. Am J Med, **53**, 315.

LONDERO, A. T., AND RAMOS, C. D. 1972 Paracoccidioidomycosis; a clinical and mycologic Study of Forty-One Cases Observed in Santa Maria, RS, Brazil. Am J Med, **52**, 771.

MARSHALL, J. 1973. Tropical Dermatoses. Practitioner, **211**, 620.

McCORNICK, W. F., SCHOCHET, S. S., JR., WEAVER, P. R., AND McCRARY, J. A., III. 1975 Disseminated Aspergillosis. Arch Pathol, **99**, 353.

MEYER, R. D., AND KAPLAN, M. H. 1973 Cutaneous Lesions in Disseminated Mucormycosis. JAMA, 325, 737.

MEYERS, B. R., WORRISER, G., HIRSCHMAN, S. Z., AND BLITZER, A. 1979 Rhinocerebral Mucormycosis; Postmortem Diagnosis and Therapy. Arch Intern Med, **139**, 557.

MONTES, L. F. 1971 Oral Amphotericin B in Superficial Candidiasis. Clin Med, **78**, 14.

MONTES, L. F., CARTER, R. E., MORELAND, N., AND CEBALLOS, R. 1968 Generalized Cutaneous Candidiasis Associated with Diffuse Myopathy and Thymoma. JAMA, **204**, 351.

MONTES, L. F., KRUMDIECK, C., AND CORNWELL, P. E. 1973 Hypovitaminosis A in Patients with Mucocutaneous Candidiasis. J Infect Dis, **128**, 227.

MOYE, T. D., AND CAUDILL, R. J. 1980 Rhinocerebral Phycomycosis; Report of Case. J Oral Surg, **38**, 132.

MURRAY, H. W., LITTMAN, M. L., AND ROBERTS, R. B. 1974 Disseminated Paracoccidioidomycosis (South American Blastomycosis) in the United States. Am J Med, **56**, 209.

NAIRN, R. I. 1975 Nystatin and Amphotericin B in the Treatment of Denture-related Candidiasis. Oral Surg, **40**, 68.

OZATO, K., AND UESAKA, I. 1974 The Role of Macrophages in *Candida albicans* Infection *in Vitro*. Jpn J Microbiol, **18**, 29.

PICKARD, R. E., AND KOTZEN, S. 1973 Histoplasmosis of the Larynx. South Med J, **66**, 1311.

POWELL, K. E., DAHL, B. A., WEEKS, R. J., AND TOSH, F. E. 1972 Airborne *Cryptococcus neoformans*. J Infect Dis, **125**, 412.

RAYNER, C. R. W. 1973 Disseminated Candidiasis in a Severely Burned Patient. Plast Reconstr Surg, **51**, 461.

REBELL, G., AND TAPLIN, D. 1970 *Dermatophytes: Their Recognition and Identification*, Ed. 2. University of Miami Press, Coral Gables, Fla.

RENNER, R. P., LEE, M., ANDORS, L., AND NAMARA, T. F. 1979. The Role of *C. albicans* in Denture Stomatitis. Oral Surg, **47**, 323.

RENSTRUP, G. 1970 Occurrence of Candida in Oral Leukoplakias. Acta Pathol Microbiol Scand, **78**, 421.

REESE, M. C., AND COLCLASURE, J. B. 1975 Cryptococcosis of the Larynx. Arch Otolaryngol, **101**, 698.

RESTREPO, A., AND DE URIBE, L. 1976 Isolation of Fungi Belonging to the Genera Geotrichum and Trichosporum from Human Dental Lesions. Mycopathologia, **59**, 3.

RIST, T. E., AND CAVES, J. M. 1973 Fluorescent Technique for Identification of *Candida albicans* from Skin Scrapings. Arch Dermatol, **108**, 426.

ROBERTS, G. D. 1976 Laboratory Diagnosis of Fungal Infections. Hum Pathol, **7**, 161.

ROBINSON, E. D. 1974 The Diagnosis and Treatment of Fungal Infections. JAMA, **229**, 709.

SAGEL, S. S. 1973 Common Fungal Diseases of the Lungs; I. Coccidioidomycosis. Radiol Clin North Am, **11**, 153.

SAKULA, A. 1974 Fungous Infection of the Lung. Practitioner, **212,** 335.

SALES, J. L., AND MUNDY, H. B. 1973 Renal Candidiasis; Diagnosis and Management. Can J Surg, **16,** 139.

SAROSI, G. A., HAMMERMAN, K. J., TOSH, F. E., AND KRONENBERG, R. S. 1974 Clinical Festures of Acute Pulmonary Blastomycosis. N Engl J Med, **290,** 540.

SAUER, G. C. 1974 Monilial Vaginitis. JAMA, **227,** 941.

SHORNE, S. K., SIRKAR, D. K., AND GUGNANI, H. C. 1973 Changing Spectrum of Cryptococcosis in Dehli. Indian J Med Res, **61,** 23.

SIEVERS, M. K. 1974 Disseminated Coccidioidomycosis among Southwestern American Indians. Am Rev Respir Dis, **109,** 602.

SIMPSON, J. R. 1974 Tinea Barbae Caused by *Trichophyton erinacei. Br J Dermatol,* **90,** 697.

SMITH, J. D., MURTISHAW, W. A., AND McBRIDE, M. E. 1973 White Piedra (Trichosporosis). Arch Dermatol, **107,** 439.

SORENSEN, R. H., PETERSON, E. T., AND WALDMANN, W. J. 1972 Survey Participation by Practitioners; the Key to Establishing Endemic Boundaries of North American Blastomycosis. Clin Med, **79,** 19.

SOTGUI, G., MANTOVANI, A., AND MAZZONI, A. 1970 Histoplasmosis in Europe. Mycopathol Mycol Appl, **40,** 53.

SPELLACY, W. N., ZAIAS, N., BUCHI, W. C., AND BIRK, S. A. 1971 Vaginal Yeast Growth and Contraceptive Practices. Obstet Gynecol, **38,** 349.

STIFF, R. 1963 Histoplasmosis; Report of a Case. Oral Surg, **16,** 140.

SWATEK, F. E. 1970 Ecology of *Coccidioides immitis.* Mycopathol Mycol Appl, **40,** 3.

TASCHDJIAN, C. L. 1970 Opportunistic Yeast Infections, with Special Reference to Candidiasis. Ann NY Acad Sci, **174,** 606.

THEOLOGIDES, A. 1970 Opportunistic Infections in Neoplastic Diseases. Geriatrics, **25,** 126.

TRUNK, G., LEAVEY, R., AND BYRD, R. B. 1976 Acute Histoplasmosis in a Military Housing Area; Case Reports with Pulmonary Function Studies. Milit Med, **141,** 333.

UTZ, J. P., AND SHADOMY, S. 1974 Fungal Infections. Clin Pharmacol Ther, **16,** 912.

WARDER, F. R., CHIKES, P. G., AND HUDSON, W. R. 1975 Aspergillosis of the Paranasal Sinuses. Arch Otolaryngol, **101,** 683.

WARNOCK, M. L., FENNESSY, J., AND RIPPON, J. 1974 Chronic Eosinophilic Pneumonia, a Manifestation of Allergic Aspergillosis. Am J Clin Pathol, **62,** 73.

WERNER, S. B., PAPPAGIANIS, D., HEINDL, I., AND MICKEL, A. 1972 An Epidemic of Coccidioidomycosis among Archeology Students in Northern California. N Engl J Med, **286,** 507.

WHITING, D. A., AND BISSET, E. A. 1974 The Investigation of Superficial Fungal Infections by Skin Surface Biopsy. Br J Dermatol, **91,** 57.

YOUNG, L. L., DOLAN, C. T., SHERIDAN, P. J., AND REEVE, C. M. 1972 Oral Manifestations of Histoplasmosis. Oral Surg, **33,** 191.

---

chapter **35**

General Principles of Virology

Memory Elvin-Lewis

HISTORICAL OVERVIEW

At the close of the 19th century it was discovered that some agents that caused disease were smaller than bacteria. These entities that passed through bacteriological filters were referred to as "*contagium vivum fluidum*" since such infectious filtrates could cause disease in susceptible hosts. This phenomenon, first described in plants, was shortly followed by the discovery of similar "viruses or poisons" in animals, bacteria and finally fungi.

During the early period it was only possible to identify animal viruses by the pathological changes they produced in infected cells, no instrument was then available that had the capability to further distinguish them. However, types of virus-induced intracellular structures termed inclusions were recognized that aided in the pathodiagnosis of some viral diseases, for example, the intracytoplasmic Guarnieri bodies of smallpox and Negri bodies of rabies.

In many ways viruses did not act like "living entities" since they were readily manipulated chemically to the point of being "crystallized," were dependent on an intracellular environment (obligate intracellular parasitism), contained only one type of nucleic acid, DNA or RNA, and often the only other component was a protein coat. Furthermore, it was difficult to assay them in animals, since host responses interfered with accurate measurement of response. By using the tissues of the embryonated egg it was possible to circumvent the problems of studying infections in the adult animal,

and thus in the early 1930s definitive studies with animal viruses began (fig. 35/1A). For example, it was soon found that the pox viruses and herpes simplex viruses could elicit discrete lesions on the surface of the chorioallantoic membrane of eggs, and viral assay techniques were subsequently evolved (fig. 35/1B). Other viruses such as influenza could be propagated in cells lining the allantoic and amniotic cavities, and virus-containing allantoic fluid served as the source of material for study.

When bacterial viruses or bacteriophage were first discovered during World War I, it was presumed that they could be used to control bacterial diseases, but it was soon shown that this was not feasible. Thus studies with them were essentially abandoned and not resumed until after World War II when it became apparent that bacteriophages were valuable tools in understanding the biology of viruses themselves. When studies on the fundamental biology of bacterial viruses were resumed, particularly with those infecting *Escherichia coli* and other members of Enterobacteriaceae, the roles of protein and nucleoprotein were elucidated and the complexities of virulent and latent replicative cycles unraveled. Also, temperate phages that had the ability to integrate into the host genome were found to participate in a number of genetic phenomena. For example, in *lysogenic conversion*, the presence of the integrated prophage changes the genome so that new antigens or toxins are manifest (*e.g.*, diphtheria toxin) and in *transduction*, the bacteriophage acts as the vector for the interchange of bacterial genes between host bacteria.

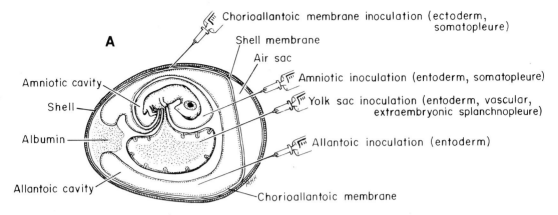

A

Chorioallantoic membrane inoculation (ectoderm, somatopleure)

Shell membrane

Air sac

Amniotic inoculation (entoderm, somatopleure)

Yolk sac inoculation (entoderm, vascular, extraembryonic splanchnopleure)

Allantoic inoculation (entoderm)

Amniotic cavity

Shell

Albumin

Allantoic cavity

Chorioallantoic membrane

Figure 35/1 *A.* Sites at which virus may be inoculated into embryonated eggs.

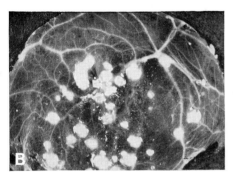

Figure 35/1 *B.* Lesions produced by vaccinia virus growing on the chorioallantoic membrane of the chick embryo (AFIP AMS 1060-19.)

When visualization of virus particles was finally achieved through advances in electron microscopy, recognition of viral components and distinctive morphological features permitted their use in classification schemes.

With the advent of practical tissue culture procedures, animal viruses that had eluded culture in the fertile hen's egg could be studied. At first, only viruses that caused total cell destruction or cytophathogenic effect werc isolated in tissue culture; however, as new types of cell cultures were developed, and techniques such as hemadsorption, cell fusion and interference were employed, more elusive viruses were discovered. The golden era of medical virology had arrived and during the 1960s and 1970s many of the viruses known to cause human disease were isolated, and a number of vaccines developed to control infections.

Development of more sophisticated biochemical techniques permitted definition of the replicative cycles of animal viruses. These data have been used in conjunction with morphologic and biochemical criteria for purposes of classification, and for the study of antiviral chemotherapeutic agents. In these studies it also became evident that, like bac-

teriophages, certain animal viruses could replicate in a virulent fashion or integrate into the host genome. Some of these integrated viruses were found to have the ability to transform cells into those with malignant capabilities, leading to a new understanding of tumorigenesis.

VIRUS STRUCTURE AND REPLICATION

Definition of a Virus

Viruses are small infectious agents ranging in size from 20 to 300 nm. They are differentiated from higher organisms by their possession of an autonomously replicating DNA or RNA genome; their dependance on living cells for replication; and their lack of energy-producing Lipmann enzymes. Viruses do not divide and grow as do bacteria but have the ability to direct the synthesis of their component parts and assemble them in the cells they parasitize. Thus they are considered "alive" although, extracellularly, they are metabolically inert.

Structure and Composition of Viruses

The virus particle, or virion, is composed of a protein coat or capsid that surrounds a nucleic acid core; together these structures are referred to as a nucleocapsid. Also associated with the nucleocapsid can be enzymes needed for replication. Members of certain virus groups are naked nucleocapsids but many are surrounded by various types of envelopes that are derived in part from the host cell and contain proteins, carbohydrates and lipids. Glycoprotein spikes or peplomers may protrude from this envelope and aid in attachment, cell fusion or release of the virus particles (fig. 35/2).

Viral Nucleic Acids. Nucleic acids function as the genome and can possess neutral proteins or histones that serve to link the loops of the molecule together. In the virion, the RNA and DNA can be double- or single-stranded, linear, circular or seg-

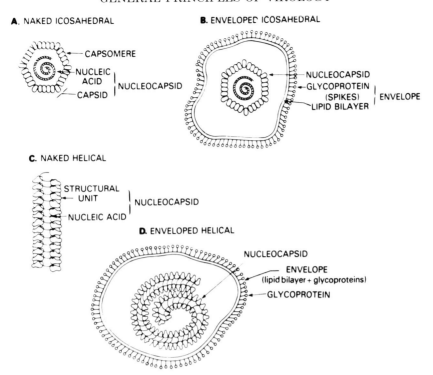

A. NAKED ICOSAHEDRAL

CAPSOMERE

NUCLEIC ACID
NUCLEOCAPSID
CAPSID

B. ENVELOPED ICOSAHEDRAL

NUCLEOCAPSID
GLYCOPROTEIN (SPIKES)
LIPID BILAYER
ENVELOPE

C. NAKED HELICAL

STRUCTURAL UNIT
NUCLEOCAPSID
NUCLEIC ACID

D. ENVELOPED HELICAL

NUCLEOCAPSID
ENVELOPE (lipid bilayer + glycoproteins)
GLYCOPROTEIN

Figure 35/2. Schematic representation of morphological groups of viruses. (Reproduced with permission from B. A. Freeman, *Burrows Textbook of Microbiology* Ed. 21. Saunders, Philadelphia, Pa.

mented and of either minus or plus polarity. The amount of genetic information per virion varies for different viruses. Small viruses contain about three or four genes while large viruses may contain several hundred. With the exception of the retroviruses, the virions contain only a single copy of the nucleic acid.

Double-stranded DNA genomes may be linear, as seen with the herpes viruses, or circular, as with the papovaviruses (*e.g.,* papilloma viruses). The linear DNA molecules may have repeating sequences at the end (terminal redundancy) that may be several hundred base pairs long. In some viruses the DNAs are terminally redundant but the repeated sequences are inverted or reversed. The reasons for terminal redundancy are undoubtedly related to the mode of replication of those nucleic acids.

Single-stranded DNA genomes also may be circular, as in some bacteriophages, or linear, as in the parvoviruses. In the former the strand is the same in all virions. In some of the latter, such as adeno-associated viruses, some virions contain DNA strands that are complementary to those in other virions of the same group.

Double-stranded RNA is found in the reovirus group of animal viruses. The genome is segmented into 10 portions and replicates in a manner different from other RNA viruses.

Single-stranded RNA genomes may be in a single piece, as in picornaviruses or segmented, as in orthomyxoviruses. All have considerable secondary structure, that may have an important function in translation and replication. The retroviruses, those whose RNA genome is transcribed by a reverse transcriptase enzyme into double-stranded DNA that becomes integrated into host cell genome, are diploid, rather than haploid as are most viruses. They contain two equal RNA molecules held together near one end, a feature that may be particularly important in their replication.

Capsid. The capsid protein functions as a protection against nucleases, participates in virus attachment and determines the antigenicity of the virus. Also variations in capsid symmetry determine the morphology of the virus.

Helical Viruses. The basic polypeptide structural unit or protomer is composed of a single type of protein. These protomers are bound together by identical bonds to form a ribbon-like helical structure and they are stabilized internally by similar bonding. While the diameter of helical viruses is determined by the nature of the protomers, their length is dependent upon the size of the nucleic acid that is located in helical grooves between the protomers. Those helical viruses that possess an envelope are less rigid than those that are naked since the former have to coil within the envelope.

Icosahedral or Cubical Viruses. Protomers in these viruses can be composed of one or several protein types, depending upon the size of the viral genome that codes them. These protomers aggregate by strong covalent bonds to form morphological units termed capsomeres. The capsomeres cluster together to form the capsid. In small viruses a series of capsomeres termed pentons, comprised of five protomers, form the icosahedral surface of the capsid. In larger viruses, pentons are linked together with hexons, usually made of six protomers, that can differ in protein composition, to comprise the capsid structure. The number, arrangement and morphology of these capsomeres are distinctive taxonomic criteria. In these icosahedral viruses, the presence of histones or histone-like compounds in the nucleic acid allows it to be looped and tightly packed in the central core of the virion. The association of structural proteins and the nucleic acid is diagrammatically represented for an adenovirus in figure 35/3.

Complex Viruses. Some large DNA bacteriophages have what is termed binal symmetry in that their heads are icosahedral and their tails helical in structure. Poxviruses also are complex in structure.

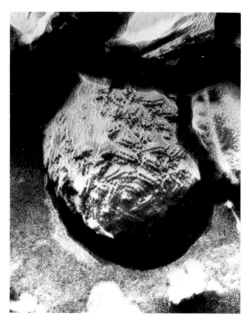

Figure 35/4. Freeze-etched vaccinia virion showing subunits and the thread-like, double-ridged, beaded structures that appear to wrap around the virion (× 148,000). (Reproduced with permission from E. L. Medzon and H. Bauer. 1970. Virology **40**, page 860.)

They are brick-shaped and are covered with a layer of coarse fibrils. The DNA is enclosed in a biconcave disc-shaped nucleoid (fig. 35/4). Thus a precise symmetry is not defined.

Enzymes. Enzymes are an integral part of some viruses. Most function in the replication of the virion, such as transcribing the viral genome into messenger RNA, adding specific terminal groups to viral m-RNA, copying virion RNA into DNA, or processing or replicating the nucleic acid. Others of host origin, or induced early in infection, include nucleases, nucleotide phosphorylases, protein kinases and capping enzymes of mRNA. Some enzymes affecting interaction of virions with host cells are an integral part of the envelope and will be discussed below.

Envelopes. Envelopes that surround the nucleocapsid of many viruses are derived in part from the host cell and are acquired during the final stage of assembly either at the nuclear-limiting or cytoplasmic membrane. The proteins, carbohydrates and lipids that the envelope contains confer on the virion various distinctive characteristics. For example, the shape of enveloped viruses often is dependent upon the liquid or solid state of the complex mixture of neutral lipids, phospholipids and glycolipids or the presence or absence of connections between envelope proteins, such as a nonglycosylated matrix protein sometimes found at the inner layer of the envelope surface. Glycoprotein

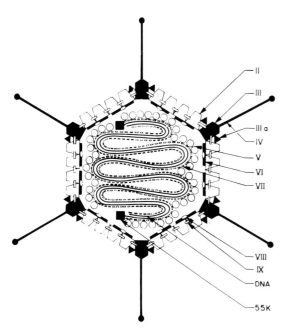

Figure 35/3. Model of an adenovirus particle showing the apparent architectural interrelationships of the structural proteins (*roman numerals*) and the nucleoprotein core. The capsid is composed of the hexon (*II*) the penton base (*III*) and fiber (*IV*) and the hexon-associated proteins (*IIIa, VI, VIII* and *IX*). Proteins *V* and *VII* are core proteins associated with viral DNA. The *55k* protein is covalently linked to the 5′ end of the DNA. (Reproduced with permission from: B. D. Davis, *et al.* 1980 *Microbiology* Ed. 3 Harper & Row, Hagerstown, Md.)

spikes or peplomers function as attachment sites to tissue receptors or certain erythrocytes (hemagglutinins), contain neuraminidase that facilitates virus release from cells, and through a fusion factor have both hemolytic capabilities and the ability to form multinucleate syncytia. The envelope contains antigenic glycoproteins that can bind specific antibodies. If this occurs it may neutralize or block viral infectivity. Also the envelope is readily lysed by cell membrane lysing disinfectants such as phenol and lipid solvents.

Virus Classification

Criteria usually used for classifying viruses include the nature of the nucleic acid (type, strandedness, linear, segmented or circular); the virus size (in nanometers) and shape (symmetry); the presence or absence of an envelope (fig. 35/5); the site of assembly; and the physical and chemical nature of the virion (table 35/1). Further differentiation may be made by distinctive physical and chemical properties (*e.g.*, low pH lability; ether sensitivity); the form of intracellular replication; or antigenic differences. This is discussed more fully in Chapter 1.

VIRAL REPLICATION

In general terms virus replication can be divided into a number of phases. During primary infection of cells virus attachment occurs through electromagnetic forces and chemical affinities between the virus and specific cell receptors on the cell surface. The initial attachment is reversible and temperature independent, followed by irreversible attachment which is temperature dependent. The presence of receptors accounts for specific cell tropisms, to some extent. Whether or not receptors for a particular virus are present depends on the species and tissue from which the cell is derived and on its physiological state.

After attachment, the virus may penetrate the

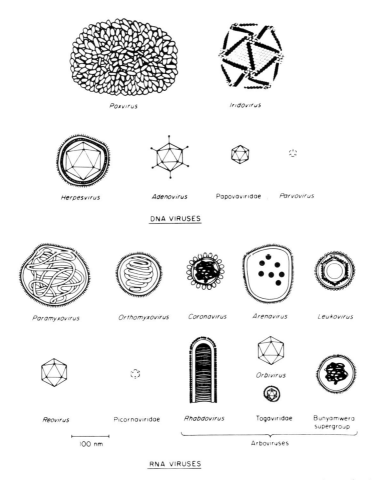

Poxvirus   Iridovirus

Herpesvirus   Adenovirus   Papovaviridae   Parvovirus

DNA VIRUSES

Paramyxovirus   Orthomyxovirus   Coronavirus   Arenavirus   Leukovirus

Reovirus   Picornaviridae   Rhabdovirus   Orbivirus   Togaviridae   Bunyamwera supergroup

100 nm   Arboviruses

RNA VIRUSES

Figure 35/5. Diagram illustrating the shapes and relative sizes of animal viruses of the major taxonomic groups. (Reproduced with permission from: F. Fenner. 1974 *The Biology of Animal Viruses*, Ed. 2, Academic Press, New York.)

Table 35/1
Distinguishing features of animal virus families

Nucleic Acid Type*	Symmetary of Nucleocapsid	Enveloped or Naked Virion	Virus Particle Size	Virus Family
			nm	
DNA-DS	Complex	Complex	230 × 400	Poxviridae
DNA-DS	Icosahedral	Enveloped	180–200	Herpesviridae
DNA-DS	Icosahedral	Naked	79–90	Adenoviridae
DNA-DSO	Icosahedral	Naked	40–50	Papovaviridae
DNA-SS	Icosahedral	Naked	18–22	Paravoviridae
RNA-SS-S	Complex or ?	Enveloped	50–300	Arenaviridae
RNA-SS	Complex or ?	Enveloped	80–160	Coronaviridae
RNA-SS	Complex or ?	Enveloped	100	Retroviridae
RNA-SS-S	Helical	Enveloped	90–100	Bunyaviridae
RNA-SS-S	Helical	Enveloped	80–120	Orthomyxoviridae
RNA-SS	Helical	Enveloped	150–300	Paramyxoviridae
RNA-SS	Helical-B	Enveloped	70–80	Rhabdoviridae
RNA-SS	Icosahedral	Enveloped	30–90	Togaviridae
RNA-SS	Icosahedral	Naked	35–39	Caliciviridae
RNA-SS	Icosahedral	Naked	21–30	Picornaviridae
RNA-DS-S	Icosahedral	Naked	75–80	Reoviridae

* DS, double stranded; DSO, double stranded circular; SS, single stranded; S, segmented; B = bullet shaped .

host cell membrane by invagination into phagocytic vesicles (viropexis). Nonenveloped viruses may penetrate morphologically intact through the plasma membrane into the cytoplasm, while some viruses which are surrounded by a lipoprotein envelope enter after fusion of the viral envelope and host cell membrane (principally the paramyxoviruses). Following penetration, uncoating and the eclipse phase occur. Uncoating, the opening of the protein coat to free the viral genome, is complex and varies with the particular virus-host cell system studied. It is mediated by the action of lytic enzymes on the capsid, although the origin of the enzymes may be different. For example, poliovirus, a small nonenveloped virus is easily stripped of its protein coat by the host cell's proteolytic enzymes, releasing the RNA into the cytoplasm. A complex virus such as vaccinia requires a more involved uncoating process. The outer membrane of this virus, located in a vesicle within the cell cytoplasm, is broken down by cellular hydrolytic enzymes. Following this an RNA polymerase, carried by the virus in its core, mediates the synthesis of mRNA. This virus-directed messenger is transcribed within the virus core, then released into the cell cytoplasm where it codes for a protein that directs the release of viral DNA from the core. After the virus is uncoated it is said to be in eclipse phase that is characterized by loss of recoverable viral infectivity. Transcription into appropriate mRNAs occurs by the presence of viral or host enzymes and, if polycistronic, these may be cleaved before they are translated on host ribosomes into early proteins, such as enzymes, for viral genome replication and/or tumor antigens.

Once the virus is uncoated, the synthetic phase of the virus replication begins. This encompasses replication of viral genome and synthesis of viral proteins. In the case of RNA viruses, most genetic information is expressed soon after uncoating. In the case of double-stranded DNA viruses, the multiplication cycle can be divided into early and late phases. Onset of viral DNA replication marks the beginning of the late period. The early period of the synthetic phase is devoted mainly to onset of reactions necessary for initiating viral genome replication. This may involve inhibition of host metabolic steps such as DNA, RNA and protein synthesis and formation of enzymes, especially RNA and DNA polymerases. During the late period, late viral functions occur. These include formation of structural proteins that are components of the progeny particles, and formation of enzymes and other nonstructural proteins that function during viral morphogenesis. The late viral mRNAs and subsequent proteins are transcribed from different sequences of the viral genome than early ones, and furthermore, are transcribed from progeny genomes. The details of genome replication will be described in a subsequent section.

After progeny genomes and capsid proteins are formed, they are assembled into progeny virus particles (assembly). This is a spontaneous process since most of the information necessary resides in the amino acid sequences of the capsid polypeptides: nucleic acid performs no essential function during morphogenesis of most animal viruses.

Release of the newly formed progeny virus particles varies with the nature of the virus and its site of maturation, *i.e.*, nuclear or cytoplasmic. Cell lysis is the most simple method of release. Replication of the virus kills the cell, it undergoes lysis, and the progeny virions are released into the extracellular area. Some viruses are extruded from the cells without lysis. Other viruses are released slowly, by budding or reverse phagocytosis from the host cell. They first direct alterations in the structure and/or composition of host cell membrane, in a nonrandom fashion, necessary for their release. The viral membrane is formed by aggregation of viral proteins and cell lipids, followed by addition of carbohydrates. The virions are then slowly extruded from the cell, acquiring a membrane envelope in the process. Some viruses which replicate in the nucleus can acquire a coat from the nuclear membrane, or perhaps even two coats, one from the nuclear and one from the cytoplasmic membrane. Viruses which bud into cytoplasmic vacuoles are released when the vacuole fuses with the cell membrane. Those viruses which bud from the nuclear membrane into the cytoplasm may reach the outside through cytoplasmic channels.

MOLECULAR EVENTS OF VIRAL REPLICATION

The replication of RNA and DNA viruses differs depending upon the type of nucleic acid, the enzymes utilized for transcription and replication, depending on whether they are inherent to the virus or derived from the host cell, and the site of replication and assembly.

DNA-Containing Viruses

DNA viruses belong to one of three major classes, determined by their nucleic acid composition.

Class I virus genomes are double-stranded linear DNA, and families within the group are further distinguished by the type of repetitions, redundancies or linkages that characterize the molecule, and whether or not they utilize host enzymes or carry or encode their own for purposes of transcription and DNA replication. For example, poxviruses carry their own transcriptase for the formation of mRNAs and encode their own polymerases for DNA replication; herpesviruses utilize host enzymes for primary transcription but encode their own polymerase for DNA replication, while adenoviruses utilize both host replicases and DNA polymerases for replication. Transcription of Class I DNAs involves early and late transcription of the genome into polycistronic mRNAs that are later cleaved to produce monocistronic RNAs that are translated to produce viral proteins in a sequential order. Translation of early transcripts results in the formation of enzymes required for replication and some antigens while translation of late transcripts yields those proteins needed for viral structural components.

Class II viruses, represented by papovaviruses, have circular, double-stranded DNA genomes. Early mRNAs are transcribed, using host enzymes, from one strand of the genome whereas late transcripts are obtained from the complementary strand. These transcripts are polycistronic, and are cleaved into monocistronic messengers. Early proteins include tumor antigens and enzymes required for replication whereas late proteins are for structural purposes. Replication of the cyclic DNAs is bidirectional and symmetric and the unwinding of parental DNA is carried out by a swivel enzyme.

Class III viruses, containing single-stranded DNA, replicate by producing a DNA strand complementary to the strand in the parent virion so that following replication of the DNA by base pairing the genome of the progeny particle will be identical to that of the parent. These parvoviruses utilize host enzymes for replication and require that the host cell be in its S phase (replicating its own DNA) for replication to proceed. Defective (adenoassociated virus, AAV) can only replicate when helper adenoviruses are replicating simultaneously but do not require S phase cells. Thus, due to the dependence of host enzymes found in the nucleus, all families of DNA viruses except the poxviruses replicate in the nucleus or at the nuclear membrane.

RNA-Containing Viruses

RNA viruses belong to five major classes determined by their genome composition, the polarity of their genomic strands, enzymes that are utilized for transcription, be they inherent to the virus or to host cell, and the site of translation, replication and assembly.

Class I viruses, represented by the picornaviruses, contain a single strand of RNA which is termed a *positive* strand because it can and does act as messenger RNA. The entire length of the infecting RNA is translated as if it were monocistronic, resulting in a polyprotein which is subsequently cleaved into smaller functional proteins including replicating enzyme(s) and structural proteins. The genome of the togaviruses that also belongs to this group is transcribed into two messenger RNAs that act to translate proteins for replication and structural components.

Class II viruses, represented by the enveloped paramyxoviruses, contain a *minus*-stranded RNA genome (one that does not act as a messenger). By virtue of a virus-contained transcriptase, this is transcribed into positive RNA strands. These serve as messengers for the translation of enzymes for the replication of additional negative strands required for the progeny virus and for structural and envelope proteins. Rhabdoviruses also replicate in a similar manner but differ from paramyxoviruses in basic structure and by the fact that they enter the cell by viropexis rather than envelope-cell membrane fusion.

Class III viruses, represented by the orthomyxoviruses, contain segmented, negative-stranded genomes that, following priming by newly capped cellular RNAs, are transcribed by a viral transcriptase in the host nucleus to form eight mRNAs. These are translated into separate proteins that serve as enzymes of replication, enzymes that facilitate virus release (*e.g.*, neuraminidase) and as structural components of the capsid and envelope. Both Class II and III viruses are released from the cytoplasmic membrane by budding or reverse pinocytosis. It should be apparent that any minus-strand RNA virus, Class II or Class III, must contain an active RNA polymerase if replication is to occur.

Class IV viruses, represented by the reoviruses, contain 10 double-stranded RNA segments which are surrounded by a double-layered capsid. When reovirus infects a susceptible cell, the outer capsid is partially degraded by host enzymes to form a subviral particle. This activates an RNA polymerase (transcriptase) within the subviral particle which transcribes all 10 genome segments into mRNA molecules. These messengers are translated into protein. The parental double-stranded RNA never leaves the subviral particle which persists throughout the multiplication cycle. After a time the single-stranded mRNA molecules begin to associate with proteins to form complexes within which they are transcribed into minus strands. The strands remain associated, giving rise to the progeny double-stranded RNA molecules. Subsequent mRNAs are translated into more proteins which associate with immature virus particles resulting in complete progeny.

Class V viruses, represented by the oncogenic retroviruses, contain a positive-stranded RNA genome that, following entrance into the cell, is transcribed by an enzyme, a reverse transcriptase, into a DNA strand that circularizes and becomes integrated into the host genome. Subsequently, it transcribes into mRNA that serves as progeny viral genome and translates into the appropriate replication enzymes and structural proteins.

CULTIVATION OF VIRUSES

Methods

Virus susceptibility is dependent upon such factors as compatible receptor sites on the virus and host cell surface and the metabolic potential of the cell to allow replication to proceed. Permissive cells have this inherent capability, nonpermissive cells lack factors for complete viral gene expression and can only allow replication to continue at a slower pace or incompletely, whereas resistant cells are capable of blocking replication and are refractory to infection. In the animal, immune mechanisms also can affect successful infection. Therefore the use of tissue cultures, the embryonated egg or neonatal animals is frequently employed for viral cultivation.

Animal cultivation is limited to those viruses with unknown tissue culture cell susceptibilities or where cell culture does not yield satisfactory growth. For example, neonatal mice are still employed for the isolation of certain Coxsackie A viruses and togaviruses; mice are used for rabies and encephalomyocarditis virus; neonatal hamsters for the production of tumors by oncogenic adenoviruses; and adult simians for studies with hepatitis A and B viruses, and slow viruses that cause Creutzfeldt-Jakob disease and kuru.

The embryonated egg, long a staple of viral cultivation, is now being replaced by appropriate tissue culture cell lines; however some viruses such as influenza viruses and the 17D strain of yellow fever virus are still propagated in the allantoic cavity for vaccine production in spite of the ability of egg proteins to elicit allergy.

Tissue culture cultivation of a virus is dependent upon its specific cell tropism. Primary cell lines are established from normal tissues of humans or animals. For example, for cultivation of some viruses infecting humans, the kidneys of simians are preferred. Since they are already differentiated, these cell lines have a limited capacity to divide, but they often have greater virus susceptibility than diploid cell lines that can be propagated for longer time periods or those derived from malignant cells whose divisions are limitless. Primary cell lines also are preferred for the propagation of attenuated viruses for vaccines since they are less likely to contain latent viruses with oncogenic potential. However, in diagnostic laboratories a number of cell lines representing all these types usually are employed to ensure optimal virus recovery from clinical specimens.

In infected monolayers, viruses can be detected by the specific cell destruction they cause (cytopathic effect, CPE) (fig. 35/6) or their ability to interfere with indicator viruses that do cause cell destruction (*e.g.*, rubella virus interferes with CPE caused by some enteric viruses); they can change the cytoplasmic membrane of the cells so that they will adsorb specific erythrocytes (hemadsorption) in the same manner as the infecting hemagglutinating virion (*e.g.*, paramyxoviruses), or cause the loss of contact inhibition to produce "minitumors"

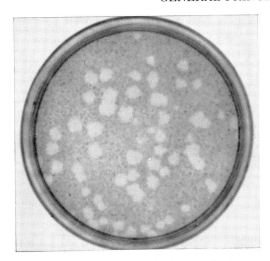

Figure 35/6. Plaques formed by herpes simplex virus on monolayer culture of rabbit kidney cells in a Petri dish. Actual size. (Courtesy of W. K. Ashe.)

among cells on a monolayer. Infected cells placed on slides or grown on coverslips can be stained with fluorescent dyes conjugated to specific antibody to detect virus antigens and inclusions on or in the cells.

Plaque techniques that serve to limit the spread of viruses growing in cell monolayers by using an agar overlay are useful for quantitating or titrating virus particles. The viruses produce localized areas of cell destruction or plaques, and by counting the number of plaques produced by various dilutions of virus, the number of infectious units may be determined.

Also recovery of viruses replicating incompletely in nonpermissive cells can be achieved by cell fusion with permissive cells.

VIRAL DIAGNOSIS

Rationale

Most virus infections are diagnosed by clinical criteria since often by the time isolation and determination of the virus has been made the patient has either recovered or died. However, a clinical syndrome may have many etiologies, and when those of a bacterial or fungal nature have been eliminated it may be important for the management of the patient, their contacts, or the control of the disease to know the specific virus involved. For example, the determination of rubella as the cause of a viral exanthem in a patient in the first trimester of pregnancy may favor an elective abortion. Prophylactic treatment of influenza A contacts with amantadine has prevented spread of this disease and determination of the cause of viral encephalitis is useful in knowing if those chemotherapeutic agents available are useful for its treatment (e.g., Ara-A for herpes encephalitis). Also, extra protec-

tive precautions or curtailment of the practice of dentists who have been found to be subclinical carriers of hepatitis B have prevented the spread of the disease to their patients. Moreover, surveillance to determine the effectiveness of immunization is important with diseases such as influenza and polio. For example, antigenic drift is a common phenomenon with strains of influenza, and is responsible for new outbreaks of the disease annually; constant monitoring of present serotypes is essential if current vaccines are to be effective. Also, when immunization is not possible, insect vector control of certain togavirus carriers (e.g., mosquito with dengue virus) is an effective way to control increased virus activity that has been detected.

Always at the forefront of virus diagnosis are those diseases of unknown etiology, and isolation and characterization is necessary if appropriate control measures are to be developed.

Virus Diagnostic Techniques

For diagnostic purposes it is important to know when optimal recovery of a virus, its antigens, or its antibodies can be achieved from clinical specimens. Usually viruses are more likely to be retrieved at the onset of symptoms or during the acute stage, and less frequently during the prodromal or recovery periods. In contrast, an immune response develops later, and occurs during the acute and convalescent periods. Tests to detect IgM antibodies that occur early in infection are oftentimes more diagnostically significant than those devised to detect IgG, that reflects the development of persistent immunity.

Immunofluorescent techniques are useful in detecting viral inclusions, antigens or antibodies. By using specifically labeled antiserum, rabies inclusions (Negri bodies) can be found in infected brain tissue or corneal impressions; and viral antigens for herpes simplex, herpes zoster and adenoviruses in exudates or eye scraping; enteroviruses in the buffy coat of cerebrospinal fluid or brain biopsy material; hepatitis B virus in liver biopsy tissue and Epstein-Barr virus antigens (EBV) in lymphocytes from patients with infectious mononucleosis. Also, by utilizing indirect immunofluorescent techniques, antibodies to EBV antigens can be detected in patients with Burkitt's lymphoma and nasopharyngeal carcinoma.

Electron microscopic examination of stool specimens is useful to detect the reovirus-like agents (rotaviruses) that cause a sometimes fatal infantile gastroenteritis. These are difficult to culture with commonly available cell cultures.

Solid-phase immunoassays like the radioimmunoassay (RIA) are helpful in detecting antigens and antibodies to hepatitis B virus. Where radioactive materials and radiation counters are unavailable, the use of the enzyme-linked immunosorbent assays (ELISA) are viable alternatives. Indirect ELISA tests also have been applied to the detection of specific antibodies during the course of virus infections e.g., herpesvirus. Similarly counterimmunoelectrophoresis (CIE) has been used to detect antibodies to hepatitis B virus.

Tissue culture isolation can be successful if care is taken to prepare and preserve the specimens prior to inoculation in an appropriate tissue culture line. If there is a time interval between collection and culture, the specimens are best preserved in a suitable transport medium and kept at deep freezing temperatures obtained with dry ice or in a deep freeze at −76 C. All specimens should be treated with antibiotics to eliminate bacterial contamination and put in culture as soon as possible.

The choice of the tissue culture cell line depends upon the virus family one expects to isolate. Both the human diploid line (MRC-5 and primary cynomolgous monkey kidney (CMK) will support to a greater or lesser degree the growth of enteroviruses, rhinoviruses, orthomyxoviruses, paramyxoviruses, herpesviruses, and adenoviruses. Cytopathogenic effects may be distinctive enough to aid in presumptive diagnosis and can vary from rapid cell destruction (e.g., picornavirus) to formation of multinucleate syncythia (e.g., paramyxovirus), grapelike clusters (e.g., adenovirus), cell rounding and formation of clear plaques (e.g., poxvirus); or ballooning degeneration (e.g., herpesvirus). Enteroviruses can be distinguished from rhinoviruses by their resistance to pH 3; nonenveloped viruses can be distinguished from enveloped viruses by their resistance to ether or chloroform; and rubella virus can be identified in green monkey tissue culture by interfering with ECHO 11 virus replication. Serotyping of the virus isolates then can be achieved by the neutralization test, which involves adding specific antiserum to a virus isolate prior to cell culture inoculation for the purpose of inhibiting CPE. Infection of monkey kidney cells with either orthomyxoviruses or paramyxoviruses can be detected earlier than the development of CPE by the addition of guinea pig erythrocytes that attach to infected cells (hemadsorption) to the culture medium. Hemadsorption can be prevented by specific antiserum and such specific hemadsorption inhibition (Had-I) is useful for virus typing as well.

Serodiagnostic tests usually involve the detection of antibodies to specific virus antigens in convalescent sera. Sometimes this is done by detecting IgM antibodies in convalescent serum, complement-fixing antibodies, or more commonly those that will inhibit or cause the hemagglutination of specific erythrocytes. Hemagglutination inhibition tests have been developed for paramyxoviruses, orthomyxoviruses, togaviruses and rubella viruses. In infectious mononucleosis, the development of heterophile antibodies that agglutinate sheep cells is the basis for presumptive diagnostic tests. Radioimmunoassays, ELISA assays and counterimmune electrophoresis already have been discussed.

VIRUS INFECTIONS AT HOST LEVEL

The outcome of a virus infection depends upon properties of the virus, the host cell and the environment in which the viral-host cell interaction occurs. Viruses must have the ability to spread from one cell to another, and if virulent, also have the capacity to cause functional alterations in the cells they parasitize. In the cell, the response to virus infection is recognized under three major categories; cytolytic, steady state and integrated.

Cytolytic reactions result from rapid viral replication that causes destruction of cells. In the host, this can result in tissue damage that is manifest as a localized (e.g., respiratory infection) or systemic (e.g., smallpox) type of disease. Even slow virus infections, such as kuru that have a long incubation period, eventually cause specific cell damage and ultimately tissue dysfunction.

Steady state infection may or may not cause cell death and is characterized by extracellular release of virus through membrane-associated budding processes. In these types of infections it also is possible for the infected cells to divide and carry out normal functions. When immunity develops and prevents the spread of viruses by the normal route, carrier types of infections may ensue that limit virus spread, such as through cytoplasmic bridges between cells e.g. herpes virus. In a congenital steady state, symptoms may be inapparent, intermittent, or appear after a considerable time although virus can be shed and contacts infected (e.g., rubella).

Integrated infections result when virus nucleic acid is physically integrated into the host genome in an analagous fashion to lysogenization. In this state, virus particles are not produced, and may not be recovered unless "capture techniques" are employed; a function usually only possible with RNA but not DNA tumor viruses. Acquisition of such an integrated virus may convey to the cell properties such as specific "tumor" antigens, loss of topoinhibition, and the ability to divide and metabolize rapidly, all characteristics of a malignant cell. Integration is more likely to occur in nonpermissive cells that do not allow lytic infection.

In the whole animal, most virus infections cause acute diseases with a well defined period of symptoms and the development of a long lasting immunity; only in a few instances is a chronic course usual. Clinical symptoms may not always be apparent, and subclinical infections are common with a number of virus diseases. For example, poliovirus in the nasopharynx or mumps virus in the saliva ould be a source of contagion to the unsuspecting dentist. The convalescent patient also can be a carrier of those infections with this potential. Hepatitis B virus is known to sometimes result in a carrier state. The situation with recurrent herpes simplex infections is somewhat different. Although virus may be shed intermittently, apparent symptoms only occur during periods of exacerbation, since usually, in the quiescent stage, the virus resides in an incomplete state in adjacent ganglion cells. Following some acute infections, a virus may enter semipermissive cells and replicate slowly over a period of time. This results in the development of serious sequelae, such as those described with the slow infection known as subacute sclerosing panencephalitis possibly associated with measles virus. Serious consequences also can occur if a virus like rubella infects a developing fetus. Should the fetus survive, a tolerant state is created through antibody-virus complexes that confer upon the neonate the capability of shedding virus in the absence of acute symptoms. This type of phenomenon is the cause of nursery-outbreaks among susceptible nurses. Viruses also may remain in an occult state for years, and are only caused to replicate under an appropriate stimulus. This phenomenon, referred to as occult infection, was first described with swine flu virus, and its exciting agent, the lungworm. The same type of inference may be made with occult or latent oncoviruses and cocarcinogens that could excite them.

Immunological Mechanisms in Viral Infections

The immune response to virus infections depends upon the extent and duration of the disease. For example, local cytolytic infections may only elicit regional IgA production, whereas generalized infections may involve both cellular and humoral systems. With the development of a steady-state or chronic infection, cellular immunity is particularly important since the infected cells may elicit an immunopathological response that, in the process of eliminating such cells, results in significant tissue damage and impairment of infection.

Interferon

Interferons are a group of low molecular weight (15,000 to 30,000 MW) glycoproteins that confer upon cells the ability to resist virus infection, activate killer cells or serve in an immunoregulatory capacity. Although the majority of cells possess the genetic potential to elicit interferons, most are made by specific producer cells of the reticuloendothelial system. Three specific types have been described that differ in antigenicity, stability, stimulus of induction, phylogenetic specificity, mechanism of cell action and mode of action.

Interferons with antiviral activity are elicited by either cells of fibroepithelial (fibroblast, epithelial cell, macrophage) or leukocytic origin. These are produced through the activation of genes on chromosomes 5 and 2 in response to the presence of double-stranded RNA, or other replicative or synthetic polynucleotides, especially with a high helical content and in a glycosylated form, accumulate in vacuoles at the time that virus maturation is achieved. Because mRNA and protein synthesis must continue in a cell for large amounts of interferon to be produced, viruses that block these cellular processes are poor interferon producers.

Following release from the cell the interferon interacts with membranes of surrounding cells to derepress genes on chromosome 21 that encode for cellular antiviral protein(s). For example, the activation of proteases and kinases can block the initiation of protein synthesis or polypeptide elongation and cause changes in viral RNAs related to function or nucleolytic destruction of mRNA, depletion of specific tRNAs or methylation changes in viral RNA. These activities affect virion uncoating and assembly as well. Generally, these glycoproteins are active only with cells of the same or closely related species (e.g., humans and simians) but are not virus specific. A somewhat larger molecule, referred to as preformed interferon, also is released during cellular infections with rickettsiae, chlamydiae or by contact with bacterial endotoxin.

Leukocytic interferon elicited by foreign or transformed cells can increase the cytotoxic activity of natural killer cells, inhibit tumor cell growth and stimulate cell-mediated immunity. Thus positive antitumor effects have been demonstrated for this form of interferon in the successful treatment of a number of osteosarcomas.

An "immune" or α-interferon is excreted by lymphocytes that are stimulated to divide by mitogenic or antigenic sensitization. This interferon is believed to regulate the proliferation of lymphoid cells which are stimulated to divide in response to antigenic stimulus. It has the capacity to cause a shift from humoral to cellular immunity, by causing a reduction of antibody production in B cells and an enhancement of T cell activity. Also, this immune interferon has been shown to kill tumor cells, and in high concentrations is known not only to exert an anticell proliferative effect on tumor but also on certain normal cells. Because of this latter capacity it has been proposed that its primary function is to regulate the expression of cellular mRNAs, and only secondarily acts as an antiviral defense mechanism.

Since artificial polynucleotides, like poly I:C have been found to be too toxic as therapeutic agents, except on topical application; and the production of interferon in cultured leukocytes too costly, the products of genetic engineering should prove valuable in the near future. In limited trials, interferon has been successfully used in the treatment of influenza and other respiratory infections, for the clearance of hepatitis B antigen from the blood of chronic carriers, to lessen the pain in herpes zoster and to limit the spread of herpes keratitis.

VIRUS VACCINES

Virus vaccines belong to three categories. Incomplete or subparticle vaccines are used for hepatitis B and influenza; killed virus vaccines are used for rabies, influenza A and B and polio (Salk vaccine); and attenuated vaccines are used for smallpox (vaccinia), yellow fever (17-D), polio (Sabin vaccine); mump, measles, rubella and varicella.

Incomplete or subparticle vaccines have been devised to reduce the potential for infectivity due to incomplete inactivation of the virion (*e.g.*, hepatitis B) or toxicity (influenza A and B) related to the whole virion. Hepatitis B vaccine, made of capsid antigen harvested from infected blood, is currently available for use among individuals in high risk professions such as dentistry and surgery.

Treatment of the influenza virion with lipid solvents yields subvirion or split product vaccines that are recommended for use in some persons.

Killed virus vaccines are still used for rabies and the current strains of influenza A and B, and others are available. The use of the new diploid cell vaccine for rabies is effective and prevents the development of postinfection encephalitis caused by vaccines made in rabbit nerve tissue. On the other hand, the Salk polio vaccines are available but are not administered routinely in the United States, since they do not elicit coproantibodies that prevent infection in the intestine. Also, for institutional or military use, Japanese B and adenovirus A vaccines are available.

Attenuated vaccines are made from live, attenuated, viruses that can replicate but have lost their pathogenicity for humans. They are available for the childhood infections of mumps, measles and rubella and for the three serotypes of poliovirus (trivalent vaccine of Sabin). Their use has dramatically reduced the number of cases seen annually among the pediatric age group, and outbreaks of these diseases now reported are more often in un-

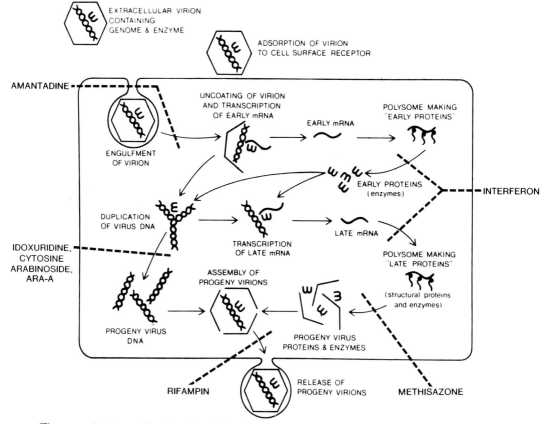

The steps in the replication of a DNA virus.

Figure 35/7. Possible interruption of viral replication by various antiviral agents. (Reproduced with permission from W. L. Drew (Ed.) 1976 *Viral Infections, A Clinical Approach* F. A. Davis, Philadelphia.

immunized adolescents or adults. Recently an outbreak of rubella among dental students underscores the necessity for immunization among this group.

Individuals with immune deficiencies are particularly prone to fatal or serious complications following immunization with proliferative vaccines. For example, the slow infection, subacute sclerosing panencephalitis (SSPE), can result from either wild type or vaccine strains of measles proliferating in semipermissive cells of the brain, and occasionally encephalitis has developed following administration of mumps vaccine. Rarely, reversion to virulence of the trivalent polio vaccine has resulted in paralytic poliomyelitis, but the risk in its use is low. However, arthralgia and arthritis can develop in a significant number of adults receiving rubella vaccine.

Immune globulins, sometimes obtained from hyperimmune individuals can be administered to individuals with defective immune responses such as premature infants, children with primary immunodeficiency or patients undergoing steroid treatment. Immune globulin has been found to modify the severity of measles, and prevent the development of clinical symptoms of hepatitis A and hepatitis B. Immune serum globulins also are useful in preventing varicella or zoster in the immune-compromised patient.

VIRAL INHIBITION AND CHEMOTHERAPY

The ability to inactivate viruses by agents used to kill bacteria is variable. For example, larger quantities of chlorine are required to inactivate poliovirus than the typhoid bacillus (*Salmonella typhi*) and contaminating organic material can significantly reduce the effect of iodine compounds. The range of virucidal activity of most commercial disinfecting solutions (phenolics, oxidants, etc.) usually are limited to enveloped viruses, although formaldehyde and 2% glutaraldehyde are generally effective (see Chapter 7).

A few agents, selected for low toxicity, have the ability to inhibit virus adsorption or replication. These include agents such as the nucleoside analogues idoxuridine, cytosine arabinoside, and adenosine arabinoside and the antiinfluenza agent, amantadine. Generally, they are still used under restricted conditions since they are not without side reactions. However, for topical use, for prophylaxis or under life-threatening conditions, they have value (*e.g.*, herpetic infections). The majority are still undergoing clinical analysis and, although many have promise, none are yet available that are in general use in dentistry (fig. 35/7).

ADDITIONAL READING

DAVIS, B. D., DULBECCO, R., EISEN, H. N., AND GINSBERG, H. G. 1980 *Microbiology* Ed. 3, p. 1355. Harper & Row, Hagerstown, Md.

DREW, W. L. 1976 *Viral Infections, A Clinical Approach*, p. 301. F. A. Davis, Philadelphia.

FENNER, F., McAUSLAN, B. R., MIMS, C. A., SAMBROOK, J., AND WHITE D. O. 1974 *The Biology of Animal Viruses Student Edition*, Ed. 2, p. 834. Academic Press, New York.

FREEMAN, B. A. 1979 *Burrows Textbook of Microbiology*, Ed. 21, p. 1138. Saunders, Philadelphia.

HSIUNG, G. D. 1973 *Diagnostic Virology: An Illustrated Handbook*, p. 174. Yale University Press, New Haven, Conn.

HUGHES, S. S. 1977 *The Virus, The History of the Concept*, p. 140. Heinemann Educational Books, Science History Publications, New York.

JOKLIK, W. K., WILLET, H. P., AND AMOS, D. B. 1980 *Zinsser Microbiology*, Ed. 17, p. 1539. Appleton-Century-Crofts, New York.

MELNICK, J. L. 1976 Taxonomy of Viruses. Prog Med Virol, **22**, 211.

WASHINGTON, J. A. 1981 *Laboratory Procedures in Clinical Microbiology*, p. 856. Springer-Verlag, New York.

chapter 36

Poxviruses: Molluscum Contagiosum, Yaba, Vaccinia, Smallpox, Alastrim, Milker's Nodules, and Orf

Memory Elvin-Lewis

INTRODUCTION

Poxviruses (family Poxviridae) are large, complex DNA viruses that produce vesicular skin diseases that are sometimes fatal in man and animals. Members of this virus family share a common internal antigen and are divided into specific genera and species by differences in morphology, specific antigens, and natural hosts.

Poxviruses that cause disease in man are species that belong to the *Orthopoxvirus* and *Parapoxvirus* groups or remain unclassified. Among those with primary human hosts are the unclassified poxvirus, molluscum contagiosum; and the orthopoxviruses, variola major (smallpox), variola minor (alastrim) and vaccinia, the vaccine strain (perhaps a human strain of cowpox). Animal poxviruses that are sometimes transmitted to man include the unclassified monkey poxviruses, Yaba and Tanapox; the *Orthopoxvirus*, cowpox; the Parapoxvirus, paravaccinia virus of cattle that causes milker's nodules, and orf virus of sheep and goats that elicits contagious pustular dermatitis.

Since smallpox and alastrim are believed to be eradicated, discussions of these infections are of historical interest but no longer have precedence over the more innocuous infections such as molluscum contagiosum, the most common poxvirus infection seen in man today. Second in importance are those complications associated with the use of vaccinia for the purposes of smallpox immunization or possible prophylaxis of recurrent herpes simplex. Poxvirus infections derived from animals are of minor significance, since they are rare and occur only sporadically.

Causative Agents

The virions are brick-shaped and asymmetrical, measure 300 × 240 × 100 nm and have a whorled surface. There is an internal nucleoid with a dumbbell-shaped core surrounded by lipoprotein membranes. Between the nucleoid and outer viral coat is an elliptical body which causes a thickening in the middle of the virion.

Replication occurs primarily in epidermal cells and is initiated through phagocytic engulfment of the virus particles. In the phagocytic vacuoles, the virus is uncoated by host hydrolytic enzymes to only release a virus transcriptase (polymerase) that acts with the encased viral DNA to form mRNA that transcribes proteins necessary for the release of viral DNA from the core. After release of the viral DNA and additional viral enzymes, early translation continues to form enzymes necessary for DNA replication and some structural proteins. Following production of progeny DNA, late translation occurs to produce structural proteins and enzymes that will be incorporated into the virion. Unlike other enveloped viruses that acquire this structure at cell membranes, poxviruses form theirs *de novo*. The intracytoplasmic location of viral replication is evidenced in the inclusion bodies detected by cytochemical and immunofluoescence techniques that are often utilized in pathodiagnosis.

Poxvirus virions are generally resistant to drying and thus can remain viable on fomites for long periods of time, a factor important in the epidemiology of many poxvirus diseases. They are inactivated by autoclaving, heating for 10 minutes at 60 C or exposure to quaternary ammonium compounds, iodophores, chlorine and formaldehyde.

MOLLUSCUM CONTAGIOSUM

Molluscum contagiosum is caused by molluscum contagiosum virus and is a disease of the skin and mucous membranes characterized by the development of chronic, umbilicated papules. Histologically, the lesions are characterized by a markedly abnormal epidermis with extensive downgrowth of infected cells bearing the large eosinophilic cytoplasmic inclusion bodies.

Epidemiology

The infection is worldwide in distribution and is readily transmitted by fomites and contracted through minor abrasions. The disease is most common among children and it is an occupational hazard of athletes, barbers, beauticians, and masseurs who acquire it as a result of contact with contaminated fomites such as towels. Although avoidance of infected individuals is the best way to prevent contagion, dental treatment of infected patients may be necessary. Under these circumstances the use of surgical gloves and protective glasses are recommended over and above other good hygienic practices.

Clinical Manifestations

Following an incubation period of 14 to 50 days, discrete, pearly gray lesions of 1 to 5 mm (fig. 36/1) that can be painful and wartlike develop anywhere on the skin and mucous membranes. In the infected region the skin is generally distended and the lesion, that has a central depression through which a milky fluid exudes, is usually not surrounded by inflammation. The lesions heal without scarring in about 2 months if secondary infection is absent. However, through reinfection others may form in adjacent areas and if not treated the disease can persist from 6 months to 3 years. Multiple lesions that occur principally on the face, dorsal surfaces of the body, genitalia, and occasionally also on the oral mucous membranes should be diagnostically differentiated from warts. If the eye is infected, a reactive conjunctivitis or keratitis can occur that should be differentiated from syringomas and hydrocystomas. Also, single lesions may be confused with keratoachanthomas, pyogenic granulomas and basal cell epitheliomas.

Diagnosis

Microscopic examination of exudate material will reveal the pathodiagnostic molluscum bodies. These may be seen in wet mounts prepared with 10% KOH, or as eosinophilic, cytoplasmic inclusions when stained with Giemsa stain.

Treatment

If a few lesions are present removal by surgical curettage or cryoanesthesia is recommended; however, to prevent reinfection all lesions must be removed. Scarring can occur if corrosive chemicals such as podophyllin, trichloroacetic acid, iodine, phenol or cantharidin are applied.

VACCINIA

Variolation, or the introduction of vaccinia virus (fig. 36/2) into the skin for the purposes of immunization against smallpox with attenuated, replicative poxvirus strains has been carried out for over 2 centuries. The belief by the World Health Organization that smallpox and alastrim have now been eradicated is testimony to its effectiveness. Immunization against smallpox is no longer recommended for the civilian population and is restricted mainly to laboratory workers directly involved with smallpox or closely related orthopoxviruses (e.g., monkeypox, vaccinia). It also is available for indi-

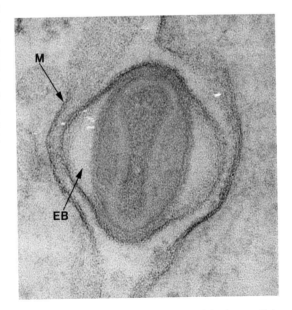

Figure 36/2. Thin section of intact vaccinia virus particle showing the inner nucleic acid core and surrounding membranes. The elliptical body (EB) on either side of the nucleoid causes a prominent central bulging of the virion. The particle is located between two cells (M) (× 120,-000). (Reproduced with permission from S. Dales. Journal of Cell Biology 18, 51, 1963.)

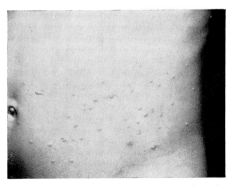

Figure 36/1. Cutaneous manifestations of molluscum contagiosum (AFIP 7757–37.)

viduals entering countries like Democratic Kampuchea (Cambodia), Madagascar, Djibouti and Chad where immunization is still required. Since smallpox vaccination carries with it a small but measurable risk of serious complications to both vaccinees and their contacts, there is no justification for its continued use. Unfortunately cases of complications from vaccination are still being reported where vaccine is being used for unnecessary immunizations, or incorrectly used to try to prevent recurrent episodes of herpes simplex.

Vaccination Technique

Jennerian vaccination or variolation requires the introduction of the vaccine into the skin (usually the arm or scapular region) by scratching or intradermal jet injection. On primary vaccination a papule develops in about 3 days. This becomes a vesicle, then a pustule in 7 to 10 days and forms a scab by the 21st day. When this falls off, it leaves a scar about 1 cm in diameter. During the evolution of the lesion some fever and regional lymphadenopathy may occur and is associated with moderate swelling and tenderness at the site of the vaccination, although this rarely leads to complications. Revaccination may produce an acclerated reaction in 1 to 2 days following vaccination, a response that varies from a small papule to formation of a vesicle, but scarring is unusual. Some local dermal hypersensitivity also may be elicited on revaccination. Both humoral and cellular immunity develop within 5 days of immunization. When vaccination against smallpox was a routine procedure, revaccination was recommended every 3 years to maintain a protective level of immunity.

Complications from Vaccination

The type of complication that develops is often dependent upon the age of the recipient, their immune status, *e.g.*, immunosuppression or malignancy, or presence of dermatological disease.

In infants eczema vaccinatum is the most common complication. This is due to the local spread and dissemination of the infection as a consequence of eczema or other form of active dermatitis (fig. 36/3). In this state the viremia associated with immunization results in the development of secondary vesicles over the entire body. These lesions may resolve but if organ systems are involved, or secondary bacterial infection takes place, the infection may be life threatening. A history of prior vaccination may not affect the course of the illness.

Accidental inoculation from the primary lesion to the eyes, nose, mouth or anus also can produce cellulitis, edema and residual scar formation.

Infants vaccinated prior to the 1st year of life also may develop a generalized vaccinia 7 to 12 days after immunization, but unlike eczema vaccinatum

no virus can be isolated from the small vesicular lesions that develop or from the patient's blood. Since the patient is often nontoxic and frequently febrile, this condition may be some form of hypersensitivity reaction.

In adults a similar type of hypersensitivity reaction may be manifest as a postvaccinal encephalitis. It has been associated with primary vaccinations and to a lesser degree with revaccination. It is fatal in 10 to 30% of the cases. Depending upon the strain of vaccinia and the country reporting, the incidence of primary vaccinees developing this condition has been as high as 1:4000 and as low as 1:1000,000. However, when vaccinia immune globulin (VIG) was administered at the time of immunization it was found that a reduction in the number of cases was achieved.

In individuals with impaired cell-mediated immunity, a progressive necrosis beginning at the site of the vaccination can develop without accompanying signs of regional lymphadenopathy or erythema. This disease, called vaccinia gangrenosa, can metastasize and be fatal. Usually this type of complication occurs where immunization has occurred before the immune-deficient state was detected. Examples of susceptible individuals include infants, cancer victims on immunosuppressant chemotherapy and immunologically compromised individuals with chronic recurrent herpes infections who are seeking relief by "prophylactic" vaccinations. The administration of VIG, β-thiosemicarbazone or rifampin has sometimes arrested the progress of the disease but these therapeutic measures are not always successful.

Other complications include the development of myocarditis, thrombocytopenia, arthritis and pericarditis. Other rare but severe and sometimes fatal reactions include erythema multiforme bullosum, overwhelming viremia resulting in sudden infant death and, as a result of pregnant women being immunized, the almost always fatal fetal vaccinia.

SMALLPOX AND ALASTRIM

Smallpox is an acute exanthematous disease that is frequently fatal. It is caused by the variola virus (poxvirus variolae or variola major) that produces a generalized rash with rapidly successive papules, vesicles, and pustules that form a crust in 14 days, followed by scarring. Alastrim, produced by a less virulent strain called variola minor, is a milder disease and is rarely fatal like smallpox. Due to successful immunization practices, in May 1980 the World Health Organization declared the world to be free of both forms of smallpox.

Epidemiology

Prior to its eradicaton, variola was readily transmitted from one patient to the other by contami-

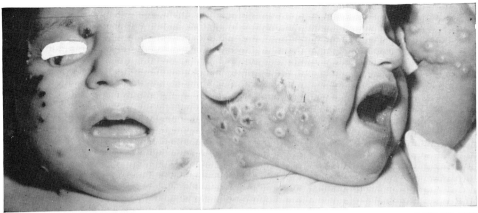

Figure 36/3. Disseminated vaccinia of a child with eczema of the face and oral manifestations. (AFIP 53–728 9–10.)

nated fomites and through respiratory discharges and exudates from lesions of the skin and mucous membranes. The virus is particularly resistant to drying and could persist for long lengths of time in contaminated bedding and clothing, facilitating transmission.

Pathogenesis

Smallpox is acquired through the respiratory tract and during the incubation period of approximately 2 weeks the following course of infection takes place. Replication first occurs in the respiratory epithelium and regional lymphoid tissue. The virus is then disseminated through the reticulendothelial system by the blood stream (primary viremia). The secondary viremia that develops heralds the prodromal illness when the virus is spreading to organs and tissues. The lesions first begin as a macular rash. In the second or papular stage capillary dilatation and edema of the papillary layer of the corium is observed, and with a thickening of the epithelial layer, the vesicle develops. Perivascular inflammation with lymphocytic and histiocytic infiltration results in pustule formation which then is resolved by crusting and epithelial migration across the lesion site. A hypersensitivity response to viral antigen also may contribute to lesion formation. Ulceration is more pronounced when lesions occur in the mucosa of the upper respiratory and digestive tracts. Although not as vesiculated as skin lesions, focal necrosis of the epithelial cells causes sloughing and results in dissemination of the virus. Pathological changes also may be apparent in the liver, kidneys and heart.

Clinical Manifestations

Smallpox can take many forms, from a mild type without lesions to a severe, widely disseminated exanthem that can be hemorrhagic and fatal. Onset begins with a toxemia phase that is characterized by fever, chills, vomiting, severe backache, and prostration, which continue for 3 to 6 days. During this time a flat, erythematous macular rash often develops in the groins, axillae and on the flanks. Such rashes are indicative of prognosis: if erythematous the disease is mild, if petechial the disease is severe and if hemorrhagic, almost always fatal. At the end of the prodromal period, the characteristic single crop of lesions develops. These progress through stages from papule, to vesicle, pustule, scab and scar. Lesion development is centrifugal and they first appear on the back, followed by rapid appearance on the trunk and extremities. Lesions also can appear in the oral cavity especially on the buccal mucosa, tongue, soft palate and in the mucosa of the upper respiratory and digestive tracts. The prognosis is poor if discrete lesions become confluent. The temperature rises and falls during the early course of the exanthemous period, and again on the 9th day when the pustules finally form scabs then desquamate.

Variola minor follows the same pattern of symptoms however they are less severe, the skin lesions more superficial and the course of the disease shorter. The electron micrograph in figure 36/4 is of variola minor, obtained from the last case reported: it occurred in East Africa on October 26, 1977.

Following an attack of these infections immunity is often permanent, and if secondary attacks occur these are often mild and without a rash, as are the modified forms of smallpox that occur in individuals rendered partially immune by vaccination. When clinical smallpox occurred, the mortality rate of nonimmunized patients with variola major was from 20 to 80% and with variola minor less than 5%.

Treatment

When smallpox was a clinical problem, patients and their contacts were given β-thiosemicarbazone to reduce the severity or prevent infection. In some cases rifampin also was found useful. To further

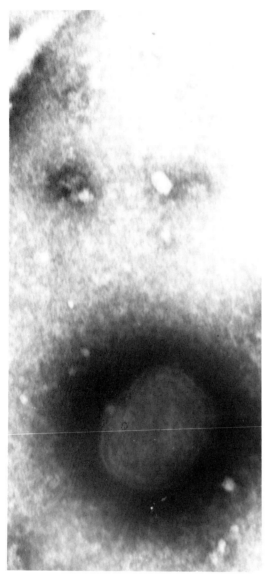

Figure 36/4. Variola minor virus from world's last endemic case, Merka, Somalia, 1977. (×115,000). (Courtesy of Dr. J. Nakano.)

reduce the severity of the symptoms VIG also was administered.

ANIMAL POXVIRUSES CONTAGIOUS TO MAN

Cattle are the source of two poxvirus diseases that are acquired by milking infected cows. The disease due to the *Orthopoxvirus*, cowpox, usually appears on the hands and develops like primary vaccinia. It is accompanied with some fever and constitutional symptoms. Infection with the *Parapoxvirus*, paravaccinia virus, that causes milker's nodules, occurs in the same manner as cowpox, however, the lesions that develop are initially small papules that grow over a period of a week into red to brown or purplish nodules 1 to 2 inches in diameter. In time the nodules become verrucoid crusted or granulomatous. Regional lymphadenopathy, allergic rash and secondary infections can occur. Usually the primary lesions are not painful and subside within 1 to 2 months. Immunization with vaccinia will protect against cowpox but not infection with paravaccinia virus.

Sheep, particularly lambs, develop contagious pustular dermatitis ("scabby mouth") or orf, a papulovesicular eruption that is confined to the lips and surrounding skin. Sheep herders can acquire a single lesion on their face, arms or hands that develops through six stages, each lasting 6 days, ending uneventfully about 35 days following initial symptoms. The papular phase is a red, elevated lesion; the target stage then develops into a nodule with a red center, a white middle ring and red periphery: the surface may be red and weeping. The nodule then develops a thin dry crust with black dots; small papillomas appear over the surface in the papillomatous stage; and during the regressive stage a thick crust develops on the surface of the lesion. A reduction in size and elevation of the papillomas then occurs. Excision and cautery promote healing in 2 to 3 weeks and antibiotics for secondary infections are also of value.

Monkeys from Africa can carry Yaba virus, a poxvirus that produces in them, and humans that handle them, benign tumors. Also Tanapox virus, probably transmitted by an insect, can produce solitary skin lesions associated with a general feeling of malaise.

ADDITIONAL READING

Advisory Committee on Immunization Practices. 1978 Smallpox Vaccine. Morbidity and Mortality Weekly Reports, **27**, 156.

Departments of the Army, the Navy, the Air Force and Transportation: 1977 *Medical Services Immunization Requirements and Procedures.* Washington, D.C.

Jawetz, E., Melnick, J. L., and Adelberg, E. A. 1980 Poxvirus Family. *Medical Microbiology,* Ed. 14, 468. Lange Medical Publications, Los Altos, Calif.

Kern, A. B., and Schiff, B. L. 1959 Smallpox Vaccinations in the Management of Recurrent Herpes Simplex: A Controlled Evaluation. J Invest Dermatol, **33**, 99.

Lane, J. M., Ruben, F. L., Abrutyn, E., and Millar, J. D. 1970 Deaths Attributable to Smallpox Vaccination. JAMA, **212**, 441.

Mandell, G. L., Douglas, R. G., Jr., and Bennett, J. E. (Eds.) 1979 *Principles and Practice of Infectious Diseases.* John Wiley & Sons, New York.

Morbidity and Mortality Weekly Reports. 1979 Adverse Reactions to Smallpox Vaccination—1978, **28**, 265.

Morbidity and Mortality Weekly Reports. 1979 Smallpox Certification—East Africa. **28**, 497.

Morbidity and Mortality Weekly Reports. 1980 Fatal Reaction to Smallpox Vaccination—California. **29**, 117.

Morbidity and Mortality Weekly Reports. 1980 Smallpox Vaccine. **29**, 417.

Washington, J. A. (Ed.), 1981 *Lab Procedures in Clinical Microbiology.* Springer-Verlag, New York.

chapter 37

Herpesviruses: Herpes Simplex 1 and 2, *Herpesvirus simiae*, Varicella-Zoster Virus, Epstein-Barr Virus, and Cytomegalovirus

Memory Elvin-Lewis

INTRODUCTION

Herpesviruses (family Herpetoviridae) are enveloped, icosahedral, DNA-containing viruses with dermatotropic, neurotropic and lymphotropic predilections. They characteristically produce diseases with latent, recurrent and sometimes teratogenic or malignant tendencies. Members of this virus family which share a common group antigen and are morphologically similar are further divided into genera, species and serotypes by specific antigens, the characteristic disease conditions they elicit and the host range of cells they infect.

Within the animal kingdom, the potential of this family to produce disease is widespread and those Herpetoviridae that cause disease in man belong to three subfamilies. Represented in the Alphaherpesvirinae (herpes simplex virus group) are the herpes simplex viruses types 1 and 2, the varicella-zoster virus and the herpes B virus of monkeys; within the Betaherpesvirinae (cytomegalovirus group) is the human cytomegalovirus; and in the Gammaherpesvirinae (lymphoproliferative virus group) the Epstein-Barr virus.

Causative Agents

The virions have an icosahedral capsid composed of 162 capsomeres, arranged as 150 elongated hexagonal and 12 pentagonal prisms, with a central axial hole. The capsid encloses a double-stranded DNA genome wrapped around associated proteins as on a spool and referred to as a toroidal core. The nucleocapsids (100 nm) are surrounded by a zone composed of globular proteins called a tegument and encompassed by a lipoprotein envelope with periodic short projections. The diameters are from 150 to 250 nm depending on the particular virus.

The virions enter the cells by either pinocytosis or fusion of the envelope with the cell membrane and are then uncoated; the virus DNA proceeds to the nucleus, where replication begins. Host transcriptases are utilized to form early and late mRNAs that are translated in the cytoplasm into proteins and then are transported into the nucleus where they are used for replicative and structural purposes. For example, viral-induced DNA polymerases and thymidine kinases are utilized in progeny DNA formation. Intranuclear inclusions referred to as Cowdry type A are the sites of initial virus assembly. However, the mature inclusion does not contain virions since envelopment is completed at the nuclear membrane where virions then transverse the cytoplasm through the endoplasmic reticulum or vacuoles to be released at the cell surface (fig. 37/1). Pathodiagnostic features of *Herpesvirus*-infected cells include the eosinophilic intranuclear inclusions and the formation of large syncytial giant cells or nonsyncytial giant cells; ballooning degeneration of epithelial cells also can occur.

Viral Latency

The latent state that can develop in herpesvirus infections is related to the ability of these viruses to travel along sensory nerve pathways to specific sensory ganglia; with herpes simplex 1 (HSV-1), it is usually the trigeminal nerve ganglion; with herpes simplex 2 (HSV-2) the thoracic, lumbar and sacral dorsal root ganglia are frequent sites of latency; and with varicella-zoster, sensory ganglia of the vagal, spinal or cranial nerves. Although the means by which herpesviruses remain sequestered in ganglion cells is not completely understood, it has been hypothesized that the virion DNA remains in these cells as a type of episome, plasmid or nonreplicating form that has the potential to spread peripherally to other sensory nerves (fig. 37/2).

The latter two alternatives seem more likely

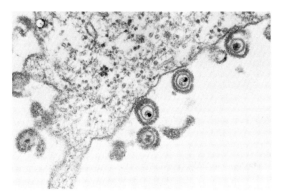

Figure 37/1. Herpes simplex virus type 1 in extracellular space. The nucleocapsid is surrounded by an envelope at least partly derived from host cell membranes. × 80,000. Courtesy Dr. H. D. Mayor. (Reproduced with permission from H. D. Mayor, S. Drake, and L. Jordan. 1975 The Replication of Adeno-Associated Satellite Virus. The Three-Component System, Satellite, Herpes Virus, and Adenovirus. Journal of Ultrastructure Research, **52**, 52.)

since complete virus particles cannot be detected unless ganglion cells are cultured, and the DNA synthesis required for most types of genome integration is absent in nondividing neurons. It has been further proposed that only viral DNA is produced within the neuron and that final viral replication and assembly takes place in epithelial cells. The role of the exacerbating factors such as fever, hormonal changes of menses, irradiation, or immune suppression have yet to be elucidated, although in different ways they may inactivate inhibitors that prevent complete virus replication in a manner similar to that proposed for ultraviolet induction of prophage in lysogenized bacteria. Reactivation is dependent upon the integrity of the anterior root and peripheral nerve pathways. Cytomegalovirus also has a latent potential since it can be retrieved from normal tonsillar tissue through tissue culture.

Viral Transformation

Transformation is another phenomenon associated with viruses of this group. Herpes simplex 2 has been implicated in cervical carcinoma by serologic studies and the virus or its T antigen also has been isolated from cervical carcinomas following several passages in cell culture. Similar studies have suggested a similar relation between HSV-1 and lip cancers. The association of Epstein-Barr virus with nasopharyngeal carcinoma and African Burkitt's

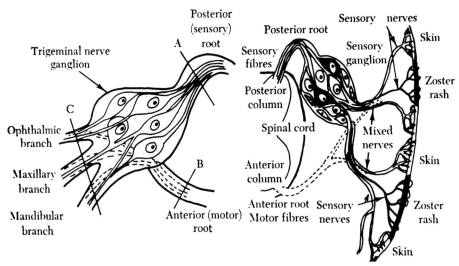

Figure 37/2. Diagram illustrating the probable pathogenesis of recurrent herpes simplex (*left*) and herpes zoster (*right*). *Left*, herpes simplex virus is presumed to be latent in the sensory nerve cells of the trigeminal nerve ganglion. Recurrent viral activity is triggered by fever, ultraviolet light, etc., and also by nerve injury. Section of posterior (sensory) root of trigeminal nerve (*A*) produces herpes simplex lesions in skin innervated by maxillary and mandibular branches of that nerve. Section of the motor root (*B*) or the branches (*C*) has no such effect. *Right*, varicella virus is presumed to become latent in sensory cells of the dorsal root ganglion. Upon activation, the virus grows down the sensory nerve and infects the skin to produce the vesicles of herpes zoster. (Latter modified from Hope-Simpson, 1965, and reproduced with permission from F. Fenner *et al.* 1974 *The Biology of Animal Viruses*, Ed. 2. Academic Press, New York.)

lymphoma is better established and will be discussed in that section.

HERPES SIMPLEX TYPES 1 AND 2

Herpes simplex infections are caused by two serologically related types, 1 and 2, that differ somewhat in cultural characteristics, cell predilections and oncogenic potential. The diseases include vesicular eruptions of the skin and mucous membranes often characterized by recurrent episodes, and by disseminated infections involving the viscera or nervous system. Since the viruses have oncogenic potential they have been implicated in cervical carcinomas and, to a lesser degree, in lip carcinomas.

Epidemiology

Herpes simplex infections are worldwide in distribution and acquired by individuals by direct contact of infected secretions such as saliva or genital lesion exudates from active cases, or subclinical carriers. Although there is no marked sexual or seasonal variation, rates of infection are related to socioeconomic status, and with HSV-2 also to the degree of promiscuity. Surveys have shown that up to 90% of individuals in a lower socioeconomic status will have had HSV-1 infection, whereas only 30 to 50% of those from higher strata will have been infected. The incidence of HSV-2 is somewhat less. Moreover, there is an expected age difference in the acquisition of both types. For example, neonates are more likely to acquire HSV-2 infections of the eye or central nervous system during birth, whereas other HSV-2 infections occur after puberty, following the initiation of sexual activity, and are usually confined to the genitalia. HSV-1 infections can be easily transmitted by casual contact, and young children, especially under crowded conditions, are more likely to acquire primary gingivostomatitis and pharyngitis than others, college-age students that develop this infection often present with tonsillitis and posterior pharyngitis rather than the labial disease. The axiom that HSV-1 infections are found primarily from the waist up, and HSV-2 infections from the waist down does not now hold since changes in sexual practices also have changed the pattern of serotypes found at the site of primary infection. Accidental inoculation into the fingers is an occupational hazard of dentists, physicians and medical auxiliaries, but whitlow is not a prevalent affliction. Nosocomial outbreaks of *Herpesvirus* infection in hospital personnel, neonatal nurseries or among laboratory personnel have been reported.

Pathogenesis

On the mucous membranes of the oral cavity, genitalia or eye, or through traumatic inoculation into the skin, the herpes simplex virus gains access to the parabasal and intermediate epithelial cells where it initiates infection. Multinucleated cells that contain the typical inclusions are formed and these show ballooning degeneration. As these cells are lysed, a local inflammatory response develops that appears first as a small patch of erythema, then evolves into a vesicle filled with a clear fluid. Virus is more likely to be recovered from this vesicle fluid than the crusts that develop as it heals. Additional virus replication may result in a viremia and dissemination to the viscera such as the lungs and liver or through peripheral nerves to the central nervous system. Usually individuals with impaired cellular immune responses develop more severe disease than others and it has been postulated that those that develop recurrent infections also have an altered cellular response. The development of neutralizing antibody, sensitized killer lymphocytes and interferon all play a role in the resolution of the herpes simplex infections. During this period a latent state can develop, with a nonreplicating form of the virus residing in adjacent nerve ganglia. Since recurrent infection can develop in the presence of high titers of neutralizing antibody that acts to prevent the extracellular spread of the virus, other factors are clearly involved with its exacerbation, control or resolution. For example, the basis for the use of vaccinia immunization in the prophylaxis of recurrent herpes was to stimulate nonspecific cellular responses such as interferon production. However, since results of this procedure were equivocal and the hazards of giving vaccinia are great, this practice has been abandoned. Similarly, use of other immune-stimulating agents such as levamisole and the tuberculosis vaccine, BCG, also have proven disappointing.

Clinical Manifestations

Herpes simplex virus causes both primary and recurrent infections of the skin, mucous membranes, eyes, the nervous system, and occasionally a generalized infection. The diseases arising from these infections are herpetic eczema, traumatic infections, herpes genitalis, keratitis, keratoconjunctivitis, herpetic meningoencephalitis, and infections associated with trigeminal neuralgia.

Herpetic Gingivostomatitis

Primary herpetic gingivostomatitis is the most common type of herpes simplex infection seen and is a systemic infection with characteristic oral lesions (figs. 37/3 and 37/4). It usually is initiated by the virus entering the body through the nonkeratinized cells of the oral mucosa or at the site of trauma. Following an incubation period of 2 to 14 days (average 4 days) soreness of the mouth and excessive salivation are accompanied by fever, ma-

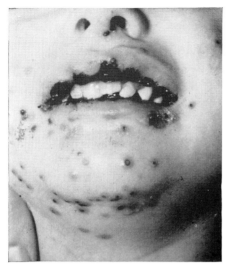

Figure 37/3. Primary herpetic gingivostomatitis in a child. (AFIP 53-728-5).

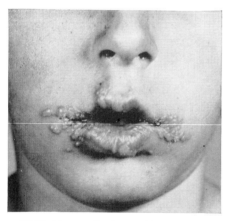

Figure 37/4. Herpes simplex and herpetic gingivostomatitis in a youth. (AFIP AN 2049.)

laise and irritability. In the initial phase the cervical lymph nodes enlarge, the mouth and throat are painful and the temperature rises to as high as 105 F, but the average is about 101 F. Then a generalized vesicular eruption develops throughout the oral cavity, especially on the tongue and buccal mucosa, but lesions also can develop on the tonsillar region and soft palate. The vesicles are often modified by eating to appear as grayish yellow plaques. The gingivae are almost always involved. In mild cases the gingival margins appear bright red whereas in more severe cases the gingivae are swollen, hypertrophic, and bleed easily. Pain and fever accompany this and it is not uncommon for young children to refuse to eat, become dehydrated and develop a fetid breath. The initial infection is usually self-limiting, and after 6 to 15 days the lesions begin to heal and resolve within another week. Also, generalized symptoms gradually disappear as immunity develops. Gingival lesions and regional lymphadenopathy are frequently the last symptoms to disappear.

Herpes Labialis

Recurrent herpes labialis that occurs in 20 to 40% of the population is usually mild, without fever, and the lesions are limited to a few isolated areas on the vermillion borders of the lips (fig. 37/5), on the tongue or in the oral cavity: only rarely are other sites such as the nose, chin or cheek involved. Prodromal symptoms often occur. These include burning and itching at the site of the lesion and they can last from 6 to 24 hours before vesicle development. The vesicles frequently occur at identical sites during each exacerbation. They are extremely painful and develop to the crusting stage in 48 hours, unlike the more slowly evolving lesions of the primary disease. Although a local adenopathy may accompany these symptoms other systemic signs are absent. Usually the episode resolves within 7 to 10 days.

Ocular Infections

Ocular herpes simplex infections can result from primary inoculation, extension of infection from elsewhere on the face, or as a consequence of exacerbation and extension via the trigeminal nerve. Primary inoculation of infants can occur at birth and is characteristically an HSV-2 infection manifest as a chorioretinitis. More commonly HSV-1 is the causative agent and produces an unilateral follicular conjunctivitis, blepharitis on the margin of the eyelid and a regional lymphadenopathy that resolves in 2 to 3 weeks. If the cornea becomes involved, dendritic ulcers or coarse punctate epithelial opacities may develop that may persist in an acute phase for 2 to 3 weeks. This is followed by a keratitis of several weeks duration. Should the infection be severe the cornea may rupture, then heal

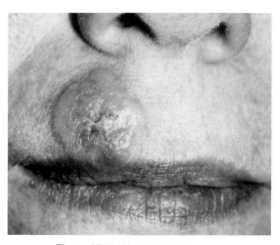

Figure 37/5. Herpex labialis lesion.

with scar formation causing visual impairment. Secondary bacterial infection is common in herpes simplex infections of the eye.

Recurrent ocular infections can occur as unilateral, or less frequently bilateral, blepharitis or keratoconjunctivitis. When dendritic ulcers occur, there frequently is a loss in corneal sensation and visual acuity. Should stromal involvement take place, often as a consequence of steroidal therapy, uveitis can develop. Following a number of recurrent episodes loss of sight can occur due to the formation of dense scars, corneal thinning and neovascularization, and in some cases, there may be actual rupture of the globe.

Genital Infections

Herpes genitalis is usually a consequence of venereal transmission with HSV-2 and less frequently with HSV-1. Ninety percent of the primary infections are subclinical and commonly occur in young adults. This acute inflammatory disease results in the formation of vesicles on the genital area accompanied by fever, malaise, anorexia and bilateral lymphadenopathy. Most lesions in men occur on the penis and can persist for several days. In women they can occur on the external and internal genitalia and surrounding skin, and usually ulcerate and become covered by a grayish white exudate. Urethral involvement also may result in dysuria, urinary retention and associated neuralgias.

Recurrent herpes genitalis is usually associated with a milder course of events, with less systemic involvement and fewer genital lesions. It is sometimes referred to as herpes progenitalis. In women, exacerbation in the cervix may be asymptomatic. As a consequence of repeated attacks, urethral stricture or labial fusion can occur. In rare instances meningitis also may develop.

Traumatic Infections

Traumatic or inoculation herpes occurs following entrance of the virus into the skin usually through some minor abrasion or accidental inoculation. A common form among dentists, medical and paramedical personnel is herpetic whitlow, caused by HSV-1. It is characterized by prodromal itching and the sudden appearance about the nails and at the ends of the fingers of deep vesicles that can coalesce. The development of these lesions is associated with intense pain and some neuralgia and axillary adenopathy. If the syndrome is not mistaken for a pyogenic paronychia and excised, it will resolve in 2 to 3 weeks. With surgical intervention, however, healing is delayed and often associated with secondary bacterial infection. In other members of the community, HSV-2 may be responsible for a similar type of infection. Recurrences are uncommon but do occur, although symptoms are usually less severe. Accidental infection that occurs on skin of the extremities may cause primary symptoms similar to whitlow or a more superficial infection. With recurrent infections, however, a severe local neuralgia, local edema and lymphangitis is characteristic.

Eczema

Eczema herpeticum (fig. 37/6) is an extreme and potentially dangerous form of herpes simplex infection that is also known as Kaposi's varicelliform eruption. The infection occurs throughout eczematous parts of the skin and adjacent areas. Vesicles that can be confluent and hemorrhagic persist for a week and are accompanied by high fever. Like other herpetic infections, recurrences can occur, and the severity of the attack is dependent upon the underlying condition of the skin. The illness can be fatal if bacterial infections such as *Pseudomonas aeroginosa* are superimposed.

Encephalitis

Encephalitis may be a consequence of acquisition of HSV-2 at birth, or later in life due to extension by neural routes of a primary or recurrent attack of either HSV-2 or HSV-1. Although a rare event,

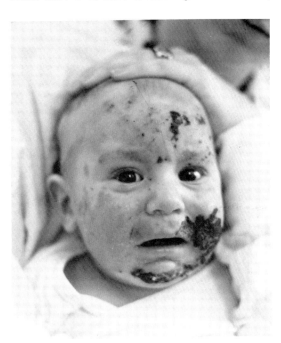

Figure 37/6. Four-month-old child with eczema herpeticum, on 5th day of treatment with topical methylene blue and light. Lesions on treated side of face (*right side*) are healed, while untreated ones (*left side*) are covered with eschar. Courtesy Dr. T. Chang. (Reproduced with permission from T. Chang and L. Weinstein. 1975 Eczema Herpeticum. Treatment with Methylene Blue and Light. Archives of Dermatology, **111**, 1174. © 1975, American Medical Association.)

herpes encephalitis is more common than any other nonepidemic viral disease. Headache, fever and flu-like symptoms are followed by behavioral disorders, speech difficulties and focal seizures. The temporal lobes are commonly involved, and a necrotizing hemorrhagic encephalitis develops that, if untreated, can be fatal in 80% of the cases, with those that survive having neurologic sequelae.

Neonatal Infections

Neonatal infections may be acquired at birth as a result of maternal genital infection with HSV-2, or by contact with hospital personnel with active HSV-1 disease. These infections can result in local ocular or oral infections or become disseminated and fulminant and invade the central nervous system or viscera with perhaps a fatal outcome. Recent studies have shown that the incidence of HSV infection acquired *in utero* increases the nearer the mother is to parturition when disease develops. Thus, only 10% of infants will acquire infection at the 8th month of gestation whereas 40% are affected if virus excretion is detected at birth. As a rule, severe congenital disease is more likely to occur if the mother has primary rather than recurrent disease. In some instances, maternal viremia has been responsible for fetal wasting or birth defects. Congenital infection is evidenced at birth by the appearance of vesicular lesions and ocular manifestations, but also by symptoms that indicate visceral and central nervous system involvement. Should this occur the fatality rate is high (65%) and the number surviving without serious sequelae is low. Injury of the liver is reflected by swelling and jaundice: in fatal cases the liver has been found to be necrotic. Splenomegaly and necrosis of the adrenals also can occur. Central nervous system disease can cause seizures, palsies, temperature instability, microcephaly and coma. Destructive encephalitis or disseminated intravascular coagulation can develop in survivors.

Other Herpetic Infections

In the compromised host, serious herpetic infections are likely to occur. Thus, infections of the respiratory tract can result from extensions of HSV-1 disease in the oral cavity, in those immunosuppressed for transplantation or in debilitated individuals subject to eosophageal or respiratory tract instrumentation. Severe, chronic or progressive mucocutaneous infections have developed in individuals with malignancies or thymic disorders, and disseminated disease in those who are debilitated by pregnancy or age. Burned areas of the skin are also susceptible to herpetic infection, appearing as an erosive, discolored or vesicular area in the healing wound: these infections also have the capacity to become disseminated.

Diagnosis

On a clinical basis alone, diagnosis of oral or genital infections may be confused with a number of other diseases. For example, the pharyngitis evident in oral herpes is similar to that of streptococcal origin, to diphtheria, herpangina, Vincent's infection, infectious mononucleosis and Stevens-Johnson syndrome. Also, genital herpes may be confused with chancroid, syphilis, Behçet's syndrome, erythema multiforme and candidiasis.

Scrapings of exudates from lesions on the skin or eye may yield the multinucleated giant cells with typical inclusions. However, to differentiate HSV from lesions of varicella, or to differentiate HSV-1 from HSV-2, specific antibody must be used in immunofluorescent techniques.

Cell culture of HSV can result in characteristic cytopathogenic effect (CPE) or cell behavior patterns. Virus strain differentiation usually requires immunological procedures.

Serological techniques are only useful if primary infection can be proven. Detection of specific IgM antibodies is particularly useful with the neonate, but cannot distinguish between recurrent and primary infection in the older individual. In order to circumvent brain biopsy in encephalitis, the uses of radioimmunoassays or enzyme-linked immunosorbent assays (ELISA) to detect viral glycoproteins or viral specific enzymes in the CSF are being investigated.

Prevention

The widespread prevalence of herpes simplex viruses makes it impossible to completely avoid the acquisition of this disease. However, certain precautions can be taken. For example, dentists and medical personnel who must treat infected patients should wear surgical gloves and protective glasses. Also, patients with extensive herpetic skin infections should be isolated and individuals with active HSV infections should be prevented from contacts with neonates. Present data suggests that mothers with genital lesions during parturition should have delivery by caesarian section if feasible.

Control and Treatment

Herpes simplex virus is relatively stable, particularly in the presence of proteins. While it is heat sensitive and remains infectious at 37 C for only a few hours, it can be preserved by storage at low temperature for long periods of time. However, the virus is sensitive to acid (pH less than 6.8), lipid solvents, cationic detergents, proteolytic enzymes and ultraviolet irradiation.

Although a variety of drugs exist that have the potential for use against herpes infections, in practice only a few are utilized. Thus 5-iododeoxyuridine (IUDR) has been used with equivocal success as a topical medication for herpetic infections of the eye and lip, and trifluorothymidine and interferon have shown some promise in the treatment of herpetic keratitis. Because of its superior therapeutic to toxic ratio adenine arabinoside (Ara-A or vidarabine) is effective in treating some cases of herpetic encephalitis. Nonspecific immune enhancers such as Bacillus Calmette-Guerin (BCG), and levamisole have not proved as valuable in controlled studies as initial investigation indicated. More importantly, the use of photoactive dyes is not recommended since they may increase the malignant transforming potential of the virus.

Topical antibiotics are sometimes prescribed to decrease secondary bacterial infections. For oral lesions, especially before meals, topical anesthetics can be used. Also with infants, fluids may be administered to compensate for reduced intake during severe cases of gingivostomatitis.

VARICELLA-ZOSTER (V-Z) VIRUS

Varicella (chickenpox), and zoster (shingles) are caused by infection with the varicella-zoster (V-Z) virus. Although similar to herpes simplex viruses in morphology, ability to produce Cowdry type A inclusions and to elicit a disease with vesicular, latent and neurotropic aspects, V-Z differs from these species by being larger in size (180 to 200 nm), unable to cause disease in animals or chick embryos, more cell-associated in cell cultures, and possessing different antigens.

Varicella is a highly contagious exanthematous disease that is characterized by successive lesions. Usually a disease of childhood, it can recur in partially immune adults as Zoster where vesicles are restricted to areas of the skin supplied by sensory nerves of a single or associated dorsal root ganglion. One type of manifestation can follow the other.

Epidemiology

Varicella is primarily a disease of childhood (fig. 37/7) and is common throughout the world. It has been estimated that most adults in the United States have acquired either a clinical or subclinical infection by the time they reach middle age. In temperate regions it has a higher incidence of occurrence in the winter and spring. Infection is acquired through contact with infected secretions from patients with varicella or zoster, but unlike variola, scabs are not infective. Congenital infection is possible. If acquired early in gestation, infants may develop various forms of the varicella syndrome. However, if infection occurs late in gestation, symptoms are not evident at birth, but subsequently a zoster-type disease may evolve.

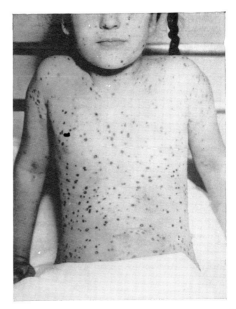

Figure 37/7. Varicella (chickenpox). (AFIP AMH 10529E.)

Pathogenesis

Although the exact route of invasion of V-Z virus is uncertain, it is presumed that the virus enters the body through the respiratory tract, where it multiplies and invades the blood stream to be carried to the skin or other organs. Lesions are similar to herpes simplex in that ballooning degeneration in cells of the epidermis, and to a lesser degree the corium, occurs with focal cellular destruction: vesicle fluid is predominantly polymorphonuclear leukocytic. Multinucleated giant cells are formed that contain Cowdry type A intranuclear inclusions. Following primary infection a latent state develops in the dorsal ganglion and is probably maintained by cellular immunity. On exacerbation of the zoster syndrome the initial cutaneous lesions are similar to those of varicella, but dorsal root ganglia also show cell infiltration, focal hemorrhages and degeneration. Nerve destruction may extend back to the posterior column of the cord and forward to the skin.

Clinical Manifestations

Varicella is a highly contagious disease, and after an incubation period of 2 to 3 weeks, a prodromal period of 1 to 2 days with fever and malaise heralds the onset of clinical illness. The appearance of successive crops of lesions is sudden. This occurs over a period of 2 to 5 days. The lesions progress from macules to papules to vesicles within a few hours, remain for 3 to 4 days and leave a granular, blood-colored scab. Pruritis and scratching can lead to secondary bacterial infection. The exanthem usually involves first the trunk, then the neck and face, with less involvement of the extremities. Vesicles that occur in the mouth, nose and larynx are often quite painful, and stomatitis may accompany the more severe forms of the disease.

Complications are not common but may include abscesses, conjunctivitis, otitis media, pharyngitis, tonsillitis, myocarditis, pancarditis, nephritis, septicemia, ulcerative gastritis, gastrointestinal bleeding, orchitis and appendicitis. When pneumonia supervenes, this occurs 3 to 5 days after the rash, and concomitant with this manifestation, varicella hepatitis may occur to further complicate the illness. Central nervous system disease may occur anytime after the onset of the exanthem and may be manifest as encephalitis, transverse myelitis, neuritis, or meningitis. Bleeding may appear on or before the development of skin lesions and is sometimes associated with coagulation abnormalities.

Congenital varicella is usually acquired by the fetus from an infected mother during the first trimester of pregnancy. Symptoms vary widely and can include growth retardation that results in atrophy of the extremities, often with the development of associated cicatricial lesions, cerebrocortical atrophy or microcephaly that leads to mental retardation and deafness, and various types of eye involvement like microophthalmia, chorioretinitis, or cataracts.

Herpes zoster or shingles occurs in 0.5 to 2.0% of the population, but rarely in children or individuals over 60 years of age. The incubation period is from 1 to 3 weeks, and is frequently exacerbated in partially immune adults by exposure to X-rays, immunosuppressive therapy, drugs such as sulfonamides, or to a case of varicella. If also may be secondary to another febrile illness or occur without any apparent incitement. The infection produces lesions of the nervous system and is accompanied by a systemic response characterized by headache, fever, malaise and regional lymphadenopathy. Neuritis pain is prominent. The exacerbation is frequently unilateral (fig. 37/8). Cutaneous lesions are usually localized and appear as vesicles with an erythematous base located in the area innervated by infected peripheral sensory nerves or dorsal root ganglia. These lesions also may appear in crops in an irregular fashion along nerve pathways and are more deeply seated than those of varicella. The lesions vesiculate in 12 to 24 hours and become pustules by 72 hours, then develop crusts. The severity of zoster varies considerably. A few lesions may appear and regress within 7 to 10 days, or the lesions may persist for several weeks. On occasion, the lesions can become gangrenous and secondarily infected.

Constant or intermittent pain described as stabbing, burning, or aching is characteristic of zoster. It may appear during the prodromal period, during

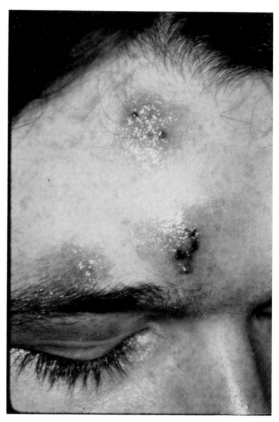

Figure 37/8. Herpes zoster involving the ophthalmic branch of the trigeminal nerve. Note that the lesions do not cross the midline.

the acute stage, during healing, or even after the lesions disappear. The severity of the pain is not related to the severity of the disease.

Zoster has a predilection for certain sites, including the thoracic, lumbar, and sacral regions, or cephalic (including cervical, oral, opthalmic or auricular) regions. When the lingual, facial, and auditory regions are involved, temporary or permanent paralysis can result.

A variety of complications can occur. Encephalitis following herpes zoster is usually self-limiting. As with varicella, it can occur before the rash but usually begins around the second week following onset of the rash. Eye infections can vary from a superficial conjunctivitis to scleritis, keratitis, iridocyclitis, or to development of glaucoma. Following an attack of zoster, neuroparalytic ulceration, corneal anestheis or proptosis may develop. In rare cases disseminated zoster can develop about a week after the appearance of the original lesions, and include the lungs, central nervous system, liver and pancreas. Death is rare, but is usually a result of overwhelming pulmonary involvement. Varicella-zoster also may result in the development of a number of other neurological disorders such as the

Guillain-Barré syndrome, Bell's palsy or Ramsay Hunt syndrome.

Diagnosis

The distinctive symptoms of either varicella or zoster facilitate diagnosis on a clinical basis. It is possible, using specific immune sera, to differentiate V-Z virus from HSV by immunofluorescent staining of exudates that contain inclusion-bearing multi-nucleated cells. The virus also will produce a distinctive CPE in some cell cultures. A rise in complement-fixing antibody from acute to convalescent sera also is helpful in confirming zoster or varicella infection.

Treatment

Treatment is usually symptomatic. Pruritis may be treated with topical calamine solutions or by the administration of trimeprazine. Pain associated with zoster may be treated with analgesics or some type of tricyclic antidepressant. High-dose interferon holds some promise for therapy since in trials its use has diminished postherpetic neuralgia, new vesicle formation, and the frequency of visceral complications. Ara-A (vidarabine) also has been found to reduce the persistence of virus in skin lesions and diminish duration of pain. Also, among the immune compromised, zoster-immune globulin or plasma (ZIG, ZIP) is helpful in reducing the severity of the disease. A live varicella vaccine is now undergoing evaluation.

CYTOMEGALOVIRUS

Cytomegaloviruses (CMV) cause a variety of infections. These viruses are about 180–250 nm in diameter and produce characteristic large eosinophilic nuclear inclusions and smaller, basophilic, paranuclear, cytoplasmic inclusions. The virus is antigenically distinct from other herpesviruses and like V-Z virus is primarily cell associated. It can only replicate slowly in diploid fibroblast cells where it produces a characteristic plaque-like CPE.

Cytomegalovirus infections are typically latent and subclinical in adults or occasionally result in an infectious mononucleosis syndrome. This also may occur in infants that acquire the infection perinatally. Congenital infection is classically fulminant, with viscerotropic and neurotropic features that may result in death or a variety of neurologic sequelae in the survivors.

Epidemiology

In the general population acquisition of this infection is apparently ubiquitous and inapparent. Studies on seroconversion rates suggest that infants at the age of 1 to 2 years and adults from 16 to 50 years are more likely to be infected than others. Congenital infection may occur anytime during pregnancy but is more likely during the third trimester from a mother that is undergoing primary infection, or from one that has had CMV infection in the past and has developed a carrier state. Also, cervical excretion can be high during the third trimester of pregnancy and infection acquired by the infant at birth may not be detected, and is frequently asymptomatic. Since the virus is shed also in the saliva, respiratory secretions and urine, as well as colostrum, these are other possible sources of contagion. In a carrier, many tissues must be involved since recipients of kidneys, bone marrow, and blood from seropositive donors have been shown to acquire infection by this route. Cytotoxic immunosuppressants can cause CMV viremias that sometimes result in clinical evidence of the disease, e.g., interstitial pneumonia. Immunosuppression related to malignancies also predisposes to exacerbation of latent infection or to the acquisition of infection. Venereal transmission also has been implicated.

Clinical Manifestations

Clinical manifestations vary with the age, immune status and route of infection of the individual.

Neonatal infection results in the development of the classic fulminant syndrome at birth or shortly thereafter that is referred to as cytomegalic inclusion disease (CID). The onset is associated with lethargy, respiratory distress, convulsive seizures, development of a petechial rash, jaundice resulting from hepatosplenomegaly, and chorioretinitis. In survivors neurologic sequelae such as microcephaly, mental retardation, motor disability, and loss of hearing may become evident, and perhaps at a later time a carrier status also may evolve.

Postnatal infection is usually much less severe and visceral and nervous system involvement may be absent. Sometimes these infants may develop a mononucleosis-like illness, or a prolonged respiratory disease such as pharyngitis, bronchitis, pneumonia and croup, although the majority remain asymptomatic.

Adult infection is either subclinical or an infectious mononucleosis-like illness that can develop spontaneously, or as a result of blood transfusion, organ transplantation or immune suppression. The disease is characterized by prolonged fever (9 to 35 days) and mild elevation of liver function tests. Hepatosplenomegaly, adenitis, tonsillitis or pharyngitis are usually not striking features. Complications that occur only rarely include interstitial pneumonitis, hepatitis, granulomatous hepatitis, Guillain-Barré syndrome, meningoencephalitis, myocarditis, thrombocytopenia, hemolytic anemia, rubelliform rash, and chorioretinitis.

Diagnosis

Typical large inclusion-containing cells found in urine sediment are pathodiagnostic. They also are often found in tissues of asymptomatic individuals on routine autopsy. A characteristic CPE can be demonstrated in cell cultures when urine, tissues, or swabs from the oral cavity or cervix are cultured. A number of serodiagnostic tests are available and are valuable under certain circumstances. For example, the complement-fixation test is useful in detecting infection in the immunosuppressed patient and the macroglobulin immunofluorescent test in the diagnosis of congenital CMV when maternal IgG is present. Otherwise detection of antibody by anticomplement immunofluorescent or indirect immunofluorescent techniques is considered more sensitive.

EPSTEIN-BARR

Epstein-Barr Virus (EBV) is 180 to 200 nm in diameter and is characterized by its transforming and lymphoproliferative effects and ability to cause abnormal lymphocytes in infected individuals.

Epstein-Barr virus infections may be subclinical or manifest in a variety of acute or malignant illnesses depending upon the age, health and race of the individual. In children it may appear as a recurrent tonsillitis, or Burkitt's lymphoma, in adolescents and young adults as infectious mononucleosis (IM) and possibly in orientals as nasopharyngeal carcinoma.

Epidemiology

EBV is present in the nasopharynx and is transmitted by kissing or other contact with oral secretions. In many third world countries where hygiene is poor, infection can occur at a very young age (*e.g.*, 3 to 5 years).

The majority of individuals that become infected with EBV do so during adolescence or as young adults, and it is unusual to find primary infection occurring later. Subclinical convalescent carriers are an important source of contagion since the virus is excreted from the nasopharynx for at least 18 months following infection. In southeast Asia, the predisposition for nasopharyngeal carcinoma among certain groups of orientals, also has been associated with some HLA haplotypes and infection with EBV. Transmission by blood transfusion also occurs and may cause posttransfusion mononucleosis and sometimes postransfusion hepatitis.

Clinical Manifestations

The predominant disease associated with EBV infection is infectious mononucleosis. Others, such as recurrent tonsillitis, do not as yet enjoy the same etiological recognition. Correlative evidence has been established for the malignancies of African Burkitt's lymphoma and nasopharyngeal carcinoma although certain susceptibility patterns require further elucidation.

Infectious mononucleosis can develop following a prolonged incubation period that may be from 1 to 3 months but is somewhat less following transfusion, perhaps 3 to 5 weeks (fig. 37/9). The onset of the illness is insidious and is heralded by mild headache, sore throat, prolonged irregular fever and a pharyngitis that can be mild, as a follicular tonsillitis or severe, as an exudative pharyngitis. Some signs may be similar to acute necrotizing ulcerative gingivitis. However, the hallmark of this disease is the tender and enlarged lymph nodes that can involve the anterior and posterior cervical chains as well as the axillary, epitrochlear, inguinal, mediastinal and mesenteric nodes. Their size may vary and they are firm, discrete, and tender on palpation. Also, in approximately half of the patients splenomegaly is found, and another 10% of the patients may develop hepatomegaly, jaundice, rash and a palatal exanthem that is located at the junction of the hard and soft palates. Usually the sore throat persists for 3 to 5 days. The patients remain febrile for 10 to 14 days, following which the fever usually becomes low grade. Most patients recover after a 2 to 3 week period. As the illness resolves it is not unusual for symptoms to recrudesce between periods of well being.

Complications that can arise include development of an autoimmune hemolytic anemia that resolves in 2 months, and a usually mild, but sometimes severe, thrombocytopenia. Splenic rupture is a rare but painful consequence of IM that can be fatal. Only 1% of cases will develop neurologic complications and the most common is an acutely evolving and severe encephalitis distinguished as a cerebellitis, that clinically resembles aseptic meningitis. The majority of patients recover. Involvement of the liver is indicated by jaundice and elevation of hepatic enzymes, whereas ECG abnormalities, pericarditis and fatal myocarditis are seen with cardiac disease.

Recurrent cases of IM reported in the literature are few, however anecdotal evidence suggests that most go unreported. Known periods between exacerbation can vary from 18 months to 10 years. In one rare instance, IM has been antecedent to the development of Burkitt's lymphoma and in another, to leukemia. Thus the development of the malignant forms of EBV infection may not always be completely separate from the milder, self-resolving forms.

Recurrent exudative tonsillitis caused by EBV is characterized as recurring at least three times a year. Since the tonsils appear to be the nidus for latent infection with EBV it is noteworthy that

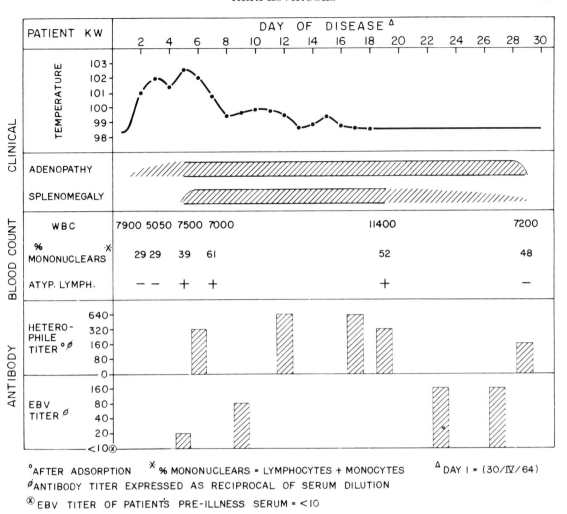

Figure 37/9. Time relationships between clinical features, hematologic changes, and antibody levels (Epstein-Barr virus and heterophile) in a typical case of infectious mononucleosis in an 18-year-old male patient. (Reproduced with permission from J. C. Niederman, R. W. McCollum, G. Henle, and W. Henle. 1968 Journal of the American Medical Association, **203**, 205–209).

there is a statistically significant difference between those individuals who acquire IM in later life and have tonsils, and those who have had tonsillectomies and remain refractory.

Postperfusion syndrome (posttransfusion mononucleosis) can occur following massive blood exchange, e.g., following heart surgery. Rather than the usual spectrum of symptoms the disease is more commonly characterized by fever, atypical lymphocytes and splenomegaly.

Posttransfusion hepatitis associated with EBV infection has occurred in patients in hemodialysis units, but is rarer than non-A, non-B hepatitis, cytomegalovirus-induced hepatitis, or that due to hepatitis B virus.

Burkitt's lymphoma (BL) has been associated with EBV infection in Africa, and less so in the United States. This phenomenon is not well under-stood but it is possible that a number of serotypes of EBV exist that not only differ in their oncogenic potential but also in their ability to be recovered from malignant cells. Also, since inherent predisposition exists for nasopharyngeal carcinoma, genetics may play a role in Burkitt's lymphoma. Age and health also may be factors in predisposition. Most children in Africa that acquire BL are young and sometimes malnourished and/or suffering from malaria and the disease that is evoked is predominantly that of oral tumors. In the United States, affected children may be older, generally healthier, are most often white, and usually present with abdominal rather than oral tumors. Whatever the underlying reasons may be, only with African BL is an association with EBV established.

Nasopharyngeal carcinomas are most commonly found in male Asians that possess the HLA haplotypes Bw46 and A9-B18. Patients not only produce an antibody response to EBV antigens but also contain EBV in their tumors. In North America, where the Chinese population tends to be more heterotypic, the incidence of this malignancy is less than in areas of Malaya, Singapore, and Hong Kong where these haplotypes predominate.

Diagnosis

Diagnosis of IM can be made by clinical, hematological and serological criteria that are pathognomonic for the disease. For example, the epidemic nature of this infection especially among adolescents and college students is a guideline to diagnosis when the typical clinical manifestations of IM appear in this age group. Presumptive diagnosis is usually readily made by detecting heterophile antibodies and atypical lymphocytes. When more definitive diagnosis is required, the detection of antibodies to EBV-associated antigens by indirect immunofluorescent or ELISA tests is possible. Diagnostic conclusions from these techniques are shown in table 37/1, and clinical and laboratory features of a typical case are illustrated in fig. 37/9.

Table 37/1
Interpretation of results of Epstein-Barr virus serology[a]

Serology				Interpretation
Capsid Ig	Capsid IgM	EBNA[b] Ig	EA Ig	
−				No evidence of infection, past or current
+				Past or current infection
↑*				Current primary infection
+	−			Probable past infection
+	+			Probable current or recent primary infection; or endogenous reactivation of a latent infection?
+		−		Current or recent primary infection
+		+		Probable past infection
+			+	Current or recent infection?
+	+	+	+	Endogenous reactivation of latent infection?
−	+			Technical error or current primary infection
−		+		Technical error or new finding?
−			+	Technical error or new finding?

[a] Reproduced with permission from R.S. Chang. 1980 *Infectious Mononucleosis.* G.K. Hall, Boston, Mass.
[b] EBNA Ig = antibody against the EBV-associated nuclear antigen; EA Ig = antibody against the EBV early antigen; + = positive; − = negative.
* Seroconversion.

Treatment

Supportive treatment such as salicylates or acetaminophen to relieve pain and fever are useful.

African BL responds well to combinations of cancer chemotherapeutics. Surgical intervention that is more frequently done in American BL may contribute to the poorer prognosis of cases treated in the United States.

HERPESVIRUS SIMIAE (B VIRUS)

Macaque monkeys (old world monkeys) carry *Herpesvirus simiae* in their saliva and other tissues, often without associated symptomology. Human acquisition is rare but almost always fatal. These have occurred through a monkey bite, or by contact with cell cultures derived from these animals. If immune globulin is not administered shortly after the injury the following typical symptoms may occur approximately 3 days after exposure. Vesicles develop at the site of the injury and regional lymphangitis and adenitis follow. About a week later neurological involvement is evident by motor and sensory abnormalities, development of an acute ascending paralysis, involvement of the respiratory center and death.

ADDITIONAL READING

APPELBAUM, E., KREPS, S., AND SUNSHINE, A. 1962 Herpes Zoster Encephalitis. Am J Med, **32**, 25.

BARINGER, J. R., AND SWOVELAND, P. 1973 Recovery of Herpes-Simplex Virus from Human Trigeminal Ganglions. N Engl J Med, **288**, 648.

BARTON, B. W., AND TOBIN, J. O. H. 1970 The Effect of Idoxuridine on the Excretion of Cytomegalovirus in Congenital Infection. Ann N Y Acad Sci, **173**, 90.

BETTS, R. F., GEORGE, S. D., RUNDELL, B. R., FREEMAN, R. B., AND DOUGLAS, R. G., JR. 1976 Comparative Activity of Immunofluorescent Antibody and Complement-Fixing Antibody in Cytomegalovirus Infection. J Clin Microbiol, **4**, 151.

BONKOWSKY, H. L., LEE, R. V., AND KLATSKIN, G. 1975 Acute Granulomatous Hepatitis: Occurrence in Cytomegalovirus Mononucleosis. JAMA, **233**, 1284.

BRUNELL, P. A. 1967 Varicella-Zoster Infections in Pregnancy. JAMA, **199**, 315.

CHANG, T. W. 1977 Genital Herpes and Type 1 Herpesvirus Hominis. JAMA, **238**, 155.

CRABTREE, J. A. 1968 Herpes Zoster Oticus. Laryngoscope, **78**, 1853.

DANIELS, C. A., LEGOFF, S. G., AND NOTKINS, A. L. 1975 Shedding of Infectious Virus/Antibody Complexes from Vesicular Lesions of Patients with Recurrent Herpes Labialis. Lancet, **2**, 524.

DIENSTAG, J. L., FEINSTONE, S. M., AND PURCELL, R. H. 1975 Experimental Infection of Chimpanzees with Hepatitis A Virus. J Infect Dis, **132**, 532.

DOUGLAS, R. G., JR. AND COUCH, R. B. 1970 A Prospective Study of Chronic Herpes Simplex Virus Infection and Recurrent Herpes Labialis in Humans. J Immunol, **104**, 289.

EAGLSTEIN, W. H., KATZ, R., AND BROWN, J. A. 1970 The Effects of Early Corticosteroid Therapy on the Skin Eruption and Pain of Herpes Zoster. JAMA, **211**, 1681.

ERON, L., KOSINSKI, K., AND HIRSCH, M. S. 1976 Hepatitis in an Adult Caused by Herpes Simplex Virus Type 1. Gastroenterology, **71**, 500.

FELDMAN, S., HUGHES, W. T., AND DANIEL, C. B. 1975 Varicella in Children with Cancer: Seventy-Seven Cases. Pediatrics, **56**, 388.

GHATAK, N. R., AND ZIMMERMAN, H. M. 1973 Spinal Ganglion in Herpes Zoster. Arch Pathol, **95**, 411.

GINSBERG, H. 1980 Cytomegalovirus (Salivary Gland Virus) Group. In *Microbiology*, Ed. 3, p. 1071, edited by B. D. Davis, R. Dulbecco, H. N. Eisen, and H. S. Ginsberg. Harper & Row, Hagerstown, Md.

HANSHAW, J. B. 1970 Developmental Abnormalities Associated with Congenital Cytomegalovirus Infection. In *Advances in Teratology*, Vol. 4, edited by D. H. M. Wollam. Academic Press, New York.

HARRIS, A. L., MEYER, R. J., AND BRODY, E. A. 1975 Cytomegalovirus-Induced Thrombocytopenia and Hemolysis in an Adult. Ann Intern Med, **83**, 670.

HAYES, K., DANKS, D. M., GIBAS, H., AND JACK, I. 1972 Cytomegalovirus in Human Milk. N Engl J Med, **287**, 177.

HO, H. 1979 Cytomegalovirus. In *Principles and Practice of Infectious Diseases*, p. 1307, edited by G. L. Mandell, R. G. Douglas Jr., and J. E. Bennett. John Wiley & Sons, New York.

JOHNSON, R., AND MILBOURNE, P. E. 1970 Central Nervous System Manifestations of Chickenpox. Can Med Assoc J, **102**, 831.

KANICH, R. E., AND CRAIGHEAD, J. E. 1966 Cytomegalovirus Infection and Cytomegalic Inclusion Disease in Renal Homotransplant Recipients. Am J Med, **40**, 874.

KLEMOLA, E. 1970 Hypersensitivity Reactions to Ampicillin in Cytomegalovirus Mononucleosis. Scand J Infect Dis, **2**, 29.

KLEMOLA, E., KAARIAINEN, L., VON ESSEN, R., HALTRA, K., KOIVUNIEMI, A., AND VON BONSDORFF, C. H. 1967 Further Studies on Cytomegalovirus Mononucleosis in Previously Healthy Individuals. Acta Med Scand, **182**, 311.

KLEMOLA, E., AND KAARIAINEN, L. 1965 Cytomegalovirus as a Possible Cause of a Disease Resembling Infectious Mononucleosis. Br Med J, **2**, 1099.

KLEMOLA, E., STENSTROM, R., AND VON ESSEN, R. 1972 Pneumonia as a Clinical Manifestation of Cytomegalovirus Infection in Previously Healthy Adults. Scand J Infect Dis, **4**, 7.

LANG, D. J., AND KUMMER, J. F. 1972 Demonstration of Cytomegalovirus in Semen. N Engl J Med, **287**, 756.

LAYZER, R. B. 1974 Neuralgia in Recurrent Herpes Simplex. Arch Neurol, **31**, 233.

LEONARD, J. C., AND TOBIN, J. O. H. 1971 Polyneuritis Associated with Cytomegalovirus Infections. Q J Med, **40**, 435.

LIGHT, L. J., AND LINNEMANN, C. C., JR. 1974 Neonatal Herpes Simplex Infection Following Delivery by Cesarean Section. Obstet Gynecol, **44**, 496.

MORBIDITY AND MORTALITY WEEKLY REPORTS. 1977 Zoster Immune Globulin and Varicella-Zoster Immune Globulin. October 28, 359.

MURRAY, H. W., KNOW, D. L., AND GREEN, W. R. 1977 Cytomegalovirus Retinitis in Adults: A Manifestation of Disseminated Viral Infection. Am J Med, **63**, 574.

NAHMIAS, A. J., JOSEY, W. E., AND OLESKE, J. M. 1975 Epidemiology of Cervical Cancer. In *Viral Infections of Humans—Epidemiology and Control*, p. 501, edited by A. Evans. Plenum Press, New York.

NAHMIAS, A. J., JOSEY, W. E., NAIR, Z. M., LUCE, C. F., AND DUFFEY, A. 1970 Antibodies to Herpesvirus Hominis Types 1 and 2 in Humans. I. Patients with Genital Herpetic Infections. Am J Epidemiol, **91**, 539.

NAHMIAS, A. J., SHORE, S. L., AND DELBUONO, I. 1974 Diagnosis by Immunofluorescence of Human Viral Infections with Emphasis on Herpes Simplex Virus. In *Viral Immunodiagnosis*, p. 157, edited by E. Kurstak, and R. Morissett. Academic Press, New York.

NISENBAUM, C., WALLIS, K., AND HERCZEG, E. 1969 Varicella Pneumonia in Children. Helv Paediatr Acta, **24**, 212.

OLSEN, L. C., KETUSINHA, R., MANSUWAN, P., AND SNITBHAN, R. 1970 Respiratory Tract Excretion of Cytomegalovirus in Thai Children. J Pediatr, **77**, 499.

RAO, N., WARUSZEWSKI, D. T., ARMSTRONG, J. A., ATCHISON, R. W., AND HO, M. 1977 Evaluation of the Anti-Complement Immunofluorescence Test in Cytomegalovirus Infection. J Clin Micro, **6**, 633.

ROIZMAN, B. 1974 Herpesvirus, Latency and Cancer: A Biochemical Approach. J Reticuloendothel Soc, **15**, 312.

SCHOOLEY, R. T., AND DOLIN, R. 1979 Epstein-Barr Virus (Infectious Mononucleosis). In *Principles and Practice of Infectious Diseases*, p. 1324, edited by G. L. Mandell, R. G. Douglas, Jr., and J. E. Bennett. John Wiley, New York.

SIEGEL, M. 1973 Congenital Malformations Following Chickenpox, Measles, Mumps and Hepatitis. JAMA, **226**, 1521.

SRABSTEIN, J. C., MORRIS, N., LARKE, R. P. B., DE SA, D. J., CASTELINO, B. B. AND SUM, E. 1974 Is there a Congenital Varicella Syndrome? J Pediatr, **84**, 239.

SUWANSIRIKUL, S., RAO, N., DOWLING, J. N., AND HO, M. 1977 Clinical Manifestations of Primary and Secondary Cytomegalovirus Infection. Arch Intern Med, **137**, 1026.

TIULA, E., AND LEINIKKI, P. 1972 Fatal Cytomegalovirus Infection in a Previously Healthy Boy with Myocarditis and Consumption Coagulopathy as Presenting Signs. Scand J Infect Dis, **1**, 57.

WARIS, E., RASANEN, O., KREUS, K. E., AND KREUS, R. 1972 Fatal Cytomegalovirus Disease in a Previously Healthy Adult. Scand J Infect Dis, **4**, 61.

WASHINGTON, J. A., (ED.) 1981 *Lab Procedures in Clinical Microbiology*, p. 855. Springer-Verlag, New York.

WILSON, J. F., MARSA, G. W., AND JOHNSON, R. E. 1972 Herpes Zoster in Hodgkin's Disease: Clinical, Histologic, and Immunologic Correlations. Cancer, **29**, 461.

WONG, T. W., AND WARNER, N. E. 1962 Cytomegalic Inclusion Disease in Adults. Arch Pathol, **74**, 403.

chapter 38

Adenoviruses and Parvoviruses

Memory Elvin-Lewis

INTRODUCTION

Adenoviruses (Adenoviridae) of the genus *Mastadenovirus* were originally isolated from respiratory secretions and adenoid tissues of man and animals. Human adenoviruses are characterized by their ability to induce latent infections in lymphoid tissues, particularly the tonsils and adenoids, to elicit tumors in unrelated animal hosts *e.g.*, baby hamsters, and to aid those parvoviruses referred to as adeno-associated viruses in their replication. Depending upon the age and immune status of the individual, specific serotypes have been associated with syndromes like acute respiratory disease (ARD), pharyngoconjunctival fever, conjunctivitis, epidemic keratoconjunctivitis, pneumonia, hemorrhagic cystitis, acute infectious diarrhea, and encephalitis and other diseases (table 38/1)

Causative Agents

Adenoviruses are relatively stable. They are resistant to ether and chloroform, and remain infective for weeks at −4 C, and for months at −25 C. They can be inactivated by heat (56 C for 5 minutes), formalin and treatment with trypsin or deoxyribonuclease.

The naked virions are icosahedral in symmetry, range in size from 60 to 90 nm and contain double-stranded DNA surrounded by a capsid with 252 capsomeres arranged as 12 pentons, from which projects a fiber, and 240 hexons. The fiber contains a major type-specific antigen and also is termed a toxin since it can cause cells in culture to clump, round up and detach from the growth surface. It also impairs their biosynthetic mechanisms so they are incapable of supporting the replication of related or unrelated viruses. However, antibodies to this fiber will only weakly neutralize viral infectivity. The hexons contain type-specific antigens that are important in differentiation of the adenoviruses into 35 distinct serotypes.

Viral Replication

Adenoviruses enter the cell by pinocytosis and release of the viral DNA occurs in the cytoplasm from which it is transported to the nucleus for replication. Utilizing host transcriptases, early mRNAs are transcribed from five parts of the genome and are translated in the cytoplasm into T antigens and enzymes necessary for nucleic acid replication. DNA replication is semiconservative and is initiated at either end of the molecule. As these replicates are formed a polycistronic late mRNA strand is transcribed that is cleaved and processed into monocistronic segments to be translated into structural proteins. Inclusions that appear in the nucleus represent accumulations of unassembled virions. With some serotypes (types 3, 4 and 7) crystalline lattices of adenoviruses can be detected in basophilic intranuclear inclusions, whereas with others (types 5 and 6) the eosinophilic crystals are only arginine-rich proteins.

Epidemiology

Adenoviruses are ubiquitous and usually are acquired by contact with infected respiratory secretions, often early in life. They may establish asymptomatic latent infections in the tonsils and adenoids of those they infect and this serves as a reservoir for contagion to susceptible individuals. Specific serotypes that are associated with particular disease syndromes differ somewhat in their epidemiology; for example, strains causing acute respiratory disease in young adults are readily transmitted in the crowded conditions often found in military camps. Those that cause respiratory or eye infections may be transmitted to dental personnel by aerosols generated during dental treatment.

Clinical Manifestations

Since adenovirus infections can be quite specific their various syndromes will be discussed separately.

Table 38/1
Diseases caused by Adenoviruses[a]

Group Effected	Syndromes	Common Causal Adenovirus Serotypes
Infants	Coryza, pharyngitis (most asymptomatic)	1,2,5
Children	Upper respiratory disease	1,2,4–6
	Pharyngoconjunctival fever	3,7
	Hemorrhagic cystitis	11,21
Young adults	Acute respiratory disease and pneumonia	3,4,7
Adults	Epidemic keratoconjunctivitis	8,19
Immunocompromised	Pneumonia with dissemination	34,35
	CNS disease including encephalitis	7,7a,12

[a] Reproduced with permission from G. L. Mandell, R. G. Douglas, Jr. and J. E. Bennett. 1979 *Principles and Practice of Infectious Diseases* John Wiley, New York.

Respiratory infections that occur in children usually appear as a mild pharyngitis or tracheitis, however, adenovirus type 7 infection in infants may cause a fulminant bronchiolitis and pneumonia. In young adults the illness known as "acute respiratory disease," or ARD, is a tracheobronchitis caused by adenoviruses types 4 and 7 and is prevalent among army recruits. Cough, fever, sore throat and rhinorrhea persist for 3 to 5 days and are accompanied by pharyngitis and rales.

Pharyngoconjunctival fever occurs in small epidemics among children, particularly those residing in groups, as in summer camps. It is characterized by an acute onset with symptoms of conjunctivitis, pharyngitis, rhinitis, and cervical adenitis with a mild fever of 38 C that last for 3 to 5 days.

Epidemic keratoconjunctivitis was once referred to as "shipyard workers conjunctivitis" because of its prevalence among these workers. This was due to ocular trauma from paint and rust chips. Following an incubation period of 4 to 24 days there is sudden onset of conjunctivitis with excessive lacrimation, periorbital edema and later superficial corneal opacity, but there is no ulceration and recovery is usually complete.

Adenovirus types 3 and 7 may produce a bilateral conjunctivitis (fig. 38/1) with associated preauricular adenopathy, excessive lacrimation and serous exudation, that may last from 1 to 4 weeks. As this resolves, a keratitis with corneal involvement can develop that may cause temporary visual disturbances that can last for months or even years.

Adenovirus types 11 and 21 may cause a hemorrhagic cystitis in children. It is more common among males than females. The condition is characterized as a gross hematuria that persists for about 3 days with symptoms of dysuria and urinary frequency continuing somewhat longer.

Adenoviruses have been associated with other syndromes, but to a lesser degree. These include acute infectious diarrhea, pericarditis, chronic interstitial fibrosis, rubelliform illness, congenital anomalies, and neurologic disease.

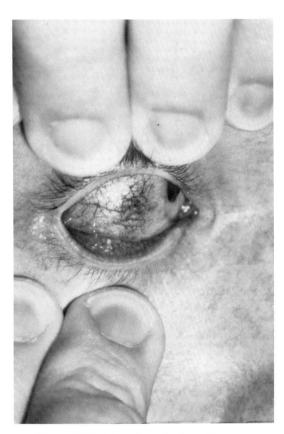

Figure 38/1. Adenovirus infection of the eye.

Diagnosis

The distinctive symptoms associated with specific epidemiological events are often helpful in diagnosing adenovirus infections on a clinical basis alone. For purposes of verification, the viruses are readily retrieved from specimens from the eye, nasopharynx or urine by culture in primary and diploid simian and human cell lines where they elicit a characteristic cytopathogenic effect (CPE). They can be typed by specific neutralizing antisera. To detect infection rapidly, especially with ocular infections, specifically labeled fluorescent antibody is used for staining of conjunctival or corneal scrapings.

Treatment

There are no specific drugs utilized in the treatment of adenovirus infections. In the military, adenovirus types 4 and 7 are administered to recruits in an enteric capsule for the purposes of immunization. By this alternate route of administration, these strains have proven excellent immunogens without causing respiratory symptoms. This technique has decreased the amount of ARD in the military.

ADENO-ASSOCIATED VIRUS AND OTHER PARVOVIRUSES

Adeno-associated viruses (AAV) are members of the parvovirus group. They are small (18 to 26 nm) icosahedral, naked virions containing a single-stranded DNA that may exist as a positive or negative strand. These viruses can only replicate in cells infected with helper adenoviruses, although they inhibit the replication of this helper once they initiate their own replication. Four serotypes of AAV have been distinguished and, although frequently associated with their helper viruses and the diseases they cause, they do not appear to affect the disease process except perhaps to diminish the quantity of the adenovirus produced.

Unlike AAV, other parvoviruses are not defective in their natural hosts, but instead require concurrent replication of host DNA as it occurs in the S phase. In animal models, such as pregnant mice and rats, they have been found to elicit a variety of congenital defects like mongolism in the offspring. Animals infected soon after birth may show a variety of dental abnormalities including cementomas, odontomas and absent or malformed third molars.

PARVOVIRUS-LIKE AGENTS

A parvovirus-like agent known as the Norwalk-like agent has been associated with a very common acute gastrointestinal disease of worldwide distribution. These agents are 23 to 25 nm in diameter, and are naked, icosahedral virions. Nucleic acid has not been isolated from these agents, however, their resistance to heat, acid and ether suggest a relationship to parvoviruses. A number of antigenic types have been distinguished in this group.

Epidemiology

The disease occurs most frequently from September to March, and affects all age groups and any type of population. Person-to-person transfer likely occurs by the fecal-oral route.

Pathogenesis

Infection acquired by ingestion is restricted to the jejunum where villi are blunted, and round cells and polymorphonuclear leukocytes infiltrate the lamina propria. This histopathology develops about 24 hours after infection and disappears after 2 weeks or more. There is a transient malabsorption syndrome affecting D-xylose and fat. Also brush-border enzymes are affected during this period. The precise mechanisms of viral induction of diarrhea and vomiting are unknown.

Clinical Manifestations

Following an incubation period of 24 to 48 hours, symptoms of nausea and abdominal cramps develop gradually or abruptly. Vomiting and diarrhea occurs and may be accompanied by myalgia, malaise, headache, and low grade fever.

Diagnosis

Clinical and epidemiological data aid in the diagnosis, and confirmation can be done by utilizing immune adherence assays or radioimmunoassays.

Treatment

The disease usually resolves without serious consequences and thus most forms of therapy are supportive to control the headache, diarrhea and vomiting. In the debilitated patient, fluid replacement orally is usually adequate, although sometimes intravenous replacement therapy may be necessary. Since the disease may be waterborne, measures to prevent contamination from these sources may help control the spread of the infection.

ADDITIONAL READING

BAER, P. N., AND KILHAM, L. 1974 Comparison of Dental Defects in Hamsters Infected with MVM and H-1 Viruses. J Dent Res, **53**, Special Issue, 158.

BAUM, S. G. 1979 Adenovirus. In *Principles and Practice of Infectious Diseases*, p. 1353, edited by G. L. Mandell, R. G. Douglas, Jr., J. E. Bennett. John Wiley, New York.

BRANDT, C. D., HYUN, W. K., VARGOSKO, A. J., *et al.* 1969 Infections in 18,000 Infants and Children in a Controlled Study of Respiratory Tract Disease. I. Adenovirus Pathogenicity in Relation to Serologic Type and Illness Syndrome. Am J Epidemiol, **90**, 484.

BUCHTA, R. M. 1974 Membranous Conjunctivitis Due to Adenovirus Type 7 Infection. Clin Pediatr, **13**, 232.

DOLIN, R. 1979 Norwalk-Like Agents of Gastroenteritis. In *Principles* and *Practice of Infectious Diseases*, p. 1364, edited by G. L. Mandell, R. G. Douglas, Jr., J. E. Bennett. John Wiley, New York.

HIERHOLZER, J. C., AND PUMAROLA, A. 1976 Antigenic Characterization of Intermediate Adenovirus 14-11 Strains Associated with Upper Respiratory Illness in a Military Camp. Infect Immun, **13**, 354.

HUEBNER R. J., ROWE, W. P., WARD T. G., *et al.* 1954

Adenoidalpharyngeal-Conjunctival Agents: A Newly Recognized Group of Common Viruses of the Respiratory System. N Engl J Med, **251,** 1077.

HUEBNER R. J., ROWE, W. P., AND LANE W. T. 1962 Oncogneic Effects in Hamsters of Human Adenoviruses Types 12 and 18. Proc Natl Acad Sci USA, **48,** 2051.

LIPTON, H., NATHANSON, N., AND HODOUS, J. 1973 Enteric Transmission of Parvoviruses: Pathogenesis of Rat Virus Infection in Adult Rats. Am J Epidemiol, **96,** 443.

OTSUKI, Y. 1973 Virus-Like Particles Observed in Normal Tissues and Adenovirus 12-Induced Tumors in Hamsters. Gann, **64,** 609.

PHILIPSON, L., PETTERSSON, U., LINDBERG, U. 1975 Molecular Biology of Adenoviruses. *Virology Monographs 14.* Springer-Verlag, New York.

ROWE, W. P., HUEBNER, R. J., GILLMORE L. K., *et al.* 1953 Isolation of a Cytopathogenic Agent from Human Adenoids Undergoing Spontaneous Degeneration in Tissue Culture. Proc Soc Exp Biol Med, **84,** 570.

SAHLER, O. J., AND WILFERT, C. M. 1974 Fever and Petechiae with Adenovirus Type 7 Infection. Pediatrics, **53,** 233.

SCHLESINGER, R. W. 1969 Adenoviruses: The Nature of the Virion and Controlling Factors in Productive or Abortive Infection and Tumorigenesis. Adv Virus Res, **14,** 1.

SCHWARTZ, H. S., VASTINE, D. W., YAMASHIROYA, H., AND WEST, C. E. 1976 Immunofluorescent Detection of Adenovirus Antigen in Epidemic Keratoconjunctivitis. Invest Ophthalmol, **15,** 199.

SOBEL, G., ARONSON, B., AND ARONSON, S. 1956 Pharyngoconjunctival fever. Am J Dis Child, **92,** 596.

TOOLAN, H. W. 1972 The Parvoviruses. Progr Exp Tumor Res, **16,** 410.

chapter 39

Papovaviruses: Papilloma Virus and Polyoma Virus

Memory Elvin-Lewis

INTRODUCTION

Papovaviruses (Papoviridae) are small, naked icosahedrons 45 to 55 nm in diameter that contain circular, double-stranded DNA enclosed in a capsid with 72 capsomeres. Members of this family are very resistant to heat inactivation and formalin, which explains why the potentially oncogenic monkey strain SV40 survived in what were thought to be formalin-killed virus vaccines against various viral infections. Two genera have been isolated in man and animals. The papilloma viruses are responsible for causing warts in humans and papillomatosis in a number of animals. Other papovaviruses, of the genus *Polyomavirus*, are known to have oncogenic potential in animals and those isolated from man have been associated with a slow virus infection, progressive multifocal leukoencephalopathy (PML), from Wiskott-Aldrich syndrome, and as a viruria in immunosuppressed individuals.

PAPILLOMA VIRUSES

The human *Papillomavirus* can produce flesh-colored, small hyperplastic papules that are flat or filiform in shape and depending on their location are referred to as plane warts, verruca vulgaris, or plantar warts, and condylomata acuminata.

Epidemiology

Warts are a common infection, primarily of childhood, acquired through direct contact: the virus enters through minor abrasions of the skin. Warts may be found on the fingers (fig. 39/1), the palms (palmar), the soles of the feet (plantar), or other exposed flat surfaces of the body. In adults, they also can appear on the genitalia as condylomata acuminata and are spread through venereal contact.

Pathogenesis

Papilloma viruses gain entrance to the keratinized layers of the skin through minor abrasions where they infect single epidermal cells which are stimulated to divide to form a well delineated hyperplastic papule that extends to the depth of the basal layer. Acanthosis, parakeratosis and hyperkeratosis are evident and viruses can be located in the cytoplasm and nuclei of infected cells. Large vacuolated cells that appear in the upper stratum Malpighi and granular layer are pathodiagnostic since they do not occur in nonviral papillomas. Their location also renders them free from most of the immune mechanisms of the body.

Clinical Manifestations

Clinical evidence of infection usually does not occur until the virus has replicated for 1 to 6 months. Common warts (verruca vulgaris) are more common on the dorsal surfaces of the hands or periungual regions, appear gray, brown or flesh-colored and can reach a size of 1 to 10 mm, but they also can coalesce to form a larger lesion. Filiform warts are a variant of this type and protrude from the skin of the neck and face in small, 1 to 10 mm projections. Flat warts (verrucae planae) are smaller than the other types, and occur on the face or extensor surfaces of the arm as discrete, multiple, flesh-colored or slightly brown, papules. They may be spread by shaving. Plantar and palmar warts are elevated or flat lesions which can be quite painful. Capillaries that appear as punctate dots may be scattered over their surface, which distinguishes these warts from corns and callouses. Condylomata acuminata, or venereal warts, are apparent on the genitalia or perineum. They coalesce to form large pink-to-brown masses and should not be confused with the moist gray sessile lesions, condylomata lata, or secondary syphilis. Unlike other types of

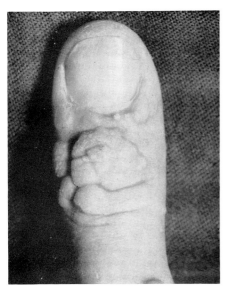

Figure 39/1. Verruca vulgaris in a child. (AFIP AMH 10737-B.)

warts, condylomata acuminata have a tendency to undergo malignant transformation.

Diagnosis

Warts are usually diagnosed on a clinical basis only. In young lesions, the large vacuolated cells may be seen in biopsies. They should be distinguished from seborrhaic keratosis or molluscum contagiosum and also condylomata lata. The virus will grow in monkey kidney and human embryo fibroblast cells which they transform into epithelioid cells; however this is not done for diagnostic purposes.

Treatment

Warts may spontaneously disappear leaving no trace. Electro- or cryosurgery often is used to remove the wart, or corrosive topical agents like salicyclic acid are used to expose the virus to the immune system of the body. For the treatment of condylomata acuminata that are refractory to this substance, topical podophyllum is useful. Warts resistant to either of these medicaments may respond to topical 5-fluorouracil.

POLYOMA VIRUSES

Strains of the genus *Polyomavirus*, designated JC, COL and a hybrid SV40-PML virus, have been associated with a relatively uncommon demyelinating disease, progressive multifocal leukoencephalopathy, of the brain of adults who have some concurrent chronic condition that impairs their immune responses.

Epidemiology

Apparently these viruses, that are somewhat smaller than papilloma viruses, are ubiquitous agents that are acquired early in life and remain in some latent form, or slowly replicate in semipermissive cells when conditions are appropriate. Most patients are predisposed by concurrent myeloproliferative neoplasms such as Hodgkin's disease or chronic lymphocytic leukemia; other cases have occurred in patients with concurrent carcinomas, sarcoid, tuberculosis, Whipple's disease or systemic lupus erythematosis; whereas another was found following immunosuppression prior to transplantation. With the elimination of SV40 from poliovirus vaccines, exposure to this virus has been diminished.

Pathogenesis

The actual pathogenesis of the infection(s) has not been elucidated, however, in diseased brains altered oligodendrocytes, usually at the border between the white matter and the cortex of the cerebrum are observed. The early lesions enlarge, coalesce and may become necrotic. Late lesions contain few oligodendrocytes but the virus can, by immunofluorescent techniques, be located in astrocytes, macrophages and giant astrocytes that are pleomorphic with hyperchromatic nuclei that resemble pleomorphic glioblastomas.

Clinical Manifestations

Most patients that develop the disease are hyperergic adults. The condition develops rapidly and, following a variety of neurologic symptoms that progressively become more and more severe, results in death in 2 to 4 months. Only in rare instances, in the more prolonged cases, do remissions occur. The symptoms are initially like those of other slow infections, and can include partial paralysis, difficulty in speaking, swallowing, or walking, cortical blindness and certain personality changes. As the disease progresses quadriparesis, severe dementia and coma are usual.

Treatment

Some cases have gone into remission by the use of adenine or cytosine arabinoside, but there are no controlled studies to establish their efficacy.

ADDITIONAL READING

AHMED, M. M., AND MUKHERJEE, D. K. 1974 Virus-Like Particles in Human Laryngeal Papilloma. An Ultrastructural Study. Experientia, **30,** 361.

BOYLE, W. F., RIGGS, J. L., OSHIRO, L. S., AND LENNETTE, E. H. 1973 Electron Microscopic Identification of Papovavirus in Laryngeal Papilloma. Laryngoscope, **83,** 1102.

DAVIS, B. D., DULBECCO, R., EISEN, H. N., AND GINS-

BERG, H. S. 1980 *Microbiology*, Ed. 3, p. 1355. Harper & Row, New York.

FENNER, F. J., AND WHITE, D. O. 1976 *Medical Virology*, Ed. 2, p. 485. Academic Press, New York.

GREER, K. 1979 *Papillomavirus* (Warts). In *Principles and Practice of Infectious Diseases*, p. 1362, edited by G. L. Mandell, R. G. Douglas, Jr. and J. E. Bennett. John Wiley, New York.

KOVI, J., TILLMAN, R. L., AND LEE, S. M. 1974 Malignant Transformation of Condyloma Acuminatum. A Light Microscopic and Ultrastructural Study. Am J Clin Path, **61,** 702.

LEHRICH, J. R. 1979 *Polyomavirus* (Progressive Multifocal Leukoencephalopathy). In *Principles and Practice of Infectious Diseases*, p. 1436, edited by G. L. Mandell, R. G. Douglas, Jr. and J. E. Bennett. John Wiley, New York.

MENDELSON, C. G., AND KLIGMAN, A. M. 1961 Isolation of Wart Virus in Tissue Culture. Successful Reinoculation into Humans. Arch Derm, **83,** 559.

chapter 40

Viral Hepatitis:Hepatitis A, Hepatitis B and Hepatitis C (Non-A, Non-B)

Memory Elvin-Lewis

INTRODUCTION

Hepatitis may be caused by several different viruses, all of which produce illnesses that are very similar clinically. The names of the various forms were originally derived from the supposed routes of transmission, but since it has been shown that the different forms may be transmitted by multiple routes, it is preferable to use the terms hepatitis A for what was previously called infectious hepatitis, hepatitis B for what was called serum hepatitis and non-A, non-B hepatitis for a form that is caused by neither hepatitis A nor B viruses and frequently follows transfusion with infected blood.

HEPATITIS A

Causative Agent

Infectious hepatitis or hepatitis A (HAV) is caused by a small (27 nm), naked, icosahedral virus that contains single-stranded linear RNA and resembles a picornavirus. It elicits an acute febrile illness, usually characterized by jaundice, that may range from a mild to a severely disabling form with several months of convalescence.

Hepatitis A virus has physical and morphological properties similar to an enterovirus. It replicates in the cytoplasm but unlike picornaviruses is difficult to grow in cell cultures. It is similar to the enteroviruses in being stable to pH 3.0, ether and alcohol, but is somewhat more resistant to most disinfection procedures in that it requires treatment with chlorine at 10 to 15 ppm or 1:400 formalin for 3 days at 37 C before it is inactivated. However, it is readily destroyed by normal autoclaving, boiling and dry heat regimens.

Epidemiology

Epidemics of hepatitis A occur in cyclical waves (as susceptibles accumulate) in communities throughout the world. It is usually transmitted by the fecal-oral route and widespread outbreaks have been linked to fecal contamination of water supplies, contaminated shellfish or to infected food handlers. Only rarely has this virus been transmitted parenterally and, as such, it differs in its primary mode of transmission from other hepatitis viruses.

Outbreaks are prevalent in young school-age children, particularly in communities or institutions where sanitation may be poor and crowding prevalent. Also secondary outbreaks within a family unit exposed to the infectious child are common, since studies have shown that virus is usually shed in the prodromal stage and first 2 weeks of the disease. Unlike hepatitis B, long-term, chronic carriers are unknown.

Seroconversion rates vary, depending upon the socioeconomic status of the individual. For example, in rural areas of the developing third world most individuals are seroconverted by the time they are adults, whereas in the United States the incidence may be as low as 20%. Generally, as sanitation improves, the seroconversion rates are lowered.

Pathogenesis

The incubation period may be from 2 to 7 weeks. Early in this period (1 to 2 weeks) the virus can be found in the cytoplasm of liver hepatocytes where it presumably replicates. During the early icteric stage examination of liver biopsies shows hepatocytes that are acidophilic and swollen, Kupffer cells are prominent, the lobular architecture distorted, and there is a marked monocytic infiltration at the portal areas and cellular degeneration. In about one-half of the cases, bilary thrombi are present and virus is excreted through the bile ducts to the feces. At about the same time, serum transaminase levels are elevated. Visceral involvement also may be evident in the pathological changes that can be seen in the kidney, stomach and intestine. In the

413

acute phase, antibodies to the virus antigen are predominantly IgM. During convalescence IgG predominates.

Clinical Manifestations

After the incubation period, a preicteric stage develops that lasts for 2 weeks and is followed by a 1- to 3-week icteric period. During the preicteric state, symptoms such as fatigue, anorexia, nausea, abdominal discomfort and low grade fever are prominent along with a swollen liver and spleen. The transition to the icteric stage is gradual; the patient may be afebrile, and in 20% of the cases the liver and spleen are palpable. The feces is beige to light brown and liver function tests are abnormal (*e.g.*, transaminase, bilirubin, thymol turbidity, cephalin flocculation and alkaline phosphatase). Recovery usually takes a month or more and fatalities are unusual (about 1%) except when the course is fulminant.

The typical course of hepatitis A virus excretion, symptoms, and antibody development is illustrated in figure 40/1.

Diagnosis

Under usual conditions diagnosis is made using clinical criteria and the demonstration of abnormal values in liver function tests consistent with this type of infection. For experimental purposes a number of serological tests are available that include determination of anti-HA titers (especially of the IgM class) by complement fixation, immune adherence hemagglutination, immune electron microscopy and radioimmunoassay. Differential diagnosis should eliminate hepatitis B, infectious mononucleosis, leptospirosis, relapsing fever and malaria. Table 40/1 illustrates the differentiating characteristics of hepatitis types A and B.

Treatment and Prevention

Most cases recover uneventfully within a period of 7 weeks and only a few individuals develop chronic, active hepatitis.

The administration of immune globulin has been found to reduce the severity of symptoms and, if given at onset, may prevent development of the icteric stage. In contacts, immunoglobulin prophylaxis is useful in preventing the development of the disease. Usually this type of prophylactic therapy is restricted to close contacts such as household members.

Although isolation of ill persons is not necessary, care must be taken in the proper decontamination of exposed utensils, bedding and clothing. Medical

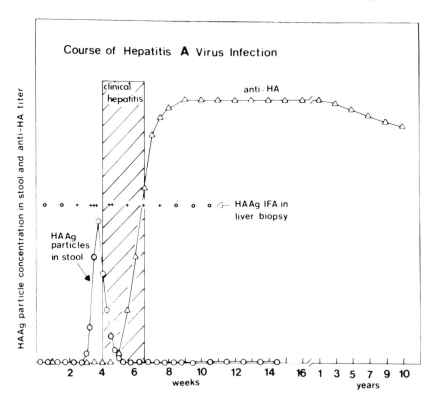

Figure 40/1. Schema of hepatitis A viral markers in blood, feces and liver during the course of HAV infection. (Reproduced with permission from G. L. Mandell *et al.* 1979 *Principles and Practice of Infectious Diseases*. John Wiley, New York.)

Table 40/1
Differentiating characteristics of hepatitis types A and B[a]

Property	Type A	Type B
Usual transmission	Fecal-oral	Parenteral inoculation[b]
Characteristic incubation period[c]	15–40 days	60–160 days
Type of onset	Acute	Insidious
Fever >38°	Common	Uncommon
Seasonal incidence	Autumn and winter	Year-round
Age incidence	Commonest in children and young adults	All ages; commonest in adults
Size of virus	27 nm	42 nm
Viruses in feces	Incubation period and acute phase	Not demonstrated
Virus in blood	Incubation period and acute phase	Incubation period and acute phase; may persist for years
Appearance of HBsAg	Absent	30–50 days after infection
Detection of HBsAg		Blood (less often in feces, urine, semen, and bile)
Duration of HBsAg		60 days to years
Prophylactic Value of γ-globulin	Good	Good if titer of anti-HBsAg is high

[a] Reproduced with permission from B. D. Davis *et al.* 1980 *Microbiology*, Ed. 3. Harper & Row, Hagerstown, Md.
[b] Parental injection is probably not the predominant mode of transmission in developing countries where the means of spread is unknown.
[c] Considerable overlapping in the duration of incubation periods for types A and B has been noted in volunteers as well as in patients during epidemics, *i.e.*, as long as 85 days for type A hepatitis and as short as 20 days for type B hepatitis.

personnel should wear gloves to handle excreta and to take blood. It also is recommended that medical or dental personnel with active hepatitis A infection curtail their professional activities until the illness has completely resolved.

HEPATITIS B

Causative Agent

Serum hepatitis or hepatitis B (HBV) infection is caused by a small (42 nm) enveloped, icosahedral virus that contains a circular, double-stranded DNA, although one strand is shorter than the other leaving a single-strand region of perhaps one third of the circle length. Hepatitis B virus produces an insidious infection that varies in severity from subclinical to an fulminant form of hepatic necrosis that can be fatal (fig. 40/2).

The infectious form of the virus is believed to be the Dane particle that is about 42 nm in diameter. Its envelope contains hepatitis B surface antigen (HBsAg) and surrounds an inner core with icosahedral symmetry that contains DNA, hepatitis B core antigen (HBcAg) and a DNA polymerase. Virion replication that takes place in hepatocytes is usually incomplete, and core antigen can be detected in the nucleus, whereas surface antigen is found in the cytoplasm. Predominant forms appearing in the blood of infected persons are those aggregations of subunits containing surface antigens that appear as either small 22-nm spherical particles or filaments about 200 nm long, but of the same diameter; the Dane particle is the least com-

mon form. The surface antigen is a complex molecule that contains at least four polypeptides and four glycoproteins of various molecular sizes and lipid, and alterations in these are responsible for the antigenic differences that have been detected among strains. Antibodies to this antigen (HBsAg) are protective in nature. A large protein (probably a complex of many antigens) referred to as the "e" antigen (HBeAg) also occurs in infected blood and sera of chronic carriers and may represent an antigen-antibody complex. Hepatitis B virus has not been cultured in tissue culture and thus the nature of its replicative cycle is not known.

The resistance of HBV to many disinfection and sterilization regimens has made its destruction paramount in the development of sterilization procedures in dentistry. This problem is usually complicated by the protection provided by blood on instruments. Thus, the time for autoclaving at 121 C has been extended to 30 minutes in spite of the claims that 100 C for 10 minutes will destroy virus infectivity. The use of disinfection agents is discouraged. Sterilization procedures have been discussed in Chapter 7.

Epidemiology

It has been estimated that at least 300,000 cases of clinical hepatitis occur each year in the United States, although only about 20% are reported. Also, it is likely that 5 to 10 times more cases are subclinical and remain undetected. In a normal population, the overall seroconversion rate approximates 3%, however, in the age group between 15 and 29

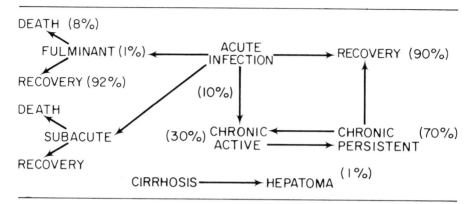

Figure 40/2. Possible outcome of Hepatitis B virus infection. (Reproduced with permission from L. S. Barker, R. J. Gerety and E. Tabor. 1978 The Immunology of the Hepatitis Viruses. In *Advances in Internal Medicine*, Vol. 23, edited by G. H. Stollerman *et al.* Copyright © 1978 by Year Book Medical Publishers, Chicago.)

years, the estimated attack rate is approximately 80/100,000. In American populations it has been found that at least 0.3% carry the specific surface antigen (HBsAg) and an additional 4 to 14% carry its antibody (anti-HBs). However, in tropical Africa, Southeast Asia and Oceania, most adults carry the antibody, and at least 20% are possible carriers.

Also studies among United States medical and dental personnel indicate that seroconversion rates among them are higher than the general population, but vary with the study reporting the data. Therefore, 13 to 21% of dentists, 21% of oral surgeons and 22% of general surgeons surveyed have been found seropositive. Epidemiological data also has suggested that carriers within the dental and medical professions have been responsible for transmitting their infection to multiple patient contacts.

Acquisition of the virus is usually by contact with blood, and, in the absence of parenteral exposure, through contact with other body fluids such as saliva, semen, vaginal secretions, feces, urine, menstrual blood and breast milk. Testing for HBsAg in blood used for transfusion has eliminated most, but not all, cases acquired through blood transfusion. Sporadic cases can result from individuals who have received blood products, employees of renal dialysis centers, drug addicts, and among surgeons and dentists who accidentally injure themselves during surgery. Infants can acquire infection perinatally, especially during the third trimester and, if chronically infected, can serve as reservoirs. Another type of chronic carrier is created when an individual is infected with a low dose of the virus and develops a mild disease. It is therefore possible for a dentist who acquires infection through minor trauma to develop a subclinical or mild, undiagnosed infection and thus become an inadvertent carrier.

The means by which institutionalized children and the mentally infirm are prone to infection with HBV is not understood. The fecal-oral route has been implicated but fecal excretion of the virus is low in the absence of gastrointestinal bleeding. However, those that are institutionalized frequently have poor oral hygiene, and if gingival bleeding is induced by periodontal disease, xerostomia due to medication or poor toothbrushing habits, the predisposition to spurious contagion exists. Seizures are not uncommon among certain types of institutionalized individuals and saliva is readily disseminated during this event. Should patients with a predisposition for hepatitis come in contact with contaminated saliva of a carrier in this condition, infection could be achieved simply from hand to mouth. Also, although care is taken to prevent toothbrush exchanges in these types of institutions, should it occur, this could be another mechanism by which infection takes place. At least in monkeys, the simple act of toothbrushing followed by oral exposure to hepatitis virus has elicited the disease.

Clinical Manifestations

The incubation period of hepatitis B depends upon the dose of virus acquired by the patient. The general axiom is the higher the dose, the shorter the incubation period and the more likely that icteric hepatitis will develop. The incubation period can vary from 1 to 7 months, but most often hepatitis will develop anytime between 2 to 4 months. Acute hepatitis can take several forms. Approximately 20% of the cases will develop a maculopapular rash, urticaria, arthralgias, arthritis, and fever several days to weeks before liver disease is evident. These may disappear in 48 hours or remain for over a week. Others will develop a mild nonicteric form of hepatitis that is characterized by anorexia, headache, malaise, nausea and vomiting, and a slightly elevated temperature. These symptoms may be associated with pain in the right upper quadrant, dark urine and light clay-colored stools. Should an icteric phase develop, jaundice and scleric icterus can develop that is also sometimes accompanied by pruritis and arthralgia. The liver and spleen are palpable, and cervical lymph nodes may be enlarged. Recovery can vary with age; in adults it can be as long as 4 to 6 weeks, whereas in children it can be as short as 2 weeks. On rare occasions a fulminant disease develops resulting in hepatic failure, encephalopathy, and death. Chronic active hepatitis is another grave syndrome that can progress to cirrhosis, hepatic failure and death. In milder cases, hepatitis can persist for 3 to 4 months. A number of predisposing factors such as alcoholism, corticosteroid therapy during acute illness or early ambulation may cause relapses to develop. Usually the prognosis becomes more unfavorable as the age of the patient and the severity of the infection increase.

Pathogenesis and Pathology

Three types of HBV infections exist that are characterized by the antigens and antibodies that are detected and whether or not clinical or subclinical disease occurs. When clinical hepatitis results HBsAg, HBeAg and Dane particles can be detected prior to symptoms and during the clinical disease. During this interval, HBsAg is present longer than

HBeAg, while Dane particle reaches its peak titer at the onset of symptoms and falls off rapidly thereafter. During the clinical disease anti-HBc appears and rises to its highest titer; during convalescence it slowly diminishes, but may be detectable for several years. Also during convalescence, anti-HBs appears and reaches a peak about 10 weeks after infection, which is the same time that anti-HBe makes a brief appearance. Like anti-HBc, anti-HBs antibodies can persist for several years (fig. 40/3).

Two types of subclinical infections are known. In self-limited infections where HBsAg is not detected, antibodies to HBs and HBc begin to appear shortly before disease is indicated by changes in transaminase levels. These antibodies continue to rise until after symptoms disappear, and remain detectable for several years thereafter. Unlike patients with clinical disease, anti-HBs can be detected earlier and achieve a higher titer than those of anti-HBc (fig. 40/4). In patients with persistent infection, HBsAg rises to a higher titer before subclinical hepatitis develops (fig. 40/5), and remains at this level indefinitely. Unlike other types of hepatitis, antibodies to this antigen cannot be detected alone but may be present as an antigen-antibody complex. Also, the Dane particle that is detected prior

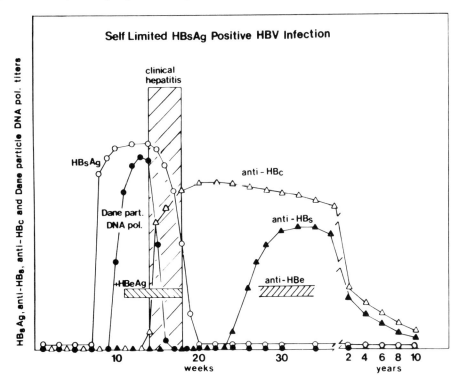

Figure 40/3. Schema of hepatitis B viral markers in the blood during the course of self-limited HBsAg-positive infection. (Reproduced with permission from G. L. Mandell *et al.* 1979 *Principles and Practice of Infectious Diseases* John Wiley, New York.)

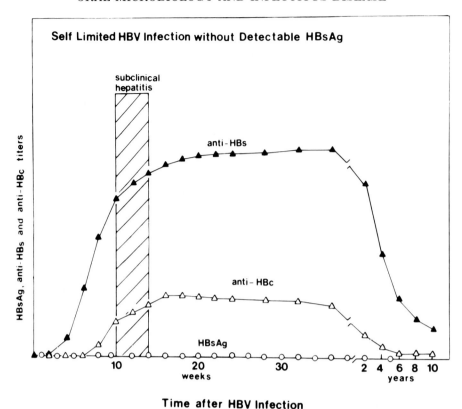

Figure 40/4. Schema of hepatitis B viral markers in the blood during the course of self-limited HBV infection without the appearance of detectable HBsAg in the blood. (Reproduced with permission from G. L. Mandell *et al.* 1979 *Principles and Practice of Infectious Diseases.* John Wiley, New York.)

to subclinical disease and reaches its highest titer at the onset of symptoms rapidly drops to lower levels and is present in varying amounts during convalescence and may persist for years. Antibody-to-core antigen (anti-HBc) begins to rise at the beginning of subclinical symptoms, reaching its highest titer in convalescence and is a marker for persistent infection, since it is always present in these cases. The presence of HBeAg around the period when subclinical infection occurs, and its intermittent occurrence in the presence or absence of its antibody during the convalescent period, is another indicator of the carrier state. The duration of carrier state can vary from individual to individual, but as a rule one is established if virus can be detected 4 months after infection.

Following second exposure to HBV, a marked rise in titer to anti-HBs occurs without concurrent rise in anti-HBc. This pattern suggests that reinfection has not occurred, but an anamestic response to the protective anti-HBs has developed.

The pathology of hepatitis B is morphologically indistinguishable from hepatitis A. Various degrees of parenchymal degeneration, necrosis and regeneration are evident as is the presence of a mononuclear exudate. Persistent infections may not cause changes in liver pathology always, but some can produce a chronic portal inflammatory infiltration with various degrees of fibrosis, leading to necrosis, adjacent lobular involvement and cirrhosis in the more severe active form. It has been proposed that the localization of HBsAg in the cytoplasm of hepatocytes in persistently infected patients may be due to the effect of anti-HBs that prevents its release from the cell. The role of antibodies to hepatic antigens in persistently infected individuals is not understood; cellular immune mechanisms may, however, elicit an autoimmune reaction that is responsible for hepatocellular injury evident in chronic cases.

In some parts of the world, chronic carriers of HBsAg frequently develop hepatocellular carcinoma.

Diagnosis

Liver function tests are useful in diagnosing the degree of liver damage that has occurred, and often help in detecting subclinical disease. The serum may appear yellow, and when the bilirubin level exceeds 2.5 mg%, scleral icterus is usually evident. Serum transaminase levels may become elevated prior to symptoms and can reach 1000 units/ml

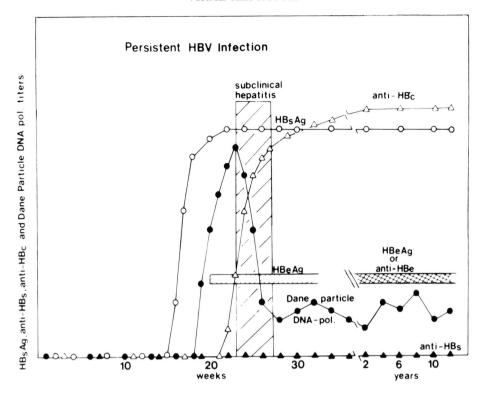

Figure 40/5. Schema of hepatitis B viral markers in the blood during the course of HBV infection which becomes persistent. (Reproduced with permission from G. L. Mandell *et al.* 1979 *Principles and Practice of Infectious Diseases.* John Wiley, New York.)

during the first week of symptoms. Serum alkaline phosphatase is normal or slightly elevated, and glucose tolerance may be decreased.

Differential diagnosis should eliminate non-A, non-B hepatitis (HBC), hepatitis A hepatitis, Epstein-Barr virus, cytomegalovirus, yellow fever virus, leptospirosis and toxic hepatitis due to ethanol, halothane and industrial chemicals.

A number of serological tests are available to detect antigens and antibodies that are present. The most sensitive are the radioimmunoassays and reverse passive hemagglutination for the detection of HBsAg, and anti-HBc. Less sensitive tests are rheophoresis, counterelectrophoresis, complement-fixation, and reverse passive latex agglutination.

Table 40/2 illustrates the various serological responses that may be expected with various types of hepatitis B.

Treatment

Bed rest and convalescence twice the duration of the acute attack is advised. In patients with chronic active hepatitis, corticosteroids and azothioprine have been helpful in preventing the development of cirrhosis. Individuals with chronic hepatitis have been given human leukocyte interferon or adenine

arabinoside (Ara-A) to reduce the blood levels of Dane particles. The use of hyperimmune hepatitis B globulin (HBIG) and standard serum globulin (Ig) can sometimes afford protection. Individuals who would be candidates for either are outlined in table 40/3.

Vaccines consisting of purified and formalin-treated HBsAg from the plasma of chronic HBsAg carriers have recently become available. The prospects of utilizing these types of vaccine among high-risk individuals to prevent hepatitis is encouraging.

Dentist and Hepatitis B

It is advisable that the dentist determine periodically, by the simple serodiagnostic tests available, his status with regard to possible hepatitis B infection. While in the general population the infectivity rate is 0.5%, at least 2% of dentists may be carriers. Studies also indicate that over 25% of all dentists have at one time or another been infected but only one-quarter of these have ever had clinical hepatitis. Although a temporary cessation of a dentist's practice may be recommended during convalescence, it usually is not necessary to cease practicing if a carrier state is recognized. However, care must be taken to avoid contact with open wounds and

Table 40/2
Four patterns of serologic responses to hepatitis B virus exposures[a]

Pattern	HBsAG	Anti-HBs	Anti-HBc
Typical acute type B hepatitis	Transient (<6 mo)	Detectable after clearance of HBsAg	Appears shortly after HBsAg; titer falls gradually after recovery
Chronic type B hepatitis	Persistent (>6 mo)	Not usually detected	Appears shortly after HBsAg and persists in high titer
Primary antibody response	Not detected	Appears after exposure (>2 weeks) and persists, often in high titer	Appears transiently and in low titer or not detected
Anamnestic antibody response	Not detected	Usually present prior to exposure; titer rises rapidly within 2 weeks after exposure	Either not detected or, if present prior to exposure, titer unchanged following exposure

[a] Reproduced with permission from L. F. Barker, R. J. Gerety and Tabor, E. 1978 The Immunology of the Hepatitis Viruses. In *Advances in Internal Medicine*, Vol. 23, edited by G. H. Stollerman *et al.* Copyright © 1978 by Year Book Medical Publishers, Inc., Chicago.

Table 40/3
Possible target populations for immunization against type B hepatitis

Preexposure or chronic exposure prophylaxis

Patients and staff in dialysis units, adult oncology units and custodial institutions with endemic hepatitis B
Physicians, dentists, particularly oral surgeons, and other health care personnel
Spouses and other family members of acute cases or chronic carriers
Infants of acutely or chronically infected mothers
Individuals requiring long-term therapy or massive therapy with blood and blood products, *e.g.*, hemophiliacs, thalassemics
Drug addicts, homosexuals and prostitutes
Travelers to or inhabitants of endemic areas

Postexposure prophylaxis

Single, acute exposure, *e.g.*, accidental inoculation ("needle stick") or oral ingestion
Accidental transfusion of HBsAg positive blood or blood component, *e.g.*, platelets
Transfusion of high-risk pooled plasma derivatives, *e.g.*, factor IX complex, antihemophilic factor or fibrinogen
Spouses and other family members of acute cases and chronic carriers
Infants of acutely or chronically infected mothers

Therapeutic

Acute hepatitis, type B
Chronic hepatitis, type B
Fulminant hepatitis, type B

[a] Reproduced with permission from L. F. Barker, R. J. Gerety and Tabor, E. 1978 The Immunology of the Hepatitis Viruses. In *Advances in Internal Medicine*, Vol. 23, edited by G. H. Stollerman *et al.* Copyright © 1978 by Year Book Medical Publishers, Inc., Chicago.

gloves should always be worn. Moreover the dentist should understand that he places his patients in jeopardy of contagion if he elects to treat them while he is a carrier.

Should treatment of a hepatitis B patient be unavoidable, protective clothing such as gloves, gowns, masks and glasses should be worn. Even when gloves are worn, careful handwashing should be undertaken following contact with a known infectious patient. Items such as tourniquets, blood pressure cuffs, marking pens used on the skin, containers with antiseptics and skin care lotion, should not be used on HBsAg-negative patients until they are decontaminated. Also, surface decontamination of the operatory should be scrupulously carried out so that any blood or saliva is removed as quickly as possible. If the patient is particularly infectious, *e.g.*, at the onset of clinical disease, it is advised that all dental personnel also be given prophylactic immunoglobulin as an added preventitive measure. Since the HBV vaccines are now available, it is advisable that all dental personnel, especially those in oral surgery, become immunized as soon as feasible.

HEPATITIS C, OR NON-A, NON-B HEPATITIS

The etiologic agent(s) of Hepatitis C (HBC) of hepatitis have not been identified, but since recurrent episodes following transfusions have been recorded, several serotypes or viruses may be involved. The disease is usually a mild form of hepatitis that in some instances can become fulminant or evolve into a chronic form with cirrhosis.

Epidemiology

The majority of individuals that develop hepatitis following blood transfusion are infected with the virus(es). Like hepatitis B, parenteral transmission through contaminated needles used by drug abusers, tattooers or medical personnel have been implicated in cases of multiple contact disease. Other forms of transmission have yet to be determined.

Pathogenesis

The degree and duration of altered liver enzymes and bilirubin levels are usually not as severe nor as long as with HAV and HBV infections. The axiom still holds that the higher the dose of virus, the shorter the incubation period and the greater the chance of developing more serious complications. Most patients that develop the chronic form usually return to normal liver function within a period of a year.

Clinical Manifestations

Following an incubation of 6 to 23 weeks (average 5 to 10 weeks) following a blood transfusion or other parenteral contact, a relatively mild acute disease develops with symptoms similar to those described for uncomplicated HAV or HBV. However, like HBV, a more fulminant variety can develop at about the same incidence as it does for HBV. The development of chronic active hepatitis is not unusual, however, in most cases it resolves within a year, and only in rare instances does it develop into the cirrhotic form.

Treatment

Patients with hepatitis C should be managed like those with other forms of viral hepatitis.

Prevention

Blood from volunteer donors are less likely to contain the virus than those obtained from commercial donors. Routine screening for increased serum transaminase levels may further reduce the risk of contagion from this source. Patients requir-

ing massive transfusions during surgery can be prevented from developing the icteric or cirrhotic forms of the disease by prophylactic administration of immunoglobulin.

ADDITIONAL READING

ALTER, H. J., CHALMERS, T. C., FREEMAN, B. M., et al. 1975 Healthcare Workers Positive for Hepatitis B Surface Antigen: Are Their Contacts at Risk? N Engl J Med, **292**, 454.

ALTER, H. J., PURCELL, R. H., FEINSTONE, S. M., et al. 1978 Non-A, Non-B Hepatitis: A Review and Interim Report of an Ongoing Prospective Study. In *Viral Hepatitis: A Contemporary Assessment of Etiology, Epidemiology, Pathogenesis and Prevention*, p. 359, edited by G. N. Vyas, S. N. Cohen, and R. Schmidt. Franklin Institute Press, Philadelphia.

ALTER, H. J., PURCELL, R. H., GERIN, J. L., et al. 1977 Transmission of Hepatitis B to Chimpanzees by Hepatitis B Surface Antigen-Positive Saliva and Semen. Infect Immun, **16**, 928.

ALTER, H. J., SEEFF, L. B., KAPLAN, P. M., et al. 1976 Type B Hepatitis: The Infectivity of Blood Positive for E Antigen and DNA Polymerase After Accidental Needlestick Exposure. N Engl J Med, **295**, 909.

BARKER, L. F., GARETY, R. J., AND TABOR, E. 1978 The Immunology of the Hepatitis Viruses. In *Advances in Internal Medicine*, Vol. 23, p. 327, edited by G. H. Stollerman et al. Year Book Medical Publishers, Chicago.

BOGGS, J. D., MELNICK, J. L., CONRAD, M. E., et al. 1970 Viral Hepatitis—Clinical and Tissue Culture Studies. JAMA, **214**, 1041.

CHERUBIN, C. E., PURCELL, R. H., LANDER, J. J., et al. 1972 Acquisition of Antibody to Hepatitis B Antigen in Three Socioeconomically Different Medical Populations. Lancet, **2**, 149.

DAVIS, B. D., DULBECCO, R., EISEN, H., AND GINSBERG, H. S. 1980 Hepatitis Viruses. In *Microbiology*, Ed 3, p. 1218. Harper & Row, New York.

DIENSTAG, J. L., FEINSTONE, S. M., KAPIKIAN, A. Z., et al. 1975 Faecal Shedding of Hepatitis-A Antigen. Lancet, **1**, 765.

GIBSON, P. E. 1976 Quantitative Analysis of the Major Subdeterminants of Hepatitis B Surface Antigen. J Infect Dis, **134**, 540.

GOLD, J. W. M., ALTER, H. J., AND HOLLAND, P. V. 1974 Passive Hemagglutination Assay for Antibody to Subtypes of Hepatitis B Antigen. J Immunol, **112**, 1100.

GOLDFIELD, M., BILL, J., AND COLOSIMO, F. 1978 The Control of Transfusion Associated Hepatitis. In *Viral Hepatitis: A Contemporary Assessment of Etiology, Epidemiology, Pathogenesis and Prevention*, p. 405, edited by G. N. Vyas, S. N. Cohen and R. Schmidt. Franklin Institute Press, Philadelphia.

GOODWIN, D., FANNIN, S. L., AND MCCRACKEN, B. B. 1976 *An Oral Surgeon-Related Hepatitis B Outbreak*. California Morbidity (California State Department of Health), April 16.

GRAF, J. P., AND MOESCHLIN, P. 1975 Risk to Contacts of a Medical Practitioner Carrying HBsAg. N Engl J Med, **293**, 197.

HAVENS, W. P. 1946 Period of Infectivity of Patients with Experimentally Induced Infectious Hepatitis. J Exp Med, **83**, 251.

HOOFNAGLE, J. H., GERETY, R. I., AND BARKER, L. F. 1975 Antibody to the Hepatitis B Surface Antigen in Immune Serum Globulin. Transfusion, **15**, 408.

JAWETZ, E., MELNICK, J. L., AND ADELBERG, E. A. 1980

Hepatitis Viruses. In *Medical Microbiology*, p. 417. Lange Publications, Los Altos, Calif., 417.

KLUGE, T. 1963 Gamma Globulin in the Prevention of Viral Hepatitis. A Study on the Effect of Medium-Sized Doses. Acta Med Scand, **174,** 469.

LANDER, J. J., HOLAND, P. V., ALTER, H. J., *et al.* 1972 Antibody to Hepatitis B-Associated Antigen: Frequency and Pattern of Response Detected by Radioimmunoprecipitation. JAMA, **220,** 1079.

LEVIN, M. L., MADDREY, W. C., WANDS, J. R., *et al.* 1974 Hepatitis B Transmission by Dentists. JAMA, **228,** 1139.

MANDELL, G. L., DOUGLAS, R. G., JR., AND BENNETT, J. E. (Eds.) 1979 *Principles and Practice of Infectious Diseases*, p. 1370. John Wiley, New York.

PANEL OF THE COMMITTEE ON PLASMA AND PLASMA SUBSTITUTES, NATIONAL ACADEMY OF SCIENCES-NATIONAL RESEARCH COUNCIL: Statement on Laboratory Screening Tests for Identifying Carriers of Viral Hepatitis in Blood-Banking and Transfusion Services. Transfusion, **10,** 1.

RAKELA, J., STEVENSON, D., EDWARDS, V., *et al.* 1977 Antibodies to Hepatitis A Virus: Patterns by Two Procedures. J Clin Microbiol, **5,** 110.

RIMLAND, D., PARKIN, W. E., MILLER, G. B., *et al.* 1977 Hepatitis B Outbreak Traced to an Oral Surgeon. N Engl J Med, **296,** 153.

ROBINSON, W. S. 1977 The Genome of Hepatitis B Virus. Ann Rev Microbiol, **31,** 357.

ROSENBERG, J. L., JONES, D. P., LIPITZ, L. R., *et al.* 1973 Viral Hepatitis: An Occupational Hazard to Surgeons. JAMA, **223,** 395.

SCHALM, S. W., SUMMERSKILL, W. H. J., GITNICK, G. L., *et al.* 1976 Contrasting Features and Responses to Treatment of Severe Chronic Active Liver Disease with and without Hepatitis Bs Antigen. Gut, **17,** 781.

SHIH, J. W., AND GERIN, J. L. 1977 Proteins of Hepatitis B Surface Antigen. J Virol, **21,** 347.

SOLOWAY, R. D., SUMMERSKILL, W. H. J., BAGGENSTOSS, A. H., *et al.* 1972 Clinical, Biochemical and Histological Remission of Severe Chronic Active Liver Disease: A Controlled Study of Treatments and Early Prognosis. Gastroenterology, **63,** 820.

SZMUNESS, W., DIENSTAG, J. L., PURCELL, R. H., *et al.* 1976 Distribution of Antibody to Hepatitis A Antigen in Urban Adult Populations. N Engl J Med, **295,** 755.

SZMUNESS, W., DIENSTAG, J. L., PURCELL, R. H., *et al.* 1977 The Prevalence of Antibody to Hepatitis A Antigen in Various Parts of the World. Am J Epidemiol, **106,** 392.

chapter 41

Orthomyxoviruses: Influenza

Memory Elvin-Lewis

INTRODUCTION

Orthomyxoviruses (Orthomyxoviridae) are the etiologic agents of influenza, an acute infectious disease characterized by sudden onset of fever, malaise, headache and myalgia. In uncomplicated cases, the disease is self-limiting and recovery occurs within a week.

Causative Agents

Influenza virus is distinguished by possessing a helical nucleocapsid with eight segments of negative-stranded RNA as the genome. It is enveloped in a monomeric matrix protein and lipid bilayer from which extends distinctive glycoprotein peplomers that possess either neuraminidase or hemagglutinating activity. The virions approximate 90 to 100 nm in size (fig. 41/1). Three genera of influenza viruses are known, *Influenzavirus A*, *Influenzavirus B*, and *Influenzavirus C*. They vary somewhat in their size, appearance, antigenic structure, and disease patterns. For example, *Influenzavirus A* is somewhat smaller than *Influenzavirus B*, and *Influenzavirus C* has fewer peplomers on its surface. Filamentous forms of the viruses do occur, especially in fresh clinical isolates.

Influenza viruses attach to cell receptors by their hemagglutinin peplomers, enter in phagocytic vesicles and are uncoated. The viral genome is transcribed in the nucleus to form mRNAs necessary for translation into replicative and structural proteins, and neuraminidase that is necessary for release from host cells. Final assembly occurs at the cell membrane, where the virion is enveloped and released by budding.

Influenza viruses are susceptible to lipid solvents and surface active compounds. The virus is relatively labile when stored at temperatures above −15 C, but is stable at −70 C. The antigenic characteristics of influenza viruses have particular epidemiologic significance and warrant detailed discussion. A particularly distinctive feature of influenza is the frequency with which antigenic changes due to mutation occur, particularly with *Influenzavirus A* and less so with *Influenzavirus B*. With human strains, changes in antigenicity are due to variations in the polypeptides of the four subtypes of hemagglutinins (H0 to H3) and two subtypes of neuramidase (N1, N2) found as peplomers on the surface of the virus. Development of antibodies to these two peplomers affords protection since the hemagglutinin is utilized by the virion for attachment to host cells during infection and the neuraminidase is utilized for the release of the virus from the infected cell. In this way antihemagglutinin antibodies prevent attachment to host cells and antineuraminidase antibodies decrease infectious virus release and also shorten the duration of illness. Thus, when major antigenic changes occur in the neuraminidase and hemagglutinin types, such as occurred in 1918 and 1957, a worldwide pandemic results, as few individuals are immune. Thereafter the virus persists in the community by subtle antigenic changes that result from a process referred to as antigenic shift. Therefore, antigenic patterns of the virions are important factors in spread of influenza.

Pathogenesis

Infection is mainly by respiratory droplets. In uncomplicated influenza the virus spreads directly in the mucous membranes of the respiratory tract; viremia is not common. During influenza there may be sufficient cell damage to the ciliated respiratory epithelium so that break-down products of dying cells are absorbed into the bloodstream, producing a toxic effect. This may explain why the symptoms are more severe than would be expected from a local infection of the respiratory tract. Also during the regeneration process there is a transitional

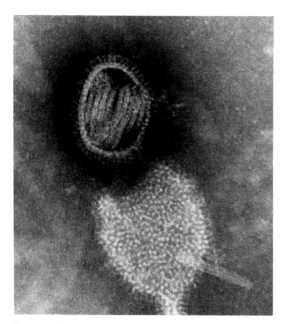

Figure 41/1. *Influenzavirus A2.* The nucleocapsid is loosely coiled inside an envelope that consists of protein and lipid, and to which glycoprotein spikes are attached. (Reproduced with permission from *Zinsser Microbiology,* Ed. 17, edited by W. K. Joklik, H. P. Willett and D. B. Amos. Appleton-Century-Crofts, New York.)

stratified squamous epithelium that results in edema, hyperemia and congestion and increased secretions.

Clinical Manifestations

The incubation period of influenza is short (1 to 3 days) and the onset is abrupt with high fever (102 to 104 F), chills, rigor and headache. Myalgia, especially of the back and limb muscles, is another prominent symptom. Cough and coryza may be scanty, although infection of the pharynx and conjunctivae occur. Fever usually abates in 3 to 4 days if secondary infections do not occur.

Influenza-infected cells permit certain bacteria of the oropharynx to adhere to them. Thus, pneumonia complicating influenza can be caused by such residents as *Hemophilus influenzae, Streptococcus pneumoniae* and *Streptococcus pyogenes.* This complication is more common in adults than children. Bronchiolitis, myocarditis and pericarditis, and the development of the ascending paralysis, Guillain-Barré syndrome with *Influenzavirus A* (including that used in vaccine) are other complications that can occur rarely. Also, *Influenzavirus B,* and less frequently *Influenzavirus A,* can elicit in children a hepatic and nervous system complication referred to as Reye's syndrome that causes lethargy or delerium, seizures and respiratory arrest; it has a mortality rate of 10 to 40%. This syndrome is not unique to influenza and also may arise following a number of upper respiratory or gastrointestinal infections and varicella. Other individuals that are particularly predisposed to serious sequelae are those with various types of heart disease, chronic diseases of the lungs and kidney, diabetes mellitus, severe anemia and the immunologically compromised. *Influenzavirus C* infections are mild and similar to the common cold.

Diagnosis

Clinical and epidemiological symptoms are helpful in diagnosing a typical case of influenza. However, for epidemiological purposes strains may be isolated from respiratory secretions in primary monkey kidney tissue culture and identified as to serotype by hemadsorption-inhibition tests. Determination of seroconversion against a specific strain is readily carried out by hemagglutination inhibition tests.

Treatment

Supportive therapy including bed rest, antipyretics and analgesics are useful. Increased fluid intake should be encouraged to compensate for loss through fever. Antibiotics may be given to prevent the development of secondary bacterial pneumonia. Amantadine has been successfully used to prevent the development of the disease in household contacts, the elderly or debilitated or in institutions when the correct vaccine is unavailable.

Epidemiology

Influenza is a highly contagious disease transmitted by exposure to virus-containing respiratory secretions. The incidence of illness that occurs in a community from one year to the next is a direct reflection of the immune status of the population for those strains that are currently in circulation. Epidemics occur when antigenic changes are sufficient to permit infection of susceptible individuals or those not resistant to closely related strains. Pandemics arise only rarely and in these instances major antigenic changes have occurred (fig. 41/2). As a rule epidemics of *Influenzavirus A* occur every 2 to 4 years and of *Influenzavirus B* every 4 to 6 years. *Influenzavirus C* only occurs sporadically and is not responsible for epidemics.

Outbreaks are more common in late autumn to early spring; and the attack rate can be as high as 40%, particularly in the 5- to 14-year-old group. The incidence of pulmonary complications is higher in adults.

Swine influenza that is a variant of *Influenzavirus A* is usually limited to sporadic cases among pig farmers. In the 1918 pandemic a particularly severe pathotype was isolated; however, it has been an insignificant cause of human disease since then.

Worldwide influenza virus surveillance occurs an-

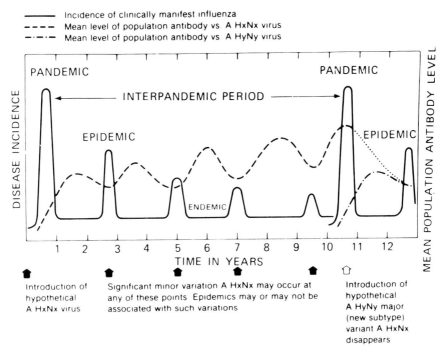

Figure 41/2. Schema of occurrence of influenza pandemics and epidemics in relation to the level of immunity in the population. *AHxNx* and *AHyNy* represent influenza viruses with completely different hemagglutinins and neuraminidases. (Courtesy Dr. R. G. Douglas, Jr., reproduced with permission from G. J. Glasso, T. C. Merigan, and R. A. Buchanan. 1979 *Antiviral Agents and Viral Diseases of Man.* Raven Press, New York.)

nually so that major and minor antigenic shifts in hemagglutinin and neuraminidase subtypes and the location and year in which they are first isolated can be traced. Using these techniques, changes that arise may be used in the development of current virus vaccines since if antigenic shift is great, immunization with one strain may not induce immunity to a new, although perhaps related strain. Thus, in 1979–1980 the recommended vaccine strains were influenza A/Brazil/78 (H_1N_1), A/Texas/77 (H_3N_2) and B/Hong Kong/72. The next year significant antigenic drift in A/Texas/77 and B/Hong Kong/72 resulted in their replacement with A/Bangkok/79 in the vaccine. The former strains predominated in the preceding two seasons. During 1979–1980 seasons, *Influenzavirus B* was prominent, causing scattered outbreaks and school absenteeism of from 15 to 30%, and during that season influenza-related, pneumonia-associated deaths were significant. However, early in February 1980, isolates of the Bangkok strain A (H_3N_2) were made in Australia. During the 1980–1981 flu season this strain was isolated in 16 states in the United States by February 1981 and, by March, 1982, other countries throughout the world. Thus, the changes were justified.

Prevention

Immunization for dentists and other medical personnel is recommended by public health officials since these individuals would have more opportunity to contract and spread the disease to those under greater risk of developing adverse consequences from infections of the lower respiratory tract. Since increased mortality is frequently associated with those over 65, immunization also is recommended, especially if the elderly are institutionalized. Side effects of immunization have included an influenza-like disease due to vaccine toxicity, hypersensitivity reactions and, with swine influenza strains especially, Guillian-Barré syndrome. Whole virion vaccine reflecting the current strains is recommended for adults, and subparticle vaccine for children under 5 years of age due to less toxicity.

ADDITIONAL READING

Douglas, R. G., and Betts, R. F. 1979 Influenza Virus, In *Principles and Practices of Infectious Diseases*, p. 1135, edited by G. L. Mandell, R. G. Douglas, Jr. and J. E. Bennett. John Wiley, New York.

Hoke, C. H., and Hattwick, M. A. W. 1975 Limiting the Effects of Influenza Epidemics. Postgrad Med, **58**, 59.

Mair, H. J., Sansome, D. A., and Tillett, H. E. 1974 A Controlled Trial of Inactivated Monovalent Influenza A Vaccines in General Practice. J Hyg, **73**, 317.

Murphy, B. R., Kasel, J. A., and Chanock, R. M. 1972 Association of Serum Antineuraminidase Antibody with Resistance to Influenza in Man. N Engl J Med, **286**, 1329.

Morbidity and Mortality Weekly Reports. 1979 Guillian-Barré Syndrome, **28**, 22.

MORBIDITY AND MORTALITY WEEKLY REPORTS. 1978 Influenza—New York, California, **27,** 507.

MORBIDITY AND MORTALITY WEEKLY REPORTS. 1979 Influenza—Worldwide, **28,** 51.

MORBIDITY AND MORTALITY WEEKLY REPORTS. 1979 Influenza Vaccine, **28,** 231.

MORBIDITY AND MORTALITY WEEKLY REPORTS. 1979 Influenza, U.S. Worldwide, **28,** 347.

MORBIDITY AND MORTALITY WEEKLY REPORTS. 1980 Influenza Vaccine, **29,** 225.

MORBIDITY AND MORTALITY WEEKLY REPORTS. 1980 Influenza Mortality Surveillance U.S., **29,** 578.

MORBIDITY AND MORTALITY WEEKLY REPORTS. 1980 Influenza, U.S., **29,** 599.

MORBIDITY AND MORTALITY WEEKLY REPORTS. 1982 Antigenic Analysis of Recent Influenza Isolates, **31,** 110.

RUBEN, F. L., AKERS, L. S., STANLEY, E. D., AND JACKSON, G. G. 1973 Protection with Split and Whole Virus Vaccines Against Influenza. Arch Intern Med, **132,** 568.

chapter 42

Paramyxoviridae: Parainfluenza and Mumps (*Paramyxovirus*); Measles (*Morbillivirus*); Respiratory Syncytial Virus (*Pneumovirus*); Exanthems of Unknown Etiology

Memory Elvin-Lewis

PARAMYXOVIRIDAE

Paramyxoviruses (Paramyxoviridae) are the etiologic agents of a variety of illnesses that usually affect different organ systems. However, because of distinctive characteristics not associated with tissue predilection, they have been differentiated into three genera, *Paramyxovirus*, *Morbillivirus* and *Pneumovirus* (table 42/1). The diseases with which they are associated include: the acute respiratory infections of croup (parainfluenza virus) and bronchiolitis (respiratory syncytial virus); the morbilliform exanthem, measles; and infectious parotitis, mumps.

Paramyxoviruses are 125 to 250 nm in size, possess helical nucleocapsids containing one large molecule of single-stranded RNA of negative polarity; and are enveloped in a protein and lipid envelope. The latter structure possesses two distinctive glycoprotein peplomers, one of which contains hemagglutinin and neuramidase activity and the other hemolytic and cell fusion functions. The viruses enter the cells by fusing with cell membranes and are uncoated in the cytoplasm where their RNA is transcribed by their own transciptase into 5 to 8 mRNAs that translate proteins required for nucleic acid replication, structure and peplomer enzymes. Final assembly occurs at the cell membrane where they are enveloped and are released by budding.

Paramyxoviruses are inactivated in the presence of lipid solvents, surface active compounds, formalin and ultraviolet light, and temperatures above 56 C. The viruses are stable at −70 C.

PARAINFLUENZA VIRUS

Four serotypes of parainfluenza viruses are known that are distinguished by antigenic differences in their HN (hemagglutinin-neuramidase) and F (fusion-hemolysin) peplomers and their internal nucleocapsid (NP). The strains differ somewhat in the type of acute respiratory disease they cause in children, the age of individuals they infect and the length of time the virus is shed (table 42/2).

Epidemiology

Parainfluenza viruses are worldwide in distribution. Types 1 and 2 are more likely to cause epidemic disease in alternate years and type 3 tends to infect year round: the epidemiology of type 4 is unknown. Infection usually occurs in the winter months and is transmitted from person to person by inhalation of droplets containing contaminated respiratory secretions. Maternal antibody is believed to protect the newborn, and it is uncommon to see infections with type 1 and 2 until after 4 months of age; thereafter it may cause upper respiratory disease, especially croup, until about 4 to 6 years, by which time most children have been infected. In older age groups, the disease is mild, and probably represents reinfection. With type 3 serotype, young infants are particularly predisposed to develop bronchiolitis and pneumonia and probably have been infected by the age of 3.

Pathogenesis

The pathogenesis of these infections is ill defined. It is known that the virus infects the ciliated columnar epithelium of the respiratory tract; however, it causes no distinctive pathology in the lungs, nor is the mechanism for subglottic involvement known.

Clinical Manifestations

Primary infections are usually mild and some are asymptomatic. They are typically that of a "bad

Table 42/1
Characteristics of human paramyxoviruses[a]

Common Properties		Distinguishing Properties[b]			
		Parainfluenza	Mumps	Measles	Rs v
Average size	125–250 nm (range 100–800 nm)				
Nucleocapsid diameter	18 nm (except Rs v = 14 nm)				
Viral genome	5–6 × 10⁶ daltons (17–20 Kb) single negative-strand molecules				
	Hemagglutinin	+	+	+	–
	Hemadsorption[d]	+	+	+	–
	Hemolysin	+	+	+	–
Virion RNA polymerase	+				
	Neuraminidase	+	+	–	–
Reaction with lipid solvents	Disrupts				
	Antigenic types	4	1	1	1
Syncytial formation	+				
	Antigenic relationships	Mumps	Parainfluenza		
Cytoplasmic inclusion bodies	+ (Measles virus also nuclear)				
	Genus	Paramyxovirus	Paramyxovirus	Morbillivirus	Pneumovirus
Site of multiplication	Cytoplasm				

[a] Reproduced with permission from B. D. Davis et al. 1980 Microbiology, Ed. 3. Harper & Row, Hagerstown, Md.
[b] Rs v = respiratory synctial virus; + = present; – = absent.
[c] Chicken and guinea pig RBC.
[d] Infected cells adsorb guinea pig RBCs.

Table 42/2
Characteristics of parainfluenza virus infections in children[a]

Condition	Usual Age at Onset	Length of Time Virus Shed	Clinical Manifestations		
			Severe	Mild	Proportion with Fever
Primary infections					
Type 1 & 2	8–30 mo	3–12 days (range for type 1)	Croup	Cold, bronchitis	½–⅔
Type 3	1–24 mo	8 days (median) 3–16 days (range)	Croup, pneumonia, bronchiolitis	Cold	¾
Type 4 A & B	< 6 yr	NI[b]	None	Cold	NI
Reinfections					
Type 1–3	Within a few months to several years after primary; may occur in adults	1–3 days (type 3)	Rare	Cold, bronchitis	⅓

[a] Reproduced with permission from G. L. Mandell, R. G. Douglas, Jr. and J. E. Bennett. 1979 *Principles and Practice of Infectious Diseases*. John Wiley, New York.
[b] NI = no information.

cold" with fever coryza, pharyngitis, and/or bronchitis and rarely with croup or pneumonia. Reinfections are common probably because the development of specific protective IgA is not as long lasting as the circulating IgG. Reinfection, however is usually milder. If the patient is croupy it is hazardous to look into their mouths as it is possible to initate laryngospasm.

Diagnosis

Parainfluenza virus can be isolated in primary monkey kidney lines where they produce distinctive syncytia. They can be serotyped by hemadsorption-inhibition tests.

Therapy

Humidification and oxygen therapy are helpful in reducing congestion. If necessary, a tracheostomy may be performed but care must be taken to avoid any plugging of the tube by bronchial secretions. An epinephrine nebulizer may be useful for treating the symptoms of croup.

Prevention

A killed parainfluenza vaccine has been shown to prevent the development of the more severe forms of the illness; however, this remains experimental and is not readily available.

MUMPS VIRUS

Mumps virus is monotypic for its HN, F and NP antigens but it also is antigenically related to both parainfluenza virus and Newcastle disease virus of chickens. Mumps is an acute infection characterized by fever and swelling and tenderness of the salivary glands. A number of complications can occur involving especially glandular tissues or the nervous system.

Epidemiology

Mumps is primarily a disease of children throughout the world. It is endemic the year round but its prevalence is highest in the winter and early spring. Prior to the success of the attenuated vaccine, epidemics would erupt about every 4 to 6 years and local outbreaks would occur in situations that favored crowding.

Pathogenesis

The mechanism by which mumps initiates infection is unclear but it has been proposed that following contact with infected body secretions, such as saliva droplets, replication occurs initially somewhere in the upper respiratory tract epithelium. This leads to viremia with dissemination to the salivary glands and to other organs, including neural tissue. A secondary viremia is then elicited that further disseminates the virus to previously uninvolved structures.

Pathological changes in the salivary glands appear as a serofibrinous exudate and leukocytic infiltration. The ducts degenerate and cellular debris collects in the lumina. Similar changes are seen in the pancreas and testes, but they may differ in severity. In the testes the reaction is more severe with lymphocytic infiltration, congestion, hemorrhage and destruction of the seminiferous tubules. In the brain, pervenous demyelinization may or may not occur; there is usually a degree of perivascular cuffing and an increase of microglial cells.

Clinical Manifestations

After an incubation period of about 18 (12 to 25) days prodromal symptoms of myalgia, anorexia, malaise, and headache develop with low grade fever. Earache and tender parotid glands often precede swelling of the gland. The orfices of Wharton's and Stensen's ducts are often red and swollen. Salivary gland swelling may be single or bilateral, with swelling in one gland preceding that of the other side by 1 to 5 days. Difficulty in mastication may be due to trismus. After the parotid swelling reaches its peak in about 3 days, the pain and tenderness soon disappear and usually the only complication that occurs is acute or recurrent sialadenitis. Sublingual gland involvement, submandibular adenitis and tongue swelling also may develop. Usually both swelling and other constitutional signs have resolved within a week. The most common other clinical infection that develops in 20 to 30% of postpubertal males is epididymo-orchitis characterized by pain and unilateral swelling and possibly resulting in some degree of testicular atrophy. Pancreatitis also appears in about 5% of the patients and has been implicated as a possible cause of juvenile diabetes. Mumps is also one of the leading causes of unilateral neurosensory deafness in childhood. The hearing loss is complete and permanent, but fortunately is unilateral in 75% of the cases. Only rarely does a postinfectious demyelinization occur. A migratory polyarthritis or arthralgia can exist with mumps and may persist for as long as 1 month. Adults also may develop myocarditis and pericarditis (3 to 15%); oophoritis (5%) leading to impaired fertility, and as many as 60% show some form of transient impairment of renal function. Should mumps involve the nervous system it can cause a benign meningitis or a life-threatening encephalitis. Other complications that follow CNS involvement can include aqueductal stenosis, and hydrocephalus, facial palsy, transverse myelitis or Guillian-Barré syndrome. It is not known how mumps actually affects the developing fetus, but birth weights have been low in infants infected in the first trimester.

Diagnosis

Usually it is unnecessary to carry out laboratory tests for confirmation of mumps. In primary monkey tissue culture, mumps isolated from saliva produces a characteristic granular syncytium. Complement-fixation tests to detect glycoprotein antigens also are useful, although the older mumps skin test is no longer considered reliable.

Treatment

Parotitis is usually treated by analgesic and antipyretic agents such as aspirin or acetaminophen. Similarly, the treatment of orchitis is symptomatic, and ice packs have been found useful, as has procaine, to alleviate severe pain. Mumps immune globulin may prevent orchitis.

Prevention

Live mumps vaccine is recommended for children and adults alike, since its efficacy is well known and side reactions are rare. These have included allergies, rashes and CNS involvement (febrile sizures, unilateral nerve deafness and encephalitis). The vaccine should not be administered to those with immunodeficiency or malignancy, anymore than other replicative vaccines are recommended for this group. Since mumps virus is in the saliva from 6 days before to 9 days after symptoms occur, it is recommended that all dentists ensure that they are immunized. Also a perusual of the immunization and infectious disease record of the patient may help detect a potential carrier.

MEASLES

Measles virus is monotypic for its H, NP and F antigens but it is related to canine distemper and rinderpest virus of cattle. Measles, or more correctly rubeola, is a highly contagious, acute exanthem characterized by prodromal symptoms of fever, coryza, cough, conjunctivitis, and Koplik's spots on the oral mucosa followed by generalized maculopapular eruption. Complications can occur that may be life threatening.

Epidemiology

Measles is an extremely infectious disease and is readily acquired by inhalation of contaminated droplets from the respiratory tract or contact with urine of infected persons. Prior to successful immunization with the attenuated vaccine, outbreaks used to occur every 2 to 3 years, as the pool of susceptible children reached 30 to 40%. The virus has a seasonal prevalence and causes spring outbreaks.

Pathogenesis

During the incubation period of 1 to 2 weeks, the virus first replicates in the respiratory epithelium and lymph nodes, where it infects leukocytes and is spread by them throughout the reticuloendothelial system. Following replication in these sites, destruction of the infected cells results in a secondary viremia. Virus then reaches the respiratory tract where it replicates to cause the prodromal symptoms of cough and coryza, croup, bronchiolitis and pneumonia. It has been proposed that the loss of cilia from these cells and edema predisposes to secondary bacterial infections.

Koplik's spots, characteristic blue-gray lesions with a red base that appear on the buccal mucosa, originate in the submucous glands and progress to vesiculation and necrosis. Warthin-Finkeldey cells, large multinucleate giant cells, can be demonstrated among the respiratory epithelial cells found in nasal secretions. The rash (fig. 42/2) that appears on the 14th day, just prior to the appearance of circulating antibodies, may in fact represent a hypersensitivity reaction to the infection. Sometimes infection of T lymphocytes temporarily depresses cellular immunity.

Clinical Manifestations

Prodromal symptoms appear about 10 to 12 days after infection and include coryza, a persistent barking cough, keratoconjunctivitis, often with photophobia and fever. Lymphadenopathy and splenomegaly may develop. The cardinal prodromal sign of measles is the development of small, irregular spots, bright red with a white or blue-white center on the mucosa of the lower lip and on the buccal mucosa opposite the premolars that are called Koplik's spots. (This enanthem appears similar to that seen with Coxsackie virus A16 and ECHO virus 9 infections.) These lesions disappear as the skin rash reaches its peak. The rash develops approximately 2 weeks after exposure, and appears first at the hair line and behind the ears, becomes maculopapular and spreads rapidly downward over the face, neck, trunk and extremities during the next 3 days. Fever

usually abates as the rash appears. Its color may become reddish purple and may be associated with skin edema. As the rash fades, it becomes brown, and desquamates. Petechial lesions also may appear in the oral cavity without associated skin rash.

A number of complications can occur that can be life threatening. These include development of the pneumonia that is usually due to secondary infection with residents of the oropharynx. Encephalitis following measles may be acute or chronic. In acute cases fever returns and is accompanied by headache, seizures and coma. Depending upon its severity, patients may recover with residual neurological sequelae or die.

Hemorrhagic measles is a severe, rare type known also as black measles because hemorrhages occur into the skin and from the mucous membranes. With this type, high fever, pneumonia and encephalitis are often present.

Atypical measles can develop 6 months after natural disease or after attenuated measles vaccine. Prodromal symptoms are characterized by high fever, myalgia, abdominal pains and prostration. The exanthem begins on the wrists and ankles, progressing inward to the trunk, although the greatest involvement is on the feet and legs. Petechia, purpura, urticaria, vesicles or erythema multiforme, pruritis and marked hyperesthesia are all characteristics of the rash. It is believed that this syndrome represents a hypersensitivity reaction in a partially immune host.

Giant cell pneumonia can develop if children with severe combined immunodeficiency or Di George syndrome are given attenuated vaccine. Because cellular immunity is often depressed in measles, patients with concurrent tuberculosis may have an exaggerated response.

The slow infection of measles called subacute sclerosing panencephalitis (SSPE) will be discussed in Chapter 43.

Diagnosis

Clinical symptoms usually aid in the diagnosis of measles. The virus is difficult to isolate in the laboratory since it grows slowly in cell cultures, where it forms syncytia. Therefore, virus isolation is carried out only when verification of a life-threatening complication such as pneumonia develops. Of the serological tests available, hemagglutination-inhibition tests are preferred. During infection the enanthema, Koplik's spots and multinucleate Warthin-Finkeldey cells in respiratory swabs aid in presumptive diagnosis.

Prevention

Attenuated measles vaccine is now recommended for all children at 15 months of age; it is expected that immunity is conferred for 15 years. When this

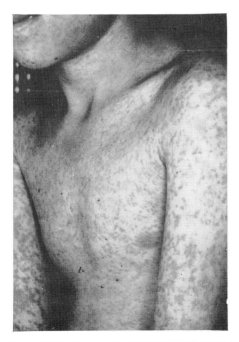

Figure 42/1. Measles (rubeola). (AFIP B 5037.)

is impossible because of concurrent immunosuppressive illness or inherent disease, prophylactic immune serum globulin may be given for known exposure. It should be remembered that measles is shed in the oropharyngeal area for several days during the prodromal period before constitutional signs develop, and thus can be a hazard to dental personnel.

RESPIRATORY SYNCYTIAL VIRUS

Three antigenic variants of respiratory syncytial virus (Rs v) have been detected in plaque neutralization tests. The virus is particularly fragile, and thus preservation of infectivity is difficult. Formation of syncytia and giant cells and prominant eosinophilic cytoplasmic inclusions in infected cells are pathognomonic. These strains are responsible for causing a significant amount of lower respiratory tract disease in infancy.

Epidemiology

This is a common infection among children, particularly during the winter and spring. Oftentimes it will be the only, or clearly predominant, respiratory infection in a community. It has been estimated that acquisition usually occurs within the 1st year or at least by the time the child enters school. Male children from lower socioeconomic families tend to be infected more frequently than other pediatric categories. Infection usually occurs by contact with contaminated respiratory secretions. A source of nosocomial contagion is often young adults with active disease.

Pathogenesis

After an incubation period of 5 days, the virus replicates in the respiratory epithelium where it incites proliferation and necrosis of bronchial epithelium. Lymphocytic infiltration is prominent, as is edema that leads to obstruction due to increased mucus excretion. A Type III hypersensitivity reaction may play a role in the more severe pulmonary manifestations that develop. In more severe cases, emphysema and lung collapse and necrotizing pneumonitis can develop.

Clinical Manifestations

The development of symptoms is often insidious following an upper respiratory episode of coryza, coughing, and fever. Pneumonia occurs in about 40% of the patients, followed in decreasing order by bronchiolitis and croup. Wheezing and difficulty in breathing are often cardinal signs of bronchiolitis; and a characteristic "whoop" and paroxysmal cough with croup. Chest roentgenograms show interstitial pneumonia and hyperinflation of the lung.

Cyanosis is frequently seen in hospitalized infants. Usually the infection resolves in 1 to 3 weeks.

A common complication of pediatric disease is the development of otitis media. Fever and earache are frequently signs of infection in older children, whereas adults usually have subclinical disease. When overt disease does occur in adults, other underlying illness may predispose to the exacerbation of symptoms. For example, hospitalized adults may develop bronchitis, pneumonia and influenza-like illness.

Respiratory syncytial virus infection only rarely involves the nervous system but it has been implicated in a number of pediatric cases of meningitis, myelitis, myocarditis and a variety of exanthems.

Children with cardiopulmonary and congenital disorders are particularly predisposed to develop life-threatening complications due to secondary bacterial pneumonia and respiratory failure.

Diagnosis

Direct immunofluorescent staining of nasal or bronchial washings will often reveal infected cells if clinical diagnosis requires confirmation. The ELISA and indirect immunofluorescent techniques may be applied in serological diagnosis. Although respiratory syncytial virus contains visible peplomers, the properties of hemagglutination, hemolysis and neuraminidase activity are not detectable.

Prevention

The development of a live attenuated vaccine is underway. Interruption of transmission particularly in hospital environments is important.

EXANTHEMS OF UNKNOWN ETIOLOGY

Erythema infectiosum (fifth disease) is a mild, exanthematous disease occurring mainly in children. It is characterized by a 5 to 14 day incubation period followed by an atypical "slapped-cheek" rash that spreads to the trunk and limbs. The maculopapular lesions have an irregular reticular pattern that fades and coalesces over a period of 10 days. Epidemics occur during the winter and springtime, and usually more among girls than boys. The prognosis is excellent.

Exanthem subitum (roseola infantum, sixth disease) is the commonest exanthem among children between 6 months and 2 years of age. The incubation period is 5 to 15 days. The illness is characterized by a high fever (105 to 106 F) for 3 to 5 days that drops suddenly before a temporary rubelliform rash appears on the neck and trunk but not on the face and limbs. The disease is self-limiting and with an excellent prognosis.

The differential diagnosis of exanthematous diseases is described in table 42/3.

Table 42/3
Differential diagnosis of exanthematous diseases

	Measles	Atypical Measles	Rubella	Roseola	Fifth Disease	Enteroviral Infections
Etiology	Measles virus	Measles virus, partially immune host	Rubella virus	? Virus	? Virus	ECHO and Coxsackie viruses
History of exposure	Usually	Usually	Often	Rare	Occasionally	Occasionally
Incubation period	10–14 days	About 10 days	12–23 days	10–15 days	4–14 days	2–7 days
Age	Children adults	Children adults	Children adults	Infants below 3 years	Children 5–14 years adults	Children adults
Season	Winter, spring	Winter, spring	Spring	Spring, fall Unusual	Winter, spring Unusual except in adults	Summer, early autumn Fever on occasion
Prodrome	3–4 days, fever, conjunctivitis, upper respiratory symptoms	1–2 days, fever, pain, cough	None in children; malaise, fever in adults			
Character of rash	Maculopapular, confluent, begins on face and moves down body	Variable: urticarial, maculopapular, petechial, purpuric, vesicular; begins peripherally	Maculopapular; may be absent	Maculopapular; appears as fever falls	Erythema of cheeks; reticular rash on extremities	Variable; if present: maculopapular, rubella-like, vesicular, petechial
Associated symptoms	Fever, cough, coryza, conjunctivitis	Fever, pneumonia, pleural effusion, edema of extremities	Posterior auricular and occipital adenopathy; arthritis in adult women	High fever, mild cervical adenopathy	Usually none	Variable: fever, sore throat, headache, aseptic meningitis, pleurodynia
Duration of illness	7–10 days	10–14 days	3–5 days	5–7 days	5–9 days	2–5 days
Complications	Bacterial superinfection, encephalitis	None reported	Uncommon—hemorrhagic manifestations, encephalitis	Very rare	Very rare	Rare

Table 42/3 (cont'd)

	Measles	Atypical Measles	Rubella	Roseola	Fifth Disease	Enteroviral Infections
Additional comments	No previous measles or vaccine. Koplik spots diagnostic	History of killed measles vaccine	No previous rubella or vaccine; teratogenic-congenital rubella syndrome	May be associated with febrile convulsions	Many adults develop fever, arthritis, adenopathy	May be confused with measles, rubella, roseola
Best method for diagnosis	Acute and convalescent serum specimens	Acute and convalescent serum specimens	Acute and convalescent serum specimens	Clinical only	Clinical only	Throat, rectal swabs, acute and convalescent sera

TOGAVIRIDAE: RUBELLA VIRUS (*RUBIVIRUS*)

Rubella virus is the cause of rubella, or German measles, an acute infection that may produce congenital damage. It belongs to the genus *Rubivirus*, and is an enveloped virus with hemagglutinin-containing peplomers and a helical nucleocapsid containing single-stranded RNA. Like other enveloped viruses it is inactivated by ether, chloroform and sodium deoxycholate and is labile at −4 C but not − 70 C. It replicates in the cytoplasm, probably in the same fashion as picornaviruses. Rubella can be described as a mild exanthematous disease common in children and young adults that may induce teratogenic effects in the developing fetus.

Epidemiology

Infection is acquired through inhalation of droplets from the respiratory tract of infected persons. Prior to the introduction of the attenuated vaccine, outbreaks would occur in 5- to 7-year cycles, especially during the winter and spring of the year. In this postvaccine era, another pattern of prevalence is occurring. Outbreaks are now being reported in postadolescent children and young adults in college who may have escaped immunization. Another source of contagion is the neonatal carrier that has caused outbreaks in nursery staff.

Pathogenesis

During the incubation period of 18 days, the virus replicates first in the upper respiratory tract mucosa and the cervical lymph nodes; it infects leukocytes and is transported in the blood to other parts of the reticuloendothelial system. Following development of the second viremia, a rash develops that is considered in part a hypersensitivity reaction, but also is considered an infection of integumentary tissue.

The extent of teratogenicity depends upon the age of the fetus when infected. Frequently a persistent and chronic viral infection is established and growth is retarded by mitotic arrest or various degrees of chromosome damage. Tissue necrosis results and hypoxia is created due to fetal vasculitis. This usually leads to spontaneous abortion or to an infant that is born as a rubella carrier, with varying degrees of congenital defects.

Clinical Manifestations

In the prodromal period, generalized lymphadenopathy may begin 7 days prior to the onset of rash and can involve the suboccipital, postauricular and posterior cervical nodes. Lymphadenopathy may be the only symptom, although others that may develop are fever, malaise, headache, mild coryza, conjunctivitis and sore throat 1 to 5 days before the rash develops. This rubella-form rash first develops at the hairline and face and spreads rapidly to involve the neck, trunk, and extremities within a 24-hour period and usually lasts for 3 to 5 days. An enanthema consisting of small red macules on the soft palate often precedes or accompanies the rash; these are referred to as Forscheimer spots. Especially in adult females, synovitis of the fingers, wrists, knees and ankle joints is a common complication and swelling may not disappear for a month. Only rarely are thombocytopenic purpura and severe encephalitis encountered.

Congenital infection can result in such teratogenic findings as malformations of the heart with patent ductus arteriosus, coarctation of pulmonary vessels and ventricular septal defects. In the eye, cataracts, glaucoma and cloudy cornea are observed. Hearing defects may develop and microcephaly and hydrocephaly can result also from disturbances of growth of the skull. Other defects that occur include enamel dysplasia of the teeth. Intra- and extrauterine growth retardation, Down's syndrome, and agammaglobulinema also may be evident (table 42/4). The fact that many adult cases occur without rash always presents a hazard to the fetus of a nonimmune mother.

Diagnosis

Clinical diagnosis is not easy unless an outbreak occurs where all forms of this mild disease can be seen. It can be confused with exanthems of infectious mononucleosis, mild rubeola, enterovirus infection, roseola, erythema infectiosum, scarlet fever, and toxoplasmosis. Laboratory diagnosis is

Table 42/4
Clinical manifestations of the expanded rubella syndrome[a]

General	Extramedullary hematopoiesis
Retardation of intrauterine growth	Hepatomegaly
Failure to thrive	Splenomegaly
Ocular	"Blueberry muffin" syndrome
Retinopathy	Generalized adenopathy
Nuclear cataract	Thymic hypoplasia[b]
Microphthalmia	Depressed humoral and cellular immunity
Glaucoma	Central nervous system
Transient corneal cloudiness	Encephalitis
Iridocyclitis	Leptomeningitis
Auditory	Microcephaly
Sensorineural hearing loss	Psychomotor retardation
Vestibular dysfunction	Spastic quadriparesis
Otitis media	Chronic progressive panencephalitis (late)
Central auditory imperception[b]	Gastrointestinal
Cardiovascular and pulmonary	Giant-cell hepatitis
Congenital heart disease[c]	Indirect inguinal hernia
Myocardial necrosis	Cholangiolytic hepatitis
Fibromuscular proliferation of arterial intima	Intestinal atresia
Stenosis or hypoplasia of pulmonary and systemic arteries	Diarrhea
Systemic hypertension	Interstitial pancreatitis[b]
Interstitial pneumonitis	Skin
Musculoskeletal	Abnormal dermatoglyphics
Myositis	Skin dimples
Metaphyseal osteoporosis	Seborrheic dermatitis
High arched palate	Vasomotor instability
Hypoplastic mandible	Dyshydrosis
Dental abnormalities	Genitourinary
Delayed eruption	Hypospadias
Enamel defects	Cryptorchidism
Minor lower extremity abnormalities	Vesicoureteral reflux[b]
Blood and reticuloendothelial system	Interstitial nephritis
Thrombocytopenic purpura	Anatomic renal abnormalities
Hemolytic anemia	Metabolic
Hypoplastic anemia	Diabetes mellitus (early onset)
	Chronic lymphocytic thyroiditis[b]

[a] Reproduced with permission from P. D. Hoeprich (Ed.). 1977 *Infectious Diseases*, Ed. 2. Harper & Row, Hagerstown, Md.

[b] Requires additional confirmation.

[c] Patent ductus arteriosus, pulmonary artery or valvular stenosis, and ventricular septal defects are most common.

readily made by detecting IgM antibodies by the ELISA test or IgG antibodies by agglutination of virus antigen-coated latex particles. Since rubella does not produce a cytopathogenic effect (CPE), its presence may be detected in the ECHO 11 interference test (Chapter 35).

Treatment

Symptoms are usually mild enough so that only salicylates are administered to treat the fever, arthritis or arthralgias. Immune globulin is not recommended for pregnant women since it might suppress symptoms but still allow a viremia to occur.

Prevention

Rubella vaccine is recommended for all children and those young adults not yet immune; however, if delayed until adulthood some individuals may develop arthritis (but not to the same degree as they would in natural infection). Since a potential risk for congenital defects due to vaccine virus exists, pregnant women should not be immunized.

Since teratogenic effects frequently result (80%) following infection of a pregnant women during the first trimester, and less frequently thereafter, elective abortions are frequently recommended.

ADDITIONAL READING

AZIMI, PH. S., SHABAN, S., HILTY, M. D., et al. 1975 Mumps Meningoencephalitis Prolonged Abnormality of Cerebrospinal Fluid. JAMA, **234**, 1161.

BEARDWELL, A. 1969 Facial Palsy due to the Mumps Virus. Br J Clin Pract, **23**, 37.

BELLANTI, J. A., SANGA, R. L., KLUTINIS, B., et al. 1969 Antibody Responses in Serum and Nasal Secretions of Children Immunized with Inactivated and Attenuated Measles-Virus Vaccines. N Engl J Med, **280**, 628.

BUESCHER, E. L. 1965 Behavior of Rubella Virus in Adult Populations. Arch Gesamte Virusforsch, **16**, 470.

DACOU-VOUTETAKIS, C., CONSTANTINIDIS, M., MOSCHOS, A., et al. 1974 Diabetes Mellitus Following Mumps: Insulin Reserve. Am J Dis Child, **27**, 890.

DOWNHAM, M. A. P. S., McQUILLIN, J., AND GARDNER, P. S. 1974 Diagnosis and Clinical Significance of Parainfluenza Virus Infections in Children. Arch Dis Child, **49**, 8.

FENNER, F. 1948 The Pathogenesis of the Acute Exanthems. Lancet, **2**, 915.

GARDNER, P. S., McQUILLIN, J., McGUCKIN, R., et al. 1971 Observations on Clinical and Immunofluorescent Diagnosis of Parainfluenza Virus Infections. Br Med J, **2**, 7.

GERSHON, A. A. 1979 Rubella Virus (German Measles). In *Principles and Practice of Infectious Diseases*, p. 1258, edited by G. L. Mandell, R. G. Douglas, Jr. and J. E. Bennett. John Wiley, New York.

GREGG, N. McA. 1941 Congenital Cataract Following German Measles in the Mother. Trans Ophthamol Soc Aust, **3**, 35.

HENLE, G., HENLE, W., WENDELL, K. K., et al. 1948 Isolation of Mumps Virus from Human Beings with Induced Apparent or Inapparent Infections. J Exp Med, **88**, 223.

KILLGORE, G. E., AND DOWDLE, W. R. 1970 Antigenic Characterization of Parainfluenza 4A and 4B by the Hemagglutination-Inhibition Test and Distribution of HI Antibody in Human Sera. Am J Epidemiol, **91**, 308.

KOPLIK, H. 1896 The Diagnosis of the Invasion of Measles from a Study of the Exanthemata as It Appears on the Buccal Mucous Membranes. Arch Pediatr, **13**, 918.

KRUGMAN, S. 1977 Present Status of Measles and Rubella Immunization in the United States: A Medical Progress Report. J Pediatr, **90**, 1.

KUSSY, J. C. 1974 Fatal Mumps Myocarditis. Minn Med, **57**, 285.

LERMAN, S. T., NANKERVIS, G. A., HEGGIE, A. D., et al. 1971 Immunologic Response, Virus Excretion and Joint Reactions with Rubella Vaccine. A Study of Adolescent Girls and Young Women Given Live Attenuated Virus Vaccine (HPV-77 DE5). Ann Inter Med, **74**, 67.

MARCY, S. M., AND KIRBRICK, S. 1977 Rubella. In *Infectious Diseases*, Ed. 2, p. 701, edited by Paul D. Hoeprich. Harper & Row, Hagerstown, Md.

MARCY, S. M., AND KIBRICK, S. 1977 Mumps. In *Infectious Diseases*, Ed. 2 p. 621, edited by P. D. Hoeprich. Harper & Row, Hagerstown, Md.

NAEYE, R. L., AND BLANC, W. 1965 Pathogenesis of Congenital Rubella. JAMA, **194**, 1277.

chapter 43

Neurologic Infections Caused by Conventional and Unconventional Viruses: Rabies and Slow Virus Infections

Memory Elvin-Lewis

INTRODUCTION

Viruses that affect the central nervous system (CNS) include those that primarily infect these tissues and those that involve it as secondary complications of primary infections elsewhere. Primary infections of the nervous system may be manifest as acute infections, exemplified by meningitis, encephalitis and rabies. They also may appear as so-called slow virus infections that are unusual manifestations of infections due to viruses that normally cause acute disease, or by unconventional viruses that are primarily neurotropic.

RHABDOVIRIDAE: *LYSSAVIRUS*

Lyssavirus is the name of the genus in the Rhabdoviridae to which rabies viruses belong. Virions of this group are characteristically bullet-shaped, enveloped, helical nucleocapsids covered with knob-like structures. The envelope consists of a lipid bilayer containing proteins, and glycoprotein peplomers, and the helical nucleocapsid contains a single, negative strand of RNA, several proteins and an RNA-dependent RNA transcriptase. Replication probably involves negative strand viral RNA transcription into mRNAs and another portion into a positive-stranded RNA to serve as a template for progeny virus RNA. Cytoplasmic inclusions termed Negri bodies represent the sites of viral replication.

Epidemiology

Rabies is primarily a zoonosis and may produce inapparent infection in vampire bats, civet cats, skunks and racoons. Disease in dogs is aberrant and results from infection by wild animals. Infection in man may be the result of a bite from a rabid dog or contact with its saliva, contact with "wild pets" like baby skunks and racoons that are incubating the disease, through the inhalation of infected bat guano, through the ingestion of (or other contact with) infected ungulates (*e.g.*, moose). It has been acquired through corneal transplants from an individual with atypical rabies. It is not known when rabies virus appears in human saliva although it can be detected for several months in bats, but only for 2 or 3 days in dogs and cats. For this reason it is not possible to ascertain the risk involved in treating a patient who is incubating the disease. Not only do prodromal symptoms mimic common respiratory or abdominal infections, but oftentimes the disease goes undetected because of atypical symptoms. Recently the Center for Disease Control has advised that all patients dying of encephalitis, particularly those from rural or semirural areas, should be suspect of having rabies. Of added concern is the fact that the number of reported cases of animal rabies has risen dramatically during the past 2 years and that rabies has been recently found in pet racoons and pet skunks that were originally captured from the wild. Therefore entire families and their friends were at risk of acquiring infection.

Pathogenesis

Rabies is an acute encephalitis, almost always fatal, that is usually acquired through the bite of a rabid animal. After a bite the virus remains localized in the connective tissue and muscle for days to months before it reaches the central nervous system by travelling along the axoplasm of the peripheral nerves to the ganglia and eventually to the central nervous system where it has a predilection for Purkinje cells. There it has been suggested that the virus causes interference with neuronal function

437

rather than neuronal destruction. Negri bodies are prominent in ganglion cells of the hippocampus and cerebellum. The pons and medulla of the brain are edematous, hemorrhagic and congested, and perivascular cuffing is evident. Pathology of the spinal cord is related to the region associated with the site of the bite.

Clinical Manifestations

Initial symptoms develop following a prolonged incubation period of weeks to months (shorter if the site of infection is closer to the head). In the prodromal period of 2 to 4 days the patient suffers from a variety of constitutional and nervous system symptoms that include fever, malaise, headache, anorexia, nausea, sore throat, nervousness, anxiety, irritability, hyperesthesia, sensitivity to light and noise, excessive salivation, lacrimation and perspiration. Facial expressions may become overactive, the pupils dilated, the pulse increased and respirations shallow. Of all of these, a change in sensation around the site of the bite is the most prominent symptom. In the excitatory phase that follows, difficulty in swallowing and respiration becomes the primary symptom, so called "hydrophobia" (morbid fear of water). Other clinical manifestation include cranial nerve malfunction such as ocular palsies, tachycardia, bradycardia, cyclic respiration, urinary retention and constipation. In the final paralytic phase, "hydrophobia" disappears as a progressive, general flaccid paralysis develops. Apathy, stupor, coma, urinary incontinence, peripheral vascular collapse and death occur.

Diagnosis

Corneal impression and brain tissue smears stained with specific antibody will demonstrate typical intracytoplasmic inclusions, Negri bodies.

Therapy

There is no specific therapy for overt rabies, and supportive therapy is given to ease the symptoms.

Following a bite or verified contact, the new diploid vaccine is administered. Patients also may receive antirabies immune globulin as an added prophylactic measure. The bite should always be well cleaned with soap and water and rabies-immune serum may be infused into the wound.

Prevention

A new diploid cell-line vaccine is available and has proven safe and efficacious. Individuals at high risk including laboratory workers, veterinarians, dog control personnel, spelunkers, Peace Corps personnel, and wildlife control personnel should receive it. Almost all communities insist that dogs be immunized and any suspect animal examined. It is extremely important to make sure that the general public is aware of the risks of befriending wild animals.

VIRAL SLOW DISEASES

A slow infection caused either by "typical" viruses or unconventional agents is defined as a host-parasite relationship in which the parasite fails to cause acute disease, the host fails to eliminate the parasite and, ultimately, the parasite's effect on the host or the host's response results in pathologic changes and clinical disease.

Some viruses that are capable of causing acute infections may cause slow infections as well. They may be found among many virus groups and, through their ability to selectively localize in specific cells of the CNS, produce the disease symptoms observed. Other viruses do not fall in this category and are only manifest as slowly evolving diseases involving primarily the central nervous system. Differences between conventional and unconventional slow agents are outlined in table 43/1. The immune status of the host may or may not predispose to slow virus disease. Although progressive multifocal leukoencephalopathy only occurs in the immunologically compromised host, subacute sclerosing panencephalitis is able to produce progressive disease in the face of an accentuated normal response. Table 43/2 illustrates those slow infections of man caused by conventional viruses and the viruses implicated.

Morbillivirus: Measles

Subacute sclerosing panencephalitis (SSPE) is a chronic, fatal encephalitis of children and adolescents which usually develops several years after initial exposure to natural measles virus or possibly live measles vaccine. The relationship between this syndrome and the measles virus appears to be well established. The virus can be detected in the brains of patients with SSPE by histological, electron microscopic, fluorescent antibody and culture techniques. Studies with multiple sclerosis patients suggest a similar etiology.

Unconventional Virus Infections

It has been suggested that the unconventional etiologic agents of these infections are, in fact, animal virioids. These are circular single-stranded RNA molecules that replicate at the cytoplasmic membrane. Clearly, their resistance to irradiation and agents like glutaraldehyde and formaldehyde and susceptibility to surface-active agents, like iodophors, phenolics, or 5% hypochorite suggest such a composition.

Table 43/1

Differences between conventional and unconventional agents causing slow infections

Property	Conventional Agent	Unconventional Agent
Tissue tropism	Many organs and tissues	Only central nervous system
Tissue pathology	Degenerative and/or inflammatory changes	Only degenerative changes
Morphology	Definitive virus structure	No evidence of virus structure
Biochemical	Possess nucleic acid genomes; inhibited by nucleic acid inhibitors; some can be reduced (SSPE[a]); usual virus lability to autoclaving, disinfectants	No evidence of nucleic acid; usual stability; labile to *autoclaving 20 lb, 60 min*; sensitive to membrane active substances such as ether, acetone, chloroform, strong detergent, periodate, phenolics, iodophors, hypochlorite
Immunogenicity	Immunogenic, immune response elicited can modify disease expression, interferon elicited	Nonimmunogenic, interferon not elicited

[a] SSPE, subacute sclerosing panencephalitis.

Table 43/2

Slow infections of man caused by conventional viruses[a]

Disease	Virus
Subacute postmeasles leukoencephalitis	*Paramyxovirus*—defective measles
Subacute sclerosing panencephalitis (SSPE)	*Paramyxovirus*—defective measles
Subacute encephalitis	Herpetovirus—herpes simplex; Adenovirus—adenotypes 7 and 32
Progressive congenital rubella	Togavirus—rubella
Progressive panencephalitis as a late sequela following congenital rubella	Togavirus—defective rubella
Progressive multifocal leukoencephalopathy (PML)	Papovavirus—JC:SV40
Cytomegalovirus brain infection	Herpetovirus—cytomegalovirus
Epilepsia partialis continua (Kojewnikoff's epilepsy) and progressive bulbar palsy in U.S.S.R.	Togavirus—RSSE[b] and other tick-borne encephalitis viruses
Chronic meningoencephalitis in immunodeficient patients	Picornaviruses—poliomyelitis; ECHO virus
Crohn's disease	Unclassified—RNA virus
Homologous serum jaundice	Unclassified—hepatitis B; Dane particle
Hepatitis	Hepatitis A; Unclassified—hepatitis B; Dane particle; Unclassified—hepatitis C

[a] From: Gajdusek, Unconventional Viruses and the Origin and Disappearance of Kuru, Science, Sept. 2, 1977, Vol. 197, No. 4307, reprinted with permission of the American Association for the Advancement of Science, Washington, D.C.

[b] Russian spring-summer encephalitis.

The most important disease of this group to dentists is that of Creutzfeldt-Jakob, since it has the potential of being transmitted to the dentist, or by the dentist to other patients. The other slow infection, kuru, is of historical significance, but worthy of note.

Kuru and Creutzfeldt-Jakob disease viruses produce a similar basic cellular lesion that is characterized by progressive vacuolation in the dentritic and axonal processes of the neurons, with associated stimulation of the elements to hypertrophy and hyperplasia. The neuronal vacuolation produces ballooning and destruction of the cells and reduction of gray matter to a spongioform state in which the finer architecture is destroyed. Pathology in organs other than the brain is notably absent. There is extensive neuron loss and minimal secondary myelin degeneration but no primary demyelination. Amyloid plaques are apparent in both of these human diseases.

Creutzfeldt-Jakob Disease

This transmissible spongioform encephalopathy has an incubation period that can range from 1½ years to several decades and usually affects individuals in middle age and beyond. It appears as a rapidly evolving cerebral disease in which profound dementia is combined with ataxia and diffuse myoclonic jerking. The duration of the disease is usually 6 months, and its initiation is evidenced by symptoms such as memory loss and changes in behavior. This progresses to the more severe forms that result in dysarthria, stupor and coma. Overall it is estimated that the prevalence is about 1 to 2 million/year, with 200 deaths probably occurring annually.

A number of mechanisms of transmission of this unconventional virus have been postulated based on particular associations. Familial clustering in at least 10% of the cases suggests autosomal susceptibility. Occupational association with meat that could be contaminated with scrapie virus has been suggested in an additional third of the cases. However, case-to-case transmission, including iatrogenic spread, or activation of latent infection through trauma or surgery is implied in a significant number of cases. Iatrogenic spread has been implicated in disease following corneal transplantation, and in two cases following electroencephalography. In the latter instance, the electrodes had been "sterilized" in benzene, 70% alcohol and formaldehyde vapor; a procedure that will not inactivate the virus. Contamination through neurosurgery was linked to three cases, although only two of these who had craniotomies within a month of each other may have acquired the disease through contaminated instruments. In the third instance, there was no clear association with the surgical procedure. Similar data has been associated with dental procedures wherein dental surgery was antecedent to development of the disease 3 years later. Other cases have been associated with surgical removal of teeth and orthodontic manipulation, further implicating iatrogenic transfer or surgical trauma as an exciting cause. Individuals in the dental profession also have acquired this disease at a slightly higher frequency than physicians, although at this time it is unclear how significant these findings are.

It has been suggested that individuals with acute psychiatric disturbances or those presenting with behavior patterns suggestive of the early stages of Creutzfeldt-Jakob disease be treated with the potential of contagion in mind.

Kuru

Kuru is confined to the Fore tribe in New Guinea and its incidence is decreasing since the cessation of ritualistic cannibalism in the late 1950s. It is presumably acquired by ingestion of contaminated brain tissue or by other means of self-inoculation (cutaneous, conjunctival and nasal), during opening of the cranial vault during mourning rites for deceased family members. Genetic susceptibility also may be a factor in its higher incidence, especially among females, in certain villages. The incubation period in man is from 5 to 20 years and symptoms include ataxia, tremor and behavioral changes.

ADDITIONAL READING

BARINGER, J. R., GAJDUSEK, D. C., GIBBS, C. J., MASTERS, C. L., STERN, E., AND TERRY, R. D. 1980 Transmissible Dementias: Current Problems in Tissue Handling. Neurology, **30**, 302.

BERNOULLI, C., SIEGRIED, J., BAUMGARTNER, G., REGLI, F., RABINOWICZ, T., GAJDUSEK, D. C., AND GIBBS, C. J. 1977 Danger of Accidental Person-to-Person Transmission of Creutzfeldt-Jakob Disease by Surgery. Lancet, **2**, 478.

BROWN, P. 1980 An Epidemiologic Critique of Creutzfeldt-Jakob Disease. Epidemiol Rev, **2**, 113.

BROWN, P., CATHALA, F., AND GAJDUSEK, D. C. 1979 Creutzfeldt-Jakob Disease in France. III. Epidemiologic Study of 170 Patients Dying During the Decade 1968–1977. Ann Neurol, **6**, 438.

CATHALA, F., CHATELAIN, J., BROWN, P., DUMAS, M., AND GAJDUSEK, D. C. 1980 Familial Creutzfeldt-Jakob Disease. J Neurol Sci, **47**, 343.

DUFFY, P., WOLF, J., COLLINS, G., DEVOE, A. G., STREETEN, B., AND COWEN, D. 1974 Possible Person-to-Person Transmission of Creutzfeldt-Jakob Disease. N Engl J Med, **290**, 692.

GAJDUSEK, D. C., GIBBS, C. J., ASHER, D. M., BROWN, P., DIWAN, A., HOFFMAN, P., NEMO, G., ROWER, R., AND WHITE, L. 1977 Precautions in Medical Care of and in Handling Materials from Patients with Transmissible Virus Dementia (Creutzfeldt-Jakob Disease). N Engl J Med, **297**, 1253.

GAJDUSEK, D. C., GIBBS, C. J., COLLINS, G., AND TRAUB, R. D. 1976 Survival of Creutzfeldt-Jakob Disease Virus in Formol-Fixed Brain Tissue. N Engl J Med, **294**, 553.

GIBBS, C. J., GAJDUSEK, D. C., AND LATARJET, R. 1978 Unusual Resistance to Ionizing Radiation of the Viruses of Kuru, Creutzfeldt-Jakob Disease and Scrapie. Proc Natl Acad Sci, **75**, 6268.

GIBBS, C. J., GAJDUSEK, D. C., AND MASTERS, C. L. 1978 Considerations of Transmissible Subacute and Chronic Infections with a Summary of the Clinical Pathological and Virological Characteristics of Kuru, Creutzfeldt-Jakob Disease and Scrapie. J Infect Dis, **142**, 205.

HOUGH, S. A., BURTON, R. C., WILSON, R. W. *et al.* 1979 Human-to-Human Transmission of Rabies Virus by a Corneal Transplant. N Engl J Med, **300**, 603.

MANDELL, G. L., DOUGLAS, R. G., JR., AND BENNETT, J. E. (Eds.) 1979 *Principles and Practice of Infectious Diseases.* John Wiley, New York.

MASTERS, C. L., HARRIS, J. O., GAJDUSEK, D. C., GIBBS, C. J., BERNOULLI, C., AND ASHER, D. M. 1978 Creutzfeldt-Jakob Disease Patterns of Worldwide Occurrence and the Significance of Familial and Sporadic Clustering. Ann Neurol, **5**, 177.

MASTERS, C. L., GAJDUSEK, D. C., GIBBS, C. J., BERNOULLI, C., AND ASHER, D. M. 1979 Familial Creutzfeldt-Jakob Disease and Other Familial Dementias: and Inquiry into Possible Modes of Transmission of Virus-Induced Familial Diseases. In *Slow Transmissible Disease of the Nervous System*, Vol. 1, edited by S. B. Prusiner and W. J. Hadlow. Academic Press, New York.

MORBIDITY AND MORTALITY WEEKLY REPORTS, Human Rabies—U.S. 1980, **30**, 97.

MORBIDITY AND MORTALITY WEEKLY REPORTS, Rabies in Skunks—Arkansas, 1978, **28**, 481.

TRAUB, R., GAJDUSEK, D. C., AND GIBBS, C. J. 1977 Transmissible Virus Dementia: The Relation of Transmissible Spongiform Encephalopathy to Creutzfeldt-Jakob Disease, In *Aging and Dementia*, p. 91, edited by L. W. Smith and M. Kinsbourne Spectrum Publications, Jamaica, N.Y.

chapter 44

Arthropod-Borne Togaviruses, Bunyaviruses, Arenaviruses and Their Infections

Memory Elvin-Lewis

TOGAVIRUSES

Togaviruses (Togaviridae) are RNA viruses whose capsids have icosahedral symmetry. They are surrounded by lipid and glycoprotein envelopes that contain glycoprotein peplomers with hemagglutinating potential. Aside from the genus *Rubivirus* already discussed, the genera, *Alphavirus* and *Flavivirus*, which are transmitted by insects, cause disease in man. They are differentiated by their size and the nature of their monocistronic, single-stranded RNA genome. For example, *Flavivirus* is 37 to 50 nm in size, contains one positive-stranded RNA that is translated to form one large protein that is cleaved in the fashion described for picornaviruses. *Alphavirus* is 45 to 75 nm in size and contains two positive-stranded RNA molecules. One strand is translated into structural and the other into nonstructural proteins. Replication is intracytoplasmic and proceeds like the picornaviruses, and envelopment takes place at the cytoplasmic membrane. A large number of species are represented in each genus and differ in their ability to be neurotropic, viscerotropic, myelotropic, or dermatotropic.

TOGAVIRIDAE: *ALPHAVIRUS*

Two subgroups are known within the genus; Subgroup I contains viruses of the mosquito-borne equine encephalitides and Subgroup II contains viruses that are primarily African and Australasian in origin and cause syndromes characterized by headache, fever, rash and myalgias. Since Subgroup I are viruses that occur in the western hemisphere they will be discussed as an example of this genus.

The equine encephalitides are eastern equine encephalitis (EEE) virus, western equine encephalitis (WEE) virus and Venezuelan equine encephalitis (VEE) virus. The infections differ in their geographical distribution (table 44/1).

Epidemiology

These infections are primarily zoonoses that are accidentally transmitted to man. In their natural state, the viruses survive in infection cycles involving biting arthropods and various vertebrates, especially birds, rodents and sometimes reptiles. During the extrinsic incubation period in the insect, the virus multiplies in the gut, disseminates in the hemolymph, and ultimately arrives in the salivary gland where it is transmitted through an insect bite to the vertebrate host (fig. 44/1). Insect control is important in preventing outbreaks in human populations, although vaccines are available for equine and human populations during an outbreak. VEE is also highly infectious by aerosol and has caused infections in laboratory workers by this unusual route.

Pathogenesis

Following percutaneous deposition, the virus replicates in lymphatic tissue and other organs before it elicits a viremia that results in viral involvement of the CNS. During the period of primary viremia, fever and other constitutional symptoms may be evident. Once the virus enters the brain, infection can be widespread and causes neuronal destruction, glial cell infiltration, and perivascular cuffing. Lesions in the basal nuclei may occur with EEE and in the cortex with WEE.

Clinical Manifestations

The incubation period of these encephalitides can vary from 1 to 3 weeks. Usually infections are subclinical and clinical disease may vary somewhat with the species. At onset, fever, chills, malaise,

441

Table 44/1. Classification and description of togaviruses[a] and clinically related viruses of humans[b]

Family	Genus (group)	Subgroup	Viral species	Vector	Clinical Diseases in Man	Geographic Distribution
Togaviridae	*Alphavirus*	I	Eastern equine encephalitis (EEE)	Mosquito	Encephalitis	Eastern USA, Canada, Brazil, Cuba, Panama, Philippines, Dominican Republic, Trinidad
			Venezuelan equine encephalitis (VEE)	Mosquito	Encephalitis	Brazil, Colombia, Ecuador, Trinidad, Venezuela, Mexico, Florida, Texas
			Western equine encephalitis (WEE)	Mosquito	Encephalitis	Western USA, Canada, Mexico, Argentina, Brazil, British Guiana
			Sindbis	Mosquito	Subclinical	Egypt, India, South Africa, Australia,
		II	Chikungunya	Mosquito	Headache, fever, rash, joint and muscle pains	East Africa, South Africa, southeast Asia
			Semliki Forest	Mosquito	Fever or none	East Africa, West Africa
			Mayaro	Mosquito	Headache, fever, joint and muscle pains	Bolivia, Brazil, Colombia, Trinidad
			(13 others named)	Mosquito	Subclinical or none known	
	Flavivirus	I	St. Louis encephalitis	Mosquito	Encephalitis	USA, Trinidad, Panama
			Japanese B encephalitis	Mosquito	Encephalitis	Japan, Guam, Eastern Asian mainland, Malaya, India
			Murray Valley encephalitis	Mosquito	Encephalitis	Australia, New Guinea
			Ilheus	Mosquito	Encephalitis	Brazil, Guatemala, Trinidad, Honduras,
			West Nile	Mosquito	Headache, fever, myalgia, rash, lymphadenopathy	Egypt, Israel, India, Uganda, South Africa
		II	Dengue (4 types)	Mosquito	Headache, fever, myalgia, prostration, rash (sometimes hemorrhagic)	Pacific islands, south and southeast Asia, northern Australia, New Guinea, Greece, Caribbean islands, Nigeria, Central and South America
		III	Yellow fever	Mosquito	Fever prostration, hepatitis, nephritis	Central and South America, Africa, Trinidad
			(18 other viruses)	Mosquito		

Table 44/1 (*cont'd*)

Family	Genus (group)	Subgroup	Viral species	Vector	Clinical Diseases in Man	Geographic Distribution
		IV	Tick-borne group (Russian spring-summer encephalitis group) 14 viruses	Tick	Encephalitis, meningoencephalitis, hemorrhagic fever	Russian spring-summer encephalitis, USSR, Canada, USA, others; Japan, Siberia, Central Europe, Finland, India, Malaya, Great Britian (louping ill)
			Rio Bravo (bat salivery (gland) (15 others)	Unrecognized Unrecognized	Encephalitis	California, Texas
Bunyaviridae	*Bunyavirus* (Bunyamwera super-group)	C group	Marituba and 10 others	Mosquito	Headache, fever	Brazil (Belem), Panama, Trinidad, Florida
		Bunyamwera group	Bunyamwera and 17 others	Mosquito	Headache, fever, myalgia, fever only, or none	Uganda, South Africa, India, Malaya, Columbia, Brazil, Trinidad, West Africa, Finland, USA
		California group	California encephalitis and 10 others	Mosquito	Encephalitis or none	USA, Trinidad, Brazil, Canada, Czechoslovakia, Mozambique
		7 other subgroups (7 ungrouped members of genus)	46 viruses			
	(At least 2 others)	Phlebotomus fever group	20 viruses	Phlebotomus	Headache, fever, myalgia	Italy, Egypt
		Uukuniemi group	Uukuniemi and 6 others	Ticks		Finland
		(8 others)	21 viruses	Mosquitoes, ticks		
			8 unassigned viruses			
Arenaviridae	Arenavirus	Tacaribe,	Tacaribe, Junin Tamiami, Machupo, Pichinde, and 3 others Lymphocytic choriomeningitis Lassa		Headache, fever, myalgia, hemorrhagic signs	South and Central America
Ungrouped			Silverwater Rift Valley fever	Tick Mosquito	None known Headache, fe-	Canada Africa

Table 44/1 (*cont'd*)

Family	Genus (group)	Subgroup	Viral species	Vector	Clinical Diseases in Man	Geographic Distribution
					ver, myalgia, joint pains, hemorrhagic signs, rash	
			Crimean hemorrhagic fever	Tick	Headache, fever, myalgia, hemorrhagic signs	Southern USSR
Others			36 others	Mosquito	None known	
			48 viruses (14 groups of 2–8 viruses)	Mosquito tick	None known in most cases	

[a] *Rubivirus* (rubella, or German measles virus), also a togavirus is discussed in Chapter 42.
[b] Reproduced with permission from B. D. Davis *et al.* 1980 *Microbiology*, Ed. 3. Harper & Row, Hagerstown, Md.

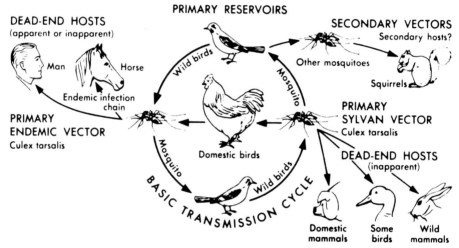

Figure 44/1. Epidemiology pattern for western equine encephalitis (WEE) virus infections. The chains for rural St. Louis encephalitis are similar, except that horses are inapparent, rather than apparent, hosts. Eastern equine encephalitis (EEE) infections also have a similar summer infection chain, but a few significant differences exist: 1) the identity of the vector infecting man is unknown, 2) domestic birds do not appear to be a significant link in the chain, and 3) it has a bird-to-bird secondary cycle in pheasants whose role is unclear. (Reproduced with permission from A. D. Hess and P. Holden. 1958 Annals of the New York Academy of Science, **70**, 294.)

nausea and vomiting are evident. These are followed by neurological symptoms that suggest meningeal involvement (stiff neck and back) and slowly evolve to show evidence of neuronal damage (drowsiness, coma, paralysis, convulsions, ataxia and organic psychoses). Fatality rates for WEE are as high as 70%, whereas with EEE they are low, (about 10%). VEE differs somewhat in its clinical presentation in that, in addition to those constitutional symptoms just presented, myaglias and pharyngitis may be present so that it is usually diagnosed as a benign influenza-like disease unless a fulminant form develops that leads to coma and death.

Diagnosis

If these infections are suspected, serological tests including hemagglutination-inhibition, complement fixation and neutralization may be employed.

TOGAVIRIDAE: *FLAVIVIRUS*

Flaviviruses are divided into subtypes depending on whether they are mosquito- or tick-borne, and grouped further according to their antigenic relationships and the distinctive diseases they cause in man.

Subgroup I: St. Louis Encephalitis

St. Louis encephalitis virus is representative of Subgroup I. It is transmitted by a variety of mosquito vectors, and retains its natural cycle in birds and rodents. Infection in children is frequently subclinical, and clinical cases are usually seen in middle-aged or older individuals. The course of infection is similar to that described for *Alphavirus* encephalitides. The clinical manifestations may include fever and headache, aseptic meningitis or severe encephalitis, with disorientation, tremors, photophobia, visual impairment and convulsions, but permanent sequelae are uncommon. The mortality rate is about 20% and usually increases with age. Fatal cases are characterized by a leptomeningeal mononuclear infiltration.

Subgroup II: Dengue

Dengue is representative of Subgroup II.

Epidemiology

Man or monkeys may serve as the reservoir of infection, and *Aedes aegypti* and *Aedes albopictus* mosquitos serve as vectors. Endemic areas include parts of the southern United States, especially Florida and Texas, and the Carribean Islands. It is also found in the southwest Pacific, southeast Asia, the Philippine Islands, Indonesia, India and Pakistan. Vector control is essential; the intrinsic period in mosquitos has been estimated as 8 to 11 days.

Pathogenesis

During the incubation period of 5 to 8 days the virus replicates in the reticuloendothelial system, and increased vascular permeability and intravascular coagulation are primary features of the infection. Petechial hemorrhage and perivascular edema can occur in a number of organs and the maculopapular rash is a result of injury to small dermal blood vessels.

Clinical Manifestations

After a brief incubation period of 2 to 5 days, the onset of symptoms is sudden and is characterized by biphasic fever that lasts for 5 to 7 days, intense headache, rapid pulse, postorbital pains, joint and muscle pains, lymphadenopathy, and rash. The rash usually appears after 3 to 4 days of fever and is either maculopapular or scarlatiniform in appearance. Petechiae also may occur on the feet, legs, axillae or palate on the last day of fever or shortly thereafter. Recovery is associated with prolonged fatigue and depression and fatalities are rare. However, in severe cases circulatory failure may result, and this dengue shock syndrome results in death of 20% of those infected.

Diagnosis

Serodiagnostic tests including complement fixation and hemagglutination-inhibition are usually adequeate to differentiate the infection from murine typhus, yellow fever, Rocky Mountain spotted fever, leptospirosis, typhoid fever, and other insect-borne viral infections such as the *Orbivirus*-induced, Colorado tick fever.

Subgroup III: Yellow Fever

Yellow fever virus is representative of Subgroup III and because of its worldwide tropical significance also is discussed in detail.

Epidemiology

The virus is transmitted from man to man (epidemic yellow fever) or from simian to man (endemic yellow fever) or from simian to simian (enzootic yellow fever) by the *A. aegypti* mosquito that is infective following a 9 to 12 day intrinsic period. Since the widespread use of the attenuated virus vaccine began, epidemic outbreaks of yellow fever are rare. Endemic zones occur in enzootic areas that include much of northern South America and sub-Saharan Africa.

Pathogenesis

The virus is mainly viscerotropic and affects the liver, kidney, heart and gastrointestinal tract. In the liver it causes an acute coagulative necrosis, and intracellular deposits known as Councilman bodies. In the kidneys, fatty degeneration is evident in the proximal tubules; and the pericardium has petechial hemorrhages. Black vomit is a result of such hemorrhages of the stomach and duodenum; petechial hemorrhages also may be evident in the mucous membranes and skin.

Clinical Manifestations

The incubation period is usually from 3 to 6 days. The infection may be asymptomatic or arise abruptly with fever, muscular aching, lack of appetite, nausea and vomiting. These symptoms may persist for 1 to 7 days. Jaundice occurs around the 3rd day, if it appears at all. In severe infections bleeding occurs from the nose, gingivae and gastrointestinal tract due to oozing petechial hemorrhages and the effects of impaired clotting factor production by a diseased liver. The frequency of some of the classical symptoms is a defining feature, and is a reflection of the genotype involved. Mortality is usually about 5%.

Diagnosis

Hemagglutination-inhibition and complement-fixation tests are useful only if other cross-reacting viruses are excluded during differential diagnosis. In this regard, the infection must be differentiated from dengue, influenza, hepatitis, malaria, typhoid, leptospirosis and carbon tetrachloride poisoning.

Prevention

The 17-D Theiler vaccine prepared in the chick embryo is an excellent attenuated strain that affords protection for 10 or more years. Persons allergic to egg proteins may be immunized by scarification.

BUNYAVIRUSES

Bunyaviruses (Bunyaviridae) contain a helical nucleocapsid with three negatively-stranded RNA molecules, and a polymerase (transcriptase). They are surrounded by a lipid-containing envelope 90 to 100 nm in size that has projecting filamentous-like glycoprotein peplomers with hemagglutinating properties. Its replication cycle is unknown. The species that belong to this family typically cause diseases that are characterized by headache, fever and myalgias. Infection may be more severe and present symptoms of joint pain, encephalitis, or hemorrhagic fever. California encephalitis virus is a representative species of this group and strains have been isolated in the United States, Czechoslovakia and Mozambique.

In nature, the forest dwelling mosquito *Aedes triseriatus* transmits the virus to rodent reservoirs. Man acquires the infection through a mosquito bite, and develops classical symptoms of encephalitis, initiated by headache, fever and lethargy. Convulsions may be the initial sign in children and are accompanied by nausea, vomiting, and neurological symptoms such as incoordination, aphasia and paralysis, suggestive of neuronal damage. Although most individuals recover completely, sequelae such as personality changes and learning disabilities have been seen. Diagnosis is achieved by hemagglutination-inhibition and complement fixation tests.

ARENAVIRUSES

Arenaviruses (Arenaviridae) are 80 to 130 nm in size and are similar in structure to the bunyaviruses, except that the peplomers are regularly spaced and club shaped. Within the envelope, dense granules presumed to be host ribosomes are entrapped, and thus give the structure a unique appearance. The virion is known to contain three negatively-stranded RNA molecules and the envelope proteins and glycoproteins. The status of this group awaits further definition.

Small rodents, mice, rats and hamsters are reservoirs of diseases that are transmitted to humans and can cause the mild influenza-like illness of lymphocytic choriomeningitis; the more severe hemorrhagic fevers of the Tacaribe complex with associated oral lesions; or the fatal Lassa fever with its fever, oral lesions, rash, myalgia, heart and kidney damage.

ADDITIONAL READING

CASALS, J., AND BUCKLEY, S. M. 1974 Lassa Fever. Progr Med Virol, **18**, 111.

DARNELL, M. B., KOPROWSKI, H., AND LAGERSPETZ, K. 1974 Genetically Determined Resistance to Infection with Group B Arboviruses. J Infect Dis, **129**, 240.

DE MADRID, A. T., AND PORTERFIELD, J. S. 1974 The Flaviviruses (Group B Arboviruses): A Cross-Neutralization Study. J Gen Virol, **23**, 91.

DOHERTY, R. L. 1977 Viral Encephalitides. In *Infectious Diseases*, Ed. 2, p. 919, edited by P. D. Hoeprich. Harper & Row, Hagerstown, Md.

LORD, R. D., CALISHER, C. H., CHAPPELL, W. A., METZGER, W. R., AND FISCHER, G. W. 1974 Urban St. Louis Encephalitis Surveillance through Wild Birds. Am J Epidemiol, **99**, 360.

MANDELL, G. L., DOUGLAS, R. G. JR., AND BENNETT, J. E. (Eds.) 1979 *Principles and Practice of Infectious Diseases*. John Wiley, New York.

MILLER, J. R., AND HARTER, D. H. 1972 Acute Viral Encephalitis. Med Clin North Am, **56**, 1393.

MURPHY F. A., HARRISON, A. K., AND WHITFIELD, S. G. 1973 Bunyaviridae: Morphologic and Morphogenetic Similarities of Bunyamwera Serologic Supergroup Viruses and Several Other Arthopod-borne Viruses. Intervirology, **1**, 297.

PECK, R. O., BROWN, A., AND WUST, C. J. 1975 Preliminary Evidence for Cell-Mediated Immunity in Cross-Protection Among Group A Arboviruses. J Immunol, **114**, 581.

PFAU, C. J. 1974 Biochemical and Biophysical Properties of Arenaviruses. Progr Med Virol, **18**, 64.

PORTERFIELD, J. S., CASALS, J., CHUMAKOV, M., GAIDAMOVIC, S. Y., HANNOUN, C., HOLMES, I. H., HORZINER, M. C., MUSSGAY, M., AND RUSSEL, D. K. 1974 Bunyaviruses and Bunyaviridae. Intervirology, **2**, 170.

SIMPSON, D. I. 1972 Arboviruses Diseases. Br Med Bull, **28**, 10.

WATTS, D. M., AND ELDRIDGE, B. F. 1975 Transovarial Transmission of Arboviruses by Mosquitoes; A Review. Med Biol, **53**, 271.

chapter 45

Picornaviruses: *Enterovirus, Aphthovirus, Cardiovirus* and *Rhinovirus* Infections; Coronaviruses and Their Infections

Memory Elvin-Lewis

INTRODUCTION

Picornaviruses comprise a large number of virus strains pathogenic for humans and many animal species. They are divided into four genera: *Enterovirus*, that includes polio and Coxsackie viruses; *Rhinovirus*, that includes the viruses of the common cold; *Aphthovirus*, that includes foot and mouth disease virus; and Mengo and encephalomyocarditis viruses of mice that belong to the genus, *Cardiovirus*.

Causative Agents

Picornaviruses (Picornaviridae) are small, naked icosahedral viruses (22 to 30 nm) that contain a monocistronic single-stranded RNA within a capsid containing 32 capsomeres. The genera are divided by differences in their physical properties and the major diseases that they cause. Generally, species within the genus *Enterovirus* are unstable at 50 C, but are ether resistant and tolerate a pH ranging from 3.8 to 8.5. Furthermore, they are slowly inactivated by such disinfectants as alcohol, phenol, formaldehyde, and chlorine. They are susceptible to oxidizing agents and drying. They elicit diseases with visceral, neural, and sometimes dermal and cardiac manifestations. Conversely the genus *Rhinovirus* is noted for its acid lability. It is unstable at pH 3.0. Its species are responsible in part for the syndrome known as the common cold. Similarly, cardioviruses are acid stable while aphthoviruses are acid labile.

Picornaviruses enter the cell by pinocytosis, losing one polypeptide in the process. The virion is uncoated to release its monocistronic RNA. This is translated into a large protein that is cleaved to form enzymes such as an RNA polymerase for nucleic acid replication and others for virion structure. Viral replication and encapsulation take place in the cytoplasm and the virions are released on cell lysis. Most species of picornaviruses readily cause cytopathogenic effect (CPE) in cell cultures with the exception of certain Coxsackie A strains that can only be propagated in newborn mice.

ENTEROVIRUS: POLIOVIRUS

Poliovirus belongs to a group of enteroviruses that have encephalomyalgic tendencies. Three serotypes are known (Types 1 to 3) that have the potential to cause an acute illness that can range from subclinical to a form involving the nervous system and producing symptoms of aseptic meningitis, encephalitis and paralysis in a disease referred to as poliomyelitis, polio or infantile paralysis.

Epidemiology

Within temperate climates the incidence of infection is highest in summer and early fall; in tropical areas outbreaks occur throughout the year. Transmission is by the fecal-oral route and is facilitated by fecal-contaminated food, water or sewage. Flies also have been implicated as mechanical carriers.

Susceptibility patterns have changed markedly since the advent of the polio vaccines. In the pre-vaccine era, children usually developed an ubiquitous disease in childhood without the development of paralysis. However, as the standard of living increased, infection was often delayed until individuals were adults and, thus, more prone to develop the paralytic form. Following the introduction of the attenuated trivalent vaccine (Sabin), that unlike its formalin-inactivated predecessor (Salk vaccine), prevents intestinal replication, the disease has virtually disappeared except in isolated communities, where inadequate immunization usually can be proved. Rarely, recipients of the vaccine develop apparent disease, but usually these patients have some form of inherent immune deficiency.

Pathogenesis

Following ingestion, the virus first replicates in lymphatic tissue such as the tonsils, and lymphoid tissues of the gut, and after spreading to the deeper lymph nodes initiates a viremia where it reaches cells of the reticuloendothelial system. In subclinical infection, it may remain there to elicit a primary antibody response, or replicate and give rise to a second viremia that corresponds to the clinical symptoms known as abortive poliomyelitis. Virus may be excreted in the stool and nasopharynx at this point. With a persistent viremia, virus may pass through capillary walls and enter the central nervous system (CNS). The virus also may spread to the CNS from peripheral ganglia by transmission along nerve fibers. Destruction of neurons, especially in the anterior horn cells of the spinal cord and motor nuclei of the pons and medulla and elsewhere result in paralysis. In the medulla and brain stem (bulbar polio) this reaction can be fatal since respiratory or cardiac failure can result. In fatal cases, necrosis of a number of visceral organs and lymph nodes is apparent in addition to involvement of cerebellar nuclei, the hypothalamus, the thalamus, and cerebral hemispheres. Also edema and lymphocytic and neutrophilic infiltration are pronounced in the perivascular spaces.

It has been suggested that possession of either HL-A3 or HL-A7 histocompatibility types predisposes to the paralytic form. Also, fatigue, trauma, pregnancy, age and drug injection may affect the frequency and severity of paralysis. Those that have undergone tonsillectomies are more likely to succumb and individuals lacking tonsils are more prone to bulbar involvement.

Clinical Manifestations

The incubation period of poliomyelitis can vary from 1 to 7 weeks but most clinical cases develop within the 2nd week. The disease may proceed through several stages or terminate at any point.

The abortive form develops with fever, headache, vomiting, constipation, coryza and sore throat that lasts for 2 to 6 days before subsiding permanently or temporarily. If patients become excessively fatigued or undertake strenous exercise during the period of these initial symptoms they are more likely to develop paralytic disease; however, these predisposing factors are by no means the only reason why neurological involvement takes place.

In the second or preparalytic phase, fever returns and is accompanied by irritability, motor disturb-

ance, sweating, muscle pain, spasms, and symmetrically accentuated tendon reflexes and stiffness of the neck and back. These symptoms of aseptic meningitis may occur with any of the encephalomyalgic enteroviruses; however, they are earliest in paralytic poliomyelitis.

Paralytic poliomyelitis may follow the earlier stages and loss of motor function is characteristically asymmetric and noncontiguous. For example, in 60% of the patients, one or both legs are involved; and in 25% of patients, one or both arms are involved. In this regard, an arm is particularly predisposed to paralysis if it has received any type of intramuscular injection for 2 weeks prior to the onset of illness. Breathing may be impaired when the diaphragm and intercostal muscles are involved.

Approximately 95% of all infections with polioviruses result in subclinical infection; in the remainder, most develop the abortive form and only about 1% have neurologic involvement that leads to paralysis in 0.1% of cases.

In bulbar paralysis, when there is involvement of the 9th and 10th cranial nerves, facial and extraocular enervations result that affect the soft palate, pharynx and larynx and cause difficulty in speaking or swallowing. Should the 5th nerve also be involved, chewing is difficult and trismus may result. When lower cranial nerves are affected, respiratory obstruction, regurgitation, and aspiration problems develop and death can occur if the medullary respiratory center is involved.

Complications that develop include encephalitis with seizures that are difficult to distinguish from other types of viral encephalitis, respiratory failure, aspiration pneumonia, pulmonary embolism, myocarditis, gastrointestinal hemorrhage and a paralyzed ileus.

Diagnosis

The CSF will at first show a leukocytosis that eventually evolves into a lymphocytosis with about 100 to 500 cells/ml.

Nonparalytic poliomyelitis cannot be diagnosed clinically and requires serological or tissue culture isolation for verification. Unlike poliomyelitis, other enteroviruses rarely cause permanent paralysis. Neutralization tests are helpful in distinguishing the cytopathogenic enteroviruses, including polioviruses from each other.

Treatment and Prevention

Since no specific antiviral agents are available for treatment, management of cases is supportive and symptomatic. Heat is helpful in relieving the pain of myalgias, and respirators are available for those unable to breathe. The trivalent attenuated vaccines have proved effective in preventing poliomyelitis and are commonly used in the United States. In other countries the inactivated vaccine also is used.

ENTEROVIRUSES: COXSACKIE VIRUS

Coxsackie viruses can cause a variety of symptoms that are outlined in table 45/1. Two groups are differentiated by their ability to cause a distinctive pathology in suckling mice and their ability to be propagated in tissue culture. Coxsackie A viruses produce a generalized myositis of skeletal muscle and due to hyaline degeneration result in flaccid paralysis; most strains cannot be propagated in tissue culture. Coxsackie B viruses produce a focal myositis and, because of central nervous system involvement, cause a focal paralysis. Infection of the myocardium, pancreas and brown fat also occur. These viruses can readily be propagated in tissue culture. Strains of Coxsackie A and B are differentiated into serotypes by neutralization tests.

Epidemiology

The fecal-oral nature of Coxsackie virus transmission, like that of other enteroviruses, produces a seasonal periodicity to infections of summer and autumn in temperate climates, and a year-round occurrence in the tropics. Outbreaks that are more common in young children of lower socioeconomic status usually are caused by specific serotypes currently present in the community. Respiratory-oral transmission is suggested as an alternate means of transmission and occurs in all populations.

Pathogenesis

Coxsackie viruses are acquired by ingestion of contaminated material and, depending on the dose, initiate replication in the lymphoid tissue of the gut and nasopharynx. Following primary replication at these sites, it is usual for fecal shedding to occur but nasopharyngeal involvement is dependent upon a higher infecting dose. After replication occurs in

Table 45/1
Clinical spectrum of infection with Coxsackie viruses and ECHO viruses. [a][b]

Condition	Coxsackie Viruses Group A	Coxsackie Viruses Group B	ECHO Viruses
Illness associated with many enteroviruses	Asymptomatic infection Febrile illness with or without respiratory symptoms Aseptic meningitis (1, 2, 4–7, 9, 10, 14, 16, 22, 24) Paralysis (4, 7, 9) or encephalitis	Asymptomatic infection Febrile illness with or without respiratory symptoms Aseptic meningitis (1–6) Paralysis (1–5) or encephalitis	Asymptomatic infection Febrile illness with or without respiratory symptoms Aseptic meningitis (all except 24, 26, 27, 29, 32) Paralysis (1, 2, 4, 6, 7, 9, 11, 16, 18, 30) or encephalitis
Illness more characteristic of particular groups or immunotypes	Herpangina (2–6, 8, 10, 22) Hand-foot-mouth syndrome (5, 10, 16) Lymphonodular pharyngitis (10) Exanthem (9) Epidemic conjunctivitis (24)	Pleurodynia (1–5) Pericarditis (1–5) Myocarditis (1–5) Generalized disease of newborn Orchitis Hepatitis	Exanthem (especially 9, 16 but also 1–8, 11, 14, 18, 19, 25, 30, 32) Generalized disease of newborn Neonatal diarrhea (11, 14, 18) Chronic meningoencephalitis in agrammaglobulinemics
Etiologic role undefined or uncertain	Diarrhea Hemolytic-uremic syndrome (4) Chronic myopathy (9) or myositis of skeletal muscle Guillain-Barré syndrome Reye's syndrome Mononucleosis-like syndrome (5, 6) Infectious lymphocytosis	Diarrhea Chronic cardiomyopathy Endocarditis Diabetes mellitus Hemolytic-uremic syndrome Mononucleosis-like syndrome (5) Reye's syndrome	Diarrhea Reye's syndrome

[a] Reproduced with permission from G. L. Mandell, R. G. Douglas, Jr., and J. E. Bennett (Eds.) 1979 *Principles and Practice of Infectious Diseases.* John Wiley, New York.
[b] Most commonly implicated immunotypes designated in parentheses.

submucosal lymphatic tissue it continues in deep cervical and mesenteric nodes. A primary, minor viremia develops that causes seeding of the cells of the reticuloendothelial system, and following replication there, a secondary viremia disseminates the virus to target organs such as the meninges, heart, skin, muscles or mucosa.

Clinical Manifestations

Coxsackie virus serotypes may elicit well defined disease syndromes, cause illnesses indistinguishable from other enteroviruses or play an undefined role in other infections.

Hand, foot and mouth disease is a herpetiform exanthem caused by Coxsackie A16 (less commonly A5, A10, B2 and B5) that is defined as a mild illness, often occurring in epidemics or families that produces vesicles in the oral mucosa and on the hands and feet. It occasionally is accompanied by a generalized erythematous rash and rarely by paralysis, myocarditis and aseptic meningitis.

After a short incubation period of 3 to 5 days, a low grade fever occurs, followed by a sore throat and mouth. Vesicles develop typically in the oral cavity on the buccal mucosa, gingiva, soft palate, tongue (fig. 45/1) and pharynx that can coalesce to form vesicles, and rapidly break down to leave shallow, whitish ulcerations with red areolae. These oral lesions are accompanied by mixed papules and clear vesicles, surrounded by a zone of erythema, appearing on the dorsum of the fingers, the toes, heel margins and also occasionally on the palms and soles and elsewhere (fig. 45/2). Following development of these typical symptoms, the patient usually recovers within a week.

A herpetiform exanthem due to Coxsackie A19 may develop on the head, trunk and extremities, appearing as crops of vesicles that do not scab or scar, during a febrile period. A maculopapular rash and urticarial lesions also may be evident.

Purpuric rashes resembling meningococcemia occur with some Coxsackie virus A9 infections, as can

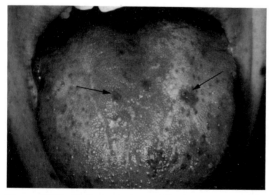

Figure 45/1. Vesicular lesions of the tongue caused by Coxsackie virus.

a rubelliform rash on the flexor and extensor surfaces of the limbs. It is accompanied by fever, malaise and cervical and occipital lymphadenopathy.

Herpangina is a febrile illness of seasonal incidence and pediatric predilection. The majority of cases are caused by Coxsackie A viruses 1 to 6, 8, 10, 16, and 22 and less commonly from Coxsackie virus B 1 to 5 and ECHO viruses 3, 6, 9, 17, 25 and 30. After a short incubation period of 3 to 5 days a high fever (101 to 105 F) develops and lasts for 1 to 4 days. This febrile episode is accompanied by sore throat and development of gray-white, papulovesicular oral lesions 1 to 2 cm in diameter that rupture leaving large, punched out ulcers of 5 mm. These lesions typically appear on the soft palate, uvula, and tonsillar pillars, and occasionally on the oropharynx, and buccal mucosa. They are surrounded by a zone of erythema and are painful. The lesions resolve in 2 to 3 days. Other symptoms may include excessive salivation, anorexia, malaise, and sometimes vomiting and abdominal pain. Systemic symptoms usually disappear along with the fever in 4 to 5 days and recovery is complete within a week.

Acute lymphonodular pharyngitis is a variant of herpangina. In these cases, the lesions consist of tiny nodules of packed lymphocytes which recede without vesiculation or ulceration.

An acute respiratory disease characterized as a common cold is frequently caused by Coxsackie viruses A 21 and A 24, and less commonly by ECHO viruses 4, 8, 9, 11, 20, 22, and 25. Coxsackie virus B respiratory infections appear to be more severe and include laryngotracheobronchitis, bronchiolitis and pneumonia.

Epidemic pleurodynia is primarily caused by the group B Coxsackie viruses and rarely other enteroviruses like Coxsackie A 4, 6 and 10 and ECHO viruses 1, 6, 9, 16, and 19. The disease usually occurs in childen from 5 to 15 and their parents, and it is characterized by fever, chest pain and sometimes headache and sore throat.

Onset is sudden with low grade fever and spasmodic pain over the lower rib cage and upper abdomen that lasts for 2 to 10 hours. Depending on whether the pain is mild or severe, the patient will be ambulatory or require bed rest. Intermittent periods of pain may occur for 5 or 6 days, although relapses can occur for up to a month. Pleuritis, aseptic meningitis, orchitis, pericarditis and pneumonia are possible complications.

Myocarditis and pericarditis are primarily caused by Coxsackie virus groups B 1 to 6, and less commonly by other Coxsackie viruses and some ECHO viruses. Myocarditis usually occurs in the neonate where it is fulminant and fatal in 50% of the cases. It is frequently associated with nursery outbreaks.

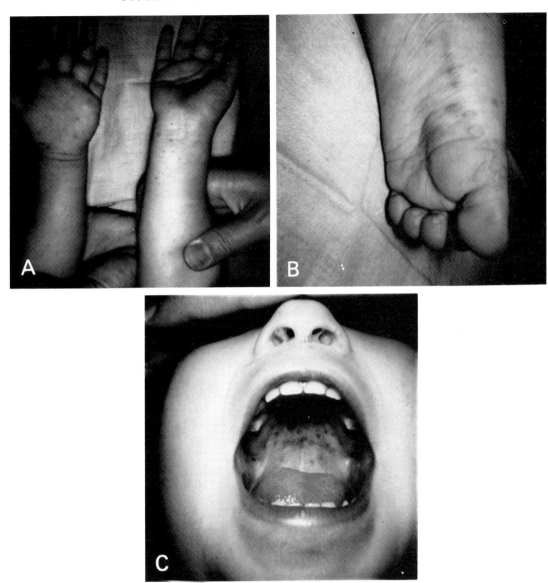

Figure 45/2. (*A*) Ventral surface of hands and forearms of a child with hand, foot, and mouth disease. Note multiple vesicular lesions; some lesions have ulcerated. (*B*) Foot of child with hand, foot, and mouth disease. Vesicular lesions are present along the plantar surface of the foot and toes. (*C*) Palate of child showing initial lesions of hand, foot, and mouth disease. Some vesicular lesions have ruptured, leaving painful ulcerated areas that are surrounded with erythematous halos. Notice the exudative rhinitis in the nares. This occurred at the same time as the onset of the lesions. (Photos courtesy of Dr. R. V. McKinney. Reproduced with permission from R. V. McKinney. 1975 Hand, Foot, and Mouth Disease: A Viral Disease of Importance to Dentists. Journal of the American Dental Association, **91**, 122. Copyright by the American Dental Association.)

Onset typically occurs during the 1st week of age and for 2 days the child is feverish, listless and anorectic; symptoms may disappear and recur again in a week's time. When myocarditis develops it is characterized by tachycardia, systolic murmur, and ECG evidence of myocardial injury. Cyanosis, visceral involvement and circulatory collapse occurs in fatal cases.

In pericarditis of children, and especially in male adults, cardiac symptoms are usually preceded by upper respiratory illness. Symptoms include dyspnea, malaise, chest pain and fever, associated with ECG abnormalities and elevated serum enzymes and white blood count. the illness can resolve or develop into a chronic, recurrent form that can persist for a year or more.

A variant of Coxsackie virus A 24 has been associated with outbreaks of epidemic conjunctivitis in the Far East. It is similar to the more widespread disease caused by *Enterovirus* 70.

Diagnosis

The herpetiform exanthems of hand, foot and mouth disease and A 19 infection must be differentiated from herpes simplex and varicella by the predominance of intraoral lesions, and from herpangina by the location of the lesions in the oral cavity. The symptoms of pleurodynia, myocarditis and pericarditis are usually typical but can be confused with other major illnesses that cause abdominal or chest pain. For abdominal pain, differential diagnosis should exclude peptic ulcer, pancreatitis, and peritonitis and for chest pain, the diagnosis should exclude pneumonia, pulmonary lesions and myocardial ischemia. For verification, complement-fixation tests and isolation of the virus in the appropriate cell cultures or in neonatal mice, and typing by neutralization can be carried out.

ENTEROVIRUS: ECHO VIRUS AND NEW ENTEROVIRUSES

ECHO virus is the acronym for enteric cytopathic human orphan virus. This group of 34 viruses, and other enteroviruses, were first isolated with unknown etiological significance, but eventually a pattern evolved that designated some as the causative agents of specific illnesses while others produce diseases similar to other enteroviruses or remain undefined (table 40/1).

Epidemiology

Like other enteroviruses, ECHO viruses and undesignated enteroviruses are transmitted by the fecal-oral route, with a summer-fall prevalence in temperate regions and year round prevalence in the tropics. Infections usually occur in children, and the adults that live with them.

Pathogenesis

The pathogenesis of ECHO viruses and enteroviruses is much like that described for polioviruses and Coxsackie viruses. Those that are neurotropic produce infection much like that described for abortive poliomyelitis. Others are dermatotrophic, oculotrophic, rhinotropic or have other tissue predilections. They can be isolated from feces and throat or eye swabs, and during viremia, from the blood.

Clinical Manifestations

A variety of illnesses are associated with ECHO viruses.

ECHO 9 rubelliform exanthem is a biphasic infection characterized by fever, anorexia, vomiting and mild sore throat. This is followed by a period of quiesence and then development of a maculopapular rash that first appears on the malar prominances and neck and within 6 to 8 hours descends over the trunk and extremities. Sometimes an exanthem occurs on the buccal mucosa that resembles Koplick's spots of measles. Petichiae may also develop that are reminiscent of meningococcemia. Occasionally aseptic meningitis may occur as well. In addition rubelliform rashes are known to be formed with ECHO virus types 2, 4, 11, 19, and 25 infections.

ECHO 16 roseoliform or "Boston" exanthem is a febrile illness associated with headache, sore throat and gastrointestinal symptoms, a maculopapular rash of the face and thorax and oral lesions similar to herpangina. The disease is more severe in adults and also may involve higher fever, prostration and signs of aseptic meningitis. The infection usually resolves in a week's time.

Chronic meningoencephalitis can develop in patients with hereditary B cell dysfunction anytime between their 2nd and 24th year. The infection with ECHO virus types 2, 3, 9, 11, 24, 25, 30 and 33 is characterized by chronic meningeal irritation or encephalitis. A dermatomyositis-like syndrome also may accompany the neurological involvement. In fatal cases, focal loss of neurons lymphocytic perivascular cuffing and gliosis of the white and gray matter are evident.

Acute aseptic meningitis occurs frequently in infants under the age of 1 year, but also in children and young adults. ECHO viruses that have been implicated most often are types 4, 6, 9, 11, 16, and 30. Less commonly, Coxsackie virus types are B2, B5, A7, and A9, and the poliovirus serotypes are involved. On rare occasions the *Cardiovirus*, encephalomyocarditis virus, also has been implicated. The onset is heralded by fever and chills, followed by frank signs of meningitis such as stiffness of the neck and back with muscle spasm. If the disease is biphasic, an episode of nausea and vomiting is followed by a perid of defervescence before fever and headache resume with other signs of meningitis. *Enterovirus* meningitis also may produce a transitory weakness of skeletal muscle and the Kernig and Brudzinski signs may or may not be excitable. Recovery from viral meningitis usually begins a few days after the illness and is complete within a week or so thereafter.

Acute hemorrhagic conjunctivitis is a disease caused by newly identified picornaviruses termed *Enterovirus* types 70 and 71 that have worldwide distribution. The disease begins abruptly with symptoms of a burning sensation, swelling of the eyelids, ocular pain, photophobia and a watery discharge. In some patients fever, malaise, headache and swelling of the preauricular lymph nodes are seen. The disease is distinctive in the production of subconjunctival hemorrhage. Follicle formation, punctate keratoconjunctivitis and corneal erosion may be evident in the first 24 hours and can, in rare instances, lead to scarring. Should the disease be biphasic in nature, motor paralysis associated with aseptic meningitis may be a further complication.

Diagnosis

The ECHO virus exanthems should be differentiated from other exanthematous diseases with which they can be confused. Similarly, a number of other viruses can cause aseptic meningitis, including togaviruses, mumps virus, herpes simplex virus, lymphocytic choriomeningitis virus, hepatitis viruses, adenoviruses, varicella, rabies, influenza and infectious mononucleosis.

ECHO viruses and enteroviruses are readily isolated in cell culture and differentiated into serotypes by neutralization techniques. Serotyping is particularly important if an outbreak is expected. It is not unusual to have a number of related enteroviruses with the same potential circulating in a community simultaneously.

APHTHOVIRUS

Foot and mouth disease is primarily a zoonosis and is an infection that is rare in man except cattlemen, butchers, and dairymen that may come in contact with infected cattle or contaminated meat, bones, hides, or milk. The disease is characteristically biphasic and following an incubation period of 2 to 18 days lesions appear at a primary site on the skin or mucous membranes. They ulcerate and heal without scarring. Following a period of quiescence, fever occurs and is followed by a more generalized outbreak of vesicles, particularly on the soles, palms, digits and interdigital areas. Lesions in the oral cavity may be seen on the tongue, pharynx and lips, and are usually painful. The virus can be isolated in tissue culture, or diagnosis may be facilitated by serologic procedures. In order to prevent the disease in man, care must be taken when handling infected animals or their by-products.

CARDIOVIRUS

Encephalomyocarditis virus of mice has occasionally been implicated in an aseptic meningitis. It is probably contracted through contact with contaminated mouse feces.

RHINOVIRUS

Rhinovirus serotypes number approximately 100, and are one of the major causes of the common cold, defined as a self-limiting nasal catarrh that may be followed by sinusitis, pharyngitis and lower respiratory tract infections.

Epidemiology

Rhinoviruses are found throughout the world, and circulate randomly in a community or area. Studies with transmission of rhinoviruses have indicated that peak prevalence occurs during the rainy periods of spring and fall or during the rainy season in the tropics. Acquisition depends upon some sort of exposure to infectious secretions over a short distance, thus contamination of the hands, with subsequent autoinoculation of the nasal and conjunctival mucosa is a more likely route of infection than inhalation of virus particles. Thus, during dental treatment, stringent hand washing procedures may offer more protection than the mask alone. Children are considered the reservoir for most rhinoviruses, and annually they acquire six to eight infections per year whereas adults average two to four. For this reason adults who are parents of young children, or dentists who treat large numbers of children, are likely to have more colds per year than others. Although rhinoviruses can confer lasting immunity, large virus challenges can overcome it. Also, little cross-protection among the many types occurs.

Pathogenesis

The viruses enter and multiply in the nasal passages and pharynx. Within 24 hours, inflammatory changes with hyperemia, edema, and leukocyte infiltration are apparent. Desquamation of ciliated columnar epithelium reaches a maximum on the 2nd to 5th day of a cold and regeneration of these cells is not complete until the 14th day. During acute illness nasal secretions rich in glycoproteins are produced in excessive amounts. If inflammatory changes are severe, and marked swelling of the nasal mucosa occurs, sinus ostia, paranasal sinusitis or otitis media may develop.

Clinical Manifestations

Within 24 to 72 hours after contact, nasal stuffiness, sneezing, mild headache, lacrimation, chilliness and malaise develop and persist for 2 to 7 days thereafter. If tracheobronchitis develops, cough and sternal discomfort are seen and, in severe cases, symptoms can be prolonged for up to 2 weeks. A severe cold may spread and lead to sinusitis, otitis media and bronchitis.

Diagnosis

Symptoms of a common cold are usually sufficient to differentiate it from other infections, however, allergic rhinitis and in infants *Streptococcus pyogenes* rhinorrhea may cause similar symptoms.

Treatment

Supportive therapy, including decongestants, syrup or lozenges for sore throat, and cough and antipyretics are recommended. Antipyretics other than aspirin are recommended, since its use may promote congestion.

CORONAVIRUS

Coronaviruses (Coronaviridae) are 80 to 160 nm, possess a helical nucleocapsid containing a single-stranded RNA genome that is surrounded by a spiked envelope that contains lipid, glycoprotein, and protein. There are three distinct serotypes.

Coronaviruses and rhinoviruses are responsible for the majority of upper respiratory infections classified as the common cold.

Epidemiology

It has been estimated that at least 15% of adult common colds are caused by coronaviruses. They have a seasonal prevalence of winter and spring in temperate climates but there are strain differences in epidemic prevalence. Also, the immunity that is conferred following an attack is poor, and reinfections, particularly among children, are common. Coronaviruses also have been isolated from the stools of cases of infantile gastroenteritis and thus certain strains also may be involved in this syndrome.

Pathogenesis

The precise pathogenesis of *Coronavirus* infections in the human respiratory tract has not been described, however, it is likely that it follows a similar pattern to that found for rhinoviruses in causing infection and desquamation of ciliated columnar epithelium.

Clinical Manifestations

Slight differences between *Rhinovirus* and *Coronavirus* common colds exist, although in general terms the symptoms are indistinguishable. With coronaviruses subclinical infections are more common; the incubation period is somewhat longer and the duration of symptoms, shorter. Also the development of pneumonia, pleural reactions and exacerbations of chronic bronchitis are complications more often associated with *Coronavirus* infections.

Diagnosis

Isolation of coronaviruses is not routinely carried out since they are not readily isolated from clinical specimens. For epidemiological surveys, complement-fixation tests on patient's sera are sometimes used.

Treatment

Those measures described for *Rhinovirus* colds apply to *Coronavirus* infections.

ADDITIONAL READING

Bradburne, A. F., and Somerset, B. A. 1972 Coronavirus Antibody Titres in Sera of Health Adults and Experimentally Infected Volunteers. J Hyg Camb, **70,** 235.

Gump, D. W., Phillips, C. A., Forsyth, B. R., et al. 1976 Role of Infection in Chronic Bronchitis. Am Rev Respir Dis, **113,** 465.

McIntosh, K. 1974 Coronaviruses: A Comparative Review. Curr Top Microbiol Immunol, **63,** 85.

McIntosh, K., Chao, R. K., Krause, H. E., et al. 1974 *Coronavirus* Infection in Acute Lower Respiratory Tract Disease in Infants. J Infect Dis, **130,** 502.

McIntosh, K. 1979 *Coronavirus.* In *Principles and Practice of Infectious Diseases*, p. 1212, edited by G. L. Mandell, R. G. Douglas, Jr., and J. E. Bennett. John Wiley, New York.

Wenzel, R. P., Hendley, J. O., Davies, J. A., et al. 1974 *Coronavirus* Infections in Military Recruits: Three-Year Study with *Coronavirus* Strains OC43 and 229E. Am Rev Respir Dis, **199,** 621.

chapter 46

Reoviruses and Their Infections

Memory Elvin-Lewis

INTRODUCTION

The virions of the *Reovirus* group (Reoviridae) contain segmented double-stranded RNA as a genome and a transcriptase for replication. They are 70 to 80 nm in size and are surrounded by a double capsid. Three genera are known that differ antigenically, in the number of genomic RNA segments they possess, and the distinct diseases they cause; of these *Rotavirus* and *Orbivirus* cause disease in man. Replication proceeds in the cytoplasm associated with lysosomes whose proteolytic enzymes partially hydrolyze the outer capsid. The genome segments are not released free in the cytoplasm. Transcription of some of the virion RNA produces early mRNA strands necessary to encode uncoating enzymes followed by additional transcription that allows for genome replication. The double-stranded genome replicates conservatively rather than semiconservatively, unlike double-stranded DNA.

ROTAVIRUSES

Rotaviruses are responsible for the disease called sporadic acute enteritis in infants. It is assumed that these viruses are transmitted by the fecal-oral route although, unlike enteroviruses, their seasonal peak is in the cooler months of the year. Infection can be subclinical, or mild to severe with occasionally fatal diarrhea. Virus is detected in stool specimens by electron microscopy since it cannot be propagated in tissue culture. Treatment involves the maintenance of electrolyte balance.

ORBIVIRUSES

The *Orbivirus* responsible for Colorado tick fever is transmitted to man from rodent reservoirs during the spring and summer by ticks such as *Dermacentor andersonii*. Colorado tick fever is an acute illness characterized by chills, biphasic fever, retrobulbar headache, malaise, anorexia and nausea. Pharyngeal and conjunctival erythema may be present and petechial rashes have been reported on the extremities and macular rashes on the trunk. Neurological involvement may be manifest as meningitis, meningoencephalitis, or encephalitis and can be life threatening in children under 10. However, it is a self-limiting disease. Other organs can become involved producing pericarditis, myocarditis, orchitis, pleuritis and arthritis, however these symptoms are believed to be immunopathic in origin.

Treatment is primarily supportive and symptomatic and usually involves analgesics and antipyretics.

ADDITIONAL READING

BISHOP, R. F., DAVIDSON, G. P., HOLMES, I. H., AND RUCK, B. J. 1974 Detection of a New Virus by Electron Microscopy of Faecal Extracts from Children with Acute Gastroenteritis. Lancet **1,** 149.

GOMEZ-BARRETO, J., PALMER, E. L., NAHMIAS, A. J., AND HATCH, M. H. 1976 Acute Enteritis Associated with *Reovirus*-Like Agents. JAMA **235,** 1857.

JARUDI, N. H., HUGGETT, D. O., AND GOLDEN, B. 1973 *Reovirus* Keratoconjunctivitis. Can J Ophthalmol, **8,** 371.

KILHAM, L., AND MARGOLIS, G. 1973 Pathogenesis of Intra-uterine Infections in Rats Due to Reovirus Type 3. I. Virologic Studies. Lab Invest **28,** 597.

MIDDLETON, P. J., SZYMANSKI, M. T., ABBOTT, G. D., BORTOLUSSI, R., AND HAMILTON, J. R. 1974 *Orbivirus* Acute Gastroenteritis of Infancy. Lancet **1,** 1241.

MANDELL, G. L., DOUGLAS, R. G., JR., AND BENNETT, J. E. (Eds.) 1979 *Principles and Practice of Infectious Diseases.* John Wiley, New York.

PARROTT, R. H. 1976 Human Reoviruslike Agent As the Major Pathogen Associated with "Winter" Gastroenteritis in Hospitalized Infants and Young Children. N Engl J Med **294,** 965.

RAINE, C. S., AND FIELDS, B. N. 1973 Reovirus Type 3 Encephalitis—A Virologic and Ultrastructural Study. J Neuropathol Exp Neurol **32,** 19.

Index